Reviewers

Susan Beggs, RN, MSN
Associate Professor, Nursing Faculty
Austin Community College
Austin, Texas

MaryAnn Cosgarea, RN, BSN, BA
Nurse Administrator, Practical Nursing
Health Coordinator, Adult Education
Portage Lakes Career Center
W. Howard Nicol School of Practical Nursing
Green, Ohio

Nancy T. Hatfield, RN, BSN, MA
Director/Department Chairperson
Health Occupations/Practical Nursing
Albuquerque Public Schools
Career Enrichment Center
Albuquerque, New Mexico

Debra Menshouse, RN, BSN
Nursing Faculty
Ashland Technical College
Ashland, Kentucky

Esther Salinas, RN, MSN, MS Ed
Associate Professor, Nursing
Vocational Nursing and Registered Nursing Departments
Del Mar College
Corpus Christi, Texas

Julie A. Slack, RN, MSN
Nursing Faculty
Mohave Community College
Colorado City, Arizona

Bonnie J. Smith, RN, BSN
Coordinator, Practical Nurse Program
Sikeston Public Schools—Health Occupations
Hayti, Missouri

Ginger White, RN, ADN
Instructor, Vocational Nursing Program
Wharton County Junior College
Wharton, Texas

W9-BPJ-617

Preface

The seventh edition of *Introductory Clinical Pharmacology* reflects the ever-changing science of pharmacology and the nurse's responsibilities in administering pharmacologic agents. All information has been updated and revised according to the latest available information to prepare nurses to meet the challenges of safely administering medications. The text prepares the nurse to meet the challenges of the 21st century by promoting critical thinking and problem solving when administering medications.

PURPOSE

This text is designed to provide students with a clear, concise introduction to pharmacology. The basic explanations presented in this text are *not* intended to suggest that pharmacology is an easy subject. Drug therapy is one of the most important and complicated treatment modalities in modern health care. Because of its importance and complexity and the frequent additions and changes in the field of pharmacology, it is imperative that health care professionals constantly review and update their knowledge.

CURRENT DRUG INFORMATION

The student and practitioner should remember that information about drugs, such as dosages and new forms, is constantly changing. Likewise, there may be new drugs on the market that were not approved by the Federal Drug Administration (FDA) at the time of publication of this text. The reader may find that certain drugs or drug dosages available when this textbook was published may no longer be available. For the most current drug information and dosages, the practitioner is advised to consult references such as the most current *Physician's Desk Reference* or *Facts and Comparison* and the package inserts that accompany most drugs. If reliable references are not available, the hospital pharmacist or physician should be contacted for information concerning a specific drug, including dosage, adverse reactions, contraindications, precautions, interactions, or administration.

SPECIAL FEATURES

A number of features have proven useful for students in their study of basic pharmacology. The following features appear in the seventh edition:

- **Key Terms**—lists the important words defined in the chapter
- **Nursing Process**—used as a framework in most chapters for presenting care of the patient as it relates to the drug and the drug regimen. *Preadministration* and *Ongoing Assessments* are included in the assessment phase of the nursing process. These assessments are divided in order to highlight the important assessments to perform before administering a specific drug and those important during the entire time the drug is being administering. In the implementation phase of the nursing process, most chapters contain sections *Promoting an Optimal Response to Therapy* and *Monitoring and Managing Adverse Reactions*. These sections provide invaluable information needed to ensure that the drug is properly administered and nursing interventions to use when certain adverse reactions occur.
- **Nursing Alerts**—short segments that identify urgent nursing considerations in the management of the patient receiving a specific drug or drug category
- **Gerontologic Alerts**—short segments to alert the nurse about specific problems for which the older adult is at increased risk. As the number of the older adults in our society increases, it becomes imperative that nurses recognize the necessity of specialized care.
- **Contraindications, Precautions, and Interactions**—of the most commonly used drugs in the category under discussion. While space prevents every contraindication, precaution, and interaction to be listed, the more common ones are included in the text. Pregnancy categories are identified for many drugs discussed within the chapter.
- **Home Health Care Checklists**—highlight specific issues that the patient or family may

http://connection.LWW.com

Get Connected...

To a one-of-a-kind educational resource!

connection

Register in 3 easy steps...

1. Visit the connection website and click log-on...

2. Set up a new user profile

3. Enter your name and e-mail address, and create a user name and password.

With registration you'll receive e-mail notification whenever this site is updated.

Resource Centers include

for Faculty...
- Supplemental content on substance abuse.
- Links to updated drug information.
- Author Profile

for Students....
- Supplemental content on substance abuse
- Sample Study Guide Content
- Links to updated drug information
- Author Profile

connect today

http://connection.LWW.com/go/lpnresources

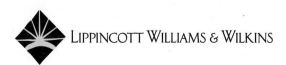
LIPPINCOTT WILLIAMS & WILKINS

G452-01   N1NXG452

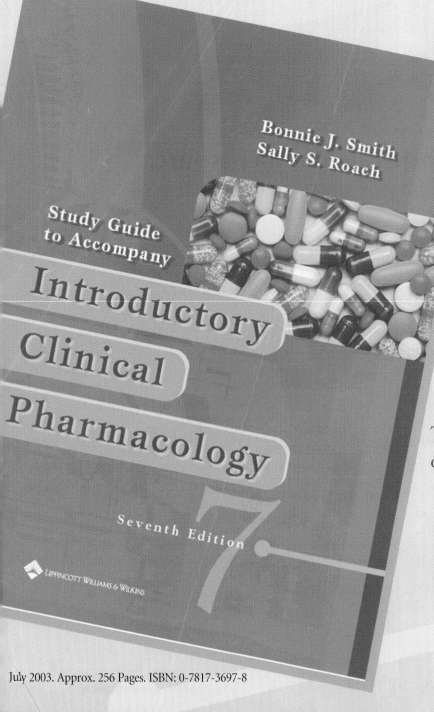
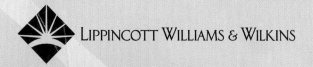

Introductory Clinical Pharmacology

Seventh Edition

Sally S. Roach, MSN, RN

Associate Professor

University of Texas at Brownsville and Texas Southmost College

Brownsville, Texas

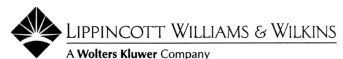

LIPPINCOTT WILLIAMS & WILKINS

A **Wolters Kluwer** Company

Philadelphia • Baltimore • New York • London
Buenos Aires • Hong Kong • Sydney • Tokyo

...gnton
...ter
...ussa Olson
...g Manager: William Alberti
...r: Michael Ferreira
Compositor: TechBooks
Printer: Quebecor/World—Dubuque

7th Edition

9 8 7 6 5 4 3 2

Library of Congress Cataloging-in-Publication Data
Roach, Sally S.
  Introductory clinical pharmacology / Sally S. Roach.— 7th ed.
    p. ; cm.
  Includes index.
  ISBN 0-7817-3696-X (alk. paper)
  1. Clinical pharmacology.   2. Nursing. I. Title: Clinical pharmacology. II. Title.
  [DNLM: 1. Pharmacology, Clinical—Nurses' Instruction.   2. Drug Therapy—Nurses'
  Instruction.   3. Pharmaceutical Preparations—administration & dosage—Nurses' Instruction.
QV 38 R628i 2004]
RM301.28.S34 2004
615.5′8—dc21

                                                      2002043393

Care has been taken to confirm the accuracy of the information presented and to describe generally accepted
practices. However, the author, editors, and publisher are not responsible for errors or omissions or for any consequences from application of the information in this book and make no warranty, express or implied, with
respect to the content of the publication.

The author, editors, and publisher have exerted every effort to ensure that drug selection and dosage set forth
in this text are in accordance with the current recommendations and practice at the time of publication.
However, in view of ongoing research, changes in government regulations, and the constant flow of information
relating to drug therapy and drug reactions, the reader is urged to check the package insert for each drug for any
change in indications and dosage and for added warnings and precautions. This is particularly important when
the recommended agent is a new or infrequently employed drug.

Some drugs and medical devices presented in this publication have Food and Drug Administration (FDA)
clearance for limited use in restricted research settings. It is the responsibility of the health care provider to
ascertain the FDA status of each drug or device planned for use in his or her clinical practice.

encounter while undergoing drug therapy in the home setting. As more and more patients are cared for outside the hospital, it becomes increasingly important for the nurse to know what information the patient or family needs to obtain an optimal response the drug regimen.

- **Patient and Family Teaching Checklists**—highlight teaching points relating to specific pharmacologic techniques and most-know information for the patient undergoing drug therapy. This empowers the family to participate knowledgeably and accurately in the patient's drug regimen.
- **Summary Drug Tables**—contain commonly used drugs representative of the class of drugs discussed in the chapter. Important drug information is provided, including the generic name, pronunciation guide for generic names, trade names, adverse reactions, and dosage ranges. In these tables, generic names are followed by trade names; when a drug is available under several trade names, several of the available trade names are given. The more common or serious adverse reactions associated with the drug are listed in the table's adverse reaction section. It should be noted that any patient may exhibit adverse reactions not listed in this text. Because of this possibility, the nurse, when administering any drug, should consider any sign or symptom as a *possible* adverse reaction until the cause of the problem is determined by the primary health care provider.

   The adverse reactions are followed by the dose ranges for the drug. In most cases, the adult dose *ranges* are given in these tables because space does not permit the inclusion of all possible dosages for various types of disorders. Likewise, space limitation does not permit an inclusion of pediatric dose ranges due to the complexity of determining the pediatric dose of many drugs. Many drugs given to children are determined on the basis of body weight or body surface area and have a variety of dosage schedules. When drugs are given to the pediatric patient, the practitioner is encouraged to consult references that give complete and extensive pediatric dosages.

- **Critical Thinking Exercises**—realistic patient care situations that help the student apply the material contained in the chapter by exploring options and making clinical judgments related to the administration of drugs
- **Abbreviations**—important pharmacologic and general medical abbreviations the nurse needs to know when caring for the patient undergoing drug therapy are spelled out in the back of the text.
- **Glossary**—key terms and other drug-related terms are listed and defined in the back of the text

NEW FEATURES

- **Four-Color Illustrations**—the text is beautifully illustrated throughout with new four-color illustrations. Each illustration highlights and explains an important pharmacologic concept, technique, or idea.
- **New Chapters**—new chapters are included, such as Chapter 33, Cholinesterase Inhibitors, and Chapter 18, Nonsteroidal Anti-Inflammatory Drugs. Several of the chapters in previous editions have been divided. For example, the chapter on antiviral and antifungal drugs was divided into two chapters: Chapter 14, Antiviral Drugs, and Chapter 15, Antifungal Drugs.
- **Herbal or Health Supplement Alerts**—provide important information on common herbs and supplements not regulated under the auspices of the Federal Drug Administration. **Appendix B** gives a listing of select herbs with examples of their common and scientific name(s). While not all of the common or scientific names are given, the more common names (both common and scientific) are included. With more and more individuals using herbs as a part of their health care regimen, it is critical that the nurse be aware of the more common herbs currently in use. The nurse must consult appropriate sources when patients indicate they are using herbs as part of their health care regimen.
- **Review Questions**—several questions, reviewing important information covered in the chapter, can be found at the end of each chapter. The questions are written in PN-NCLEX format and provide the student an opportunity to answer questions specifically about the drugs covered in the chapter. Space does not permit more questions of this type, but provides the student practice in answering questions concerning medication therapy and administration of drugs.
- **Medication Dosage Problems**—Calculation of medication dosage is an important aspect of medication administration. Chapter 3 reviews the mathematics involved in dosage calculation and formulas used in the calculate medication dosages. To ensure the student's understanding and application of this type of problem, two or more medication dosage problems are included at the end of most chapters dealing with specific medications discussed in the chapter. This provides the student an opportunity for immediate application in medication administration. As an added benefit, several current medication labels are used throughout the text to help the student learn to read these labels and solve medication dosage problems using the information found on these labels.

- **Drug and Health Care Information Sources on the World Wide Web**—The inside back cover provides a listing of websites dealing with pharmacology and medication administration. The student can use these sites as valuable resources to identify new drugs and important new information on current drugs.

ORGANIZATION

The text contains 58 chapters, which are divided into 11 units. Organization of the text in this manner allows the student to move about the text when these general areas are covered in the curriculum. While pharmacologic agents are presented in specific units, a disease may be treated with more than one type of drug, which may require consulting one or more units.

Unit I presents a foundation for the study of pharmacology and covers general principles of pharmacology, the administration of drugs, a review of arithmetic and calculation of drug dosages, a discussion of the nursing process as applicable to pharmacology, and a review of the teaching learning process and general areas of consideration when educating the patient and family.

Unit II contains 11 chapters that present the antiinfective drugs, grouped according to classification. These shorter chapters allow for more inclusive coverage of the different types of anti-infectives and the appropriate nursing considerations for each classification.

Unit III includes four chapters covering the various types of drugs used to manage pain: the nonnarcotic analgesics (Salicylates, Nonsalicylates, and Nonsteroidal Anti-Inflammatory Drugs), the narcotic analgesics, and the narcotic antagonists.

Unit IV has been expanded to 15 chapters covering the many classifications of drugs that affect the nervous system and the neuromuscular system. These chapters include the following types of drugs: drugs that affect the musculoskeletal system, adrenergic drugs, adrenergic blocking drugs, cholinergic drugs, cholinergic blocking drugs, sedatives and hypnotics, central nervous system stimulants, anticonvulsants, antiparkinsonism drugs, antianxiety drugs, antidepressant drugs, antipsychotic drugs, cholinesterase inhibitors, antiemetic and antivertigo drugs, and anesthetic drugs.

Unit V has three chapters concerning drugs that affect the respiratory system. The first chapter in this unit discusses antihistamines and decongestants, the second chapter in the unit covers bronchodilators and antiasthma drugs, and the last chapter of the unit deals with antitussives, mucolytics, and expectorants.

Unit VI covers drugs that affect the cardiovascular system. This unit is divided into five chapters: cardiotonics and miscellaneous inotropic drugs, antiarrhythmic drugs, antianginal and peripheral dilating drugs, antihypertensives, and antihyperlipidemics.

Unit VII consists of two chapters dealing with drugs that affect the hematological system: anticoagulants and thrombolytic drugs, and agents used in the treatment of anemia.

Unit VIII has been expanded to cover drugs that affect both the gastrointestinal and urinary systems. The unit consists of three chapters: uretics, urinary anti-infectives and miscellaneous urinary drugs, and drugs that affect the gastrointestinal system.

Unit IX discusses drugs that affect the endocrine system and consists of five chapters: antidiabetic drugs, pituitary and andrenocortical hormones, thyroid and antithyroid drugs, male and female hormones, and drugs acting on the uterus.

Unit X discusses drugs that affect the immune system. The unit consists of two chapters: immunologic agents and antineoplastic drugs.

Unit XI consists of three chapters that discusses types of drugs not previously discussed or that are not members of a particular class or group. Chapters in this unit include topical drugs used in the treatment of skin disorders, otic and ophthalmic preparations, and fluids and electrolytes.

CHAPTER CONTENT

Each chapter opens with learning objectives and a listing of key terms used and defined in the chapter. Less commonly used medical terms are also defined within the chapter and may be found in the Glossary. Chapters 1 to 5 provide introductory information concerning general principals of pharmacology, medication administration, a review of arithmetic and calculation of drug dosages, the nursing process, and patient and family teaching. Each chapter ends with critical thinking questions and several chapter review questions.

The remaining chapters discuss specific drug classifications and contain a common format. In addition to the learning objectives and key terms, the remaining chapters contain a table indicating the drug classifications and drugs discussed in the chapter. The body of each chapter contains the actions, uses, adverse reactions, contraindications, precautions and interactions of the class or type of drug being discussed, followed by a section devoted to the nursing process. These chapters end with critical thinking questions, several chapter review questions, and two or more medication dosage problems. To promote easy retrieval of information, each area is identified by a large type heading.

- Actions—a basic explanation of how the drug accomplishes its intended activity
- Uses—the more common uses of the drug class or type are provided. No unlabeled or experimental

uses of drugs are given in the text (unless specifically identified as an unlabeled use) because these uses are not approved by the FDA. Students should be reminded that, under certain circumstances, some physicians may prescribe drugs for a condition not approved by the FDA or may prescribe an experimental drug.

When discussing the use of antibiotics, this text does not list specific microorganisms. Microorganisms can become resistant to antibiotic drugs very rapidly. Because of this, the author feels that listing specific microorganisms or types of infections for an antibiotic may be misleading to the user of the text. Instead, when antibiotics are needed, the author recommends consulting culture and sensitivity studies to indicate which antibiotic has the most potential for controlling the infection.

- Adverse Reactions—the most common adverse drug reactions are listed under this heading
- Contraindications—contraindications for administration of the drug or drugs discussed in the chapter
- Precautions—precautions to take before, during, or after administration
- Interactions—more common interactions between the drug(s) discussed in the chapter and other drugs
- Nursing Process—with a few exceptions, the nursing process is used in every chapter of the test and geared specifically to the administration of the drugs discussed in the chapter. The assessment phase is divided into two distinct parts to include a preadministration and ongoing assessment. This assists the reader in determining what assessments to perform before administration of specific drugs of drug categories and what important assessments to perform during the entire time the drug is administered. Nursing diagnoses related to the administration of the drug are highlighted in a nursing diagnoses checklist. Under "Implementation," three sections are included when applicable: "Promoting an Optimal Response to Therapy," "Monitoring and Managing Adverse Reactions," and "Educating the Patient and Family."
- Critical Thinking Questions—each chapter includes critical thinking questions that provide the student with the challenge of applying chapter content to specific clinical situations
- Review Questions—several PN-NCLEX review questions are found at the end of each chapter
- Medication Dosage Problems—when applicable, the chapter contains real medication dosage prescriptions and the medication available for dispensing. The student solves medication dosage problems using the information provided. Several current medication labels are used to help the student learn to read these labels and solve medication dosage problems using the information found on these labels.

APPENDICES

Seven appendices containing important pharmacologic information are located at the back of the text.

Appendix A contains a MedWatch form, which is used by health care professionals for voluntary reporting of adverse reactions and problems with the drug product. Is also contains advice about voluntary reporting. This form is a part of the FDA medical products reporting program.

Appendix B is a table of Select Herbs and Natural Products Used for Medicinal Purposes.

Appendix C contains a United States Pharmacopeia (USP) medication errors reporting program form, which is used by health care professionals for sharing information of medication errors to prevent them from occuring again. Also included is text explaining medication error and the USP.

Appendix D provides metric–apothecary equivalents and conversions. This guide covers liquid measurements; weights; Celsius and Fahrenheit temperatures; and a comparative scale of measures, weights, and temperatures.

Appendix E contains two body surface area nomograms—one for infants and young children and one for older children and adults.

Appendix F is a Vaccine Adverse Event Reporting Form.

Appendix G contains answers to the review and dosage calculation exercises appearing at the end of the chapters.

Appendix H lists examples of combination drugs.

TEACHING/LEARNING PACKAGE

- Student Study Guide—the *Study Guide to Accompany Introductory Clinical Pharmacology,* 7th Edition, correlates with the textbook chapter by chapter. For each chapter in the textbook, the *Study Guide* contains a corresponding chapter and includes three or more of the following components: a crossword puzzle featuring important terms of the chapter, multiple-choice questions, short-answer questions, and critical thinking exercises derived from the textbook. Multiple-choice question have been written using the same format as currently used in the NCLEX-PN examinations. The *Study Guide* also features activities designed around specific drug-related websites. These activities promote use of the World Wide Web as an important learning tool in the study and practice of nursing pharmacology.

- Free Back of the Book CD-ROM—this learning tool provides 3-D animated depictions of pharmacology concepts, video on preventing medication errors, monographs of the 100 most commonly prescribed drugs, and a listing of the classifications and important drugs discussed compiled by chapter.
- Instructor's Resources—two CD-ROMs are available for Introductory Clinical Pharmacology. The Instructor's Resource CD-ROM contains NCLEX-PN type questions, Dosage Problems, and Critical Thinking Questions. Answers are provided for the multiple-choice questions and dosage problems. No answers are supplied for the critical thinking exercises to encourage the students to use their creative abilities rather than be confined to a predetermined answer. The Test Generator CD-ROM contains a multiple-choice test generator and PowerPoint slides for each chapter.

ACKNOWLEDGMENTS

I wish to thank everyone involved in the creation of this 7th Edition of *Introductory Clinical Pharmacology*. A special thanks to Lisa Stead, Acquisitions Editor, for her guidance and support during the preparation of the manuscript. My heartfelt gratitude goes to Joe Morita, Managing Editor, for his support and editorial assistance with manuscript preparation and development. His input was invaluable. A special thank-you to Brenda Shaffer, RPh, for her assistance with the Summary Drug Tables and to Tom Robinson for his assistance in obtaining drug labels. My gratitude to all those who worked in any way in the design, production, and preparation of this book: Debra Schiff, Senior Production Editor; Helen Ewan, Senior Production Manager; and Brett MacNaughton, Art Director.

Although not a part of the professional development of this textbook, I wish to express my love and gratitude to those who made my contribution to this book possible, my family. Their unwavering support and encouragement saw me through many difficult days, nights, and weekends of manuscript preparation.

Sally Roach, MSN, RN, CHN

Contents

chapter **1**

General Principles of Pharmacology

Key Terms

additive drug reaction
adverse reaction
agonist
allergic reaction
anaphylactic shock
angioedema
antagonist
antibodies
antigen
biotransformation
botanical medicine
controlled substances
cumulative drug effect
drug idiosyncrasy
drug tolerance
half-life
hypersensitivity

macromolecule
nonprescription drugs
pharmaceutic
pharmacodynamics
pharmacogenetic
  disorder
pharmacokinetics
pharmacology
physical dependency
polypharmacy
prescription drugs
psychological
  dependency
receptor
synergism
teratogen
toxic

Chapter Objectives

On completion of this chapter, the student will:

- Define pharmacology.
- Discuss drug development in the United States.
- Identify the different names assigned to drugs.
- Distinguish between prescription drugs, nonprescription drugs, and controlled substances.
- Discuss the laws governing the manufacture, distribution, and sale of drugs.
- Discuss the various types of drug reactions produced in the body.
- Identify factors that influence drug action.
- Define drug tolerance, cumulative drug effect, and drug idiosyncrasy.
- Discuss the types of drug interactions that may be seen with drug administration.
- Discuss the nursing implications associated with drug actions, interactions, and effects.
- Discuss the use of botanical medicines.

Pharmacology is the study of drugs and their action on living organisms. A sound knowledge of basic pharmacologic principles is essential if the nurse is to safely administer medications and to monitor patients who receive these medications. This chapter gives a basic overview of pharmacologic principles that the nurse must understand when administering medications. The chapter also discusses drug development, federal legislation affecting the dispensing and use of drugs, and the use of botanical medicines as they relate to pharmacology.

DRUG DEVELOPMENT

Drug development is a long and arduous process, taking anywhere from 7 to 12 years, and sometimes even longer. The United States Food and Drug Administration (FDA) has the responsibility of approving new drugs and monitoring drugs currently in use for adverse or toxic reactions. The development of a new drug is divided into the pre-FDA phase and the FDA

phase (Fig. 1-1). During the pre-FDA phase, a manufacturer discovers a drug that looks promising. In vitro testing (testing in an artificial environment, such as a test tube) using animal and human cells is done. This testing is followed by studies in live animals. The manufacturer then makes application to the FDA for Investigational New Drug (IND) status.

With IND status, clinical testing of the new drug begins. Clinical testing involves three phases, with each phase involving a larger number of people. All effects, both pharmacologic and biologic, are noted. Phase I lasts 4 to 6 weeks and involves 20 to 100 individuals who are either "normal" volunteers or individuals in the intended treatment population. If Phase I studies are successful, the testing moves to Phase II, and if those results are positive, to Phase III. Each successive phase has a larger subject population. Phase III studies offer additional information on dosing and safety. The three phases last anywhere from 2 to 10 years, with the average being 5 years.

A New Drug Application (NDA) is submitted after the investigation of the drug in Phases I, II, and III is

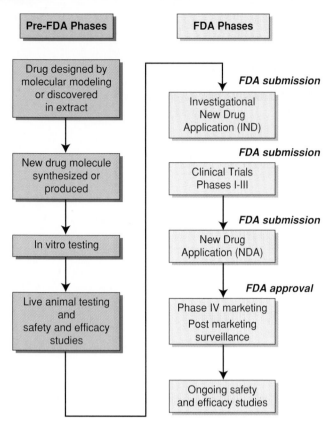

FIGURE 1-1. Phases of drug development. Adapted from (1997, Spring) *PharmPhax,* 3 (2), 2.

complete and the drug is found to be safe and effective. With the NDA, the manufacturer submits all data collected concerning the drug during the clinical trials. A panel of experts, including pharmacologists, chemists, physicians, and other professionals, reviews the application and makes a recommendation to the FDA. The FDA then either approves or disapproves the drug for use. This process of review takes approximately 2 years. After FDA approval, continued surveillance is done to ensure safety.

Postmarketing surveillance occurs after the manufacturer places the drug on the market. During this surveillance, an ongoing review of the drug occurs with particular attention given to adverse reactions. Health care professionals are encouraged to help with this surveillance by reporting adverse effects of drugs to the FDA by using MedWatch (see Display 1-1).

SPECIAL FDA PROGRAMS

Although it takes considerable time for most drugs to get FDA approval, the FDA has special programs to meet different needs. Examples of these special programs include the orphan drug program, accelerated programs for urgent needs, and compassionate use programs.

Orphan Drug Program

The Orphan Drug Act of 1983 was passed to encourage the development and marketing of products used to treat rare diseases. The act defines a "rare disease" as a condition affecting fewer than 200,000 individuals in the United States. The National Organization of Rare Disorders reports that there are more than 6000 rare disorders that affect approximately 25 million individuals. Examples of rare disorders include Tourette's syndrome, ovarian cancer, acquired immunodeficiency syndrome (AIDS), Huntington's disease, and certain forms of leukemia.

The act provides for incentives, such as research grants, protocol assistance by the FDA, and special tax credits, to encourage manufacturers to develop orphan drugs. If the drug is approved, the manufacturer has 7 years of exclusive marketing rights. More than 100 new drugs have received FDA approval since the law was passed. Examples of orphan drugs include thalidomide for leprosy, triptorelin pamoate for ovarian cancer, tetrabenazine for Huntington's disease, and zidovudine for AIDS.

Accelerated Programs

Accelerated approval of drugs is offered by the FDA as a means to make promising products for life-threatening diseases available on the market, based on preliminary evidence before formal demonstration of patient benefit.

DISPLAY 1-1 ● How to Report Adverse Reactions

A drug must be used and studied for many years before all of the adverse reactions are identified. To help in identifying adverse reactions the nurse must be aware of reporting mechanisms. The FDA established a reporting program called MedWatch by which nurses or other health care professionals can report observations of serious adverse drug effects by using a standard form (see Appendix A). The FDA protects the identity of those who voluntarily report adverse reactions. This form also is used to report an undesirable experience associated with the use of medical products (eg, latex gloves, pacemakers, infusion pumps, anaphylaxis, blood, blood components, etc.). It is important to submit reports, even if there is uncertainty about the cause-effect relationship.

Nurses play an important role in monitoring for adverse reactions. The FDA considers serious adverse reactions those that may result in death, life-threatening illness, hospitalization, or disability or those that may require medical or surgical intervention.

Adverse drug reactions may be reported to the FDA by completing the MedWatch form and sending it to:

MedWatch
5600 Fishers Lane
Rockville, MD 20852-9787

Reports may be faxed to the following number:
1-800-FDA-0178

Forms are available online and can be downloaded, completed, and returned via mail, fax, or electronic mail. See the following website:
www.fda.gov/medwatch/index.html

The approval that is granted is considered a "provisional approval," with a written commitment from the pharmaceutical company to complete clinical studies that formally demonstrate patient benefit. This program seeks to make life-saving investigational drugs available before granting final approval to treat diseases that pose a significant health threat to the public. One example of a disease that qualifies as posing a significant health threat is AIDS. Because AIDS is so devastating to the individuals affected and because of the danger the disease poses to public health, the FDA and pharmaceutical companies are working together to shorten the IND approval process for some drugs that show promise in treating AIDS. This accelerated process allows primary care providers to administer medications that indicate positive results in early Phase I and II clinical trials, rather than wait until final approval is granted. If the drug continues to prove beneficial, the process of approval is accelerated.

Compassionate Access to Unapproved Drugs

The compassionate access program allows patients to receive drugs that have not yet been approved by the FDA. This program provides experimental drugs for patients who could benefit from new treatments but whose conditions are such that they most probably would die before the drug is approved for use. These patients are often too sick to participate in the controlled studies. Drug manufacturers make a proposal to the FDA to target patients with the disease and, at the pharmaceutical company's expense, provide the drug free to patients. The pharmaceutical company analyzes and presents to the FDA data on the treatment. This program is not without problems. Because the drug is not in full production, quantities may be limited, so the number of patients may be limited, and patients may be selected at random. Because patients receiving compassionate access often are sicker, they are at increased risk

for toxic reactions. This results in the newly developed drug running the risk of obtaining a "bad reputation," even before marketing begins.

DRUG NAMES

Throughout the process of development, drugs may have several names assigned to them: a chemical name, a generic (nonproprietary) name, an official name, and a trade or brand name. This is confusing unless the nurse has a clear understanding of the different names used. Table 1-1 identifies the different names and provides an explanation of each.

DRUG CATEGORIES

After approval of a drug, the FDA assigns the drug to one of the following categories: prescription, nonprescription, or controlled substance.

Prescription Drugs

Prescription drugs are drugs that the federal government has designated to be potentially harmful unless their use is supervised by a licensed health care provider, such as a nurse practitioner, physician, or dentist. Although these drugs have been tested for safety and therapeutic effect, prescription drugs may cause different reactions in some individuals.

In institutional settings the nurse administers the drug and monitors the patient for therapeutic effect and adverse reactions. Some drugs have the potential to be **toxic** (harmful). The nurse plays a critical role in evaluating the patient for toxic effects. When these drugs are prescribed to be taken at home, the nurse provides patient and family education about the drug.

TABLE 1-1	Drug Names

DRUG NAME AND EXAMPLE	EXPLANATION
Chemical name Example: ethyl 4-(8-chloro-5,6-dihydro-11*H*-benzo[5,6] cycloheptal[1,2-b]-pyridin-11-ylidene)-1-piperidinecardisplayylate	Gives the exact chemical makeup of the drug and placing of the atoms or molecular structure; it is not capitalized.
Generic name (nonproprietary) Example: loratadine	Name given to a drug before it becomes official; may be used in all countries, by all manufacturers; it is not capitalized.
Official name Example: loratadine	Name listed in *The United States Pharmacopeia-National Formulary;* may be the same as the generic name.
Trade name (brand name) Example: Claritin©	Name that is registered by the manufacturer and is followed by the trademark symbol; the name can be used only by the manufacturer; a drug may have several trade names, depending on the number of manufacturers; the first letter of the name is capitalized.

DEA # _____

CHARLES FULLER M.D.
SUSAN LUNGLEY R.N., A.N.
1629 TREASURE HILLS
HOUSTON, TX 79635

NAME _____

ADDRESS _____ DATE _____

R$_X$

☐ Label

Refill _____ times PRN NR

_____ M.D.

To ensure brand name dispensing, prescriber must write 'Dispense As Written' on the prescription.

FIGURE 1-2. Example of a prescription form.

Prescription drugs, also called legend drugs, are the largest category of drugs. Prescription drugs are prescribed by a licensed health care provider. The prescription (see Fig. 1-2) contains the name of the drug, the dosage, the method and times of administration, and the signature of the licensed health care provider prescribing the drug.

Nonprescription Drugs

Nonprescription drugs are drugs that are designated by the FDA to be safe (if taken as directed) and obtained without a prescription. These drugs are also referred to as over-the-counter (OTC) drugs and may be purchased in a variety of settings, such as a pharmacy, drugstore, or in the local supermarket. OTC drugs include those given for symptoms of the common cold, headaches, constipation, diarrhea, and upset stomach.

These drugs are not without risk and may produce adverse reactions. For example, acetylsalicylic acid, commonly known as aspirin, is potentially harmful and can cause gastrointestinal bleeding and salicylism (see Chap. 17). Labeling requirements give the consumer important information regarding the drug, dosage, contraindications, precautions, and adverse reactions. Consumers are urged to read the directions carefully before taking OTC drugs.

Controlled Substances

Controlled substances are the most carefully monitored of all drugs. These drugs have a high potential for abuse and may cause physical or psychological dependence. **Physical dependency** is a compulsive need to use a substance repeatedly to avoid mild to severe withdrawal symptoms; it is the body's dependence on repeated administration of a drug. **Psychological dependency** is a compulsion to use a substance to obtain a pleasurable experience; it is the mind's dependence on the repeated administration of a drug. One type of dependency may lead to the other type.

The Controlled Substances Act of 1970 regulates the manufacture, distribution, and dispensing of drugs that have abuse potential (see information under "Federal Drug Legislation and Enforcement" in this chapter). Drugs under the Controlled Substances Act are divided into five schedules, based on their potential for abuse and physical and psychological dependence. Display 1-2 describes the five schedules.

Prescriptions for controlled substances must be written in ink and include the name and address of the patient and the Drug Enforcement Agency number of the primary health care provider. Prescriptions for these drugs cannot be filled more than 6 months after the prescription

DISPLAY 1-2 ● Schedules of Controlled Substances

SCHEDULE I (C-I)
- High abuse potential
- No accepted medical use in the United States
- Examples: heroin, marijuana, LSD (lysergic acid diethylamide), peyote

SCHEDULE II (C-II)
- Potential for high abuse with severe physical or psychological dependence
- Examples: narcotics such as meperidine, methadone, morphine, oxycodone; amphetamines; and barbiturates

SCHEDULE III (C-III)
- Less abuse potential than schedule II drugs
- Potential for moderate physical or psychological dependence
- Examples: nonbarbiturate sedatives, nonamphetamine stimulants, limited amounts of certain narcotics

SCHEDULE IV (C-IV)
- Less abuse potential than schedule III drugs
- Limited dependence potential
- Examples: some sedatives and anxiety agents, nonnarcotic analgesics

SCHEDULE V (C-V)*
- Limited abuse potential
- Examples: small amounts of narcotics (codeine) used as antitussives or antidiarrheals

*Under federal law, limited quantities of certain schedule V drugs may be purchased without a prescription directly from a pharmacist if allowed under state law. The purchaser must be at least 18 years of age and must furnish identification. All such transactions must be recorded by the dispensing pharmacist.

was written or be refilled more than five times. Under federal law, limited quantities of certain schedule C-V drugs may be purchased without a prescription, with the purchase recorded by the dispensing pharmacist. In some cases state laws are more restrictive than federal laws and impose additional requirements for the sale and distribution of controlled substances. In hospitals or other agencies that dispense controlled substances, the scheduled drugs are counted every 8 to 12 hours to account for each ampule, tablet, or other form of the drug. Any discrepancy in the number of drugs must be investigated and explained immediately.

FEDERAL DRUG LEGISLATION AND ENFORCEMENT

Many laws have been enacted over the last century that affect drug distribution and administration. Those included here are the Pure Food and Drug Act; Harrison Narcotic Act; Pure Food, Drug, and Cosmetic Act; and the Comprehensive Drug Abuse Prevention and Control Act. These laws control the use of the three categories of drugs in the United States (prescription, nonprescription, and controlled substances).

Pure Food and Drug Act

This act, passed in 1906, was the first attempt by the government to regulate and control the manufacture, distribution, and sale of drugs. Before 1906, any substance could be called a drug, and no testing or research was required before placing the drug on the market. Before this time, drug potency and the purity of many drugs were questionable, and some were even dangerous for human use.

Harrison Narcotic Act

This law, passed in 1914, regulated the sale of narcotic drugs. Before the passage of this act, any narcotic could be purchased without a prescription. This law was amended many times. In 1970, the Harrison Narcotic Act was replaced with the passage of the Comprehensive Drug Abuse Prevention and Control Act.

Pure Food, Drug, and Cosmetic Act

In 1938, Congress passed this law that gave the FDA control over the manufacture and sale of drugs, food, and cosmetics. Before the passage of this act, some drugs, as well as foods and cosmetics, contained chemicals that were often harmful to humans. This law requires that these substances are safe for human use. It also requires pharmaceutical companies to perform toxicology tests before a new drug is submitted to the FDA for approval. Following FDA review of the tests performed on animals and other research data, approval may be given to market the drug (see sections on "Drug Development").

Comprehensive Drug Abuse Prevention and Control Act

Congress passed this act in 1970 because of the growing problem of drug abuse. It regulates the manufacture, distribution, and dispensation of drugs that have the potential for abuse. Title II of this law, the Controlled Substances Act, deals with control and enforcement. The Drug Enforcement Agency within the US Department of Justice is the leading federal agency responsible for the enforcement of this act.

Drug Enforcement Administration

The Drug Enforcement Administration (DEA) within the US Department of Justice is the chief federal agency responsible for enforcing the Controlled Substances Act. Failure to comply with the Controlled Substances Act is punishable by fine and/or imprisonment. With drug abuse so prevalent, nurses must diligently adhere to the regulation imposed by the FDA and the Nurse Practice Act of their state. Any violation may result in the loss of the nurse's license to practice. Nurses must also report any misuse or abuse of these substances by other nurses to their State Board of Nursing. Most states have provisions within their Nurse Practice Act to assist nurses who have problems with drug abuse.

DRUG USE AND PREGNANCY

The use of any medication—prescription or nonprescription—carries a risk of causing birth defects in the developing fetus. Drugs administered to pregnant women, particularly during the first trimester (3 months), may cause teratogenic effects. A **teratogen** is any substance that causes abnormal development of the fetus leading to a severely deformed fetus. Drugs are one type of teratogen.

In an effort to prevent teratogenic effects, the FDA has established five categories suggesting the potential of a drug for causing birth defects (Display 1-3). Information regarding the pregnancy category of a specific drug is found in reliable drug literature, such as the inserts accompanying drugs and approved drug references. In general, most drugs are contraindicated during pregnancy or lactation unless the potential benefits of taking the drug outweigh the risks to the fetus or the infant.

During pregnancy, no woman should consider taking any drug, legal or illegal, prescription or nonprescription, unless the drug is prescribed or recommended by the primary health care provider. Smoking or drinking any type of alcoholic beverage also carries risks, such as low birth weight, premature birth, and fetal alcohol syndrome. Children born of mothers using addictive drugs, such as cocaine or heroin, often are born with an addiction to the drug abused by the mother.

DRUG ACTIVITY WITHIN THE BODY

Drugs act in various ways in the body. Oral drugs go through three phases: the pharmaceutic phase, pharmacokinetic phase, and pharmacodynamic phase. Liquid and parenteral drugs (drugs given by injection) go through the later two phases only.

Pharmaceutic Phase

The **pharmaceutic** phase of drug action is the dissolution of the drug. Drugs must be in solution to be absorbed. Drugs that are liquid or drugs given by injec-

tion (parenteral drugs) do not go through the pharmaceutic phase. A tablet or capsule (solid forms of a drug) goes through this phase as it disintegrates into small particles and dissolves into the body fluids within the gastrointestinal tract. Tablets that are enteric-coated do not disintegrate until reaching the alkaline environment of the small intestine.

Pharmacokinetic Phase

Pharmacokinetics refers to activities within the body after a drug is administered. These activities include absorption, distribution, metabolism, and excretion (ADME). Another pharmacokinetic component is the half-life of the drug. **Half-life** is a measure of the rate at which drugs are removed from the body.

Absorption

Absorption follows administration and is the process by which a drug is made available for use in the body. It occurs after dissolution of a solid form of the drug or after the administration of a liquid or parenteral drug. In this process the drug particles within the gastrointestinal tract are moved into the body fluids. This movement can be accomplished in several ways: active absorption, passive absorption, and pinocytosis. In active absorption a carrier molecule such as a protein or enzyme actively moves the drug across the membrane. Passive absorption occurs by diffusion (movement from a higher concentration to a lower concentration). In pinocytosis cells engulf the drug particle causing movement across the cell.

As the body transfers the drug from the body fluids to the tissue sites, absorption into the body tissues occurs. Several factors influence the rate of absorption, including the route of administration, the solubility of the drug, and the presence of certain body conditions. Drugs are most rapidly absorbed when given by the intravenous route, followed by the intramuscular route, the subcutaneous route, and lastly, the oral route. Some drugs are more soluble and thus are absorbed more rapidly than others. For example, water-soluble drugs are readily absorbed into the systemic circulation. Bodily conditions, such as the development of lipodystrophy (atrophy of the subcutaneous tissue) from repeated subcutaneous injections, inhibit absorption of a drug given in the site of lipodystrophy.

Distribution

The systemic circulation distributes drugs to various body tissues or target sites. Drugs interact with specific receptors (see Fig. 1-3) during distribution. Some drugs travel by binding to protein (albumin) in the blood. Drugs bound to protein are pharmacologically inactive. Only when the protein molecules release the drug can the drug diffuse into the tissues, interact with receptors, and produce a therapeutic effect.

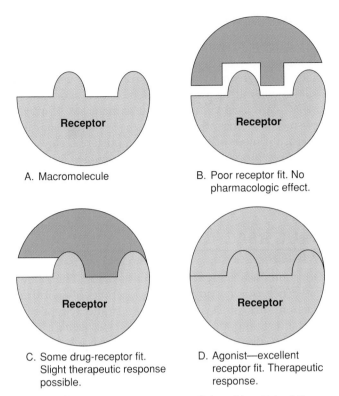

A. Macromolecule

B. Poor receptor fit. No pharmacologic effect.

C. Some drug-receptor fit. Slight therapeutic response possible.

D. Agonist—excellent receptor fit. Therapeutic response.

FIGURE 1-3. Drug-receptor interactions. (Adapted from Reiss & Evans, *Pharmacological Aspects of Nursing Care,* 3rd ed.)

As the drug circulates in the blood, a certain blood level must be maintained for the drugs to be effective. When the blood level decreases below the therapeutic level, the drug will not produce the desired effect. Should the blood level increase significantly over the therapeutic level, toxic symptoms develop. Specific therapeutic blood levels are discussed in the subsequent chapters when applicable.

Metabolism

Metabolism, also called **biotransformation,** is the process by which a drug is converted by the liver to inactive compounds through a series of chemical reactions. Patients with liver disease may require lower dosages of a drug detoxified by the liver, or the primary care provider may select a drug that does not undergo a biotransformation by the liver. Frequent liver function texts are necessary when liver disease is present. The kidneys, lungs, plasma, and intestinal mucosa also aid in the metabolism of drugs.

Excretion

The elimination of drugs from the body is called excretion. After the liver renders drugs inactive, the kidney excretes the inactive compounds from the body. Also, some drugs are excreted unchanged by the kidney without liver involvement. Patients with kidney disease may require a dosage reduction and careful monitoring of kidney function. Children have immature kidney function and may require dosage reduction and kidney function tests. Similarly, older adults have diminished kidney function and require careful monitoring and lower dosages. Other drugs are eliminated by sweat, breast milk, breath, or by the gastrointestinal tract in the feces.

Half-Life

Half-life refers to the time required for the body to eliminate 50% of the drug. Knowledge of the half-life of a drug is important in planning the frequency of dosing. For example, drugs with a short half-life (2–4 hours) need to be administered frequently, whereas a drug with a long half-life (21–24 hours) requires less frequent dosing. It takes five to six half-lives to eliminate approximately 98% of a drug from the body. Although half-life is fairly stable, patients with liver or kidney disease may have problems excreting a drug. Difficulty in excreting a drug increases the half-life and increases the risk of toxicity. For example, digoxin (Lanoxin) has a long half-life (36 hours) and requires once-daily dosing. However, aspirin has a short half-life and requires frequent dosing. Older patients or patients with impaired kidney or liver function require frequent diagnostic tests measuring renal or hepatic function.

PHARMACODYNAMIC PHASE

Pharmacodynamics deals with the drug's action and effect within the body. After administration, most drugs enter the systemic circulation and expose almost all body tissues to possible effects of the drug. All drugs produce more than one effect in the body. The primary effect of a drug is the desired or therapeutic effect. Secondary effects are all other effects, whether desirable or undesirable, produced by the drug.

Most drugs have an affinity for certain organs or tissues and exert their greatest action at the cellular level on those specific areas, which are called target sites. There are two main mechanisms of action:

1. Alteration in cellular environment
2. Alteration in cellular function

Alteration in Cellular Environment

Some drugs act on the body by changing the cellular environment, either physically or chemically. Physical changes in the cellular environment include changes in osmotic pressures, lubrication, absorption, or the conditions on the surface of the cell membrane. An example of a drug that changes osmotic pressure is mannitol, which produces a change in the osmotic pressure in brain cells, causing a reduction in cerebral edema. A drug that acts by altering the cellular environment by lubrication is sunscreen. An example of a drug that acts by altering absorption is activated charcoal, which is administered orally to absorb a toxic chemical ingested into the gastrointestinal tract. The stool softener docusate is an example of a drug that acts by altering the surface of the cellular membrane. Docusate has emulsifying and lubricating activity that causes a lowering of the surface tension in the cells of the bowel, permitting water and fats to enter the stool. This softens the fecal mass, allowing easier passage of the stool.

Chemical changes in the cellular environment include inactivation of cellular functions or the alteration of the chemical components of body fluid, such as a change in the pH. For example, antacids neutralize gastric acidity in patients with peptic ulcers.

Alteration in Cellular Function

Most drugs act on the body by altering cellular function. A drug cannot completely change the function of a cell, but it can alter its function. A drug that alters cellular function can increase or decrease certain physiologic functions, such as increase heart rate, decrease blood pressure, or increase urine output.

Receptor-Mediated Drug Action

The function of a cell alters when a drug interacts with a receptor cell. A **receptor** is a specialized **macromolecule** (a large group of molecules linked together) that attaches or binds to the drug molecule. This alters the function of the cell and produces the therapeutic response of the drug. For a drug–receptor reaction to occur, a drug must be attracted to a particular receptor. Drugs bind to a receptor much like a piece of a puzzle. The closer the shape, the better the fit, and the better the therapeutic response. The intensity of a drug response is related to how good the "fit" of the drug molecule is and the number of receptor sites occupied.

Agonists are drugs that bind with a receptor to produce a therapeutic response. Drugs that bind only partially to the receptor will most probably have some, although slight, therapeutic response. Figure 1-3 identifies the different drug–receptor interactions. Partial agonists are drugs that have some drug receptor fit and produce a response but inhibit other responses.

Antagonists join with a receptor to prevent the action of an agonist. When the antagonist binds more tightly than the agonist to the receptor, the action of the antagonist is strong. Drugs that act as antagonists produce no pharmacologic effect. An example of an antagonist is Narcan, a narcotic antagonist that completely blocks the effects of morphine, including the respiratory depression. This drug is useful in reversing the effects of an overdose of narcotics.

Receptor-Mediated Drug Effects

The number of available receptor sites influences the effects of a drug. If only a few receptor sites are occupied, although many sites are available, the response will be small. If the drug dose is increased, more receptor sites are used and the response increases. If only a few receptor sites are available, the response does not increase if more of the drug is administered. However, not all receptors on a cell need to be occupied for a drug to be effective. Some extremely potent drugs are effective even when the drug occupies few receptor sites.

DRUG REACTIONS

Drugs produce many reactions in the body. The following sections discuss adverse drug reactions, allergic drug reactions, drug idiosyncrasy, drug tolerance, cumulative drug effect, and toxic reactions. Pharmacogenetic reactions can also occur. A pharmacogenetic reaction is a genetically determined adverse reaction to a drug.

Adverse Drug Reactions

Patients may experience one or more **adverse reactions** (side effects) when they are given a drug. Adverse reactions are undesirable drug effects. Adverse reactions may be common or may occur infrequently. They may be mild, severe, or life threatening. They may occur after the first dose, after several doses, or even after many doses. An adverse reaction often is unpredictable, although some drugs are known to cause certain adverse reactions in many patients. For example, drugs used in the treatment of cancer are very toxic and are known to produce adverse reactions in many patients receiving them. Other drugs produce adverse reactions in fewer patients. Some adverse reaction is predictable, but many adverse drug reactions occur without warning.

Some texts use both terms *side effect* and *adverse reactions.* These texts distinguish between the two terms by using *side effects* to explain mild, common, and nontoxic reactions; *adverse reaction* is used to describe more severe and life-threatening reactions. For the purposes of this text only the term *adverse reaction* is used, with the understanding that these reactions may be mild, severe, or life threatening.

Allergic Drug Reactions

An **allergic reaction** also is called a **hypersensitivity** reaction. Allergy to a drug usually begins to occur after more than one dose of the drug is given. On occasion, the nurse may observe an allergic reaction the first time a drug is given because the patient has received or taken the drug in the past.

A drug allergy occurs because the individual's immune system views the drug as a foreign substance or **antigen.** The presence of an antigen stimulates the antigen–antibody response that in turn prompts the body to produce **antibodies.** If the patient takes the drug after the antigen–antibody response has occurred, an allergic reaction results.

Even a mild allergic reaction produces serious effects if it goes unnoticed and the drug is given again. Any indication of an allergic reaction is reported to the primary health care provider before the next dose of the drug is given. Serious allergic reactions require contacting the primary health care provider immediately because emergency treatment may be necessary.

Some allergic reactions occur within minutes (even seconds) after the drug is given; others may be delayed for hours or days. Allergic reactions that occur immediately often are the most serious.

Allergic reactions are manifested by a variety of signs and symptoms observed by the nurse or reported by the patient. Examples of some allergic symptoms include itching, various types of skin rashes, and hives (urticaria). Other symptoms include difficulty breathing, wheezing, cyanosis, a sudden loss of consciousness, and swelling of the eyes, lips, or tongue.

Anaphylactic shock is an extremely serious allergic drug reaction that usually occurs shortly after the administration of a drug to which the individual is sensitive. This type of allergic reaction requires immediate medical attention. Symptoms of anaphylactic shock are listed in Table 1-2.

All or only some of these symptoms may be present. Anaphylactic shock can be fatal if the symptoms are not identified and treated immediately. Treatment is to raise the blood pressure, improve breathing, restore cardiac function, and treat other symptoms as they occur.

TABLE 1-2	Symptoms of Anaphylactic Shock
Respiratory	Bronchospasm
	Dyspnea (difficult breathing)
	Feeling of fullness in the throat
	Cough
	Wheezing
Cardiovascular	Extremely low blood pressure
	Tachycardia (heart rate > 100 bpm)
	Palpations
	Syncope (fainting)
	Cardiac arrest
Integumentary	Urticaria
	Angioedema
	Pruritus (itching)
	Sweating
Gastrointestinal	Nausea
	Vomiting
	Abdominal pain

Epinephrine (adrenalin) 0.1 to 0.5 mg may be given by subcutaneous or intramuscular injection. Hypotension and shock may be treated with fluids and vasopressors. Bronchodilators are given to relax the smooth muscles of the bronchial tubes. Antihistamines may be given to block the effects of histamine.

Angioedema (angioneurotic edema) is another type of allergic drug reaction. It is manifested by the collection of fluid in subcutaneous tissues. Areas that are most commonly affected are the eyelids, lips, mouth, and throat, although other areas also may be affected. Angioedema can be dangerous when the mouth is affected because the swelling may block the airway and asphyxia may occur. Difficulty in breathing or swelling to any area of the body is reported immediately to the primary health care provider.

Drug Idiosyncrasy

Drug idiosyncrasy is a term used to describe any unusual or abnormal reaction to a drug. It is any reaction that is different from the one normally expected of a specific drug and dose. For example, a patient may be given a drug to help him or her sleep (eg, a hypnotic). Instead of falling asleep, the patient remains wide awake and shows signs of nervousness or excitement. This response is an idiosyncratic response because it is different from what the nurse expects from this type of drug. Another patient may receive the same drug and dose, fall asleep, and after 8 hours be difficult to awaken. This, too, is abnormal and describes an overresponse to the drug.

The cause of drug idiosyncrasy is not clear. It is believed to be due to a genetic deficiency that makes the patient unable to tolerate certain chemicals, including drugs.

Drug Tolerance

Drug tolerance is a term used to describe a decreased response to a drug, requiring an increase in dosage to achieve the desired effect. Drug tolerance may develop when a patient takes certain drugs, such as the narcotics and tranquilizers, for a long time. The individual who takes these drugs at home increases the dose when the expected drug effect does not occur. The development of drug tolerance is a sign of drug dependence. Drug tolerance may also occur in the hospitalized patient. When the patient receives a narcotic for more than 10 to 14 days, the nurse suspects drug tolerance (and possibly drug dependence). The patient may also begin to ask for the drug at more frequent intervals.

Cumulative Drug Effect

A **cumulative drug effect** may be seen in those with liver or kidney disease because these organs are the major sites for the breakdown and excretion of most drugs. This drug effect occurs when the body is unable to metabolize and excrete one (normal) dose of a drug before the next dose is given. Thus, if a second dose of this drug is given, some drug from the first dose remains in the body. A cumulative drug effect can be serious because too much of the drug can accumulate in the body and lead to toxicity.

Patients with liver or kidney disease are usually given drugs with caution because a cumulative effect may occur. When the patient is unable to excrete the drug at a normal rate the drug accumulates in the body, causing a toxic reaction. Sometimes, the primary health care provider lowers the dose of the drug to prevent a toxic drug reaction.

Toxic Reactions

Most drugs can produce **toxic** or harmful reactions if administered in large dosages or when blood concentration levels exceed the therapeutic level. Toxic levels build up when a drug is administered in dosages that exceed the normal level or if the patient's kidneys are not functioning properly and cannot excrete the drug. Some toxic effects are immediately visible; others may not be seen for weeks or months. Some drugs, such as lithium or digoxin, have a narrow margin of safety, even when given in recommended dosages. It is important to monitor these drugs closely to avoid toxicity.

Drug toxicity can be reversible or irreversible, depending on the organs involved. Damage to the liver may be reversible because liver cells can regenerate. However, hearing loss due to damage to the eighth cranial nerve caused by toxic reaction to the anti-infective streptomycin may be permanent. Sometimes drug toxicity can be reversed by the administration of another drug that acts as an antidote. For example, in serious instances of digitalis toxicity, the drug Digibind may be given to counteract the effect of digoxin toxicity.

Nurses must carefully monitor the patient's blood levels of drugs to ensure that they remain within the therapeutic range. Any deviation should be reported to the primary health care provider. Because some drugs can cause toxic reactions even in recommended doses, the nurse should be aware of the signs and symptoms of toxicity of commonly prescribed drugs.

Pharmacogenetic Reactions

A **pharmacogenetic disorder** is a genetically determined abnormal response to normal doses of a drug. This abnormal response occurs because of inherited traits that cause abnormal metabolism of drugs. For example, individuals with glucose-6-phosphate dehydrogenase (G6PD) deficiency have abnormal reactions to a number of drugs. These patients exhibit varying degrees of hemolysis (destruction of red blood cells) if these drugs are administered. More than 100 million people are affected by this disorder. Examples of drugs that cause hemolysis in patients with a G6PD deficiency include aspirin, chloramphenicol, and the sulfonamides.

DRUG INTERACTIONS

It is important for the nurse administering medications to be aware of the various drug interactions that can occur, most importantly drug–drug interactions and drug–food interactions. The following section gives a brief overview of drug interactions. Specific drug–drug and drug–food interactions are discussed in subsequent chapters.

Drug–Drug Interactions

A drug–drug interaction occurs when one drug interacts with or interferes with the action of another drug. For example, taking an antacid with oral tetracycline causes a decrease in the effectiveness of the tetracycline. The antacid chemically interacts with the tetracycline and impairs its absorption into the bloodstream, thus reducing the effectiveness of the tetracycline. Drugs known to cause interactions include oral anticoagulants, oral hypoglycemics, anti-infectives, antiarrhythmics, cardiac glycosides, and alcohol. Drug–drug interactions can produce effects that are additive, synergistic, or antagonistic.

ADDITIVE DRUG REACTION. An **additive drug reaction** occurs when the combined effect of two drugs is equal to the sum of each drug given alone. For example, taking the drug heparin with alcohol will increase bleeding. The equation one + one = two is sometimes used to illustrate the additive effect of drugs.

SYNERGISTIC DRUG REACTION. Drug **synergism** occurs when drugs interact with each other and produce an effect that is greater than the sum of their separate actions. The equation one + one = four may be used to illustrate synergism. An example of drug synergism is when a person takes both a hypnotic and alcohol. When alcohol is taken simultaneously or shortly before or after the hypnotic is taken, the action of the hypnotic increases. The individual experiences a drug effect that is greater than if either drug was taken alone. On occasion, the occurrence of a synergistic drug effect is serious and even fatal.

ANTAGONISTIC DRUG REACTION. An antagonistic drug reaction occurs when one drug interferes with the action of another, causing neutralization or a decrease in the effect of one drug. For example, protamine sulfate is a heparin antagonist. This means that the administration of protamine sulfate completely neutralizes the effects of heparin in the body.

Drug–Food Interactions

When a drug is given orally, food may impair or enhance its absorption. A drug taken on an empty stomach is absorbed into the bloodstream at a faster rate than when the drug is taken with food in the stomach. Some drugs (eg, captopril) must be taken on an empty stomach to achieve an optimal effect. Drugs that should be taken on an empty stomach are administered 1 hour before or 2 hours after meals. Other drugs, especially drugs that irritate the stomach, result in nausea or vomiting, or cause epigastric distress, are best given with food or meals. This minimizes gastric irritation. The nonsteroidal anti-inflammatory drugs and salicylates are examples of drugs that are given with food to decrease epigastric distress. Still other drugs combine with a drug forming an insoluble food–drug mixture. For example, when tetracycline is administered with dairy products, a drug–food mixture is formed that is unabsorbable by the body. When a drug is unabsorbable by the body, no pharmacologic effect occurs.

FACTORS INFLUENCING DRUG RESPONSE

Certain factors may influence drug response and are considered when the primary health care provider prescribes and the nurse administers a drug. These factors include age, weight, gender, disease, and route of administration.

Age

The age of the patient may influence the effects of a drug. Infants and children usually require smaller doses of a drug than adults do. Immature organ function, particularly the liver and kidneys, can affect the ability of infants and young children to metabolize drugs. An infant's immature kidneys impair the elimination of drugs in the urine. Liver function is poorly developed in infants and young children. Drugs metabolized by the liver may produce more intense effects for longer periods. Parents must be taught the potential problems associated with administering drugs to their children. For example, a safe dose of a nonprescription drug for a 4-year-old child may be dangerous for a 6-month-old infant.

Elderly patients may also require smaller doses, although this may depend on the type of drug administered. For example, the elderly patient may be given the same dose of an antibiotic as a younger adult. However, the same older adult may require a smaller dose of a drug that depresses the central nervous system, such as a narcotic. Changes that occur with aging affect the pharmacokinetics (absorption, distribution, metabolism, and excretion) of a drug. Any of these processes may be altered because of the physiologic changes that occur with aging. Table 1-3 summarizes the changes that occur with aging and the possible pharmacokinetic effect.

Polypharmacy is the taking of numerous drugs that can potentially react with one another. When practiced by the elderly, polypharmacy leads to an increase in the number of potential adverse reactions. Although multiple drug therapy is necessary to treat certain disease states, it always increases the possibility of adverse reactions. The nurse needs good assessment skills to detect any problems when monitoring the geriatric patient's response to drug therapy.

TABLE 1-3	**Factors Altering Drug Response in the Elderly**
AGE-RELATED CHANGES	**EFFECT ON DRUG THERAPY**
Decreased gastric acidity; decreased gastric motility	Possible decreased or delayed absorption
Dry mouth and decreased saliva	Difficulty swallowing oral drugs
Decreased liver blood flow; decreased liver mass	Delayed and decreased metabolism of certain drugs; possible increased effect, leading to toxicity
Decreased lipid content of the skin	Possible decrease in absorption of transdermal drugs
Increased body fat; decreased body water	Possible increase in toxicity of water-soluble drugs; more prolonged effects of fat-soluble drugs
Decreased serum proteins	Possible increased effect and toxicity of highly protein-bound drugs
Decreased renal mass, blood flow, and glomerular filtration rate	Possible increased serum levels, leading to toxicity of drugs excreted by the kidney
Changes in sensitivity of certain drug receptors	Increase or decrease in drug effect

Adapted from Eisenhauer, L., Nichols, L., Spencer, R., & Bergan, F. (1998). *Clinical pharmacology and nursing management* (5th ed., p. 189). Philadelphia: Lippincott-Raven. Used with permission.

Weight

In general, dosages are based on a weight of approximately 150 lb, which is calculated to be the "average" weight of men and women. A drug dose may sometimes be increased or decreased because the patient's weight is significantly higher or lower than this average. With narcotics, for example, higher or lower than average dosages may be necessary to produce relief of pain, depending on the patient's weight.

Gender

The gender of an individual may influence the action of some drugs. Women may require a smaller dose of some drugs than men. This is because many women are smaller than men and have a body fat-and-water ratio different from that of men.

Disease

The presence of disease may influence the action of some drugs. Sometimes disease is an indication for not prescribing a drug or for reducing the dose of a certain drug. Both hepatic (liver) and renal (kidney) disease can greatly affect drug response.

In liver disease, for example, the ability to metabolize or detoxify a specific type of drug may be impaired. If the average or normal dose of the drug is given, the liver may be unable to metabolize the drug at a normal rate. Consequently, the drug may be excreted from the body at a much slower rate than normal. The primary health care provider may then decide to prescribe a lower dose and lengthen the time between doses because liver function is abnormal.

Patients with kidney disease may exhibit drug toxicity and a longer duration of drug action. The dosage of drugs may be reduced to prevent the accumulation of toxic levels in the blood or further injury to the kidney.

Route of Administration

Intravenous administration of a drug produces the most rapid drug action. Next in order of time of action is the intramuscular route, followed by the subcutaneous route. Giving a drug orally usually produces the slowest drug action.

Some drugs can be given only by one route; for example, antacids are given only orally. Other drugs are available in oral and parenteral forms. The primary health care provider selects the route of administration based on many factors, including the desired rate of action. For example, the patient with a severe cardiac problem may require intravenous administration of a drug that affects the heart. Another patient with a mild cardiac problem may experience a good response to oral administration of the same drug.

NURSING IMPLICATIONS

Many factors can influence drug action. The nurse should consult appropriate references or the hospital pharmacist if there is any question about the dosage of a drug, whether other drugs the patient is receiving will interfere with the drug being given, or whether the oral drug should or should not be given with food.

Drug reactions are potentially serious. The nurse should observe all patients for adverse drug reactions, drug idiosyncrasy, and evidence of drug tolerance (when applicable). It is important to report all drug reactions or any unusual drug effect to the primary health care provider.

The nurse must use judgment about when adverse drug reactions are reported to the primary health care provider. Accurate observation and evaluation of the circumstances are essential; the nurse should record all observations in the patient's record. If there is any question regarding the events that are occurring, the nurse can withhold the drug but must contact the primary health care provider.

HERBAL THERAPY AND NUTRITIONAL SUPPLEMENTS

Botanical medicine or herbal therapy is a type of complementary/alternative therapy that uses plants or herbs to treat various disorders. Individuals worldwide use both herbal therapy and nutritional supplements extensively. According to the World Health Organization (WHO), 80% of the world's population relies on herbs for a substantial part of their health care. Herbs have been used by virtually every culture in the world throughout history, from the beginning of time until now. For example, Hippocrates prescribed St. Johns Wort, currently a popular herbal remedy for depression. Native Americans used plants such as coneflower, ginseng, and ginger for therapeutic purposes. Herbal therapy is part of a group of nontraditional therapies commonly known as complementary/alternative medicine (CAM). Unfortunately, CAM therapies are not widely taught in medical schools. A 1998 survey revealed that 75 of 117 US medical schools offered elective courses in CAM or included CAM topics in required courses. Complementary therapies are therapies such as relaxation techniques, massage, dietary supplements, healing touch, and herbal therapy that can be used to "complement" traditional health care. Alternative therapies, on the other hand, are therapies used in place of or instead of conventional or Western medicine. The term *complementary/alternative therapy* often is used as an umbrella term for many therapies from all over the world.

Although herbs have been used for thousands of years, most of what we know has been from observation. Most herbs have not been scientifically studied for safety and efficacy (effectiveness). Much of what we know about herbal therapy has come from Europe, particularly Germany. During the last several decades, European scientists have studied botanical plants in ways that seek to identify how they work at the cellular level, what chemicals are most effective, and adverse effects related to their use. Germany has compiled information on 300 herbs and made recommendations for their use.

Dietary Supplement Health and Education Act

Because herbs cannot be sold and promoted in the United States as drugs, they are regulated as nutritional or dietary substances. *Nutritional* or *dietary substances* are terms used by the federal government to identify substances not regulated as drugs by the FDA but that are purported to be effective for use to promote health. Herbs, as well as vitamins and minerals, are classified as dietary or nutritional supplements. Because natural products cannot be patented in the United States, it is not profitable for drug manufacturers to spend the millions of dollars and the 8 to 12 years to study and develop these products as drugs. In 1994, the US government passed the Dietary Supplement Health and Education Act (DSHEA). This act defines substances such as herbs, vitamins, minerals, amino acids, and other natural substances as "dietary supplements." The act permits general health claims such as "improves memory" or "promotes regularity" as long as the label also has a disclaimer stating that the supplements are not approved by the FDA and are not intended to diagnose, treat, cure, or prevent any disease. The claims must be truthful and not misleading and be supported by scientific evidence. Some have abused the law by making exaggerated claims, but the FDA has the power to enforce the law, which it has done, and these claims have decreased.

Center for Complementary and Alternative Health

In 1992, the National Institutes of Health established an Office of Alternative Medicine to facilitate the study of alternative medical treatments and to disseminate the information to the public. In 1998, the name was changed to National Center for Complementary and Alternative Medicine (NCCAM). This office was established partly because of the increased interest and use of these therapies in the United States. It has been estimated that approximately 40% of all individuals in the United States use some form of complementary/alternative therapy. In 1997, Americans spent more that $27 billion on these therapies. Among the various purposes of the NCCAM,

one is to evaluate the safety and efficacy of widely used natural products, such as herbal remedies and nutritional and food supplements. Although the scientific study of CAM is relatively new, the Center is dedicated to developing programs and encouraging scientists to investigate CAM treatments that show promise. The NCCAM budget has steadily grown from $2 million in 1993 to more than $68.7 million in 2000. This funding increase reflects the public's interest and need for CAM information that is based on rigorous scientific research.

Educating the Client on the Use of Herbs and Nutritional Supplements

The use of herbs and nutritional supplements to treat various disorders is common. Herbs are used for various effects, such as to boost the immune system, treat depression, and for relaxation. Individuals are becoming more aware of the benefits of herbal therapies and nutritional supplements. Advertisements, books, magazines, and Internet sites abound concerning these topics. People, eager to cure or control various disorders, take herbs, teas, megadoses of vitamins, and various other natural products. Although much information is available on nutritional supplements and herbal therapy, obtaining the correct information sometimes is difficult. Medicinal herbs and nutritional substances are available at supermarkets, pharmacies, health food stores, specialty herb stores, and through the Internet. The potential for misinformation abounds. Because these substances are "natural products," many individuals may incorrectly assume that they are without adverse effects. When any herbal remedy or dietary supplement is used, it should be reported to the nurse and the primary health care provider. Many of these botanicals have strong pharmacological activity, and some may interact with prescription drugs or be toxic in the body. For example, comfrey, an herb that was once widely used to promote digestion, can cause liver damage. Although it may still be available in some areas, it is a dangerous herb and is not recommended for use as a supplement.

When obtaining the drug history, the nurse must always question the patient about the use of herbs, teas, vitamins, or other nutritional or dietary supplements. Many patients consider herbs as natural and therefore safe. It is also difficult for some to report the use of an herbal tea as a part of the health care regimen. Display 1-4 identifies teaching points to consider when discussing the use of herbs and nutritional supplements with patients. Although a complete discussion about the use of herbs is beyond the scope of this book, it is important to remember that the use of herbs and nutritional supplements is commonplace in many areas of the country. To help the student become more aware of herbal therapy and nutritional supplements, Appendix B gives

DISPLAY 1-4 ● Teaching Points When Discussing the Use of Herbal Therapy

- If you regularly use herbal therapies, invest in a good herbal reference book such as *Guide to Popular Natural Products,* edited by Ara DerMarderosian (Facts and Comparisons Publishing Group, 2001).
- Store clerks are not experts in herbal therapy. Your best choice is to select an herbal product manufactured by a reputable company.
- Check the label for the word "standardized." This means that the product has a specific percentage of a specific chemical.
- Some herbal tinctures are 50% alcohol, which could pose a problem to individuals with a history of alcohol abuse.
- Use products with more than six herbs cautiously. It is generally better to use the single herb than to use a diluted product with several herbs.
- Do not overmedicate with herbs. The adage "If one is good, two must be better" is definitely not true. Take only the recommended dosage.
- Herbs are generally safe when taken in recommended dosages. However, if you experience any different or unusual symptoms, such as heart palpitations, headaches, rashes, or difficulty breathing, stop taking the herb and contact your health care provider.
- Inform your primary health care provider of any natural products that you take (eg, herbs, vitamins, minerals, teas, etc.). Certain herbs can interact with the medications that you take, causing serious adverse reactions or toxic effects.
- Allow time for the herb to work. Generally, 30 days is sufficient. If your symptoms have not improved within 30 to 60 days, discontinue use of the herb.

Adapted from Fontaine, K. L. (2000). *Healing practices: Alternative therapies for nursing* (pp. 126–127). Upper Saddle River, NJ: Prentice Hall. Used with permission.

an overview of selected common herbs and nutritional supplements. In addition, Herbal Alerts are placed in various chapters throughout the book, giving the student valuable information or warnings about the use of herbs.

● Critical Thinking Exercises

1. *Judy Martin, a student nurse, has just administered an antibiotic to Mr. Green. When she returns to the room about 30 minutes later, she finds Mr. Green flushed, reporting a lump in his throat, and experiencing difficulty breathing. Determine what actions the student nurse should take.*
2. *Jenny Davis, age 25, is pregnant. Jenny's primary health care provider tells her that she may not take any medication without first checking with the health care provider during the pregnancy. Jenny is puzzled and questions you about this. Discuss how you would address Jenny's concerns.*
3. *Ms. James, an 80-year-old woman, is receiving a lower dose of Demerol, a narcotic analgesic, postoperatively for pain. Her family questions the use of a lower dose. Determine what information you would give her family when they voice concerns that the dosage will not adequately relieve their mother's pain. Analyze what*

patient assessment, if any, you would need to make before talking with the family.

● Review Questions

1. Mr. Carter has a rash and pruritus. You suspect an allergic reaction and immediately assess him for other more serious symptoms of an allergic reaction. What question would be most important to ask Mr. Carter?
   A. Are you having any difficulty breathing?
   B. Have you noticed any blood in your stool?
   C. Do you have a headache?
   D. Are you having difficulty with your vision?

2. Mr. Jones, a newly admitted patient, has a history of liver disease. In planning Mr. Jones' care the nurse must consider that liver disease may result in a (an) _____.
   A. increase in the excretion rate of a drug
   B. impaired ability to metabolize or detoxify a drug
   C. necessity to increase the dosage of a drug
   D. decrease in the rate of drug absorption

3. Oxycodone is prescribed for a patient on the unit where you work. To safely administer oxycodone the nurse knows that this drug is regulated by the Controlled Substance Act, which classifies this drug as a Schedule _____.
   A. drug with a high abuse potential
   B. drug with the potential for high abuse with severe dependency
   C. drug with moderate abuse potential
   D. drug with limited abuse potential

4. A patient asks the nurse to define a hypersensitivity reaction. The nurse begins by telling the patient that a hypersensitivity reaction is also called a _____.
   A. synergistic reaction
   B. antagonistic reaction
   C. drug idiosyncrasy
   D. drug allergy

5. If a patient takes a drug on an empty stomach, the nurse is aware that the drug will be _____.
   A. absorbed more slowly
   B. neutralized by pancreatic enzymes
   C. affected by enzymes in the colon
   D. absorbed more rapidly

6. In monitoring drug therapy, the nurse is aware that a synergistic drug effect may be defined as _____.
   A. an effect greater than the sum of the separate actions of two or more drugs
   B. an increase in the action of one of the two drugs being given
   C. a neutralizing drug effect
   D. a comprehensive drug effect

The Administration of Drugs

Key Terms

buccal
drug errors
extravasation
infiltration
inhalation
intradermal
intramuscular
intravenous

parenteral
standard precautions
subcutaneous
sublingual
transdermal
unit dose
Z-track

Chapter Objectives

On completion of this chapter, the student will:

- Name the six rights of drug administration.
- Identify the different types of medication orders.
- Discuss once-a-week dosing of certain drugs.
- Describe the various types of medication dispensing systems.
- List the various routes by which a drug may be given.
- Discuss the administration of oral and parenteral drugs.
- Discuss Occupational Safety and Health Administration (OSHA) guidelines concerning needle stick injuries and precautions.
- Discuss the administration of drugs through the skin and mucous membranes.
- Discuss nursing responsibilities before, during, and after a drug is administered.

The administration of a drug is a fundamental responsibility of the nurse. An understanding of the basic concepts of administering drugs is critical if the nurse is to perform this task safely and accurately.

In addition to administering the drug, the nurse monitors the therapeutic response (desired response) and reports adverse reactions. In the home setting, the nurse is responsible for teaching the patient and family members the necessary information to administer drugs safely in an outpatient setting.

THE SIX RIGHTS AND DRUG ADMINISTRATION

The nurse preparing and administering a drug to a patient assumes responsibility for this procedure. Responsibility entails preparing and administering the prescribed drug. There are six "rights" in the administration of drugs:

- *Right* patient
- *Right* drug
- *Right* dose
- *Right* route
- *Right* time
- *Right* documentation

Right Patient

When administering a drug, the nurse must be certain that the patient receiving the drug is the patient for whom the drug has been ordered. This is accomplished by checking the patient's wristband containing the patient's name (see Fig. 2-1). If there is no written identification verifying the patient's name, the nurse obtains a wristband or other form of identification before administering the drug. In some instances the nurse may ask the patient to identify himself. However, the nurse should not ask, "Are you Mr. Jones?" Some patients, particularly those who are confused or have difficulty hearing, may respond by answering yes even though that is not their name.

Some nursing homes or extended care facilities have pictures of the patient available, which allows the nurse to verify the correct patient. If pictures are used to identify patients, it is critical that they are recent and bear a good likeness of the individual.

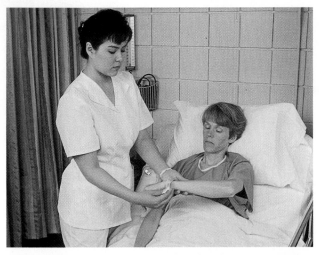

FIGURE 2-1. In following the Six "Rights" of medication administration, the nurse always verifies that the "Right Patient" is receiving the medication by checking the patient's identification bracelet. (Photograph © B. Proud.)

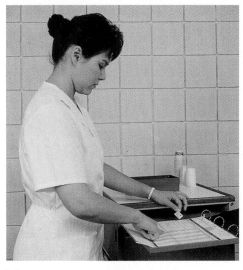

FIGURE 2-2. Prior to administering the medication, the nurse compares the medication, the container, and the medication to ensure that the patient received the "Right Drug" and the "Right Dosage." (Photograph © B. Proud.)

Right Drug

Drug names are often confused, especially when the names sound similar or the spellings are similar. Nurses who hurriedly prepare a drug for administration or who fail to look up questionable drugs are at increased risk for administering the wrong drug. Table 2-1 identifies

examples of drugs that can easily be confused. The nurse should compare medication, container label, and medication record (see Fig. 2-2).

Right Dose, Route, and Time

The nurse should obtain a primary care provider's written order for the administration of all drugs. The primary care provider's order must include the patient's name, the drug name, the dosage form and route, the dosage to be administered, and the frequency of administration. The primary care provider's signature must follow the drug order. In an emergency, the nurse may administer a drug with a verbal order from the primary care provider. However, the primary care provider must write and sign the order as soon as the emergency is over.

It is important to question any order that is unclear. This includes unclear directions for the administration of the drug, illegible handwriting on the primary care provider's order sheet, or a drug dose that is higher or lower than the dosages given in approved references.

Right Documentation

After the administration of any drug, the nurse records the process immediately (see Fig. 2-3). Immediate documentation is particularly important when drugs are given on an as-needed basis (PRN drugs). For example, most analgesics require 20 to 30 minutes before the drug begins to relieve pain. A patient may forget that he or she received a drug for pain, may not have been told that the administered

TABLE 2-1	Examples of Drugs That Are Easily Confused	
	Accupril	Accutane
	albuterol	atenolol
	Alupent	Atrovent
	Amikin	Amicar
	Bentyl	Aventyl
	Capitrol	captopril
	Cefzil	Ceftin
	Celebrex	Celexa
	DiaBeta	Zebeta
	dobutamine	dopamine
	Elavil	Mellaril
	Eurax	Serax
	Flomax	Fosamax
	Inderal	Isordil
	K-Dur	Imdur
	Klonopin	clonidine
	Lodine	codeine
	Nicobid	Nitro-Bid
	nifedipine	nicardipine
	prednisolone	prednisone
	Prilosec	Prozac
	Retrovir	ritonavir
	Taxol	Paxil
	TobraDex	Tobrex
	Versed	VePesid
	Zocor	Zoloft
	Zyvox	Vioxx

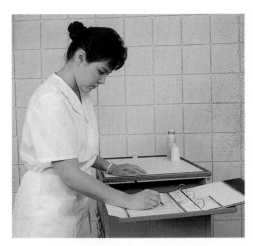

FIGURE 2-3. The nurse always documents the medication immediately after the drug is administered. (Photograph © B. Proud.)

drug was for pain, or may not know that pain relief is not immediate and may ask another nurse for drugs. If the administration of the analgesic were not recorded, the patient might receive a second dose of the analgesic shortly after the first dose. This kind of situation can be extremely serious, especially when narcotics or other central nervous system depressants are administered. Immediate documentation prevents accidental administration of a drug by another individual. Proper documentation is essential to the process of administering drugs correctly.

CONSIDERATIONS IN DRUG ADMINISTRATION

Drug Errors

Drug errors can be defined as any occurrence that can cause a patient to receive the wrong dose, the wrong drug, an incorrect dosage of the drug, a drug by the wrong route, or a drug given at the incorrect time. Errors may occur in transcribing drug orders, when the drug is dispensed, or in administration of the drug. Nurses serve as the last defense against detecting drug errors. When a drug error occurs, it must be reported immediately so that any necessary steps to counteract the action of the drug or any observation can be made as soon as possible. In most institutions, the nurse must complete an incident report and notify the primary care provider. It is important to report errors even if the patient suffers no harm.

Drug errors occur when one or more of the six "rights" has not been followed. Each time a drug is prepared and administered, the six rights must be a part of the procedure. In addition to consistently practicing the six rights, the nurse should adhere to the following precautions to help prevent drug errors:

- Confirm any questionable orders.
- When calculations are necessary, verify them with another nurse.
- Listen to the patient when he or she questions a drug, the dosage, or the drug regimen. Never administer the drug until the patient's questions have been adequately researched.
- Concentrate on only one task at a time.

Most errors are made during administration of the drug. Errors most commonly occur because of a failure to administer a drug that has been ordered, administration of the wrong dose or strength of a drug, or administration of the wrong drug. Two drugs often associated with errors are insulin and heparin.

The United States Pharmacopeia (USP) in cooperation with the Institute of Safe Medication Practices instituted a program called Medication Errors Reporting Program. This program is designed to identify the number and type of drug errors occurring around the country. The goal of this voluntary reporting system is to collect data and disseminate information that will prevent such errors in the future. A copy of the report form is included in Appendix C. Nurses are urged to participate in this important program as a means of protecting the public by identifying ways to make drug administration safer.

The Medication Order

Before a medication can be administered in a hospital or other agency the nurse must have a physician's order. Medications are ordered by the primary health care provider such as a physician, dentist, or in some cases a nurse practitioner.

Common orders include the standing order, the single order, the PRN order, and the STAT order. See Display 2-1 for an explanation of each.

DISPLAY 2-1 ● Types of Medication Orders

Standing Order: This type of order is given when the patient is to receive the drug as prescribed on a regular basis. The drug is administered until the physician discontinues the drug's use. Occasionally a drug may be ordered for a specified number of days, or in some cases a drug can only be given for a specified number of days before the order needs to be renewed.
Example: Lanoxin 0.25 mg PO QD.
Single order: An order to administer the drug one time only.
Example: Valium 10 mg IVP @ 10:00 AM.
PRN order: An order to administer the drug as needed.
Example: Demerol 100 mg IM q4h PRN for pain.
STAT order: A one-time order given as soon as possible.
Example: Morphine 10 mg IV STAT.

Once-a-Week Drugs

Soon many drugs will be available for once-a-week, or even twice-a-month, administration. The doses are designed to replace daily doses of drugs. One of the first is alendronate (Fosamax), a drug used to treat osteoporosis (see Chapter 21). In 2001, the FDA approved two new strengths for this drug to be given once a week: 70-mg and 35-mg tablets. The 70-mg tablet is used to treat postmenopausal osteoporosis, and the 35-mg tablet for prevention of osteoporosis in postmenopausal osteoporosis. In clinical trials the once-a-week dosing showed no greater adverse reactions than the once-daily regimen. Once-a-week dosing may prove beneficial for those experiencing mild adverse reactions in that the reactions would be experienced once a week, rather than every day.

Drug Dispensing Systems

There are a number of drug dispensing systems for the nurse to use to dispense medication after it has been ordered for the patient. A brief description of three methods is given below.

Computerized Dispensing System

Automated or computerized dispensing systems are used in many hospitals or agencies dispensing drugs. Drugs are dispensed in the pharmacy from drug orders that are sent from the individual floors or units. Each floor or unit has a medication cart in which medications are placed for individual patients. Medication orders are filled in the hospital pharmacy and are placed in the drug dispensing cart. When orders are filled, the cart is delivered to the unit. To administer the drugs, nurses enter the patient's name and the drug to be administered. The drug is dispensed and automatically recorded into the computerized system. After drugs are dispensed and the cart is almost empty, it goes back to the pharmacy to be refilled and for new drug orders to be placed.

Unit Dose System

The **unit dose** system is a method of dispensing medications in which drug orders are filled and medications dispensed to fill each patient's medication order(s) for a 24-hour period. The pharmacist dispenses each dose (unit) in a package that is labeled with the drug name and dosage. The drug(s) are placed in drawers in a special portable medication cart with a drawer for each patient. Many drugs are packaged by their manufacturers in unit doses. That is, each package is labeled by the manufacturer and contains one tablet or capsule, a premeasured amount of a liquid drug, a prefilled syringe, or one supposi-

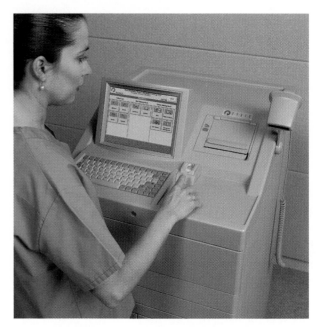

FIGURE 2-4. An automated medication system.

tory. Hospital pharmacists also may prepare unit doses. The pharmacist restocks the cart each day with the drugs needed for the next 24-hour period. The nurse takes the drug cart into each patient's room (Figure 2-4).

Some hospitals are using a bar code scanner in the administration of unit dose drugs. To use this system, a bar code is placed on the patient's hospital identification band when the patient is admitted to the hospital. The bar codes, along with bar codes on the drug unit dose packages, are used to identify the patient and to record and charge routine and PRN drugs. The scanner also keeps an ongoing inventory of controlled substances, which eliminates the need for narcotic counts at the end of each shift.

Floor Stock

Some agencies, such as nursing homes or small hospitals, use a floor stock method to dispense drugs. Some special units in hospitals, such as the emergency department, may use this method. In this situation, drugs most frequently prescribed are kept on the unit in containers in a designated medication room or at the nurses' station. The nurse takes the medication from the appropriate container and administers the drug to the patient and records the drug in the patient's administration record.

General Principles of Drug Administration

The nurse must have factual knowledge of each drug given, the reasons for use of the drug, the drug's general action, the more common adverse reactions associated with the drug, special precautions in administration (if any), and the normal dose ranges.

Some drugs may be given frequently; the nurse becomes familiar with pharmacologic information about a specific drug. Other drugs may be given less frequently, or a new drug may be introduced, requiring the nurse to obtain information from reliable sources, such as the drug package insert or the hospital department of pharmacy. *It is of utmost importance to check current and approved references for all drug information.*

It also is important for the nurse to take patient considerations, such as allergy history, previous adverse reactions, patient comments, and change in patient condition, into account before administering the drug. Before giving any drug for the first time, the nurse should ask the patient about any known allergies and any family history of allergies. This not only includes allergies to drugs but also to food, pollen, animals, and so on. Patients with a personal or family history of allergies are more likely to experience additional allergies and must be monitored closely.

If the patient makes any statement about the drug or if there is any change in the patient, these situations are carefully considered before the drug is given. Examples of situations that require consideration before a drug is given include:

- Problems that may be associated with the drug, such as nausea, dizziness, ringing in the ears, and difficulty walking. Any comments made by the patient may indicate the occurrence of an adverse reaction. The nurse should withhold the drug until references are consulted and the primary caregiver contacted. The decision to withhold the drug must have a sound rationale and must be based on knowledge of pharmacology.
- Comments stating that the drug looks different from the one previously received, that the drug was just given by another nurse, or that the patient thought the primary care provider discontinued the drug therapy.
- A change in the patient's condition, a change in one or more vital signs, or the appearance of new symptoms. Depending on the drug being administered and the patient's diagnosis, these changes may indicate that the drug should be withheld and the primary care provider contacted.

Preparing a Drug for Administration

When preparing a drug for administration, the nurse should observe the following guidelines:

- Always check the health care provider's written orders and verify any questions with the primary health care provider.
- Prepare drugs for administration in a quiet, well-lit area.
- Always check the label of the drug three times: (1) when the drug is taken from its storage area, (2) immediately before removing the drug from the container, and (3) before returning the drug to its storage area.
- Never remove a drug from an unlabeled container or from a container whose label is illegible.
- Wash hands immediately before preparing a drug for administration.
- Do not let hands touch capsules or tablets. To remove an oral drug from the container, the correct number of tablets or capsules is shaken into the cap of the container and from there into the medicine cup.
- Always observe aseptic technique when handling syringes and needles.
- Be alert for drugs with similar names. Some drugs have names that sound alike but are very different. To give one drug when another is ordered could cause serious consequences. For example, digoxin and digitoxin sound alike but are different drugs.
- Replace the caps of drug containers immediately after the drug is removed.
- Return drugs requiring special storage to the storage area immediately after they are prepared for administration. This rule applies mainly to the refrigeration of drugs but may also apply to drugs that must be protected from exposure to light or heat.
- Never crush tablets or open capsules without first checking with the pharmacist. Some tablets can be crushed or capsules can be opened and the contents added to water or a tube feeding when the patient cannot swallow a whole tablet or capsule. Some tablets have a special coating that delays the absorption of the drug. Crushing the tablet may destroy this drug property and result in problems such as improper absorption of the drug or gastric irritation. Capsules are gelatin and dissolve on contact with a liquid. The contents of some capsules do not mix well with water and therefore are best left in the capsule. If the patient cannot take an oral tablet or capsule, consult the primary care provider because the drug may be available in liquid form.
- Never give a drug that someone else has prepared. The individual preparing the drug must administer the drug.
- When using a unit dose system, do not remove the wrappings of the unit dose until the drug reaches the bedside of the patient who is to receive it. After administering the drug, the nurse charts immediately on the unit dose drug form. The method of administering drugs by the unit dose system is widely used.

ADMINISTRATION OF DRUGS BY THE ORAL ROUTE

The oral route is the most frequent route of drug administration and rarely causes physical discomfort in patients. Oral drug forms include tablets, capsules, and liquids. Some capsules and tablets contain sustained-release drugs, which dissolve over an extended period of time. Administration of oral drugs is relatively easy for patients who are alert and can swallow.

Nursing Responsibilities

The nurse should observe the following points when giving an oral drug:

- Place the patient in an upright position. It is difficult, as well as dangerous, to swallow a solid or liquid when lying down.
- Make sure that a full glass of water is readily available.
- Assess the patient's need for assistance in removing the tablet or capsule from the container, holding the container, holding a medicine cup, or holding a glass of water. Some patients with physical disabilities cannot handle or hold these objects and may require assistance.
- Advise the patient to take a few sips of water before placing a tablet or capsule in the mouth.
- Instruct the patient to place the pill or capsule on the back of the tongue and tilt the head back to swallow a tablet or slightly forward to swallow a capsule. Encourage the patient first to take a few sips of water to move the drug down the esophagus and into the stomach, and then to finish the whole glass.
- Give the patient any special instructions, such as drinking extra fluids or remaining in bed, that are pertinent to the drug being administered.
- Never leave a drug at the patient's bedside to be taken later unless there is a specific order by the primary care provider to do so. A few drugs (eg, antacids and nitroglycerin tablets) may be ordered to be left at the bedside.
- Patients with a nasogastric feeding tube may be given their oral drugs through the tube. Dilute and flush liquid drugs through the tube. However, crush tablets and dissolve them in water before administering them through the tube. Before administration, check the tube for placement. Flush the tube with water after the drugs are placed in the tube to completely clear the tubing.
- Instruct the patient to place **buccal** drugs against the mucous membranes of the cheek in either the upper or lower jaw. These drugs are given for a local, rather than systemic, effect. They are absorbed slowly from the mucous membranes of the mouth. Examples of drugs given buccally are lozenges and troches.
- Certain drugs are also given by the **sublingual** (placed under the tongue) route. These drugs must not be swallowed or chewed and must be dissolved completely before the patient eats or drinks. Nitroglycerin is commonly given sublingually.

ADMINISTRATION OF DRUGS BY THE PARENTERAL ROUTE

Parenteral drug administration means the giving of a drug by the subcutaneous (SC), intramuscular (IM), intravenous (IV), or intradermal route (Fig. 2-5). Other routes of parenteral administration that may be used by the primary care provider are intralesional (into a lesion), intra-arterial (into an artery), intracardiac (into the heart), and intra-articular (into a joint). In some instances, intra-arterial drugs are administered by a nurse. However, administration is not by direct arterial injection but by means of a catheter that has been placed in an artery.

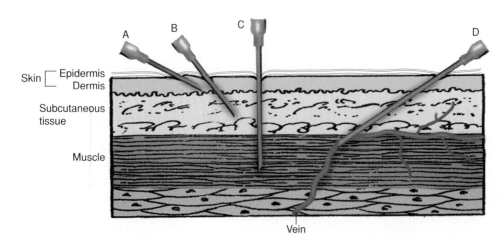

Skin [Epidermis / Dermis

Subcutaneous tissue

Muscle

Vein

FIGURE 2-5. Needle insertion for parenteral drug: (**A**) Intradermal injection: a 26-guage, ³/₈-inch long needle is inserted at a 10-degree angle. (**B**) Subcutaneous injection: a 25-guage, ¹/₂-inch long needle is inserted at an angle that depends on the size of the patient. (**C**) Intramuscular injection: a 20-gauge to 23-gauge, 1-inch to 3-inch long needle is inserted into the relaxed muscle at a 90-degree angle with a dart-throwing type of hand movement. (**D**) Intravenous injection: the diameter and length of the needle used depend on the substance to be injected and on the site of injection.

Nursing Responsibilities

The nurse should observe the following points when giving a drug by the parenteral route:

- Wear gloves for protection from the potential of a blood spill when giving parenteral drugs. The risk of exposure to infected blood is increasing for all health care workers. The Centers for Disease Control and Prevention (CDC) recommends that gloves be worn when touching blood or body fluids, mucous membranes, or any broken skin area. This recommendation is referred to as **Standard Precautions,** which combine the Universal Precautions for Blood and Body Fluids with Body Substance Isolation guidelines.
- After selecting the site for injection, cleanse the skin. Most hospitals have a policy regarding the type of skin antiseptic used for cleansing the skin before parenteral drug administration. Cleanse the skin with a circular motion, starting at an inner point and moving outward.
- After inserting the needle for IM administration, pull back the syringe barrel to aspirate the drug. If blood appears in the syringe, remove the needle so the drug is not injected. Discard the drug, needle, and syringe and prepare another injection. If no blood appears in the syringe, inject the drug. Aspiration is not necessary when giving an intradermal or SC injection.
- After inserting a needle into a vein for IV drug administration, pull back the syringe barrel. Blood should flow back into the syringe. After a backflow of blood is obtained, it is safe to inject the drug.
- After removing the needle from an IM, SC, or IV injection site, place pressure on the area. Patients with blooding tendencies often require prolonged pressure on the area.
- Do not recap syringes and dispose of them according to agency policy. Discard needles and syringes into clearly marked, appropriate containers. Most agencies have a "sharp" container located in each room for immediate disposal of needles and syringes after use.
- Most hospitals use needles designed to prevent sticks. This needle has a plastic guard that slips over the needle as it is withdrawn from the injection site. The guard locks in place and eliminates the need to recap. Other models are available as well. These newer types of methods for administering parenteral fluids provide a greater margin of safety for nurses. (See OSHA Guidelines below.)

Occupational Safety and Health Administration Guidelines

Each year between 600,000 and 1 million health care workers experience sticks from conventional needles and sharps. Needle exposures can transmit hepatitis B,

hepatitis C, and human immunodeficiency virus. Other infections, such as tuberculosis, syphilis, and malaria, also can be transmitted through needle sticks. More than 80% of needle stick injuries could be prevented with the use of safer needle devices. Nurses working at the bedside are the largest group of health care workers sustaining needle stick and sharps injuries.

Effective April 2001, the Occupational Safety and Health Administration (OSHA) announced new guidelines on needle stick prevention. Under the theory that "prevention is the best medicine," revisions were made in the Bloodborne Pathogens Standard. The revisions clarify the need for employers to select safer needle devices as they become available and to involve employees in identifying and choosing the devices. Employers with 11 or more employees must also maintain a Sharps Injury Log to include (at least) the following components:

- Type and brand of device involved in the incident (if known)
- Location of the incident
- Description of the incident

The needle stick log will help both employees and employers track all needle sticks to help identify problem areas. The log must be maintained to protect the confidentiality of the injured employee. In addition, employers must have a written Exposure Control Plan that is updated annually. During the annual review, inquiries must be made about new or prospective safer options. If new safer devices are available, they should be adopted for use in the agency. The new guidelines will help reduce needle stick injuries among health care workers and others who handle medical sharps. Safety engineered devices such as self-sheathing needles and needleless systems can be used.

Administration of Drugs by the Subcutaneous Route

A **subcutaneous** (SC) injection places the drug into the tissues between the skin and the muscle (see Fig. 2-5B). Drugs administered in this manner are absorbed more slowly than are intramuscular injections. Heparin and insulin are two drugs most commonly given by the SC route.

Nursing Responsibilities

The nurse should observe the following points when giving a drug by the SC route:

- A volume of 0.5 to 1 mL is used for SC injection. Larger volumes (eg, >1 mL) are best given as IM

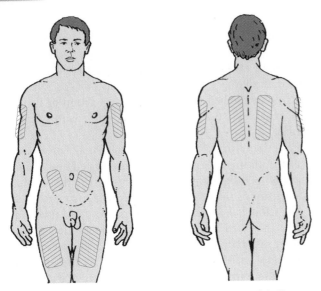

FIGURE 2-6. Sites on the body at which subcutaneous injections can be given.

injections. If a volume larger than 1 mL is ordered through the SC route, the injection is given in two sites, with separate needles and syringes.

- The sites for SC injection are the upper arms, the upper abdomen, and the upper back (Fig. 2-6). Rotate injection sites to ensure proper absorption and to minimize tissue damage.
- When giving a drug by the SC route, insert the needle at a 45-degree angle. However, to place the drug in the SC tissue, select the needle length and angle of insertion based on the patient's body weight. Obese patients have excess SC tissue, and it may be necessary to give the injection at a 90-degree angle. If the patient is thin or cachectic, there usually is less SC tissue. For such patients, the upper abdomen is the best site for injection. Generally, a syringe with a 23- to 25-gauge needle that is $1/2$ to $5/8$ inches in length is most suitable for an SC injection.

Administration of Drugs by the Intramuscular Route

An **intramuscular** (IM) injection is the administration of a drug into a muscle (see Fig. 2-5C). Drugs that are irritating to SC tissue can be given via IM injection. Drugs given by this route are absorbed more rapidly than drugs given by the SC route because of the rich blood supply in the muscle. In addition, a larger volume (1–3 mL) can be given at one site.

Nursing Responsibilities

The nurse should observe the following points when giving a drug by the IM route:

- If an injection is more that 3 mL, divide the drug and give it as two separate injections. Volumes larger than 3 mL will not be absorbed properly.
- A 22-gauge needle that is $1 1/2$ inches in length is most often used for IM injections.
- The sites for IM administration are the deltoid muscle (upper arm), the ventrogluteal or dorsogluteal sites (hip), and the vastus lateralis (thigh; Fig. 2-7). The vastus lateralis site is frequently used for infants and small children because it is more developed than the gluteal or deltoid sites. In children who have been ambulating for more than 2 years the ventrogluteal site may be used.
- When giving a drug by the IM route, insert the needle at a 90-degree angle. When injecting a drug into the ventrogluteal or dorsogluteal muscles, it is a good idea to place the patient in a comfortable position, preferably in a prone position with the toes pointing inward. When injecting the drug into the deltoid, a sitting or lying down position may be used. Place the patient in a recumbent position for injection of a drug into the vastus lateralis.

Z-Track Technique

The **Z-track** method of IM injection is used when a drug is highly irritating to SC tissues or has the ability to permanently stain the skin. The nurse should adhere to the following procedure when using the Z-track technique (Fig. 2-8):

- Draw the drug up into the syringe.
- Discard the needle and place a new needle on the syringe. This prevents any solution that may remain in the needle (that was used to draw the drug into the syringe) from contacting tissues as the needle is put into the muscle.
- Pull the plunger down to draw approximately 0.1 to 0.2 mL of air into the syringe. The air bubble in the syringe follows the drug into the tissues and seals off the area where the drug was injected, thereby preventing oozing of the drug up through the extremely small pathway created by the needle.
- Place the patient in the correct position for administration of an IM injection.
- Cleanse the skin.
- Pull the skin, SC tissues, and fat (that are over the injection site) laterally, displacing the tissue to the side.
- While holding the tissues in the lateral position, insert the needle and inject the drug.

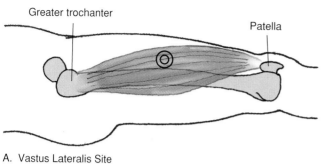

A. Vastus Lateralis Site

B. Ventrogluteal Site

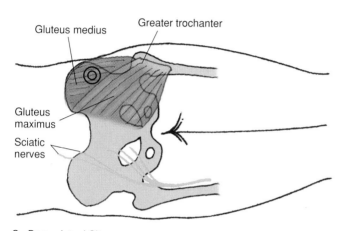

C. Dorsogluteal Site

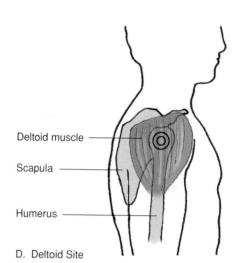

D. Deltoid Site

FIGURE 2-7. Sites for intramuscular administration. (**A**) Vastus lateralis site: the patient is supine or sitting. (**B**) Ventrogluteal site: the nurse's palm is placed on the greater trochanter and the index finger is placed on the anterior superior iliac spine; the injection is made into the middle of the triangle formed by the nurse's fingers and the iliac crest. (**C**) Dorsogluteal site: to avoid the sciatic nerve and accompanying blood vessels, an injection site is chosen above and lateral to a line drawn from the greater trochanter to the posterior superior iliac spine. (**D**) Deltoid site: the mid-deltoid area is located by forming a rectangle, the top of which is at the level of the lower edge of the acromion, and the bottom of which is at the level of the axilla; the sides are one third and two thirds of the way around the outer aspect of the patient's arm.

- After the drug is injected, release the tissues and withdraw the needle. This technique prevents the backflow of drug into the SC tissue.

Administration of Drugs by the Intravenous Route

A drug administered by the **intravenous** (IV) route is given directly into the blood by a needle inserted into a vein. Drug action occurs almost immediately.

Drugs administered via the IV route may be given:

- Slowly, over 1 or more minutes
- Rapidly (IV push)
- By piggyback infusions (drugs are mixed with 50–100 mL of compatible IV fluid and administered during a period of 30–60 minutes piggybacked onto the primary IV line)
- Into an existing IV line (the IV port)

- Into an intermittent venous access device called a heparin lock (a small IV catheter in the patient's vein connected to a small fluid reservoir with a rubber cap through which the needle is inserted to administer the drug)
- By being added to an IV solution and allowed to infuse into the vein over a longer period

When administering a drug into a vein by a venipuncture, the nurse should place a tourniquet above the selected vein. It is important to tighten the tourniquet so that venous blood flow is blocked but arterial blood flow is not. The nurse should allow the veins to fill (distend) and then should pull the skin taut (to anchor the vein and the skin) and insert the needle into the vein, bevel up, and at a short angle to the skin. Blood should immediately flow into the syringe if the needle is properly inserted into the vein.

Performing a venipuncture requires practice. A suitable vein for venipuncture may be hard to find, and some

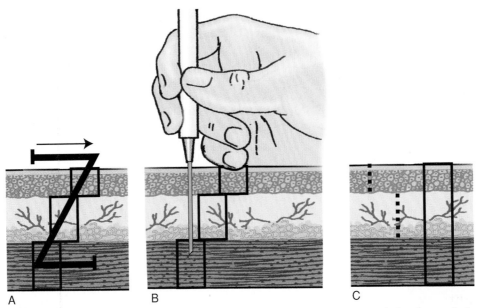

FIGURE 2-8. Z-track injection: (**A**) The tissue is tensed laterally at the injection site before the needle is inserted. This pulls the skin, subcutaneous tissue, and fat planes into a Z formation. (**B**) After the tissue has been displaced, the needle is thrust straight into the muscular tissue. (**C**) After injection, tissues are released while the needle is withdrawn. As each tissue plane slides by the other, the track is sealed.

veins are difficult to enter. The nurse should never repeatedly and unsuccessfully attempt a venipuncture. Depending on clinical judgment, three unsuccessful attempts on the same patient warrant having a more skilled individual attempt the procedure.

Some drugs are added to an IV solution, such as 1000 mL of dextrose 5% and water. The drug is usually added to the IV fluid container immediately before adding the fluid to the IV line. Whenever a drug is added to an IV fluid, the bottle must have a label attached indicating the drug and drug dose added to the IV fluid. In some hospitals, a pharmacist is responsible for adding specific drugs to IV fluids.

Intravenous Infusion Controllers and Pumps

Electronic infusion devices are classified as either infusion controllers or infusion pumps. The primary difference between the two is that an infusion pump adds pressure to the infusion, whereas an infusion controller does not. An infusion pump may be used to deliver the desired number of drops per minute. An alarm is set to sound if the IV is more than or less than the preset rate.

Controllers and pumps have detectors and alarms that alert the nurse to various problems, such as air in the line, an occlusion, low battery, completion of an infusion, or an inability to deliver the preset rate. When any problem is detected by the device, an alarm is activated to alert the nurse. Potential complications in IV therapy are the same as those with peripheral line.

Nursing Responsibilities

After the start of an IV infusion, the nurse records on the patient's chart the type of IV fluid and, when applicable, the drug added to the IV solution. It is important to check the infusion rate every 15 to 30 minutes. At this time, the nurse also inspects the needle site for signs of redness, swelling, or other problems. Swelling around the needle may indicate one of two things: extravasation or infiltration. **Extravasation** refers to the escape of fluid from a blood vessel into surrounding tissues while the needle or catheter is in the vein. **Infiltration** is the collection of fluid in tissues (usually SC tissue) when the needle or catheter is out of the vein. Both events necessitate discontinuation of the infusion and insertion of an IV line in another vein. Some drugs are capable of causing severe tissue damage if extravasation or infiltration occurs.

If extravasation or infiltration occurs, the IV must be stopped and restarted in another vein. The primary

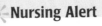

Nursing Alert

Use of an infusion pump or controller still requires nursing supervision and frequent monitoring of the IV infusion. Infiltration can progress rapidly because the increased pressure will not slow the infusion until considerable edema has occurred. Therefore, it is important to monitor frequently for signs of infiltration, such as edema or redness at the site. Careful monitoring of the pump or controller is also necessary to make sure the flow rate is correct.

care provider should be contacted if a drug capable of causing tissue damage (eg, norepinephrine [Levophed]) has escaped into the tissues surrounding the needle insertion site.

Administration of Drugs by the Intradermal Route

Drugs given by the intradermal route are usually those for sensitivity tests (eg, the tuberculin test or allergy skin testing) (see Fig. 2-5A). Absorption is slow and allows for good results when testing for allergies or administering local anesthetics.

Nursing Responsibilities

The nurse observes the following points when administering drugs by the intradermal route:

- The inner part of the forearm and the upper back may be used for intradermal injections. The area should be hairless; areas near moles, scars, or pigmented skin areas should be avoided. The nurse should cleanse the area in the same manner as for SC and IM injections.
- A 1-mL syringe with a 25- to 27-gauge needle that is $^1/_4$ to $^5/_8$ inch long is best suited for intradermal injections. Small volumes (usually <0.1 mL) are used for intradermal injections and administered with the bevel up.
- The nurse should insert the needle at a 15-degree angle between the upper layers of the skin. The nurse should not aspirate the syringe or massage the area. Injection produces a small wheal (raised area) on the outer surface of the skin. If a wheal does not appear on the outer surface of the skin, there is a good possibility that the drug entered the SC tissue, and any test results would be inaccurate.

Other Parenteral Routes of Drug Administration

The primary care provider may administer a drug by the intracardial, intralesional, intra-arterial, or intra-articular routes. The nurse may be responsible for preparing the drug for administration. The nurse should ask the primary care provider what special materials will be required for administration.

Venous access ports are totally implanted ports with a self-sealing septum that is attached to a catheter leading to a large vessel, usually the vena cava. These devices are most commonly used for chemotherapy or other long-term therapy and require surgical insertion and removal. Drugs are administered through injections made into the portal through the skin. These drugs are administered by the primary care provider or a registered nurse.

ADMINISTRATION OF DRUGS THROUGH THE SKIN AND MUCOUS MEMBRANES

Drugs may be applied to the skin and mucous membranes using several routes: topically (on the outer layers of skin), transdermally through a patch on which the drug has been implanted, or inhaled through the membranes of the upper respiratory tract.

Administration of Drugs by the Topical Route

Most topical drugs act on the skin but are not absorbed through the skin. These drugs are used to soften, disinfect, or lubricate the skin. A few topical drugs are enzymes that have the ability to remove the superficial debris, such as the dead skin and purulent matter present in skin ulcerations. Other topical drugs are used to treat minor, superficial skin infections. The various forms of topical applications and locations of use are described in Display 2-2.

Nursing Responsibilities

The nurse considers the following points when administering drugs by the topical route:

- The primary care provider may write special instructions for the application of a topical drug. For example, to apply the drug in a thin, even layer or to cover the area after application of the drug to the skin.
- Other drugs may have special instructions provided by the manufacturer, such as to apply the drug to a

---

DISPLAY 2-2 ● Topical Applications and Locations of Use

- Creams, lotions, or ointments applied to the skin with a tongue blade, gloved fingers, or gauze
- Sprays applied to the skin or into the nose or oral cavity
- Liquids inserted into body cavities, such as fistulas
- Liquids inserted into the bladder or urethra
- Solids (eg, suppositories) or jellies inserted into the urethra
- Liquids dropped into the eyes, ears, or nose
- Ophthalmic ointments applied to the eyelids or dropped into the lower conjunctival sac
- Solids (eg, suppositories, tablets), foams, liquids, and creams inserted into the vagina
- Continuous or intermittent wet dressings applied to skin surfaces
- Solids (eg, tablets, lozenges) dissolved in the mouth
- Sprays or mists inhaled into the lungs
- Liquids, creams, or ointments applied to the scalp
- Solids (eg, suppositories), liquids, or foams inserted into the rectum

clean, hairless area or to let the drug dissolve slowly in the mouth. All of these instructions are important because drug action may depend on correct administration of the drug.

Administration of Drugs by the Transdermal Route

Drugs administered by the **transdermal** route are readily absorbed from the skin and provide systemic effects. This type of administration is called transdermal drug delivery system. The drug dosages are implanted in a small patch-type bandage. The backing is removed, and the patch is applied to the skin where the drug is gradually absorbed into the systemic circulation. This type of drug system maintains a relatively constant blood concentration and reduces the possibility of toxicity. In addition, the use of drugs transdermally causes fewer adverse reactions, and administration is less frequent than when the drugs are given by another route. Nitroglycerin (used to treat cardiac problems) and scopolamine (used to treat dizziness and nausea) are two drugs given frequently by the transdermal route.

Nursing Responsibilities

The nurse observes the following points when administering drugs by the transdermal route:

- Apply transdermal patches to clean, dry, nonhairy areas of intact skin.
- Remove the old patch when the next dose is applied in a new site.
- Rotate sites for transdermal patches to prevent skin irritation. The chest, flank, and upper arm are the most commonly used sites. Do not shave the area to apply the patch; shaving may cause skin irritation.
- Ointments are sometimes used and come with a special paper marked in inches. Measure the correct length (onto the paper), place the paper with the drug ointment side down on the skin, and secure it with tape. Before the next dose, remove the paper and tape and cleanse the skin.

Administration of Drugs Through Inhalation

Drug droplets, vapor, or gas are administered through the mucous membranes of the respiratory tract with the use of a face mask, a nebulizer, or a positive-pressure breathing machine. Examples of drugs administered through **inhalation** include bronchodilators, mucolytics, and some anti-inflammatory drugs. These drugs produce, primarily, a local effect in the lungs.

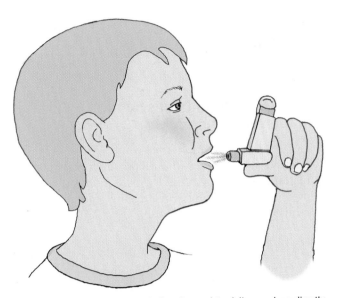

FIGURE 2-9. A respiratory inhalant is used to deliver a drug directly into the lungs. To deliver a dose of the drug, the patient takes a slow, deep breath while depressing the top of the canister. (See Chapter 37 for more information on drugs given by inhalation.)

Nursing Responsibilities

The primary nursing responsibility is to provide the patient with proper instructions for administering the drug. For example, many patients with asthma use a metered-dose inhaler to dilate the bronchi and make breathing easier. Without proper instruction on how to use the inhaler, much of the drug can be deposited on the tongue, rather than in the respiratory tract. This decreases the therapeutic effect of the drug. Instructions may vary with each inhaler. To be certain that the inhaler is used correctly, the patient is referred to the instructions accompanying each device. Figure 2-9 illustrates the proper use of one type of inhaler.

NURSING RESPONSIBILITIES AFTER DRUG ADMINISTRATION

After the administration of any type of drug, the nurse is responsible for the following:

- Recording the administration of the drug. The nurse should complete this task as soon as possible. This is particularly important when PRN drugs (especially narcotics) are given.
- Recording (when necessary) any information concerning the administration of the drug. This includes information such as the IV flow rate, the site used for parenteral administration, problems

Home Care Checklist

ADMINISTERING DRUGS SAFELY IN THE HOME

For most patients, drugs will be prescribed after discharge to be taken at home. Because the home is not as controlled an environment as a health care facility, the nurse should assess the patient's home environment carefully to ensure complete safety. It is important to keep in mind the following when making a home safety assessment:

✔ Does the home have a space that is relatively free of clutter and easily accessible to the patient or a caregiver?

✔ Do any small children live in or visit the home? If so, is there a place where drugs can be stored safely out of their reach?

✔ Does the drug require refrigeration? If so, does the refrigerator work?

✔ Does the patient need special equipment, such as needles and syringes? If so, where and how can the equipment be stored for safety and convenience? Does the patient have an appropriate disposal container? Will the refuse be safe from children and pets?

✔ If the patient needs several drugs, can the patient or caregiver identify which drugs are used and when? Do they know how to use them and why?

✔ Suggest using plastic storage containers with snap-on lids or clean, dry glass jars with screw tops for needle disposal.

✔ Advise the patient to use an impervious container with a properly fitting lid, such as a coffee can, for safe disposal of needles. A plastic milk jug with a lid or a heavy-duty, clean, cardboard milk or juice carton may be used if necessary.

✔ Explain the importance of taking precautions to make sure discarded needles do not puncture the container.

with administration (if any), and vital signs taken immediately before administration.

- Evaluating and recording the patient's response to the drug (when applicable). Evaluation may include such facts as relief of pain, decrease in body temperature, relief of itching, and decrease in the number of stools passed.
- Observing the adverse reactions. The frequency of these observations will depend on the drug administered. The nurse must record all suspected adverse reactions and report them to the primary care provider. The nurse must immediately report serious adverse reactions to the primary care provider.

ADMINISTRATION OF DRUGS IN THE HOME

Many times drugs are not administered by the nurse but in the home setting by the patient or family members serving as caregivers. When this is the case, it is important that the patient or caregivers understand the treatment regimen and are given an opportunity to ask questions concerning the drug therapy, such as why the drug was prescribed, how to administer the drug, and adverse

reactions of the drug (see Chap. 5 for information concerning patient and family education). The Home Care Checklist: Administering Drugs Safely in the Home gives some guidelines to follow when drugs are administered in the home by the patient or caregiver, rather than by the nurse.

● *Critical Thinking Exercises*

1. *Ms. Benson, a nurse on your clinical unit, tells you that the head nurse is upset with her because she has not been recording the administration of narcotics immediately after they are given. Discuss the rationales you could give to Ms. Benson to stress the importance of recording the administration of narcotics immediately after they are given.*

2. *A nurse is to give an SC injection of heparin to a patient. Determine what information the nurse needs to know about the patient before preparing the injection. Discuss how this information would affect the preparation of the injection and the technique used to give the SC injection.*

3. *After administering a drug to a patient you find that the incorrect dosage was given. The dose that you administered was two times the correct dosage. Analyze what action, if any, you would take.*

4. *Discuss why the sixth right, right documentation, is important in drug administration.*

5. *Discuss the importance in participating in the MedWatch programs and the Medication Errors Reporting Program.*

● Review Questions

1. The nurse correctly administers an intramuscular injection by _____.
   - **A.** displacing the skin to the side before making the injection
   - **B.** using a 1-inch needle
   - **C.** inserting the needle at a 90-degree angle
   - **D.** using a 25-gauge needle

2. When preparing a drug for SC administration, the nurse is aware that the usual volume of a drug injected by the SC route is _____.
   - **A.** 2 to 5 mL
   - **B.** 3 to 4 mL
   - **C.** 0.5 to 1 mL
   - **D.** <0.5 mL

3. The nurse explains to the patient receiving an IV injection that the action of the drug occurs _____.
   - **A.** in 5 to 10 minutes
   - **B.** in 15 to 20 minutes
   - **C.** within 30 minutes
   - **D.** almost immediately

4. When administering a drug the nurse _____.
   - **A.** checks the drug label two times before administration
   - **B.** is alert for any drugs with a similar name
   - **C.** may administer a drug prepared by another nurse
   - **D.** may crush any tablet that the patient is unable to swallow

5. When monitoring a patient with an IV, the nurse observes the area around the needle insertion site is swollen and red. The first action of the nurse is to _____.
   - **A.** check the patient's blood pressure and pulse
   - **B.** check further for possible extravasation
   - **C.** ask the patient if the IV site has been accidentally injured
   - **D.** immediately notify the primary health care provider

chapter 3

Review of Arithmetic and Calculation of Drug Dosages

Chapter Objective

On completion of this chapter, the student will:

- Accurately perform mathematical calculations when they are necessary to compute drug dosages.

REVIEW OF ARITHMETIC

Fractions

The two parts of a fraction are the **numerator** and the **denominator.**

$$\frac{2}{3} \begin{matrix} \leftarrow \text{numerator} \\ \leftarrow \text{denominator} \end{matrix}$$

A **proper fraction** may be defined as a part of a whole or any number less than a whole number. An **improper fraction** is a fraction having a numerator the same as or larger than the denominator.

$$\text{proper fraction} \quad \frac{1}{2}$$

$$\text{improper fraction} \quad \frac{7}{3}$$

The numerator and the denominator *must be of like entities or terms,* that is:

Correct (like terms)	Incorrect (unlike terms)
$\dfrac{2 \text{ acres}}{3 \text{ acres}}$	$\dfrac{2 \text{ acres}}{3 \text{ miles}}$
$\dfrac{2 \text{ grams}}{3 \text{ grams}}$	$\dfrac{2 \text{ grams}}{5 \text{ milliliters}}$

Mixed Numbers and Improper Fractions

A **mixed number** is a whole number and a proper fraction. A whole number is a number that stands alone; 3, 25, and 117 are examples of whole numbers. A proper fraction is a fraction whose numerator is *smaller than* the denominator; 1/8, 2/5, and 3/7 are examples of proper fractions.

These are mixed numbers:

2 2/3   2 is the whole number and 2/3 is the proper fraction

3 1/4   3 is the whole number and 1/4 is the proper fraction

When doing certain calculations, it is sometimes necessary to change a mixed number to an improper fraction or change an improper fraction to a mixed number. An improper fraction is a fraction whose numerator is *larger than* the denominator; 5/2, 16/3, and 12 3/2 are examples of improper fractions.

To change a *mixed number to an improper fraction,* multiply the denominator of the fraction by the whole number, add the numerator, and place the sum over the denominator.

EXAMPLE Mixed number 3 3/5

1. Multiply the denominator of the fraction (5) by the whole number (3) or $5 \times 3 = 15$:

$$3 \underset{\times}{\nwarrow} \frac{3}{5}$$

2. Add the result of multiplying the denominator of the fraction (15) to the numerator (3) or $15 + 3 = 18$:

$$3 \underset{\times}{\nwarrow} \nearrow \frac{3}{5}$$

3. Then place the sum (18) over the denominator of the fraction:

$$\frac{18}{5}$$

To change an *improper fraction to a mixed number,* divide the denominator into the numerator. The **quotient** (the result of the division of these two numbers) is the whole number. Then place the remainder over the denominator of the improper fraction.

EXAMPLE Improper fraction 15/4

$$\frac{15}{4} \begin{array}{l} \leftarrow \text{numerator} \\ \leftarrow \text{denominator} \end{array}$$

1. Divide the denominator (4) into the numerator (15) or 15 divided by 4 ($15 \div 4$):

$$\begin{array}{r} 3 \leftarrow \text{quotient} \\ 4\overline{)15} \\ \underline{12} \\ 3 \leftarrow \text{remainder} \end{array}$$

2. The **quotient** (3) becomes the whole number:

$$3\frac{3}{4}$$

3. The **remainder** (3) now becomes the numerator of the fraction of the mixed number:

$$3\frac{\mathbf{3}}{}$$

4. And the denominator of the improper fraction (4) now becomes the denominator of the fraction of the mixed number:

$$3\frac{3}{\mathbf{4}}$$

Adding Fractions With Like Denominators

When the denominators are the *same,* fractions can be added by adding the numerators and placing the sum of the numerators over the denominator.

EXAMPLES

$$2/7 + 3/7 = 5/7$$
$$1/10 + 3/10 = 4/10$$
$$2/9 + 1/9 + 4/9 = 7/9$$
$$1/12 + 5/12 + 3/12 = 9/12$$
$$2/13 + 1/13 + 3/13 + 5/13 = 11/13$$

When giving a final answer, fractions are *always* reduced to the lowest possible terms. In the examples above, the answers of 5/7, 7/9, and 11/13 cannot be reduced. The answers of 4/10 and 9/12 can be reduced to 2/5 and 3/4.

To reduce a fraction to the lowest possible terms, determine if any number, which always must be the same, can be divided into both the numerator and the denominator.

4/10: the numerator *and* the denominator can be divided by 2

9/12: the numerator *and* the denominator can be divided by 3

$$\text{For example: } \frac{4 \div 2 = 2}{10 \div 2 = 5}$$

If when adding fractions the answer is an improper fraction, it may then be changed to a mixed number.

2/5 + 4/5 = 6/5 (improper fraction)
6/5 changed to a mixed number is 1 1/5

Adding Fractions With Unlike Denominators

Fractions with *unlike denominators* cannot be added until the denominators are changed to like numbers or numbers that are the same. The first step is to find the *lowest common denominator,* which is the lowest number divisible by (or that can be divided by) all the denominators.

EXAMPLE Add 2/3 and 1/4

$$\left.\begin{array}{l} \dfrac{2}{3} \leftarrow \\[2mm] \dfrac{1}{4} \leftarrow \end{array}\right]$$ The lowest number that can be divided by these two denominators is 12; therefore, 12 is the lowest common denominator.

1. Divide the lowest common denominator (which in this example is 12) by each of the denominators in the fractions (in this example 3 and 4):

$$\frac{2}{3} = \frac{}{12} \quad (12 \div 3 = 4)$$

$$\frac{1}{4} = \frac{}{12} \quad (12 \div 4 = 3)$$

2. Multiply the results of the divisions by the numerator of the fractions (12 ÷ 3 = 4 × the numerator 2 = 8 and 12 ÷ 4 = 3 × the numerator 1 = 3) and place the results in the numerator:

$$\frac{2}{3} = \frac{}{12} \quad \frac{\mathbf{8}}{12}$$

$$\frac{1}{4} = \frac{}{12} \quad \frac{\mathbf{3}}{12}$$

3. Add the numerators (8 + 3) and place the result over the denominator (12):

$$\frac{8}{12}$$
$$\frac{3}{12}$$
$$\frac{11}{12}$$

Adding Mixed Numbers or Fractions With Mixed Numbers

When adding two or more mixed numbers or adding fractions and mixed numbers, the mixed number is first changed to an improper fraction.

EXAMPLE Add 3 3/4 and 3 3/4

$$3\frac{3}{4} \text{ changed to an improper fraction} \rightarrow \frac{15}{4}$$

$$3\frac{3}{4} \text{ changed to an improper fraction} \rightarrow \frac{15}{4}$$

The numerators are added $\rightarrow \dfrac{30}{4} = 7\ 2/4 = 7\ 1/2$

The improper fraction (30/4) is changed to a mixed number (7 2/4) and the fraction of the mixed number (2/4) changed to the lowest possible terms (1/2).

EXAMPLE Add 2 1/2 and 3 1/4

$$2\frac{1}{2} \text{ changed to an improper fraction} \frac{5}{2}$$

$$3\frac{1}{4} \text{ changed to an improper fraction} \frac{13}{4}$$

In the example above, 5/2 and 13/4 cannot be added because the denominators are not the same. It will be necessary to find the lowest common denominator first.

$$\frac{5}{2} \quad \text{the lowest} \quad \nearrow \frac{10}{4}$$
common
denominator
is 4
$$\frac{13}{4} \qquad \searrow \frac{13}{4}$$
$$\frac{23}{4} \text{ changed to a mixed number} = 5\frac{3}{4}$$

Comparing Fractions

When fractions with *like* denominators are compared, the fraction with the *largest numerator* is the *largest* fraction.

EXAMPLES

Compare: 5/8 and 3/8 Answer: **5**/8 is larger than **3**/8.
Compare: 1/4 and 3/4 Answer: **3**/4 is larger than **1**/4

When the denominators are *not* the same, for example, comparing 2/3 and 1/10, the lowest common denominator must first be determined. The same procedure is followed when adding fractions with unlike denominators (see above).

EXAMPLE Compare 2/3 and 1/10 (fractions with unlike denominators)

$$\frac{2}{3} = \frac{20}{30}$$
lowest common denominator
$$\frac{1}{10} = \frac{3}{30}$$

The largest numerator in these two fractions is 20; therefore, 2/3 is larger than 1/10.

Multiplying Fractions

When fractions are multiplied, the numerators are multiplied *and* the denominators are multiplied.

EXAMPLES

$$\frac{1}{8} \times \frac{1}{4} = \frac{1}{32} \qquad \frac{1}{2} \times \frac{2}{3} = \frac{2}{6} = \frac{1}{3}$$

In the above examples, it was necessary to reduce one of the answers to its lowest possible terms.

Multiplying Whole Numbers and Fractions

When whole numbers are multiplied with fractions, the numerator is multiplied by the whole number and the product is placed over the denominator. When necessary, the fraction is reduced to its lowest possible terms. If the answer is an improper fraction, it may be changed to a mixed number.

EXAMPLES

$$2 \times \frac{1}{2} = \frac{2}{2} = 1 \quad \text{(answer reduced to lowest possible terms)}$$

$$2 \times \frac{3}{8} = \frac{6}{8} = \frac{3}{4} \quad \text{(answer reduced to lowest possible terms)}$$

$$4 \times \frac{2}{3} = \frac{8}{3} = 2\frac{2}{3} \quad \text{(improper fraction changed to a mixed number)}$$

Multiplying Mixed Numbers

To multiply mixed numbers, the mixed numbers are changed to *improper fractions* and then multiplied.

EXAMPLES

$$2\frac{1}{2} \times 3\frac{1}{4} = \frac{5}{2} \times \frac{13}{4} = \frac{65}{8} = 8\frac{1}{8}$$

$$3\frac{1}{3} \times 4\frac{1}{2} = \frac{10}{3} \times \frac{9}{2} = \frac{90}{6} = 15$$

Multiplying a Whole Number and a Mixed Number

To multiply a whole number and a mixed number, *both* numbers must be changed to improper fractions.

EXAMPLES

$$3 \times 2\frac{1}{2} = \frac{3}{1} \times \frac{5}{2} = \frac{15}{2} = 7\frac{1}{2}$$

$$2 \times 4\frac{1}{2} = \frac{2}{1} \times \frac{9}{2} = \frac{18}{2} = 9$$

A whole number is converted to an improper fraction by placing the whole number over 1. In the above examples. 3 becomes 3/1 and 2 becomes 2/1.

Dividing Fractions

When fractions are divided, the *second* fraction (the divisor) is inverted (turned upside down) and then the fractions are multiplied.

EXAMPLES

$$\frac{1}{3} \div \frac{3}{7} = \frac{1}{3} \times \frac{7}{3} = \frac{7}{9}$$

$$\frac{1}{8} \div \frac{1}{4} = \frac{1}{8} \times \frac{4}{1} = \frac{4}{8} = \frac{1}{2}$$

$$\frac{3}{4} \div \frac{1}{2} = \frac{3}{4} \times \frac{2}{1} = \frac{6}{4} = 1\frac{1}{2}$$

In the above examples, the second answer was reduced to its lowest possible terms and the third answer, which was an improper fraction, was changed to a mixed number.

Dividing Fractions and Mixed Numbers

Some problems of division may be expressed as (1) fractions and mixed numbers, (2) two mixed numbers, (3) whole numbers and fractions, or (4) whole numbers and mixed numbers.

MIXED NUMBERS AND FRACTIONS. When a mixed number is divided by a fraction, the whole number is first changed to a fraction.

EXAMPLES

$$2\frac{1}{3} \div \frac{1}{4} = \frac{7}{3} \div \frac{1}{4} = \frac{7}{3} \times \frac{4}{1} = \frac{28}{3} = 9\frac{1}{3}$$

$$2\frac{1}{2} \div \frac{1}{2} = \frac{5}{2} \div \frac{1}{2} = \frac{5}{2} \times \frac{2}{1} = \frac{10}{2} = 5$$

MIXED NUMBERS. When two mixed numbers are divided, they are both changed to improper fractions.

EXAMPLE

$$3\frac{3}{4} \div 1\frac{1}{2} = \frac{15}{4} \div \frac{3}{2} = \frac{15}{4} \times \frac{2}{3} = \frac{30}{12}$$

$$= 2\frac{6}{12} = 2\frac{1}{2}$$

WHOLE NUMBERS AND FRACTIONS. When a whole number is divided by a fraction, the whole number is changed to an improper fraction by placing the whole number over 1.

EXAMPLE

$$2 \div \frac{2}{3} = \frac{2}{1} \div \frac{2}{3} = \frac{2}{1} \times \frac{3}{2} = \frac{6}{2} = 3$$

WHOLE NUMBERS AND MIXED NUMBERS. When whole numbers and mixed numbers are divided, the whole number is changed to an improper fraction and the mixed number is changed to an improper fraction.

EXAMPLE

$$4 \div 2\frac{2}{3} = \frac{4}{1} \div \frac{8}{3} = \frac{4}{1} \times \frac{3}{8} = \frac{12}{8} = 1\frac{4}{8} = 1\frac{1}{2}$$

Ratios

A ratio is a way of expressing *a part of a whole* or *the relation of one number to another*. For example, a ratio written as 1:10 means 1 in 10 parts, or 1 to 10. A ratio may also be written as a fraction; thus 1:10 can also be expressed as 1/10.

EXAMPLES

1:1000 is 1 part in 1000 parts, or 1 to 1000, or 1/1000

1:250 is 1 part in 250 parts, or 1 to 250, or 1/250

Some drug solutions are expressed in ratios, for example 1:100 or 1:500. These ratios mean that there is 1 part of a drug in 100 parts of solution or 1 part of the drug in 500 parts of solution.

Percentages

The term *percentage* or *percent* (%) means *parts per hundred.*

EXAMPLES

25% is 25 parts per hundred
50% is 50 parts per hundred

A percentage may also be expressed as a fraction.

EXAMPLES

25% is 25 parts per hundred or 25/100
50% is 50 parts per hundred or 50/100
30% is 30 parts per hundred or 30/100

The above fractions may also be reduced to their lowest possible terms:

25/100 = 1/4,   50/100 = 1/2,   30/100 = 3/10.

Changing a Fraction to a Percentage

To change a fraction to a percentage, divide the denominator by the numerator and multiply the results (quotient) by 100 and then add a percent sign (%).

EXAMPLES

Change 4/5 to a percentage

$$4 \div 5 = 0.8$$
$$0.8 \times 100 = 80\%$$

Change 2/3 to a percentage

$$2 \div 3 = 0.666$$
$$0.666 \times 100 = 66.6\%$$

Changing a Ratio to a Percentage

To change a ratio to a percentage, the ratio is first expressed as a fraction with the first number or term of the ratio becoming the numerator and the second number or term becoming the denominator. For example, the ratio 1:500 when changed to a fraction becomes 1/500. This fraction is then changed to a percentage by the same method shown in the preceding section.

EXAMPLE

Change 1:125 to a percentage

1:125 written as a fraction is 1/125

$$1 \div 125 = 0.008$$
$$0.008 \times 100 = 0.8$$
adding the percent sign = 0.8%

Changing a Percentage to a Ratio

To change a percentage to a ratio, the percentage becomes the numerator and is placed over a denominator of 100.

EXAMPLES

Changing 5% and 10% to ratios

$$5\% \text{ is } \frac{5}{100} = \frac{1}{20} \text{ or } 1{:}20$$
$$10\% \text{ is } \frac{10}{100} = \frac{1}{10} \text{ or } 1{:}10$$

Proportions

A proportion is a method of expressing equality between two ratios. An example of two ratios expressed as a proportion is: 3 is to 4 as 9 is to 12. This may also be written as:

3:4 as 9:12

or

3:4::9:12

or

$$\frac{3}{4} = \frac{9}{12}$$

Proportions may be used to find an unknown quantity. The unknown quantity is assigned a letter, usually X. An example of a proportion with an unknown quantity is 5:10::15:X.

The first and last terms of the proportion are called the *extremes.* In the above expression 5 and X are the extremes. The second and third terms of the proportion are called the *means.* In the above proportion, 10 and 15 are the means.

means
↙ ↘
5:10::15:X
↖   ↗
extremes

$$\underset{\text{mean}}{\overset{\text{extreme}}{}} \frac{5}{10} = \frac{15}{X} \underset{\text{extreme}}{\overset{\text{mean}}{}}$$

To solve for X:

1. Multiply the extremes and place the product (result) to the *left* of the equal sign.

5:10::15:X
5X =

2. Multiply the means and place the product to the *right* of the equal sign.

5:10::15X
5X = 150

3. Solve for *X* by dividing the number to the right of the equal sign by the number to the left of the equal sign (150 ÷ 5).

5X = 150
X = 30

decimal point in the divisor is moved *it must be moved* in the dividend.

Changing a Fraction to a Decimal

To change a fraction to a decimal, divide the numerator by the denominator.

EXAMPLE

$$\frac{1}{5} = 5\overline{)1.0} = .2 \qquad \frac{3}{4} = 4\overline{)3.00} = .75 \qquad \frac{1}{6} = 6\overline{)1.000} = .166$$

Changing a Decimal to a Fraction

To change a decimal to a fraction:

1. Remove the decimal point and make the resulting whole number the numerator: $0.2 = 2$.
2. The denominator is stated as 10 or a power of 10. In this example, 0.2 is read as two *tenths,* and therefore the denominator is 10.

$0.2 = \dfrac{2}{10}$ reduced to the lowest possible number is $\dfrac{1}{5}$

ADDITIONAL EXAMPLES

$$0.75 = \frac{75}{100} = \frac{3}{4} \qquad 0.025 = \frac{25}{1000} = \frac{1}{40}$$

CALCULATION OF DRUG DOSAGES

Although most hospital pharmacies dispense drugs as single doses or in a unit dose system, on occasion the nurse must compute a drug dosage because it differs from the dose of the drug that is available. This is particularly true of small hospitals, nursing homes, physicians' offices, and outpatient clinics that may not have a complete range of all available doses for a particular drug. Because certain situations may require computing the desired amount of drug to be given, nurses must be familiar with the calculation of all forms of drug dosages.

Systems of Measurement

There are three systems of measurement of drug dosages: the **metric system,** the **apothecaries' system,** and **household measurements.** The metric system is the most commonly used system of measurement in medicine. A physician may prescribe a drug dosage in the apothecaries' system, but for the most part this ancient system of measurements is only occasionally used. The household system is rarely used in a hospital setting but may be used to measure drug dosages in the home.

DISPLAY 3-1 ● Metric Measurements

WEIGHT
The unit of weight is the gram.
1 kilogram (kg) = 1000 grams (g)
1 gram (g) = 1000 milligrams (mg)
1 milligram (mg) = 1000 micrograms (mcg)

VOLUME
The unit of volume is the liter.
1 decaliter (dL) = 10 liters (L)
1 liter (L) = 1000 milliliters (mL)
1 milliliter (mL) = 0.001 liter (L)

LENGTH
The unit of length is the meter.
1 meter (m) = 100 centimeters (cm)
1 centimeter (cm) = 0.01 meter (m)
1 millimeter (mm) = 0.001 meter (m)

The Metric System

The metric system uses decimals (or the decimal system). In the metric system, the **gram** is the unit of weight, the **liter** the unit of volume, and the **meter** the unit of length.

Display 3-1 lists the measurements used in the metric system. The abbreviations for the measurements are given in parentheses.

The Apothecaries' System

The apothecaries' system uses whole numbers and fractions. Decimals are *not* used in this system. The whole numbers are written as lowercase Roman numerals, for example, x instead of 10, or v instead of 5.

The units of weight in the apothecaries' system are **grains, drams,** and **ounces.** The units of volume are **minims, fluid drams,** and **fluid ounces.** The units of measurement in this system are not based on exact measurements.

Display 3-2 lists the measurements used in the apothecaries' system. The abbreviations (or symbols) for the measurements are given in parentheses.

DISPLAY 3-2 ● Apothecaries' Measurements

WEIGHT
The units of weight are grains, drams, and ounces.

60 grains (gr) = 1 dram (ʒ)
1 ounce (ℨ) = 480 grains (gr)

VOLUME
The units of volume are minims, fluid drams, and fluid ounces.

1 fluid dram = 60 minims (♍)
1 fluid ounce = 8 fluid drams

DISPLAY 3-3 ● **Household Measurements**

3 teaspoons (tsp) = 1 tablespoon (tbsp)
2 tablespoons (tbsp) = 1 ounce (oz)
2 pints (pt) = 1 quart (qt)
4 quarts (qt) = 1 gallon (gal)

Household Measurements

When used, household measurements are for volume only. In the hospital, household measurements are rarely used because they are inaccurate when used to measure drug dosages. On occasion, the nurse may use the pint, quart, or gallon when ordering, irrigating, or sterilizing solutions or stock solutions. For the ease of a patient taking a drug at home, the physician may order a drug dosage in household measurements.

Display 3-3 lists the more common household measurements, with abbreviations in parentheses.

Conversion Between Systems

To convert between systems, it is necessary to know the equivalents, or what is equal to what in each system. Table 3-1 lists the more common equivalents.

TABLE 3-1	Approximate Equivalents	
METRIC	**APOTHECARIES**	**HOUSEHOLD**
Weight		
0.1 mg	gr 1/600	
0.15 mg	gr 1/400	
0.2 mg	gr 1/300	
0.3 mg	gr 1/200	
0.4 mg	gr 1/150	
0.6 mg	gr 1/100	
1 mg	gr 1/60	
2 mg	gr 1/30	
4 mg	gr 1/15	
6 mg	gr 1/10	
8 mg	gr 1/8	
10 mg	gr 1/6	
15 mg	gr 1/4	
20 mg	gr 1/3	
30 mg	gr ss (1/2)	
60 mg	gr 1	
100 mg	gr i ss (1 1/2)	
120 mg	gr ii	
1 g (1000 mg)	gr xv	
Volume		
0.06 mL	min (♏) i	
1 mL	min (♏) xv or xvi	
4 mL	fluidram i	1 teaspoon (tsp)
15 mL	fluidrams iv	1/2 ounce (oz)
30 mL	fluid ounce i	1 ounce (oz)
500 mL	1 pint (pt)	1 pint (pt)
1000 mL (1 liter)	1 quart (qt)	1 quart (qt)

These equivalents are only *approximate* because the three systems are different and are not truly equal to each other.

Several methods may be used to convert from one system to another using an equivalent, but most conversions can be done by using proportion.

EXAMPLES

Convert 120 mg (metric) to grains (apothecaries')

Using proportion and the known equivalent 60 mg = gr i (1 grain)

$$1 \text{ gr}:60 \text{ mg}::X \text{ gr}:120 \text{ mg}$$
$$60X = 120$$
$$X = 2 \text{ gr (grains or gr ii)}$$

Note the use of the abbreviations gr and mg when setting up the proportion. This shows that the proportion was stated correctly and helps in identifying the answer as 2 *grains*.

Convert gr 1/100 (apothecaries') to mg (metric)

Using proportion and the known equivalent 60 mg = 1 gr:

If there are 60 mg in 1 gr, there are X mg in 1/100 gr

$$60 \text{ mg}:1 \text{ gr}::X \text{ mg}:1/100 \text{ gr}$$
$$X = 60 \times \frac{1}{100} = \frac{60}{100} = \frac{3}{5}$$
$$X = \frac{3}{5} \text{ mg}$$

or

$$\frac{60 \text{ mg}}{1 \text{ gr}} = \frac{X \text{ mg}}{1/100} \text{ gr}$$
$$X = 60 \times \frac{1}{100} = \frac{60}{100} = \frac{3}{5}$$
$$X = \frac{3}{5} \text{ mg}$$

Fractions are *not* used in the metric system; therefore, the fraction must be converted to a decimal by dividing the denominator into the numerator, or $3 \div 5 = 0.6$ or

$$5)\overline{3.0} \quad .6$$

Therefore, gr 1/100 is equal to 0.6 mg.

When setting up the proportion, the apothecaries' system was written in Arabic numbers instead of Roman numerals, and their order was reversed (1 gr instead of gr i) so that all numbers and abbreviations are uniform in presentation.

Convert 0.3 milligrams (mg) [metric] to grains (gr) [apothecaries']

Using proportion and the known equivalent 1 mg = gr 1/60

$$1/60 \text{ gr:1 mg::X gr:0.3 mg}$$

$$X = \frac{1}{60} \times 0.3 = \frac{0.3}{60} = \frac{3}{600} = \frac{1}{200}$$

$$X = \frac{1}{200} \text{ grain}$$

or

$$\frac{1/60}{} = \frac{X \text{ gr}}{}$$

or

$$\frac{1/60}{1 \text{ mg}} = \frac{X \text{ gr}}{0.3 \text{ mg}}$$

$$X = \frac{1}{60} \times 0.3 = \frac{0.3}{60} = \frac{3}{600} = \frac{1}{200}$$

$$X = \frac{1}{200 \text{ gr}}$$

Therefore, 0.3 mg equals gr 1/200.

There is no rule stating which equivalent must be used. In the above problem, another equivalent (60 mg = 1 gr) also could have been used. If 60 mg = 1 gr is used, the proportion would be:

$$60 \text{ mg:1 gr::0.3 mg:X}$$
$$60X = 0.3$$
$$X = 0.005$$

or

$$\frac{60 \text{ mg}}{1 \text{ gr}} = \frac{0.3 \text{ mg}}{X \text{ gr}}$$
$$60X = 0.3$$
$$X = 0.005$$

Therefore, 0.3 mg equals 0.005 gr.

Because decimals are not used in the apothecaries' system, this decimal answer must be converted to a fraction: 0.005 is 5/1000, which, when reduced to its lowest terms, is 1/200. The final answer is now 0.3 mg = gr 1/200.

Converting Within a System

Sometimes it is necessary to convert within the same system, for example, changing grams (g) to milligrams (mg) or milligrams to grams. Proportion and a known equivalent also may be used for this type of conversion.

EXAMPLE

Convert 0.1 gram (g) to milligrams (mg)

Using proportion and the known equivalent 1000 mg = 1g

$$1000 \text{ mg:1 g::X mg:0.1 g}$$
$$X = 1000 \times 0.1$$
$$X = 100 \text{ mg}$$

or

$$\frac{1000 \text{ mg}}{1 \text{ g}} = \frac{X \text{ mg}}{0.1 \text{ g}}$$
$$X = 1000 \times 0.1$$
$$X = 100 \text{ mg}$$

Therefore, 0.1 gram (g) equals 100 milligrams (mg).

Solutions

A **solute** is a substance dissolved in a **solvent.** A solvent may be water or some other liquid. Usually water is used for preparing a solution unless another liquid is specified. Solutions are prepared by using a solid (powder, tablet) and a liquid, or a liquid and a liquid. Today, most solutions are prepared by a pharmacist and not by the nurse.

Examples of how solutions may be labeled include:

- 10 mg/mL–10 mg of the drug in each milliliter
- 1:1000–a solution denoting strength or 1 part of the drug per 1000 parts
- 5 mg/teaspoon–5 mg of the drug in each teaspoon (home use)

Reading Drug Labels

Drug labels give important information the nurse must use to obtain the correct dosage. The unit dose is the most common type of labeling seen in hospitals. The unit dose is a method of dispensing drugs in which each capsule or tablet is packaged separately. At times the drug will come to the nursing unit in a container with a number of capsules or tablets or as a solution. The nurse must then determine the number of capsules/tablets or the amount of solution to administer.

Drug labels usually contain two names: the trade (brand) name and the generic or official name (see Chap. 1). The trade name is capitalized, written first on the label, and identified by the registration symbol. The official or generic name is written in smaller print and usually located under the trade name. Although the drug has only one official name, several companies may manufacture the drug, with each manufacturer using a different trade name. Sometimes the generic or official name is so widely known that all manufacturers will simply use that name. For example, atropine sulfate is a widely used drug that is so well known that all manufacturers use the official name. In this case only the official name, atropine sulfate, will be found on the label. Drugs may be prescribed by either the trade name or the official or generic name. See Figure 3-1 for an example of a drug label showing the trade and generic names.

The dosage strength is also given on the container. The dosage strength is the average strength given to a patient as one dose. If necessary, the dosage strength is used to calculate the number of tablets or the amount of

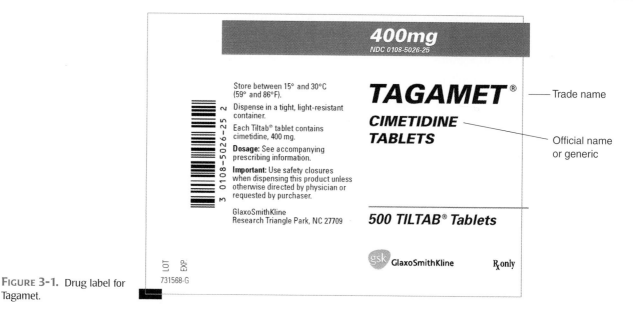

FIGURE 3-1. Drug label for Tagamet.

solution to administer. In liquid drugs there is a specified amount of drug in a given volume of solution, such as 50 mg in 2 mL.

Look at Figure 3-2. In this example, the dosage strength of the Augmentin is 125 mg/5 mL solution. If the physician orders 125 mg Augmentin, the nurse would administer 5 mL. More information on calculating drug dosages is given in the following section.

Oral Dosages of Drugs

Under certain circumstances, it may be necessary to compute an oral drug dosage because the dosage ordered by the physician may not be available, or the dosage may have been written in the apothecaries' system and the drug or container label is in the metric system.

Tablets and Capsules

To find the correct dosage of a solid oral preparation, the following formula may be used:

$$\frac{\text{dose desired}}{\text{dose on hand}} = \text{dose administered (the unknown or X)}$$

This formula may be abbreviated as

$$\frac{D}{H} = X$$

When the dose ordered by the physician (dose desired) is written in the *same system* as the dose on the drug container (dose on hand), these two figures may be inserted into the formula.

EXAMPLE

The physician orders ascorbic acid 100 mg (metric). The drug is available as ascorbic acid 50 mg (metric).

$$\frac{D}{H} = X$$

$$\frac{100 \text{ mg (dose desired)}}{50 \text{ mg (dose on hand)}} = 2 \text{ tablets of 50-mg ascorbic acid}$$

If the physician had ordered ascorbic acid 0.5 g and the drug container was labeled ascorbic acid 250 mg, a *conversion of grams to milligrams* (because the drug container is labeled in milligrams) would be necessary before this formula can be used. If the 0.5 g were *not*

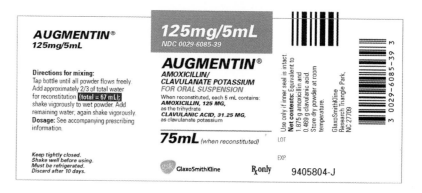

FIGURE 3-2. Drug label for Augmentin.

converted to milligrams, the fraction of the formula would look like this:

$$\frac{0.5 \text{ grams}}{250 \text{ milligrams}}$$

A fraction _must_ be stated in _like terms;_ therefore, proportion may be used to convert grams to milligrams.

$$1000 \text{ mg}:1 \text{ g}::X \text{ mg}:0.5 \text{ g}$$
$$X = 1000 \times 0.5$$
$$X = 500 \text{ mg}$$

After changing 0.5 g to mg, use the formula:

$$\frac{D}{H} = X$$

$$\frac{500 \text{ mg}}{250 \text{ mg}} = 2 \text{ tablets of 250 mg ascorbic acid}$$

As with all fractions, the numerator and the denominator must be of like terms, for example, milligrams over milligrams or grams over grams. Errors in using this and other drug formulas, as well as proportions, will be reduced if the entire dose is written rather than just the numbers.

$$\frac{100 \text{ mg}}{50 \text{ mg}} \text{ rather than } \frac{100}{50}$$

This will eliminate the possibility of using _unlike_ terms in the fraction.

Even if the physician's order was written in the apothecaries' system, the drug container most likely would be labeled in the metric system. A conversion of _apothecaries' to metric_ will now be necessary because the drug label is written in the metric system.

EXAMPLE

The physician's order reads: codeine sulfate gr 1/4 (apothecaries'). The drug container is labeled: codeine sulfate 15 mg (metric). Grains must be converted to milligrams _or_ milligrams converted to grains.

Grains to milligrams:

$$60 \text{ mg}:1 \text{ gr}::X \text{ mg}:1/4 \text{ gr}$$
$$X = 60 \times \frac{1}{4}$$
$$X = 15 \text{ mg}$$

or

$$\frac{60 \text{ mg}}{1 \text{ gr}} = \frac{X \text{ mg}}{1/4 \text{ gr}}$$
$$X = 60 \times \frac{1}{4}$$
$$X = 15 \text{ mg}$$

Therefore, 1/4 grain is approximately equivalent to 15 mg.

Milligrams to grains:

$$60 \text{ mg}:1 \text{ gr}::15 \text{ mg}:X \text{ gr}$$
$$60X = 15$$
$$X = 1/4 \text{ gr}$$

or

$$\frac{60 \text{ mg}}{1 \text{ gr}} = \frac{15 \text{ mg}}{X \text{ gr}}$$
$$60X = 15$$
$$X = \frac{1}{4} \text{ grain}$$

Therefore, 15 mg is approximately equivalent to 1/4 grain.

The formula $\frac{D}{H} = X$ can now be used

$$\frac{D}{H} = X$$

$$\frac{15 \text{ mg}}{15 \text{ mg}} = 1 \text{ tablet}$$

or

$$\frac{1/4 \text{ gr}}{1/4 \text{ gr}} = 1 \text{ tablet}$$

Liquids

In liquid drugs, there is a specific amount of drug in a given volume of solution. For example, if a container is labeled as 10 mg per 5 mL (or 10 mg/5 mL), this means that for every 5 mL of solution there is 10 mg of drug.

As with tablets and capsules, the prescribed dose of the drug may not be the same as what is on hand (or available). For example, the physician may order 20 mg of an oral liquid preparation and the bottle is labeled as 10 mg/5 mL.

The formula for computing the dosage of oral liquids is:

$$\frac{\text{dose desired}}{\text{dose on hand}} \times \text{quantity} = \text{volume administered}$$

This may be abbreviated as

$$\frac{D}{H} \times Q = X$$

The quantity (or Q) in this formula is the amount of liquid in which the available drug is contained. For example, if the label states that there is 15 mg/5 mL, 5 mL is the _quantity_ (or volume) in which there is 15 mg of this drug.

EXAMPLE

The physician orders oxacillin sodium 125 mg PO oral suspension. The drug is labeled as 250 mg/5 mL. The 5 mL is the amount (quantity or Q) that contains 250 mg of the drug.

$$\frac{D}{H} \times Q = X \text{ (the liquid amount to be given)}$$

$$\frac{125 \text{ mg}}{250 \text{ mg}} \times 5 = X$$

$$\frac{1}{2} \times 5 = 2.5 \text{ mL}$$

Therefore, 2.5 mL contains the desired dose of 125 mg of oxacillin oral suspension.

Liquid drugs may also be ordered in drops (gtt) or minims. With the former, a medicine dropper is usually supplied with the drug and is always used to measure the ordered dosage. Eye droppers are not standardized, and therefore the size of a drop from one eye dropper may be different than one from another eye dropper.

To measure an oral liquid drug in minims, a measuring glass *calibrated in minims* must be used.

Parenteral Dosages of Drugs

Drugs for parenteral use must be in liquid form before they are administered. Parenteral drugs may be available in the following forms:

1. As liquids in disposable cartridges or disposable syringes that contain a specific amount of a drug in a specific volume, for example, meperidine 50 mg/mL. After administration, the cartridge or syringe is discarded.
2. In ampules or vials that contain a specific amount of the liquid form of the drug in a specific volume. The vials may be single-dose vials or multidose vials. A multidose vial contains more than one dose of the drug.
3. In ampules or vials that contain powder or crystals, to which a liquid (called a **diluent**) must be added before the drug can be removed from the vial and administered. Vials may be single dose or multidose vials.

Parenteral Drugs in Disposable Syringes or Cartridges

In some instances a specific dosage strength is not available and it will be necessary to administer less than the amount contained in the syringe.

EXAMPLE

The physician orders diazepam 5 mg IM. The drug is available as a 2-mL disposable syringe labeled 5 mg/mL.

$$\frac{D}{H} \times Q = X$$

$$\frac{5 \text{ mg}}{10 \text{ mg}} \times 2 \text{ mL} = X$$

$$X = \frac{1}{2} \times 2 = 1 \text{ mL}$$

Note that since the syringe contains 2 mL of the drug and that *each* mL contains 5 mg of the drug, there is a total of 10 mg of the drug in the syringe. Because there is 10 mg of the drug in the syringe, half of the liquid in the syringe (1 mL) is discarded and the remaining half (1 mL) is administered to give the prescribed dose of 5 mg.

Parenteral Drugs in Ampules and Vials

If the drug is in liquid form in the ampule or vial, the desired amount is withdrawn from the ampule or vial. In some instances, the entire amount is used; in others, only part of the total amount is withdrawn from the ampule or vial and administered.

Whenever the dose to be administered is different from that listed on the label, the volume to be administered must be calculated. To determine the volume to be administered, the formula for liquid preparations is used. The calculations are the same as those given in the preceding section for parenteral drugs in disposable syringes or cartridges.

EXAMPLES

The physician orders chlorpromazine 12.5 mg IM.

The drug is available as chlorpromazine 25 mg/mL in a 1-mL ampule.

$$\frac{D}{H} \times Q = X$$

$$\frac{12.5 \text{ mg}}{25 \text{ mg}} \times 1 \text{ mL} = X$$

$$\frac{1}{2} \times 1 \text{ mL} = \frac{1}{2} \text{ mL (or 0.5 mL) volume to be administered.}$$

The physician orders hydroxyzine 12.5 mg. The drug is available as hydroxyzine 25 mg/mL in 10-mL vials.

$$\frac{D}{H} \times Q = X$$

$$\frac{12.5 \text{ mg}}{25 \text{ mg}} \times 1 \text{ mL} = \frac{1}{2} \text{ mL (or 0.5 mL)}$$

Therefore, 0.5 mL is withdrawn from the 10-mL multidose vial and administered. In this example, the amount in this or any multidose vial is *not* entered into the equation. What is entered into the equation as quantity (Q) is the amount of the available drug that is contained in a specific volume.

When the dose is less than 1 mL, it may be necessary, in some instances, to convert the answer to minims. A conversion factor of 15 or 16 minims/mL may be used.

EXAMPLES

The physician orders chlorpromazine 10 mg IM. The drug is available as chlorpromazine 25 mg/mL.

$$\frac{10 \text{ mg}}{25 \text{ mg}} \times 1 \text{ mL} = X$$

$$\frac{2}{5} \times 1 \text{ mL} = \frac{2}{5} \text{ mL}$$

$$\frac{2}{5} \times 15 \text{ minims} = 6 \text{ minims}$$

In this example 15 minims = 1 mL is used because 15 can be divided by 5.

The physician's order reads methadone 2.5 mg IM. The drug is available as methadone 10 mg/mL.

$$\frac{2.5 \text{ mg}}{10 \text{ mg}} \times 1 \text{ mL} = X$$

$$\frac{1}{4} \times 1 \text{ mL} = X$$

$$\frac{1}{4} \times 16 \text{ minims} = 4 \text{ minims}$$

Because 16 (and not 15) minims can be divided by 4, the conversion factor of 16 is used.

WARNING: ALWAYS CHECK DRUG LABELS CAREFULLY. Some may be labeled in a manner different from others.

EXAMPLE

a **2**-mL ampule labeled: **2** mL = 0.25 mg
a **2**-mL ampule labeled: **1** mL = 5 mg

In these two examples, one manufacturer states the entire dose contained in the ampule: 2 mL = 0.25 mg. The other manufacturer gives the dose per milliliter: 1 mL = 5 mg. In this 2-mL ampule, there is a total of 10 mg.

Parenteral Drugs in Dry Form

Some parenteral drugs are available as a crystal or a powder. Because these drugs have a short life in liquid form, they are available in ampules or vials in dry form and must be made a liquid (reconstituted) before they are removed and administered. Some of these products have directions for reconstitution on the label or on the enclosed package insert. The manufacturer may give

either of the following information for reconstitution: (1) the name of the diluent(s) that must be used with the drug, or (2) the amount of diluent that must be added to the drug.

In some instances, the manufacturer supplies a diluent with the drug. If a diluent is supplied, no other stock diluent should be used. Before a drug is reconstituted, the label is carefully checked for instructions.

EXAMPLES

Methicillin sodium: To reconstitute 1 g vial add 1.5 mL of sterile water for injection or sodium chloride injection. Each reconstituted mL contains approximately 500 mg of methicillin.

Mechlorethamine: Reconstitute with 10 mL of sterile water for injection or sodium chloride injection. The solution now contains 1 mg/mL of mechlorethamine.

If there is any doubt about the reconstitution of the dry form of a drug and there are no manufacturer's directions, the hospital pharmacist should be consulted.

Once a diluent is added, the volume to be administered is determined. In some cases, the entire amount is given; in others, a part (or fraction) of the total amount contained in the vial or ampule is given.

After reconstitution of any multidose vial, the following information *must* be added to the label:

- Amount of diluent added
- Dose of drug in mL (500 mg/mL, 10 mg/2 mL, etc.)
- The date of reconstitution
- The expiration date (the date after which any unused solution is discarded)

Calculating Intravenous Flow Rates

When the physician orders a drug added to an intravenous (IV) fluid, the amount of fluid to be administered over a specified period, such as 125 mL/h or 1000 mL over 8 hours, must be included in the written order. If no infusion rate had been ordered, 1 L (1000 mL) of IV fluid should infuse over 6 to 8 hours.

To allow the IV fluid to infuse over a specified period, the IV flow rate must be determined. Before using one of the methods below, the drop factor must be known. Drip chambers on the various types of IV fluid administration sets vary. Some deliver 15 drops/mL and others deliver more or less than this number. This is called the *drop factor*. The drop factor (number of drops/mL) is given on the package containing the drip chamber and IV tubing. Three methods for determining the IV infusion rate follow. Methods 1 and 2 can be used when the known factors are the total amount of solution, the drop factor, and the number of hours over which the solution is to be infused.

METHOD 1

Step 1. Total amount of solution ÷ number of hours = number of mL/h

Step 2. mL/h ÷ 60 min/h = number of mL/min
Step 3. mL/min × drop factor = number of drops/min

EXAMPLE

1000 mL of an IV solution is to infuse over a period of 8 hours. The drop factor is 14.
Step 1. 1000 mL ÷ 8 hours = 125 mL/h
Step 2. 125 ÷ 60 minutes = 2.08 mL/min
Step 3. 2.08 × 14 = 29 drops/min

METHOD 2

Step 1. Total amount of solution ÷ number of hours = number of mL/h
Step 2. mL/h × drop factor ÷ 60 = number of drops/min

EXAMPLE

1000 mL of an IV solution is to infuse over a period of 6 hours. The drop factor is 12.
Step 1. 1000 mL ÷ 6 = 166.6 mL/h
Step 2. 166.6 × 12 ÷ 60 = 33.33 (33 to 34) drops/min

METHOD 3

This method may be used when the desired amount of solution to be infused in 1 hour is known or written as a physician's order.

$$\frac{\text{drops/mL of given set (drop factor)}}{60 \text{ (minutes in an hour)}} \times \begin{array}{l}\text{total hourly} \\ \text{volume} = \\ \text{drops/min}\end{array}$$

EXAMPLE

If a set delivers 15 drops/min and 240 mL is to be infused in 1 hour:

$$\frac{15}{60} \times 240 = \frac{1}{4} \times 240 = 60 \text{ drops/min}$$

Oral or Parenteral Drug Dosages Based on Weight

The dosage of an oral or parenteral drug may be based on the patient's weight. In many instances, references give the dosage based on the weight in kilograms (kg) rather than pounds (1b). There are 2.2 1b in 1 kg.

When the dosage of a drug is based on weight, the physician, in most instances, computes and orders the dosage to be given. However, errors can occur for any number of reasons. The nurse should be able to calculate a drug dosage based on weight to detect any type of error that may have been made in the prescribing or dispensing of a drug whose dosage is based on weight.

To convert a known weight in kilograms to pounds, multiply the known weight by 2.2.

EXAMPLES

Patient's weight in kilograms is 54

$$54 \times 2.2 = 118.8 \text{ (or 119) lb}$$

Patient's weight in kilograms is 61.5

$$61.5 \times 2.2 = 135.3 \text{ (or 135) lb}$$

To convert a known weight in pounds to kilograms, divide the known weight by 2.2.

EXAMPLES

Patient's weight in pounds is 142

$$142 \div 2.2 = 64.5 \text{ kg}$$

Child's weight in pounds is 43

$$43 \div 2.2 = 19.5 \text{ kg}$$

Once the weight is converted to pounds or kilograms, this information is used to determine drug dosage.

EXAMPLES

A drug dose is 5 mg/kg/d. The patient weighs 135 1b, which is converted to 61.2 kg.

$$61.2 \text{ kg} \times 5 \text{ mg} = 306.8 \text{ mg}$$

Proportions also can be used:

$$5 \text{ mg:1 kg::X mg:61.2 kg}$$
$$X = 306.8 \text{ mg}$$

A drug dose is 60 mg/kg/d IV in three equally divided doses.

The patient weighs 143 Ib, which is converted to 65 kg.

$$65 \text{ kg} \times 60 \text{ mg} = 3900 \text{ mg/day}$$
$$3900 \text{ mg} \div 3 \text{ (dosess per day)} = 1300 \text{ mg each dose}$$

If the drug dose is based on body surface area (m²) the same method of calculation may be used.

EXAMPLE

A drug dose is 60 to 75 mg/m² as a single IV injection.
The body surface area (BSA) of a patient is determined by means of a nomogram for estimating BSA (see Appendix E) and is found to be 1.8 m². The physician orders 60 mg/m².

$$60 \text{ mg} \times 1.8 \text{ m}^2 = 108 \text{ mg}$$

Proportion can also be used:

$$60 \text{ mg: 1 m}^2\text{::X mg:1.8 m}^2$$
$$X = 108 \text{ mg}$$

Dosage Calculation Using Dimensional Analysis (DA)

When using DA to calculate dosage problems, dosages are written as common fractions. For example:

$$\frac{1 \text{ mL}}{4 \text{ mg}} \qquad \frac{5 \text{ mL}}{10 \text{ mg}} \qquad \frac{1 \text{ tablet}}{100 \text{ mg}}$$

When written as common fractions the numerator is the top number. In the example above, 1 mL, 5 mL, and 1 tablet are the numerators.

The numbers on the bottom are called denominators. In the example above, 4 mg, 10 mg, and 100 mg are denominators.

EXAMPLE

The physician orders 10 mg of diazepam. The drug comes in dosage strength of 5 mg/mL. How many mL would the nurse administer?

Step 1. To work this problem using DA, always begin by identifying the unit of measure to be calculated. The unit to be calculated will be mL or cc if the drug is to be administered parenterally. Another drug form is the solid and the unit of measure would be a tablet or capsule. In the problem above, the unit of measure to be calculated is mL. If the drug is an oral liquid drug, the measurement might be ounces.

Step 2. Write the identified unit of measure to be calculated, followed by an equal sign. In the problem above, mL is the unit to be calculated, so the nurse writes:

$$mL =$$

Step 3. Next, the dosage strength is written, with the numerator *always expressed in the same unit that was identified before the equal sign.* For example:

$$mL = \frac{1 \text{ mL}}{5 \text{ mg}}$$

Step 4. Continue by writing the next fraction with the numerator having the same unit of measure as the denominator in the previous fraction. For example, our problem continues:

$$mL = \frac{1 \text{ mL}}{5 \text{ mg}} \times \frac{10 \text{ mg}}{X \text{ mL}}$$

Step 5. The problem is solved by multiplication of the two fractions.

$$mL = \frac{1 \text{ mL}}{5 \text{ mg}} \times \frac{10 \text{ mg}}{X \text{ mL}} = \frac{10 \text{ mg}}{5X \text{ mL}} = 2 \text{ mL}$$

NOTE: Each alternate denominator and numerator cancel, with only the final unit remaining.

EXAMPLE

Ordered: 200,000 U
On hand: Drug labeled 400,000 U/mL

$$mL = \frac{1 \text{ mL}}{400,000 \text{ U}} \times \frac{200,000 \text{ U}}{X \text{ mL}} = \frac{1}{2} \text{ mL or 0.5 mL}$$

Metric Conversions Using Dimensional Analysis

Occasionally the physician may order a drug in one unit of measure, whereas the drug is available in another unit of measure.

EXAMPLE

The physician orders 0.4 mg of atropine. The drug label reads 400 mcg per 1 mL. This dosage problem is solved by expanding the DA equation by adding one step to the equation.

Step 1. As above, begin by writing the unit of measure to be calculated, followed by an equal sign.

Step 2. Next, express the dosage strength as a fraction with the numerator having the same unit of measure as the number before the equal sign.

Step 3. Continue by writing the next fraction with the numerator having the same unit of measure as the denominator in the previous fraction.

$$mL = \frac{1 \text{ mL}}{400 \text{ mcg}} \times \frac{mcg}{mg}$$

Step 4. Expand the equation by filling in the missing numbers using the appropriate equivalent. In this problem, the equivalent would be 100 mcg = 1 mg. This will convert mcg to mg.

$$mL = \frac{1 \text{ mL}}{400 \text{ mcg}} \times \frac{1000 \text{ mcg}}{1 \text{ mg}}$$

Repeat Steps 3 and 4. Continue with the equation by placing the next fraction beginning with the unit of measure of the denominator of the previous fraction.

$$mL = \frac{1 \text{ mL}}{400 \text{ mcg}} \times \frac{1000 \text{ mcg}}{1 \text{ mg}} \times \frac{0.4 \text{ mg}}{X \text{ mL}}$$

When possible, cancel out the units, leaving only mL.

Step 5. Solve the problem by multiplication. Cancel out the numbers when possible.

$$mL = \frac{1 \text{ mL}}{400 \text{ mcg}} \times \frac{1000 \text{ mcg}}{1 \text{ mg}} \times \frac{0.4 \text{ mg}}{X \text{ mL}} = \frac{400}{400 \text{ X}} = 1 \text{ mL}$$

Solve the following problems using DA. Refer to the equivalent table if necessary. (See Table 3-1.)

EXAMPLE

Ordered: 250 mg.
On hand: Drug labeled 1 gram per 1 mL

$$mL = \frac{1 \text{ mL}}{1 \text{ g}} \times \frac{1 \text{ g}}{1000 \text{ mg}} \times \frac{250 \text{ mg}}{X \text{ mL}} = \frac{1 \text{ mL}}{4} \text{ or 0.25 mL}$$

Temperatures

Two scales used in the measuring of temperatures are **Fahrenheit (F)** and **Celsius (C)** (also known as **centigrade**). On the Fahrenheit scale, the freezing point of water is 32° F and the boiling point of water is 212° F. On the Celsius scale, 0° C is the freezing point of water and 100° C is the boiling point of water.

To convert from Celsius to Fahrenheit, the following formula may be used: $F = 9/5\ C + 32$ (9/5 times the temperature in Celsius, then add 32).

EXAMPLE

Convert 38° C to Fahrenheit:

$$F = \frac{9}{5} \times 38° + 32$$
$$F = 68.4° + 32$$
$$F = 100.4°$$

To convert from Fahrenheit to Celsius, the following formula may be used: $C = 5/9\ (F - 32)$ (5/9 times the temperature in Fahrenheit minus 32).

EXAMPLE

Convert 100° F to Celsius:

$$C = \frac{5}{9} \times (100 - 32)$$
$$C = \frac{5}{9} \times 68$$
$$C = 37.77 \text{ or } 37.8°$$

(See Appendix D for Celsius (Centigrade) and Fahrenheit temperatures chart.)

Pediatric Dosages

The dosages of drugs given to children are usually less than those given to adults. The dosage may be based on age, weight, or BSA.

Body Surface Area

Charts are used to determine the BSA (see Appendix D) in square meters according to the child's height and weight. Once the BSA is determined, the following formula is used:

$$\frac{\text{surface area of the child in square meters}}{\text{surface area of an adult in square meters*}} \times \text{usual adult dose} = \text{pediatric dose}$$

(See Appendix E for Body Surface Area Nomograms.)

Weight

Pediatric as well as adult dosages may also be based on the patient's weight in pounds or kilograms. The method of converting pounds to kilograms or kilograms to pounds is explained in a previous section.

EXAMPLE

$$5 \text{ mg/kg}$$
$$0.5 \text{ mg/lb}$$

Today, most pediatric dosages are clearly given by the manufacturer, thus eliminating the need for formulas, except for determining the dose of some drugs based on the child's weight or BSA.

---

* The figure for the average BSA of an adult in square meters is 1.7.

temperature, weight, examination of the skin, examination of an intravenous infusion site, and auscultation of the lungs. Important subjective data include any statements made by the patient about relief or nonrelief of pain or other symptoms after administration of a drug.

The extent of the assessment and collection of objective and subjective data before and after a drug is administered will depend on the type of drug and the reason for its use.

Nursing Diagnosis

After the data collected during assessment are analyzed, the nurse identifies the patient's needs (problems) and formulates one or more nursing diagnoses. A **nursing diagnosis** is not a medical diagnosis; rather, it is a description of the patient's problems and their probable or actual related causes based on the subjective and objective data in the database. A nursing diagnosis identifies problems that can be solved or prevented by **independent nursing actions**—actions that do not require a physician's order and may be legally performed by a nurse. Nursing diagnoses provide the framework for selections of nursing interventions to achieve expected outcomes.

The North American Nursing Diagnosis Association (NANDA) was formed to standardize the terminology used for nursing diagnosis. NANDA continues to define, explain, classify, and research summary health statements about health problems related to nursing. NANDA has approved a list of diagnostic categories to be used in formulating a nursing diagnosis. This list of diagnostic categories is periodically revised and updated. In some instances, nursing diagnoses may apply to a specific group or type of drug or a particular patient. One example is Deficient Fluid Volume related to active fluid volume loss (diuresis) secondary to administration of a diuretic. Specific drug-related nursing diagnoses are highlighted in each chapter. However, it is beyond the scope of this book to discuss all possible nursing diagnoses related to a drug or a drug class.

Some of the nursing diagnoses developed by NANDA may be used to identify patient problems associated with drug therapy and are more commonly used when administering drugs. The most frequently used nursing diagnoses related to the administration of drugs include:

- Effective Therapeutic Regimen Management
- Ineffective Therapeutic Regimen Management
- Deficient Knowledge
- Noncompliance
- Anxiety

Because the above nursing diagnoses are commonly used for the administration of all types of drugs, they will not be repeated for each chapter. The nurse should keep these nursing diagnoses in mind when administering any drug.

Planning

After the nursing diagnoses are formulated, the nurse develops expected outcomes, which are patient oriented. An expected outcome is a direct statement of nurse–patient goals to be achieved. The **expected outcome** describes the maximum level of wellness that is reasonably attainable for the patient. For example, common expected patient outcomes related to drug administration, in general, include:

- The patient will effectively manage the therapeutic regimen.
- The patient will understand the drug regimen.
- The patient will comply with the drug regimen.

The expected outcomes define the expected behavior of the patient or family that indicates the problem is being resolved or that progress toward resolution is occurring.

The nurse selects the appropriate interventions on the basis of expected outcomes to develop a plan of action or patient care plan. Planning for nursing actions specific for the drug to be administered can result in greater accuracy in drug administration, patient understanding of the drug regimen, and improved patient compliance with the prescribed drug therapy after discharge from the hospital. For example, during the initial assessment interview, the patient may report an allergy to penicillin. This information is important, and the nurse must now plan the best methods of informing all members of the health care team of the patient's allergy to penicillin.

The **planning** phase plans the steps for carrying out nursing activities or interventions that are specific and that will meet the expected outcomes. Planning anticipates the implementation phase or the carrying out of nursing actions that are specific for the drug being administered. If, for example, the patient is to receive a drug by the intravenous route, the nurse must plan the materials needed and the patient instruction for administration of the drug by this route. In this instance, the planning phase occurs immediately before the implementation phase and is necessary to carry out the technique of intravenous administration correctly. Failing to plan effectively may result in forgetting to obtain all of the materials necessary for drug administration.

Expected outcomes define the expected behavior of the patient or family that indicates that the problem is being resolved or that progress toward resolution is occurring. Expected outcomes serve as a basis for evaluating the effectiveness of nursing interventions. For example, if the nursing intervention is to "monitor the blood pressure every hour," the expected outcome is that "the patient experiences no further elevation in blood pressure."

Implementation

Implementation is the carrying out of a plan of action and is a natural outgrowth of the assessment and planning phases of the nursing process. When related to the administration of drugs, implementation refers to the preparation and administration of one or more drugs to a specific patient. Before administering a drug, the nurse reviews the subjective and objective data obtained on assessment and considers any additional data, such as blood pressure, pulse, or statements made by the patient. The decision of whether to administer the drug is based on an analysis of all information. For example, a patient is hypertensive and is supposed to receive a drug to lower the blood pressure. Objective data obtained at the time of admission included a blood pressure of 188/110. Additional objective data obtained immediately before the administration of the drug included a blood pressure of 182/110. A decision was made by the nurse to administer the drug because the change in the patient's blood pressure was only minimal. However, if the patient's blood pressure was 132/84, and this was only the second dose of the drug, the nurse could decide to withhold the drug and contact the primary health care provider. Giving or withholding a drug or contacting the patient's health care provider are nursing activities related to the implementation phase of the nursing process.

The more common nursing diagnoses used when administering drugs are Effective Therapeutic Regimen Management, Ineffective Therapeutic Regimen Management, Deficient Knowledge, and Noncompliance. Nursing interventions applicable to each of these nursing diagnoses are discussed in the following sections. However, each patient is an individual, and nursing care must be planned on an individual basis after a careful collection and analysis of the data. In addition, each drug is different and may have various effects within the body. (For drugs discussed in subsequent chapters, some possible nursing diagnoses related to that specific drug are discussed.)

Effective Therapeutic Regimen Management

This nursing diagnosis takes into consideration that the patient is willing to regulate and integrate into daily living the treatment regimen such as the self-administration of medications. For this nursing diagnosis to be used the patient verbalizes the desire to manage the medication regimen. When the patient is willing and able to manage the treatment regimen, he or she may simply need information concerning the drug, method of administration, what type of reactions to expect, and what to report to the primary health care provider. A patient willing to take responsibility may need the nurse to develop a teaching plan that gives the patient the information needed to properly manage the therapeutic regimen (see Chap. 5 for more information on educating patients).

Ineffective Therapeutic Regimen Management

NANDA defines "ineffective therapeutic regimen management" as "a pattern of regulating and integrating into daily living a program for treatment of illness and the sequelae of illness that is unsatisfactory for meeting specific health goals." In the case of medication administration, the patient may not be taking the medication correctly or following the medication regimen prescribed by the health care provider.

The reasons for not following the drug regimen vary. For example, some people do not fill their prescriptions. Other patients skip doses, take the drug at the wrong times, or take an incorrect dose. Some may simply forget to take the drug; others take a drug for a few days, see no therapeutic effect, and quit. Some find the adverse effects so bothersome that they discontinue taking the drug without notifying the health care provider. Display 4-1 identifies some reasons for this ineffective therapeutic regimen management.

When working with a patient who is not managing the drug regimen correctly, the nurse must ensure that the patient understands the drug regimen. It is essential to provide written instructions. If possible, the nurse should allow the patient to administer the drug before he or she is dismissed from the health care facility. The nurse should determine if adequate funds are available to obtain the drug and any necessary supplies. For example, when a bronchodilator is administered by inhalation, a spacer or extender may be required for proper administration. This device is an additional expense. A referral to the social services department of the institution may help when finances are a problem.

For those who forget to take the drug, the nurse should suggest the use of small compartmentalized boxes marked with the day of the week or time the drug

---

DISPLAY 4-1 ● Possible Causes of Ineffective Management of Health Care Regimen

Extended therapy for chronic illness causes patient to become discouraged
Troublesome adverse reactions
Lack of understanding of the purpose for the drug
Forgetfulness
Misunderstanding of oral or written instructions on how to take the drug
Weak nurse–patient relationships
Lack of funds to obtain drug
Mobility problems
Lack of family support
Cognitive deficits
Visual or hearing defects
Lack of motivation

From: Carpenito, L. J. (1995). *Nursing diagnosis: Application to clinical practice* (6th ed., pp. 601–602). Philadelphia: Lippincott-Raven; Hussar, D. A. (1995, October). *Nursing95*, pp. 62–64.

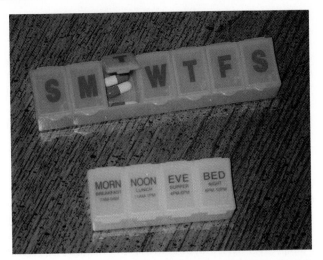

FIGURE 4-2. Various types of drug containers may be used to help individuals remember to take their medication at the correct time.

is to be taken (see Fig. 4-2). These containers can be obtained from the local pharmacy.

It is important to discuss the drug regimen with the patient, including the reason the drug is to be taken, the times, the amount, adverse reactions to expect, and reactions that should be reported. The patient needs a thorough understanding of the desired or expected therapeutic effect and the approximate time expected to attain that effect. For example, a patient may become discouraged after taking an antidepressant for 5 to 7 days and seeing no response. An explanation that 2 to 3 weeks is required before the depression begins to lift will, in many cases, promote compliance.

It is important to provide ways to minimize adverse reactions if possible. For example, many anticholinergic drugs cause dry mouth. The nurse instructs the patient to take frequent sips of water or suck on hard candy to help minimize the discomfort of a dry mouth.

Frequent follow-up sessions are needed to determine compliance with the drug regimen. If a follow-up visit is not feasible, the nurse considers a telephone call or home visit. It is vital that the nurse strive to develop a caring and nurturing relationship with the patient. Compliance is enhanced when a patient trusts the nurse and feels comfortable confiding any problem encountered during drug therapy.

Deficient Knowledge

Deficient knowledge is the absence or deficiency of cognitive information to a specific subject. In the case of self-administration of drugs the patient lacks sufficient knowledge to administer the drug regimen correctly. It may also relate to a lack of interest in learning, cognitive limitation, or the inability to remember.

Most patients, at least in the initial treatment stages, have a lack of knowledge about the drug, its possible adverse reactions, and the times and method of administration. At times, the patient may have a lack of knowledge about the disease condition. In these situations, the nurse addresses the specific deficient knowledge (ie, adverse reactions, disease process, method of administration, and so on) in words that the patient can understand. It is important for the nurse to first determine what information the patient is lacking and then plan a teaching session that directly pertains to the specific area of need. (See Chap. 5 for more information on patient education.) If the patient lacks the cognitive ability to learn the information concerning self-administration of drugs, then one or more of the caregivers should be taught to administer the proper treatment regimen.

Noncompliance

Noncompliance is defined as behavior of the patient or caregiver that fails to coincide with the therapeutic plan agreed on by the patient and the health care provider. Patients are noncompliant for various reasons, such as a lack of information about the drug, the reason the drug is prescribed, or the expected or therapeutic results. Noncompliance also can be the result of anxiety or bothersome side effects. The nurse can relieve anxiety by allowing the patient to express feelings or concerns, by actively listening as the patient verbalizes feelings, and by providing information so that the patient can be fully informed about the drug. Many patients have a tendency to discontinue use of the drug once the symptoms have been relieved. It is important to emphasize the importance of completing the prescribed course of therapy. For example, failure to complete a course of antibiotic therapy may result in recurrence of the infection. To combat noncompliance the nurse finds out the exact reason for the noncompliance, if possible. Factors related to noncompliance are similar to those listed in Display 4-1.

Anxiety

Anxiety is a vague uneasiness or apprehension that manifests itself in varying degrees from expressions of concern regarding drug regimen to total lack of compliance with the drug regimen. When anxiety is high, the ability to focus on details is reduced. If the patient or caregiver is given information concerning the medication regimen during a high anxiety state, the patient may not remember the information. This could lead to noncompliance. The anxiety experienced during drug administration depends on the severity of the illness, the occurrence of adverse reactions, and the knowledge level of the patient. Anxiety is decreased with understanding of the therapeutic regimen. To decrease anxiety before discussing the treatment regimen with the patient, the nurse takes time to talk with and actively listen to the patient. This helps to build a caring relationship and decrease patient anxiety. It is critical for the nurse to allow time for a thorough explanation and to answer all questions and concerns in language the patient can understand.

It is important to identify and address the specific fear and, if possible, reassure the patient that the drug will alleviate the symptoms or, if possible, cure the disorder. The nurse thoroughly explains any procedure. The nurse actively listens and provides encouragement as the patient expresses fears and concerns. Reassurance and understanding on the part of the nurse are required; the amount of reassurance and understanding depends on the individual patient.

Evaluation

Evaluation is a decision-making process that involves determining the effectiveness of the nursing interventions in meeting the expected outcomes. When related to the administration of a drug, this phase of the nursing process is used to evaluate the patient's response to drug therapy. The evaluation is positive if the expected outcomes have been accomplished or if progress has occurred. If the outcomes have not been accomplished, different interventions are needed. During the administration of the drug the expected response is alleviation of specific symptoms or the presence of a therapeutic effect. Evaluation also may be used to determine if the patient or family member understands the drug regimen.

To evaluate the patient's response to therapy, and depending on the drug administered, the nurse may check the patient's blood pressure every hour, inquire whether pain has been relieved, or monitor the pulse every 15 minutes. After evaluation, certain other decisions may need to be made and plans of action implemented. For example, the nurse may need to notify the primary health care provider of a marked change in a patient's pulse and respiratory rate after a drug was administered, or the nurse may need to change the bed linen because sweating occurred after a drug used to lower the patient's elevated temperature was administered.

The nurse can evaluate the patient's or family's understanding of the drug regimen by noting if one or both appear to understand the material that has been presented. Facial expression may indicate that one or both do or do not understand what has been explained. The nurse also may ask questions about the information that has been given to further evaluate the patient's or family's understanding.

● *Critical Thinking Exercises*

1. *Mr. Hatfield, age 69 years, confides to you that he is not taking the drug prescribed by his primary health care provider. He states he took the drug for a while and then quit. Explain some possible reasons Mr. Hatfield could have for not taking his drug. Discuss questions you could ask to assess the reason for Mr. Hatfield's noncompliance.*

2. *Ms. Heggan is 82 years old and lives alone. She is prescribed several drugs by the primary health care provider but is worried about taking the drugs and the side effects that might occur. She comes to the outpatient clinic after 1 week, and you learn that she has not filled her prescription and is not taking the drugs. Your nursing diagnosis is Ineffective Management of the Therapeutic Regimen related to anxiety about taking the prescribed drugs. Determine what information you would seek to obtain from Ms. Heggan. Identify important nursing interventions for this diagnosis.*

3. *Ms. Taylor is receiving three drugs for the treatment of difficulty breathing and swelling of her legs. You are giving these drugs for the first time. Discuss what questions you would ask Ms. Taylor to obtain subjective data.*

● *Review Questions*

1. A patient states that he does not understand why he had to take a specific medication. The most accurate nursing diagnosis for this man would be _____.

   A. ineffective management of therapeutic regimen
   B. anxiety
   C. noncompliance
   D. deficient knowledge

2. When the nurse enters subjective data in the patient's record, this information is obtained from _____.

   A. the primary care provider
   B. other members of the health care team
   C. the patient or family
   D. laboratory and x-ray reports

3. During the evaluation phase of the nursing process the nurse makes _____.

   A. decisions regarding the effectiveness of nursing interventions
   B. sure nursing procedures have been performed
   C. notations regarding the patient's response to medical treatment
   D. a list of all adverse reactions the patient has experienced while taking the drug

Patient and Family Teaching

Patient teaching is an integral part of nursing. When a drug is prescribed, the patient and the family must be made aware of all information concerning the drug. The nurse is responsible for supplying the patient with accurate and up-to-date information about the drugs prescribed. The teaching/learning process is the means through which the patient is made aware of the drug regimen.

THE TEACHING/LEARNING PROCESS

Teaching is defined as an interactive process that promotes learning. Both the patient and the nurse must be actively involved if teaching is to be effective. **Learning** is acquiring new knowledge or skills. When learning occurs there is a change in the patient's behavior, thinking, or both.

A patient must have **motivation** (having the desire or seeing the need) to learn. Motivation depends on the patient's perception of the need to learn. Education concerning the disease process may be necessary for the patient to become motivated to learn. Encouraging patient participation in planning realistic and attainable goals also promotes motivation. If the patient has no motivation, he or she is likely to be noncompliant.

Creating an accepting and positive atmosphere also enhances learning. Physical discomfort negatively affects the patient's concentration and, thus, the ability to learn. Making sure the patient is not in pain is vital to the teaching/learning process.

THE THREE DOMAINS OF LEARNING

Learning occurs in three domains: cognitive, affective, and psychomotor. When developing a teaching plan for the patient, the nurse must consider each domain.

Cognitive Domain

The **cognitive domain** refers to intellectual activities such as thought, recall, decision making, and drawing conclusions. In this domain the patient uses previous experiences, prior knowledge, and perceptions to give meaning to new information or to modify previous thinking. The nurse makes use of the patient's cognitive abilities when information is given to the patient or caregivers about the disease process, medication regimen, and adverse reactions. The patient uses the cognitive domain to process the information, ask questions, and make decisions.

Affective Domain

The **affective domain** includes the patient/caregiver's attitudes, feelings, beliefs, and opinions. Health care providers often ignore these aspects of patient teaching.

It is easy to pull a preprinted teaching outline off of the computer or obtain preprinted material. This type of material is often used as a checklist to teach the patient about a drug and the therapeutic regimen. Such checklists are useful in helping the nurse remember important aspects of the drug that should be covered when teaching the patients about the drug and to give to the patient for future reference. However, the use of such checklists fails to take into account the affective domain.

Perhaps the most important prerequisite to learning about the patient's affective behavior is to develop a therapeutic relationship with the patient (one that is based on trust and caring). When the nurse takes the time to develop a therapeutic relationship, the patient/family has confidence in the nurse and more confidence in the information to be taught. The nurse approaches the patient with respect and encourages the expression of thoughts and feelings. Exploring the patient's beliefs about health and illness enhances the nurse's understanding of the patient's affective behavior.

Psychomotor Domain

The **psychomotor domain** involves learning physical skills (such as injection of insulin) or tasks (such as performing a dressing change). The nurse teaches a task or skill using a step-by-step method. The patient is allowed hands-on practice under the supervision of the nurse. The nurse assesses the patient mastery of the skill by having the patient or caregiver perform a return demonstration under the watchful eye of the nurse.

ADULT LEARNING

Generally adults learn only what they feel they need to learn. Adults learn best when they have a strong inner motivation to learn a new skill or acquire new knowledge. They will learn less if they are passive recipients of "canned" educational content. Adults have a vast array of experiences and knowledge to bring to a new learning experience. Teachers who use this experience will bring about the greatest behavior change. While 83% of adults are visual learners, only 11% learn by listening. Most adults retain the information taught if they are able to "do" something with that new knowledge immediately. For example, in teaching a patient how to administer his/her own insulin, the nurse would demonstrate the technique, allow time for supervised practice, and as soon as the patient appears ready, allow the patient to prepare and inject the insulin. Most adults prefer an informal learning environment where there is mutual exchange and freedom of expression.

THE NURSING PROCESS AS A FRAMEWORK FOR PATIENT TEACHING

The nursing process is a systematic method of identifying patient health needs, devising a plan of care to meet the identified needs, initiating the plan, and evaluating its effectiveness. This process provides the necessary framework to develop an effective teaching plan. However, the teaching plan differs from the nursing process in that the nursing process encompasses all of the patient's health care needs, whereas the teaching plan focuses primarily on the patient's learning needs. Nurses must be actively involved in teaching if they are to educate their patients about the proper way to take their drugs, the possibility of adverse reactions, and the signs and symptoms of toxicity (if applicable).

Assessment

Assessment is the data-gathering phase of the nursing process. Assessment assists the nurse in choosing the best teaching methods and individualizing the teaching plan. To develop an effective teaching plan, the nurse must first determine the patient's needs. Needs stem from three areas: (1) information the patient or family needs to know about a particular drug; (2) the patient's or family member's ability to learn, accept, and use information; and (3) any barriers or obstacles to learning.

Some drugs have simple uses and, therefore, relatively little patient teaching is needed. For example, applying a nonprescription ointment to the skin requires only minimal teaching. Other drugs, such as insulin, require detailed information that may need to be given over several days.

Assessing an individual's ability to learn may be difficult. Not all adults have the same literacy level. The information to be taught should be geared to the patient's educational and reading level. When assessing language and literacy skills, it is important to remember that some patients do not have the ability to read well. The nurse must carefully assess the patient's ability to communicate. Without accurate communication, learning will not occur. If the patient has a learning impairment, a family member or friend should be included in the teaching process. Most people readily understand what is being taught, but some cannot. For example, a visually impaired patient may be unable to read a label or printed directions supplied by the primary health care provider, pharmacist, or nurse. Another means of teaching will have to be used.

Through assessment, the nurse determines what barriers or obstacles (if any) may prevent the patient or family member from fully understanding the material being presented. Taking into consideration the patient's

---

Nursing Diagnosis Checklist

✓ **Effective Therapeutic Regimen Management**

✓ **Risk for Ineffective Therapeutic Regimen Management** related to lack of knowledge, indifference, other factors

✓ **Noncompliance** with drug regimen related to indifference, lack of knowledge, other factors

✓ **Deficient Knowledge** related to the drug regimen, possible adverse reactions, disease process, other factors

---

cultural background is helpful when planning a teaching session. For example, for some patients an interpreter is needed. In other cultures a certain individual (for example, the mother or the grandmother) is the decision maker in the family. It is important for the nurse to include the decision maker and the patient in the teaching session.

Nursing Diagnoses

The nursing diagnosis is formulated after analyzing the information obtained during the assessment phase. Most often, nursing diagnoses related to the administration of drugs are associated with a risk for ineffective management, deficit knowledge, or noncompliance. Examples of nursing diagnoses related to the administration of drugs are listed in the Nursing Diagnosis Checklist.

Planning

Planning is the actual development of strategies to be used in the teaching plan and the selection of information to be taught. Planning begins with an expected outcome statement. The nurse develops a teaching plan based on the expected outcome using the information gained during the assessment. Display 5-1 identifies important information that the nurse should include in the teaching plan.

DISPLAY 5-1 ● Important Information to Include in the Teaching Plan

1. Therapeutic response expected from the drug
2. Adverse reactions to expect when taking the drug
3. Adverse reactions to report to the nurse or primary health care provider
4. Dosage and route
5. Any special considerations or precautions associated with the particular drug prescribed
6. Additional education regarding special considerations of certain drugs, such as techniques for giving injections, applying topical patches, or instilling eye drops

---

Developing an Individualized Teaching Plan

Teaching plans are individualized because patients' needs are not identical. Areas covered in an individualized teaching plan vary depending on the drug prescribed, the primary health care provider's preference for including or excluding specific facts about the drug, and what the patient needs to know to take the drug correctly. Teaching strategies must reflect individual learning needs and ability. For example, a patient who speaks and reads only Spanish will not benefit from discharge instructions given in English or from instructions written in English. Different strategies must be implemented, such as providing instructions written in Spanish or communicating through another nurse who is fluent in the Spanish language.

When developing an individualized teaching plan for patients and their families, the nurse must select information relevant to a specific drug, adapt teaching to the individual's level of understanding, and avoid medical terminology unless terms are explained or defined. Figure 5-1 is a sample form to use when developing a teaching plan. It is important to remember that repetition enhances learning. Several teaching sessions help the nurse to better assess what the patient is actually learning and provides time for clarification. The patient should be encouraged to ask questions and express feelings.

Basic Information to Consider When Developing a Teaching Plan

General material to consider when developing a teaching plan includes information on the dosage regimen, adverse reactions, family members, and basic information about drugs, drug containers, and drug storage.

DOSAGE REGIMEN. The dosage regimen is an important aspect of the teaching plan. The nurse must consider the following general points when teaching about the dosage regimen:

- Capsules or tablets should be taken with water unless the primary health care provider or pharmacist directs otherwise (eg, take with food, milk, or an antacid). Some liquids, such as coffee, tea, fruit juice, and carbonated beverages, may interfere with the action of certain drugs.
- A full glass of water is used when taking an oral drug. In some instances, it may be necessary to drink extra fluids during the day while taking certain drugs.
- It is important not to chew capsules before swallowing; they must be swallowed whole. The patient also should not chew tablets unless labeled as "chewable." Some tablets have special coatings that are required for specific purposes, such as

Patient: _____ Medical Diagnosis: _____

Nursing Diagnosis: _____

_____ Effective Therapeutic Regimen Management _____

_____ Ineffective Therapeutic Regimen Management related to _____

_____ Deficient Knowledge related to _____

Expected Outcome: Patient will _____

_____

Identified obstacles to learning: _____

_____

_____

Primary Language: _____

Cultural Considerations: _____

_____

_____

Information to include in teaching session:

Expected therapeutic drug response:

Dosage and route:

Possible adverse reactions:

Adverse reactions to report:

Special considerations:

Teaching session (s)

Date(s)	Present	Evaluation*	Comments
1.			
2.			
3.			

*return demonstration, verbalizes understanding of information, questioned by nurse, other (specify) _____ .

FIGURE 5-1. Patient and family teaching.

proper absorption of the drug or prevention of irritation of the lining of the stomach.

- The dose of a drug or the time interval between doses is never increased or decreased unless directed by the primary health care provider.
- A prescription drug or nonprescription drug recommended by a primary health care provider is not stopped or omitted except on the advice of the primary health care provider.
- If the symptoms for which a drug was prescribed do not improve, or become worse, the primary health care provider must be contacted as soon as possible because a change in dosage or a different drug may be necessary.
- If a dose of a drug is omitted or forgotten, the next dose must not be doubled or the drug taken at more frequent intervals unless advised to do so by the primary health care provider.
- All health care workers, including physicians, dentists, nurses, and health personnel must always be informed of all drugs (prescription and nonprescription) currently being taken on a regular or occasional basis.
- The exact names of all prescription and nonprescription drugs currently being taken should be kept in a wallet or purse for instant reference when seeing a physician, dentist, or other health care provider.
- Check prescriptions carefully when obtaining refills from the pharmacy and report any changes in the prescription (eg, changes in color, size, shape) to the pharmacist or primary health care provider before taking the drug because an error may have occurred.
- Wear a Medic-Alert bracelet or other type of identification when taking a drug for a long time. This is especially important for drugs such as anticoagulants, steroids, oral hypoglycemic agents, insulin, or digitalis. In case of an emergency, the bracelet ensures that medical personnel are aware of health problems and current drug therapy.

ADVERSE DRUG EFFECTS. Information about adverse drug effects of the prescribed drug must be included when the nurse develops a teaching plan for the patient. The nurse should teach the patient the following general points about adverse drug effects:

- All drugs cause adverse reactions (side effects). Examples of some of the more common adverse reactions are nausea, vomiting, diarrhea, constipation, skin rash, dizziness, drowsiness, and dry mouth. Some may be mild and disappear with time or when the primary health care provider adjusts the dosage. In some instances, mild reactions, such as dry mouth, may have to be tolerated. Some

adverse reactions are potentially serious and even life threatening.

- Adverse effects are always reported to the primary health care provider as soon as possible.
- Medical personnel must be informed of all drug allergies before any treatment or drug is given.

FAMILY MEMBERS. The nurse considers the following points concerning family members when developing a teaching plan:

- A drug prescribed for one family member is never given to another family member, relative, or friend unless directed to do so by the primary health care provider.
- The nurse makes sure that all family members or relatives are aware of all drugs, prescription and nonprescription, that are currently being taken by the patient.

DRUGS, DRUG CONTAINERS, AND DRUG STORAGE. The following are important facts about drugs, drug containers, and the storage of drugs that the nurse must consider when developing a teaching plan:

- The term *drug* applies to both nonprescription and prescription drugs.
- A drug must be kept in the container in which it was dispensed or purchased. Some drugs require special containers, such as light-resistant (brown) bottles to prevent deterioration that may occur on exposure to light.
- If any drug changes color or develops a new odor, a pharmacist must be consulted immediately about continued use of the drug.
- The original label on the drug container must not be removed while it is used to hold the drug.
- Two or more different drugs must never be mixed in one container, even for a brief time, because one drug may chemically affect another. Mixing drugs can also lead to mistaking one drug for another, especially when the size and color are similar.
- The lid or cap of the container must be replaced immediately after removing the drug from the container. The lid or cap must be firmly snapped or screwed in place because exposure to air or moisture shortens the life of most drugs.
- Drugs requiring refrigeration are so labeled. The container must be returned to the refrigerator immediately after removing the drug.
- All drugs must be kept out of the reach of children.
- Unless otherwise directed, drugs must be stored in a cool, dry place.
- Do not expose a drug to excessive sunlight, heat, cold, or moisture because deterioration may occur.

Home Care Checklist

MODIFYING DRUG ADMINISTRATION IN THE HOME

Once the patient is at home, some modifications may be necessary to ensure safe drug administration. The nurse provides written instructions, using large print (if necessary), nonglare paper, and words that the patient and caregiver can understand. In addition, it is important to modify your teaching by using the following suggestions:

✔ For patients taking more than one drug, develop a clear, easy-to-read drug schedule or a chart resembling a clock for the patient or caregiver to consult.

✔ Try using a daily calendar as an inexpensive, yet effective, means for scheduling.

✔ If the patient or caregiver has a problem with drug names, refer to the drug by shape or color. Another idea is to number bottles and use this number on the drug chart.

✔ If financially feasible, suggest the use of commercially available drug organizers. If the patient cannot afford drug organizers, egg cartons or a muffin tin can be labeled and used as drug organizers.

✔ If your patient finds it helpful to keep all drugs together, suggest using a bowl, tray, or small box to hold all the containers.

✔ If temporary refrigeration is necessary, suggest the use of a small cooler or insulated bag.

✔ If equipment items such as needles and syringes are used, suggest keeping all the supplies in one area.

✔ If the supplies came in a delivery box, suggest that the patient use it for storage. Other suggestions include using plastic storage containers with snap-on lids or clean, dry glass jars with screw tops.

✔ Advise the patient to use an impervious container with a properly fitting lid, such as a coffee can, for safe disposal. A plastic milk jug with a lid or a heavy-duty, clean, cardboard milk or juice carton may be used if necessary.

✔ Explain the importance of taking precautions to make sure discarded needles do not puncture the container.

- The entire label of the prescription or nonprescription drug container must be read, including the recommended dosage and warnings.
- All directions printed on the label (eg, "shake well before using," "keep refrigerated," "take before meals") must be followed to ensure drug effectiveness.
- In some instances, especially when an ointment or liquid drug is prescribed, some drug may remain after it is used or taken for the prescribed time. Some drugs have a short life (a few weeks to a few months) and may deteriorate or change chemically after a time. A prescription must never be saved for later use unless the primary health care provider so advises.

Implementation

Implementation is the actual performance of the interventions identified in the teaching plan. Teaching at an appropriate time for each patient fosters learning. For example,

patient teaching is not done when there are visitors (unless they are to be involved in the administration of the patient's drugs), immediately before discharge from the hospital, or if the patient has been sedated or is in pain.

Teaching is begun a day or more before discharge, at a time when the patient is alone and alert, and continued each day until dismissal. The nurse gears teaching to the patient's level of understanding and, when necessary, provides written as well as oral instructions. If much information is given, it is often best to present the material in two or more sessions. Drug administration modifications may be necessary once the patient is at home. The nurse keeps these modifications in mind when teaching the patient (see Home Care Checklist: Modifying Drug Administration in the Home).

Evaluation

To determine the effectiveness of patient teaching, the nurse evaluates the patient's knowledge of the material presented. Evaluation can be done in several ways, depending on the nature of the information.

For example, if the patient is being taught to administer insulin, several demonstrations can be scheduled, followed by a return demonstration by the patient with the nurse observing to evaluate the patient's technique.

Questions such as "Do you understand?" or "Is there anything you don't understand?" should be avoided because the patient may feel uncomfortable admitting a lack of understanding. When factual material is being evaluated, the nurse should periodically ask the patient to list or repeat some of the information presented.

● Critical Thinking Exercises

1. *Locate the clinical educator in any health care agency in your community whose job it is to do patient education. Discuss with that person his or her thoughts and feelings on patient education, as well as any problems or pitfalls he or she has identified.*
2. *Interview friends or relatives about their knowledge of the drug(s) prescribed by their primary health care provider. Discuss with them the teaching they received from nurses or other health care providers before they began taking the drugs. Determine what areas could have been included that were not discussed. Analyze how the teaching/learning process was evaluated. Identify any areas that could be improved.*
3. *Using the form in Figure 5-1, develop a teaching plan for a patient.*

● Review Questions

1. An interactive process that promotes learning is defined as _____.
   A. motivation
   B. cognitive ability
   C. the psychomotor domain
   D. teaching

2. When developing a teaching plan the nurse assesses the affective learning domain, which means that the nurse considers the patient's _____.
   A. attitudes, feelings, beliefs, and opinions
   B. ability to perform a return demonstration
   C. intellectual ability
   D. home environment

3. Actual development of the strategies to be used in the teaching plan and selections of the information to be taught occur in the _____ phase of the nursing process.
   A. assessment
   B. planning
   C. implementation
   D. evaluation

4. Unless the primary health care provider or pharmacist directs otherwise, the nurse informs patient to take oral medications with _____.
   A. fruit juice
   B. milk
   C. water
   D. food

c h a p t e r **6**

Sulfonamides

Key Terms

agranulocytosis
anorexia
antibacterial
anti-infective
aplastic anemia
bacteriostatic
crystalluria

leukopenia
pruritus
Stevens-Johnson
  syndrome
stomatitis
thrombocytopenia
urticaria

Chapter Objectives

On completion of this chapter, the student will:

- Discuss the uses, general drug actions, and general adverse reactions, contraindications, precautions, and interactions of the sulfonamides.
- Discuss important preadministration and ongoing assessment activities the nurse should perform on the patient taking sulfonamides.
- Describe the signs and symptoms associated with Stevens-Johnson syndrome.
- List some nursing diagnoses particular to a patient taking sulfonamides.
- Discuss ways to promote an optimal response to therapy, how to manage adverse reactions, and important points to keep in mind when educating patients about the use of the sulfonamides.

The sulfonamides (sulfa) drugs were the first antibiotic drugs developed that effectively treated infections. Although the use of sulfonamides began to decline after the introduction of more effective anti-infectives, such as the penicillins and other antibiotics, these drugs still remain important for the treatment of certain types of infections.

onism to para-aminobenzoic acid (PABA), a substance that some, but not all, bacteria need to multiply. Once the rate of bacterial multiplication is slowed, the body's own defense mechanisms (white blood cells) are able to rid the body of the invading microorganisms and therefore control the infection.

SULFONAMIDES

Sulfonamides are **antibacterial** agents, meaning they are active against bacteria. Another term that may be used to describe the general action of these drugs is **anti-infective** because they are used to treat infections caused by certain bacteria. Sulfadiazine, sulfisoxazole, and sulfamethizole are examples of sulfonamide preparations.

ACTIONS

The sulfonamides are primarily **bacteriostatic,** which means they slow or retard the multiplication of bacteria. This bacteriostatic activity is due to sulfonamide antag-

USES

The sulfonamides are often used to control urinary tract infections caused by certain bacteria such as *Escherichia coli, Staphylococcus aureus,* and *Klebsiella-Enterobacter.* Mafenide (Sulfamylon) and silver sulfadiazine (Silvadene) are topical sulfonamides used in the treatment of second- and third-degree burns. Additional uses of the sulfonamides are given in the Summary Drug Table: The Sulfonamides.

ADVERSE REACTIONS

The sulfonamides are capable of causing a variety of adverse reactions. Some of these are serious or potentially

SUMMARY DRUG TABLE THE SULFONAMIDES

GENERIC NAME	TRADE NAME*	USES	ADVERSE REACTIONS	DOSAGE RANGES
Single Agents				
sulfadiazine *sul-fa-dye´-a-zeen*	generic	Urinary tract infections due to susceptible microorganisms, chancroid, acute otitis media, *Hemophilus influenzae* and meningococcal meningitis, rheumatic fever	Hematologic changes, Stevens-Johnson syndrome, nausea, vomiting, headache, diarrhea, chills, fever, anorexia, crystalluria, stomatitis, urticaria, pruritus	Loading dose: 2–4 g PO; maintenance dose: 2–4 g/d PO in 4–6 divided doses
sulfamethizole *sul-fa-meth´-i-zole*	Thiosulfil Forte	Urinary tract infections due to susceptible microorganisms	Same as sulfadiazine	0.5–1 g PO tid, qid
sulfamethoxazole *sul-fa-meth-ox´-a-zole*	Gantanol, Urobak, generic	Urinary tract infections due to susceptible microorganisms, meningococcal meningitis, acute otitis media	Same as sulfadiazine	Initial dose: 2 g PO, maintenance dose: 1 g PO bid, tid
sulfasalazine *sul-fa-sal´-a-zeen*	Azulfidine, Azulfidine EN-tabs, generic	Ulcerative colitis, rheumatoid arthritis	Same as sulfadiazine; may cause skin and urine to turn orange-yellow	Initial therapy: 1–4 g/d PO in divided doses; maintenance dose: 2 g/d in evenly spaced doses 500 mg qid
sulfisoxazole *sul-fi-sox´-a-zole*	generic	Same as sulfadiazine	Same as sulfadiazine	Loading dose: 2–4 g PO; maintenance dose: 4–8 g/d PO in 4–6 divided doses
Multiple Preparations				
trimethoprim (TMP) and sulfamethoxazole (SMZ) *trye-meth´-oh-prim; sul-fa-meth-ox´-a-zole*	Bactrim, Bactrim DS, Septra, Septra DS, generic	Urinary tract infections due to susceptible microorganisms, acute otitis media, traveler's diarrhea due to *Escherichia coli*	Gastrointestinal disturbances, allergic skin reactions, hematologic changes, Stevens-Johnson syndrome, headache	160 mg TMP/800 mg SMZ PO q12h; 8–10 mg/kg/d (based on TMP) IV in 2–4 divided doses
Miscellaneous Sulfonamide Preparations				
mafenide *meph´-a-nide*	Sulfamylon	Second- and third-degree burns	Pain or burning sensation, rash, itching, facial edema	Apply to burned area 1–2 times/d
silver sulfadiazine *sil´-ver sul-fa-dye´-a-zeen*	Silvadene, Thermazene, SSD (cream)	Same as mafenide	Leukopenia, skin necrosis, skin discoloration, burning sensation	Same as mafenide

*The term *generic* indicates the drug is available in generic form.

serious; others are mild. The following hematologic changes may occur during sulfonamide therapy:

- **Agranulocytosis**—decrease in or lack of granulocytes, a type of white blood cell
- **Thrombocytopenia**—decrease in the number of platelets
- **Aplastic anemia**—anemia due to deficient red blood cell production in the bone marrow
- **Leukopenia**—decrease in the number of white blood cells

These are examples of a serious adverse reaction. If any of these occur, discontinuation of sulfonamide therapy may be required.

Anorexia (loss of appetite) is an example of a mild adverse reaction. Unless it becomes severe and pronounced weight loss occurs, it may not be necessary to discontinue sulfonamide therapy.

Various types of hypersensitivity (allergic) reactions may be seen during sulfonamide therapy, including Stevens-Johnson syndrome, **urticaria** (hives), **pruritus** (itching), and generalized skin eruptions. **Stevens-Johnson syndrome** is manifested by fever, cough, muscular aches and pains, and headache, all of which are signs and symptoms of many other disorders. However, the appearance of lesions on the skin, mucous membranes, eyes, and other organs are diagnostically significant and may be the first conclusive signs of this syndrome. Any of these symptoms must be reported to the primary health care provider immediately.

Other adverse reactions that may occur during therapy include nausea, vomiting, diarrhea, abdominal pain, chills, fever, and **stomatitis** (inflammation of the mouth). In some instances, these may be mild. Other times they may cause serious problems requiring discontinuation of the drug. Sulfasalazine may cause the urine and skin to be an orange-yellow color; this is not abnormal.

Crystalluria (crystals in the urine) may occur during administration of a sulfonamide, although this problem occurs less frequently with some of the newer sulfonamide preparations. This potentially serious problem often can be prevented by increasing fluid intake during sulfonamide therapy.

The most frequent adverse reaction seen with the application of mafenide is a burning sensation or pain when the drug is applied to the skin. Other possible allergic reactions include rash, itching, edema, and urticaria. Burning, rash, and itching may also be seen with the use of silver sulfadiazine. It may be difficult to distinguish between an adverse reaction due to the use of mafenide or silver sulfadiazine and reactions that may occur from the severe burn injury or from other agents used at the same time for the management of the burns.

CONTRAINDICATIONS

The sulfonamides are contraindicated in patients with hypersensitivity to the sulfonamides, during lactation, and in children less than 2 years old. The sulfonamides are not used near the end (at term) of pregnancy (Pregnancy Category D). If the sulfonamides are given near the end of pregnancy, significant blood levels of the drug may occur, causing jaundice or hemolytic anemia in the neonate. Additionally, the sulfonamides are not used for infections caused by group A beta-hemolytic streptococci because the sulfonamides have *not* been shown to be effective in preventing the complications of rheumatic fever or glomerulonephritis.

PRECAUTIONS

The sulfonamides are used with caution in patients with renal or hepatic impairment and bronchial asthma. These drugs are given with caution to patients with allergies. Safety for use during pregnancy has not been established (Pregnancy Category C, except at term).

INTERACTIONS

When a sulfonamide is administered with an oral anticoagulant, the action of the anticoagulant may be enhanced. The risk of bone marrow suppression may be increased when a sulfonamide is administered with methotrexate. When a sulfonamide is administered with a hydantoin, the serum hydantoin level may be increased.

Sulfonamides may inhibit the (hepatic) metabolism of the oral hypoglycemic drugs tolbutamide (Orinase) and chlorpropamide (Diabinese). This would increase the possibility of a hypoglycemic reaction.

❀**Health Supplement Alert: Cranberry**

Cranberries and cranberry juice are a commonly used remedy for the prevention of urinary tract infections (UTIs) and for the relief of symptoms from UTIs. The use of cranberry juice in combination with antibiotics has been recommended by physicians for the long-term suppression of UTIs. Cranberries are thought to act by preventing the bacteria from attaching to the walls of the urinary tract. The suggested amount is 6 ounces of the juice two times daily. Extremely large doses can produce gastrointestinal disturbances such as diarrhea or abdominal cramping. Although cranberries may relieve the symptoms of a UTI or prevent the occurrence of a UTI, their use will not cure a UTI. If an individual suspects a UTI, medical attention is necessary.

● **The Patient Receiving a Sulfonamide**

ASSESSMENT

Preadministration Assessment

Before the initial administration of the drug, it is important to assess the patient's general appearance and take and record the vital signs. The nurse obtains information regarding the symptoms experienced by the patient and the length of time these symptoms have been present. Depending on the type and location of the infection or disease, the nurse reviews the results of tests, such as a urine culture, urinalysis, complete blood count, intravenous pyelogram, renal function tests, and examination of the stool.

Ongoing Assessment

During the course of therapy, the nurse evaluates the patient at periodic intervals for response to the drug, that is, a relief of symptoms and a decrease in temperature (if it was elevated before therapy started), as well as the occurrence of any adverse reactions.

The nurse monitors the temperature, pulse, respiratory rate, and blood pressure every 4 hours or as ordered by the primary health care provider. If fever is present and the patient's temperature suddenly increases or if the temperature was normal and suddenly increases, the nurse contacts the primary health care provider immediately.

The ongoing assessment for patients receiving sulfasalazine for ulcerative colitis includes observation for evidence of the relief or intensification of the symptoms of the disease. The nurse inspects all stool samples and records their number and appearance.

When administering a sulfonamide for a burn, the nurse inspects the burned areas every 1 to 2 hours because some treatment regimens require keeping the affected areas covered with the mafenide or silver sulfadiazine ointment at all times. Any adverse reactions should be reported immediately to the primary health care provider.

NURSING DIAGNOSES

Drug-specific nursing diagnoses are highlighted in the Nursing Diagnoses Checklist. Other nursing diagnoses applicable to the drugs are discussed in depth in Chapter 4.

Nursing Diagnoses Checklist

- ✓ **Risk for Infection** related to adverse reactions of the sulfonamides
- ✓ **Risk for Impaired Skin Integrity** related to adverse drug reaction of the sulfonamides
- ✓ **Impaired Urinary Elimination** related to adverse drug reaction of the sulfonamides

---

PLANNING

The expected outcomes of the patient depend on the reason for administration of the sulfonamide but may include an optimal response to drug therapy, management of adverse drug reactions, and an understanding of and compliance with the prescribed treatment regimen.

IMPLEMENTATION

Promoting an Optimal Response to Therapy

The patient receiving a sulfonamide drug almost always has an active infection. Some patients may be receiving one of these drugs to prevent an infection (prophylaxis) or as part of the management of a disease such as ulcerative colitis.

Unless the primary health care provider orders otherwise, the nurse gives sulfonamides to the patient whose stomach is empty, that is, 1 hour before or 2 hours after meals. If gastrointestinal irritation occurs, the nurse may give sulfasalazine with food or immediately after meals. It is important to instruct the patient to drink a full glass of water when taking an oral sulfonamide and to drink at least eight large glasses of water each day until therapy is finished.

Managing Burns

When mafenide or silver sulfadiazine is used in the treatment of burns, the treatment regimen is outlined by the primary health care provider or the personnel in the burn treatment unit. There are various burn treatment regimens, such as debridement (removal of burned or dead tissue from the burned site), special dressings, and cleansing of the burned area. The use of a specific treatment regimen often depends on the extent of the burned area, the degree of the burns, and the physical condition and age of the patient. Other concurrent problems, such as lung damage due to smoke or heat or physical injuries that occurred at the time of the burn injury, also may influence the treatment regimen.

When instructed to do so, the nurse cleans and removes debris present on the surface of the skin before each application of mafenide or silver sulfadiazine and applies these drugs with a sterile gloved hand. The drug is applied approximately 1/16 inch thick; thicker application is not recommended. The patient is kept away from any draft of air because even the slightest movement of air across the burned area can cause pain. It is important to warn the patient that stinging or burning may be felt during, and for a short time after, application of mafenide. Some burning also may be noted with the application of silver sulfadiazine.

Monitoring and Managing Adverse Drug Reactions

The nurse must observe the patient for adverse reactions, especially an allergic reaction (see Chap. 1). If one or more adverse reactions should occur, the nurse withholds the next dose of the drug and notifies the primary health care provider.

The nurse monitors the patient for leukopenia and thrombocytopenia. Leukopenia may result in signs and symptoms of an infection, such as fever, sore throat, and cough. The nurse protects the patient with leukopenia from individuals who have an infection. With severe leukopenia the patient may be placed in protective (reverse) isolation. Thrombocytopenia is manifested by easy bruising and unusual bleeding following moderate to slight trauma to the skin or mucous membranes. The extremities of the patient with thrombocytopenia are handled with care to prevent bruising. Care is taken to prevent trauma when the patient is moved. The nurse inspects the skin daily for the extent of bruising and evidence of exacerbation of existing ecchymotic areas. It is important to encourage the patient to use a soft-bristled toothbrush to prevent any trauma to the mucous membranes of the oral cavity. The nurse reports any signs of leukopenia or thrombocytopenia immediately because this is an indication to stop drug therapy.

✳ Nursing Alert

Stevens-Johnson syndrome is a serious and sometimes fatal hypersensitivity reaction. The nurse must be alert for lesions on the skin and mucous membranes, a diagnostically important symptom of this syndrome. The lesions appear as red wheals or blisters, often starting on the face, in the mouth, or on the lips, neck, and extremities. This syndrome, which also may occur with the administration of other types of drugs, can be fatal. The nurse must notify the primary health care provider and withhold the next dose of the drug. In addition, the nurse must exercise care to prevent injury to the involved areas.

Maintaining Adequate Fluid Intake and Output

Because one adverse reaction of the sulfonamide drugs is altered elimination patterns, it is important that the nurse helps the patient maintain adequate fluid intake and output. The nurse can encourage patients to increase fluid intake to 2000 mL or more a day to prevent crystalluria and stone formation in the genitourinary tract, as well as to aid in the removal of microorganisms from the urinary tract. It is important to measure and record the intake and output every 8 hours and notify the primary health care provider if the urinary output decreases or the patient fails to increase his or her oral intake.

❄ Gerontologic Alert

Because renal impairment is common in older adults, the nurse should give the sulfonamides with great caution. There is an increased danger of the sulfonamides causing additional renal damage when renal impairment is already present. An increase of fluid intake up to 2000 mL (if the older adult can tolerate this amount) decreases the risk of crystals and stones forming in the urinary tract.

Educating the Patient and Family

When a sulfonamide is prescribed for an infection, some outpatients have a tendency to discontinue the drug once symptoms have been relieved. When teaching the patient and the family, the nurse emphasizes the importance of completing the prescribed course of therapy to be sure all microorganisms causing the infection are eradicated. Failure to complete a course of therapy may result in a recurrence of the infection. The nurse should develop a teaching plan to include the following information:

- Take the drug as prescribed.
- Take the drug on an empty stomach either 1 hour before or 2 hours after a meal (exception: sulfasalazine is taken with food or immediately after a meal).
- Take the drug with a full glass of water. Do not increase or decrease the time between doses unless directed to do so by the primary health care provider.
- Complete the full course of therapy. Do not discontinue this drug (unless advised to do so by the primary health care provider) even though the symptoms of the infection have disappeared.
- Drink *at least* 8 to 10 8-oz glasses of fluid every day.
- Prolonged exposure to sunlight may result in skin reactions similar to a severe sunburn (photosensitivity reactions). When going outside, cover exposed areas of the skin or apply a protective sunscreen to exposed areas.
- Notify the primary health care provider immediately if the following should occur: fever, skin rash or other skin problems, nausea, vomiting, unusual bleeding or bruising, sore throat, or extreme fatigue.
- Keep all follow-up appointments to ensure the infection is controlled.
- When taking sulfasalazine, the skin or urine may turn an orange-yellow color; this is not abnormal. If the patient wears soft contact lenses, a permanent yellow stain of the lenses may occur. It is a good idea to seek the advice of an ophthalmologist regarding corrective lenses while taking this drug.

EVALUATION

- The therapeutic drug effect is achieved.
- No evidence of infection is seen.
- The skin is intact and free of inflammation, irritation, or ulcerations.
- Adverse reactions are identified, reported to the primary health care provider, and managed successfully through appropriate nursing interventions.
- The patient verbalizes the importance of complying with the prescribed treatment regimen.
- The patient and family demonstrate an understanding of the drug regimen.

● *Critical Thinking Exercises*

1. *Ms. Bartlett, age 80, has been prescribed a sulfonamide for a urinary tract infection and is to take the drug for 10 days. You note that Ms. Bartlett seems forgetful and at times confused. Determine what problems might be associated with Ms. Bartlett's mental state and her possible noncompliance to her prescribed treatment regimen.*

2. *Mr. Garcia is receiving sulfisoxazole for a recurrent bladder infection. When keeping an outpatient clinic appointment, he tells you that he developed a fever and sore throat yesterday. Analyze the steps you would take to investigate his recent problem. Give a reason for your answers.*

3. *Ms. Watson has diabetes and is taking tolbutamide (Orinase). Her primary care provider prescribes the combination drug sulfamethoxazole and trimethoprim (Septra) for a bladder infection. Discuss any instructions/information you would give to Ms. Watson in the patient education session.*

● *Review Questions*

1. A nurse working in the clinic asks how the sulfonamides control an infection. The most correct answer is that these drugs _____.
   A. encourage the production of antibodies
   B. antagonize PABA, which some bacteria need to multiply
   C. reduce the urine output
   D. make the urine alkaline, which eliminates bacteria

2. Patients receiving sulfasalazine for ulcerative colitis are told that the drug _____.
   A. is not to be taken with food
   B. rarely causes adverse effects
   C. may cause hair loss
   D. may turn the urine orange-yellow in color

3. When mafenide (Sulfamylon) is applied to a burned area, the nurse _____.
   A. first covers the burned area with a sterile compress
   B. irrigates the area with normal saline
   C. warns the patient that stinging or burning may be felt
   D. instructs the patient to drink two to three extra glasses of water each day

4. The nurse can evaluate the patient's response to therapy by asking him if _____.
   A. he completed the entire course of therapy
   B. his symptoms have been relieved
   C. he has seen any evidence of blood in the urine
   D. has experienced any constipation

● *Medication Dosage Problems*

1. The primary health care provider prescribed sulfasalazine oral suspension 500 mg every 8 hours. The nurse has sulfasalazine oral suspension 250 mg/5 mL on hand. What dosage would the nurse give?

2. The nurse orders sulfamethoxazole 2 g PO initially, followed by 1 g PO BID. The nurse has 1000-mg tablets on hand. How many tablets would the nurse give for the initial dose?

chapter 7

Penicillins

Key Terms

anaphylactic shock	leukopenia
angioedema	nonpathogenic
bacterial resistance	normal flora
bactericidal	penicillinase
bacteriostatic	phlebitis
cross-allergenicity	prophylaxis
cross-sensitivity	pseudomembranous
culture and sensitivity	colitis
tests	stomatitis
glossitis	superinfection
hypersensitivity	thrombocytopenia

Chapter Objectives

On completion of this chapter, the student will:

- Identify the uses, general drug actions, and general adverse reactions, contraindications, precautions, and interactions of the penicillins.
- Discuss hypersensitivity reactions and pseudomembranous colitis as they relate to antibiotic therapy.
- List some nursing diagnoses particular to a patient taking penicillin.
- Identify important preadministration and ongoing assessment activities the nurse should perform on the patient taking penicillin.
- Discuss ways to promote optimal response to therapy, nursing actions to minimize adverse effects, and important points to keep in mind when educating patients about the use of penicillin.

The development of the sulfonamide antibiotics was a breakthrough in the treatment of bacterial infections. Since that time, there has been a quest to develop new and more effective antibiotic drugs. The antibacterial properties of natural penicillins were discovered in 1928 by Sir Alexander Fleming while he was performing research on influenza. Ten years later, British scientists studied the effects of natural penicillins on disease-causing microorganisms. However, it was not until 1941 that natural penicillins were used clinically for the treatment of infections. Although used for more than 50 years, the penicillins are still an important and effective group of antibiotics for the treatment of susceptible pathogens (disease-causing microorganisms).

There are four groups of penicillins: natural penicillins, penicillinase-resistant penicillins, aminopenicillins, and the extended-spectrum penicillins. See the

Summary Drug Table: Penicillins for a more complete listing of the penicillins. Display 7-1 gives examples of the various groups.

DRUG RESISTANCE

Because the natural penicillins have been used for many years, drug-resistant strains of microorganisms have developed, making the natural penicillins less effective than some of the newer antibiotics in treating a broad range of infections. Bacterial resistance has occurred within the penicillins. **Bacterial resistance** is the ability of bacteria to produce substances that inactivate or destroy the penicillin. One example of bacterial resistance is the ability of certain bacteria to produce **penicillinase,** an enzyme that inactivates penicillin. The penicillinase-resistant penicillins were developed to combat this problem.

The natural penicillins also have a fairly narrow spectrum of activity, which means that they are effective against only a few strains of bacteria. Newer penicillins have been developed to combat this problem. These penicillins are a result of chemical treatment of a biologic precursor to penicillin. Because of their chemical modifications, they are more slowly excreted

---

DISPLAY 7-1 ● Examples of Penicillins

Natural penicillins—penicillin G and penicillin V
Penicillinase-resistant penicillin—cloxacillin, dicloxacillin, nafcillin
Aminopenicillins—ampicillin, amoxicillin, bacampicillin
Extended-spectrum penicillins—mezlocillin, piperacillin, ticarcillin

---

SUMMARY DRUG TABLE PENICILLINS

GENERIC NAME	TRADE NAME*	USES	ADVERSE REACTIONS	DOSAGE RANGES
Natural Penicillins				
penicillin G (aqueous) *pen-i-sill´-in*	Pfizerpen, *generic*	Infections due to susceptible microorganisms; syphilis, gonorrhea	Glossitis, stomatitis, gastritis, furry tongue, nausea, vomiting, diarrhea, rash, fever, pain at injection site, hypersensitivity reactions, hematopoietic changes	Up to 20–30 million U/d IV or IM; dosage may also be based on weight
penicillin G benzathine	Bicillin L-A, Permapen, *generic*	Infections due to susceptible microorganisms, syphilis; prophylaxis of rheumatic fever or chorea	Same as penicillin G	Up to 2.4 million U/d IM
penicillin G procaine, IM	Wycillin	Infections due to susceptible organisms	Same as penicillin G	600,000–2.4 million U/d IM
penicillin V	Beepen VK, Pen-Vee K, Veetids, *generic*	Infections due to susceptible organisms	Same as penicillin G	125–500 mg PO q6h or q8h
Semisynthetic Penicillins				
Penicillinase-Resistant Penicillins				
cloxacillin sodium *klox-a-sill´-in*	Cloxapen, Tegopen, *generic*	Same as penicillin G	Same as penicillin G	250–500 mg PO q6h
dicloxacillin sodium *dye-klox-a-sill´-in*	Dynapen, Dycill, Pathocil, *generic*	Same as penicillin G	Same as penicillin G	125–250 mg PO q6h
nafcillin *naf-sill´-in*	Unipen, Nallpen	Same as penicillin G	Same as penicillin G	250 mg–1 g PO, 500 mg IM q4–6h; 3–6 g/d IV for 24–48 h only
oxacillin sodium *Ox-a-sill´-in*	Bactocill, *generic*	Same as penicillin G	Same as penicillin G	500 mg–1 g PO q4–6h; 250 mg–1 g q4–6h IM, IV
Aminopenicillins				
amoxicillin *a-mox-i-sill´-in*	Amoxil, Trimox, Wymox, *generic*	Same as penicillin G	Same as penicillin G	250–500 mg PO q8h or 875 mg PO BID
amoxicillin and clavulanate acid *a-mox-i-sill´-in/ klah-view-lan´-ate*	Augmentin	Same as penicillin G	Same as penicillin G	250–500 mg PO q8h or 875 mg q12h**
ampicillin, oral *am-pi-sill´-in*	Omnipen, Principen, Totacillin, *generic*	Same as penicillin G	Same as penicillin G	250–500 mg PO q6h
ampicillin sodium parenteral	Omnipen-N, *generic*	Same as penicillin G	Same as penicillin G	1–12 g/d IM, IV in divided doses of q4–6h
ampillicin/sulbactam *am-pi-sill´-in/ sull-bak´-tam*	Unasyn	Same as penicillin G	Same as penicillin G	0.5–1 g Sulbactam with 1–2 g ampicillin IM or IV q6–8h
bacampicillin *bak´-am-pi-sill-in*	Spectrobid	Same as penicillin G	Same as penicillin G	400–800 mg PO q12h, may also be given based on weight

SUMMARY DRUG TABLE PENICILLINS (*Continued*)

GENERIC NAME	TRADE NAME*	USES	ADVERSE REACTIONS	DOSAGE RANGES
Extended-Spectrum Penicillins				
mezlocillin sodium *mez-loe-sill'-in*	Mezlin	Same as penicillin G	Same as penicillin G	200–300 mg/kg/d IV or IM in 4–6 divided doses; up to 350 mg/kg/d
piperacillin sodium and tazobactam sodium *pi-per-a-sill'-in/ tay-zoe-back'-tam*	Zosyn	Same as penicillin G	Same as penicillin G	12 mg/1.5 g IV given as 3.375 g q6h
piperacillin sodium *pi-per-a-sill'-in*	Pipracil	Same as penicillin G	Same as penicillin G	3–4 g q4–6h IV or IM; maximum dosage, 25 g/d
ticarcillin disodium *ty-kar-sill'-in*	Ticar	Same as penicillin G	Same as penicillin G	150–300 mg/kg/d IV q3, 4, or 6h; maximum dosage, 24 g/d; maximum dosage IM, 2 g/d
ticarcillin and clavulanate potassium *ty-kar-sill'-in*	Timentin	Same as penicillin G	Same as penicillin G	3.1 g IV q4–6h or 200–300 mg/kg/d IV in divided doses q4–6h

*The term *generic* indicates the drug is available in generic form.
**Tablets are not interchangeable. For example, two 250-mg tablets are not equivalent to one 500-mg tablet.

by the kidneys and, thus, have a somewhat wider spectrum of antibacterial activity. Penicillin β-lactamase inhibitor combinations are a type of penicillin that have a wider spectrum of antibacterial activity. Certain bacteria have developed the ability to produce enzymes called β-lactamases, which are able to destroy a component of the penicillin called the β-lactam ring. Fortunately, chemicals were discovered that inhibit the activity of these enzymes. Three examples of these β-lactamase inhibitors are clavulanic acid, sulbactam, and tazobactam. When these chemicals are used alone, they have little antimicrobial activity. However, when combined with certain penicillins, they extend the spectrum of penicillin's antibacterial activity. The β-lactamase inhibitors bind with the penicillin and protect the penicillin from destruction. Examples of the combinations of penicillins with the β-lactamase inhibitors are seen in Display 7-2. See the Summary Drug Table: Penicillins for more information on these combinations.

DISPLAY 7-2 ● β-Lactamase Inhibitor Combinations

Augmentin—combination of amoxicillin and clavulanic acid
Timentin—combination of ticarcillin and clavulanic acid
Unasyn—combination of ampicillin and sulbactam
Zosyn—combination of piperacillin and tazobactam

Herbal Alert: Goldenseal

Goldenseal, also called Hydrastis canadensis, *is an herb found growing in the certain areas of the northeastern United States, particularly the Ohio River Valley. Goldenseal has long been used alone or in combination with echinacea for colds and influenza. However, there is no scientific evidence to support the use of goldenseal for cold and influenza or as a stimulant as there is for the use of echinacea (see Chap. 54). Similarly, goldenseal is touted as an "herbal antibiotic," although there is no scientific evidence to support this use either. Another myth surrounding goldenseal's use is that taking the herb masks the presence of illicit drugs in the urine.*

There are many traditional uses of the herb, such as an antiseptic for the skin, mouthwash for canker sores, wash for inflamed or infected eyes, and the treatment of sinus infections and digestive problems, such as peptic ulcers and gastritis. Some evidence supports the use of goldenseal to treat diarrhea caused by bacteria or intestinal parasites, such as Giardia. The herb is contraindicated during pregnancy and in patients with hypertension. Adverse reactions are rare when the herb is used as directed. However, this herb should not be taken for more than a few days to a week. Because of widespread use, destruction of its natural habitats, and renewed interest in its use as an herbal remedy, goldenseal was classified as an "endangered" plant in 1997 by the US government.

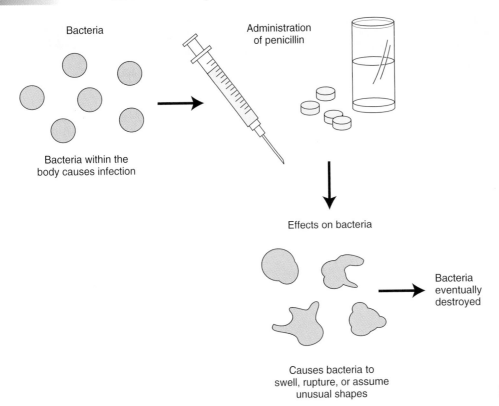

Bacteria

Administration
of penicillin

Bacteria within the
body causes infection

Effects on bacteria

Bacteria
eventually
destroyed

Causes bacteria to
swell, rupture, or assume
unusual shapes

FIGURE 7-1. Action of penicillin.

ACTIONS

The penicillins have the same type of action against bacteria. Penicillins prevent bacteria from using a substance that is necessary for the maintenance of the bacteria's outer cell wall. Unable to use this substance for cell wall maintenance, the bacteria swell, rupture, assume unusual shapes, and finally die (Fig. 7-1).

The penicillins may be **bactericidal** (destroy bacteria) or **bacteriostatic** (slow or retard the multiplication of bacteria). They are bactericidal against sensitive microorganisms (ie, those microorganisms that will be affected by penicillin) provided there is an adequate concentration of penicillin in the body. An adequate concentration of any drug in the body is referred to as the blood level. An inadequate concentration (or inadequate blood level) of penicillin may produce bacteriostatic activity, which may or may not control the infection.

Identifying the Appropriate Penicillin

To determine if a specific type of bacteria is sensitive to penicillin, **culture and sensitivity tests** are performed. A culture is performed by placing infectious material obtained from areas such as the skin, respiratory tract, and blood on a culture plate that contains a special growing medium. This growing medium is "food" for the bacteria. After a specified time, the bacteria are examined under a microscope and identified. The sensitivity test involves placing the infectious material on a separate culture plate and then placing small disks impregnated with various antibiotics over the area. After a specified time, the culture plate is examined. If there is little or no growth around a disk, the bacteria are considered sensitive to that particular antibiotic. Therefore, the infection will be controlled by this antibiotic (Fig. 7-2). If there is considerable growth around the disk, then the bacteria are considered resistant to that particular antibiotic, and the infection will not be controlled by this antibiotic.

After a culture and sensitivity report is received, the strain of microorganisms causing the infection is known, and the antibiotic to which these microorganisms are sensitive and resistant is identified. The primary health care provider then selects the antibiotic to which the microorganism is sensitive because that is the antibiotic that will be effective in the treatment of the infection.

USES

Infectious Disease

The natural and semisynthetic penicillins are used in the treatment of bacterial infections due to susceptible microorganisms. Penicillins may be used to treat infections such as urinary tract infections, septicemia, meningitis, intra-abdominal infection, gonorrhea, syphilis, pneumonia, and other respiratory infections. Examples of infectious microorganisms (bacteria) that may respond to penicillin therapy include gonococci, staphylococci,

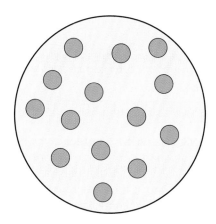

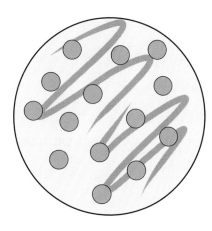

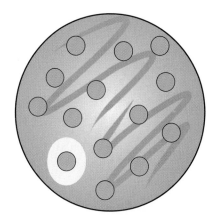

A. Culture plate with small disks containing various antibiotics.

B. Infectious material is spread on the culture plate.

C. After a specific time, the culture plate is inspected. If there is little or no growth around a disk, the bacteria is said to be sensitive to that antibiotic. That antibiotic is considered a drug that will control the infection.

FIGURE 7-2. Sensitivity testing.

streptococci, and pneumococci. Culture and sensitivity tests are performed whenever possible to determine which penicillin will best control an infection caused by a specific strain of bacteria. A penicillinase-resistant penicillin is used as initial therapy for any suspected staphylococcal infection until culture and sensitivity results are known.

Prophylaxis

Penicillin is of no value in the treatment of viral or fungal infections. However, the primary health care provider occasionally will prescribe penicillin as **prophylaxis** (prevention) against a potential secondary bacterial infection that can occur in a patient with a viral infection. In these situations the viral infection has weakened the body's defenses and the person is susceptible to other infections, particularly a bacterial infection. Penicillin also may be prescribed as prophylaxis for a potential infection in high-risk individuals, such as those with a history of rheumatic fever. Penicillin is taken several hours or, in some instances days, before and after an operative procedure, such as dental, oral, or upper respiratory tract procedures that can result in bacteria entering the bloodstream. Taking penicillin before and after the procedure will usually prevent a bacterial infection in these high-risk patients. Penicillin also may be given prophylactically on a continuing basis to those with rheumatic fever and chronic ear infections.

ADVERSE REACTIONS

Common adverse reactions include mild nausea, vomiting, diarrhea, sore tongue or mouth, fever, and pain at injection site. Penicillin can stimulate a **hypersen-**sitivity (allergic) reaction within the body. Another adverse reaction that may be seen with penicillin, as well as with almost all antibiotics, is a **superinfection** (a secondary infection that occurs during antibiotic treatment).

Hypersensitivity Reactions

A hypersensitivity (or allergic) reaction to a drug occurs in some individuals, especially those with a history of allergy to many substances. Signs and symptoms of a hypersensitivity to penicillin are highlighted in Display 7-3.

Anaphylactic shock, which is a severe form of hypersensitivity reaction, also can occur (see Chap. 1). Anaphylactic shock occurs more frequently after parenteral administration but can occur with oral use. This reaction is likely to be immediate and severe in susceptible

---

DISPLAY 7-3 ● Signs and Symptoms of Hypersensitivity to Penicillin

Skin rash
Urticaria (hives)
Sneezing
Wheezing
Pruritus (itching)
Bronchospasm (spasm of the bronchi)
Laryngospasm (spasm of the larynx)
Angioedema (also called angioneurotic edema)—swelling of the skin and mucous membranes, especially around and in the mouth and throat
Hypotension—can progress to shock
Signs and symptoms resembling serum sickness—chills, fever, edema, joint and muscle pain, and malaise

individuals. Signs of anaphylactic shock include severe hypotension, loss of consciousness, and acute respiratory distress. If not immediately treated, anaphylactic shock can be fatal.

Once an individual is allergic to one penicillin, he or she is most likely allergic to all of the penicillins. Those allergic to penicillin also have a higher incidence of allergy to the cephalosporins (see Chap. 8). Allergy to drugs in the same or related groups is called **cross-sensitivity** or **cross-allergenicity.**

Superinfections

Antibiotics can disrupt the **normal flora** (nonpathogenic microorganisms within the body) causing a superinfection. This new infection is "superimposed" on the original infection. The destruction of large numbers of **nonpathogenic** bacteria (normal flora) by the antibiotic alters the chemical environment. This allows uncontrolled growth of bacteria or fungal microorganisms, which are not affected by the antibiotic being administered. A superinfection may occur with the use of any antibiotic, especially when these drugs are given for a long time or when repeated courses of therapy are necessary. A superinfection can develop rapidly and is potentially serious and even life threatening. Bacterial superinfections are commonly seen with the administration of the oral penicillins and occur in the bowel. Symptoms of bacterial superinfection of the bowel include diarrhea or bloody diarrhea, rectal bleeding, fever, and abdominal cramping.

Fungal superinfections commonly occur in the vagina, mouth, and anal and genital areas. Symptoms include lesions of the mouth or tongue, vaginal discharge, and anal or vaginal itching. **Pseudomembranous colitis** is a common bacterial superinfection; candidiasis or moniliasis is a common type of fungal superinfection.

> ❄ **Gerontologic Alert**
>
> *Older adults who are debilitated, chronically ill, or taking penicillin for an extended period of time are more likely to develop a superinfection. Pseudomembranous colitis is one type of a bacterial superinfection. This potentially life-threatening problem develops because of an overgrowth of the microorganism* Clostridium difficile. *This organism produces a toxin that affects the lining of the colon. Signs and symptoms include severe diarrhea with visible blood and mucus, fever, and abdominal cramps. This adverse reaction usually requires immediate discontinuation of the antibiotic. Mild cases may respond to drug discontinuation. Moderate to severe cases may require treatment with intravenous (IV) fluids and electrolytes, protein supplementation, and oral vancomycin (Vancocin).*

> ☀ **Nursing Alert**
>
> *Pseudomembranous colitis may occur after 4 to 9 days of treatment with penicillin or as long as 6 weeks after the drug is discontinued.*

CANDIDIASIS OR MONILIASIS. Another type of superinfection may occur due to an overgrowth of the yeastlike fungi that usually exist in small numbers in the vagina. The multiplication rate of these microorganisms is normally slowed and kept under control because of the presence of a strain of bacteria (Döderlein's bacillus) in the vagina. If penicillin therapy destroys these normal microorganisms of the vagina (Döderlein's bacillus), the fungi are now uncontrolled, multiply at a rapid rate, and cause symptoms of a fungal infection called candidiasis (or moniliasis). Symptoms include vaginal itching and discharge.

Candida fungal superinfections also occur in the mouth and around the anal and genital areas. Signs and symptoms include lesions in the mouth or anal/genital itching.

Other Adverse Reactions

Other adverse reactions associated with penicillin are hematopoietic changes such as anemia, **thrombocytopenia** (low platelet count), **leukopenia** (low white blood cell count), and bone marrow depression. When penicillin is given orally, **glossitis** (inflammation of the tongue), **stomatitis** (inflammation of the mouth), dry mouth, gastritis, nausea, vomiting, and abdominal pain occur. When penicillin is given intramuscularly (IM), there may be pain at the injection site. Irritation of the vein and **phlebitis** (inflammation of a vein) may occur with intravenous (IV) administration.

CONTRAINDICATIONS

Penicillins are contraindicated in patients with a history of hypersensitivity to penicillin or the cephalosporins.

PRECAUTIONS

Penicillins should be used cautiously in patients with renal disease, pregnancy (Pregnancy Category C), lactation (may cause diarrhea or candidiasis in the infant), and in those with a history of allergies. Any indication of sensitivity is reason for caution. The drug is also used with caution in patients with asthma, renal disease, bleeding disorders, and gastrointestinal disease.

INTERACTIONS

Some penicillins (ampicillin, bacampicillin, penicillin V) may interfere with the effectiveness of birth control pills that contain estrogen. There is a decreased effectiveness of the penicillin when it is administered with the tetracyclines. Large doses of penicillin can increase bleeding risks of patients taking anticoagulant agents. Some reports indicate that when oral penicillins are administered with beta-adrenergic blocking drugs (see Chap. 23), the patient may be at increased risk for an anaphylactic reaction. Absorption of most penicillins is affected by food. In general, penicillins should be given 1 hour before or 2 hours after meals.

NURSING PROCESS

● The Patient Receiving Penicillin

ASSESSMENT

Preadministration Assessment

Before the administration of the first dose of penicillin, the nurse obtains or reviews the patient's general health history. The health history includes an allergy history, a history of all medical and surgical treatments, a drug history, and the current symptoms of the infection. If the patient has a history of allergy, particularly a drug allergy, the nurse must explore this area to ensure the patient is not allergic to penicillin or a cephalosporin.

The nurse should take and record vital signs. When appropriate, it is important to obtain a description of the signs and symptoms of the infection from the patient or family. The nurse assesses the infected area (when possible) and records findings on the patient's chart. It is important to describe accurately any signs and symptoms related to the patient's infection, such as color and type of drainage from a wound, pain, redness and inflammation, color of sputum, or presence of an odor. In addition, the nurse should note the patient's general appearance. A culture and sensitivity test is almost always ordered, and the nurse must obtain the results before giving the first dose of penicillin.

Ongoing Assessment

The nurse evaluates the patient daily for a response to therapy, such as a decrease in temperature, the relief of symptoms caused by the infection (such as pain or discomfort), an increase in appetite, and a change in the appearance or amount of drainage (when originally present). Once an infection is controlled, patients often look better and even state that they feel better. It is important to record these evaluations on the patient's chart. The nurse notifies the primary health care provider if signs and symptoms of the infection appear to worsen.

Additional culture and sensitivity tests may be performed during therapy because microorganisms causing the infection may become resistant to penicillin, or a superinfection may have occurred. A urinalysis, complete blood count, and renal and hepatic function tests also may be performed at intervals during therapy.

Nursing Alert

The nurse should observe the patient closely for a hypersensitivity reaction, which may occur any time during therapy with the penicillins. If it should occur, it is important to contact the primary health care provider immediately and withhold the drug until the patient is seen by the primary health care provider.

NURSING DIAGNOSES

Drug-specific nursing diagnoses are highlighted in the Nursing Diagnoses Checklist. Other nursing diagnoses applicable to these drugs are discussed in Chapter 4.

PLANNING

The expected outcomes of the patient depend on the reason for administration of penicillin but may include an optimal response to drug therapy, management of common adverse reactions, and an understanding of and compliance with the prescribed drug regimen.

IMPLEMENTATION

Promoting Optimal Response to Therapy

The results of a culture and sensitivity test take several days because time must be allowed for the bacteria to grow on the culture media. However, infections are treated as soon as possible. In a few instances, the primary health care provider may determine that a penicillin is the treatment of choice until the results of the culture and sensitivity tests are known. In many instances, the primary health care provider selects a broad-spectrum antibiotic (ie, an antibiotic that is effective against many types or strains of bacteria) for initial treatment because of the many penicillin-resistant strains of microorganisms.

Nursing Diagnoses Checklist

✓ **Diarrhea** related to adverse reaction to penicillin

✓ **Risk for Impaired Skin Integrity** related to adverse reaction to penicillin

✓ **Risk for Impaired Oral Mucous Membrane** related to adverse reaction to penicillin

✓ **Risk for Imbalanced Body Temperature**

Penicillin is ordered in units or milligrams. The exact equivalency usually is stated on the container or package insert. When preparing a parenteral form of penicillin, the nurse should shake the vial thoroughly before withdrawing the drug to ensure even distribution of the drug in the solution. Some forms of penicillin are in powder or crystalline form and must be made into a liquid (reconstituted) before being withdrawn from the vial. The manufacturer's directions regarding reconstitution are printed on the label or package insert. The manufacturer indicates the type of diluent to be used when reconstituting a specific drug. Some powdered or crystalline drugs, when reconstituted with a given amount of diluent, may yield slightly more or less than the amount of the diluent added to the vial. If there is any question regarding the reconstitution of this or any drug, the nurse consults with a pharmacist. In some health care facilities the drug is prepared in the pharmacy and delivered to the nurse for administration.

Nursing Alert

The nurse questions the patient about allergy to penicillin before administering the first dose, even when an accurate drug history has been taken. It is important to tell patients that the drug they are receiving is penicillin because information regarding a drug allergy may have been forgotten at the time the initial drug history was obtained. If a patient states he or she is allergic to penicillin or a cephalosporin, the nurse withholds the drug and contacts the primary health care provider.

Adequate blood levels of the drug must be maintained for the agent to be effective. Accidental omission or delay of a dose results in decreased blood levels, which will reduce the effectiveness of the antibiotic. It is best to give oral penicillins on an empty stomach, 1 hour before or 2 hours after a meal. Bacampicillin (Spectrobid), penicillin V (Pen-Vee K), and amoxicillin (Amoxil) may be given without regard to meals.

When administering penicillin IM, the nurse warns the patient that there may be a stinging or burning sensation at the time the drug is injected into the muscle. Discomfort at the time of injection occurs because the drug is irritating to the tissues. The nurse inspects previous areas used for injection for continued redness, soreness, or other problems. It is important to inform the primary health care provider if previously used areas for injection appear red or the patient reports pain in the area.

Monitoring and Managing Adverse Drug Reactions

Treatment of minor hypersensitivity reactions may include administration of an antihistamine such as Benadryl (for a rash or itching). Major hypersensitivity reactions, such as bronchospasm, laryngospasm,

hypotension, and angioneurotic edema, require immediate treatment with drugs such as epinephrine, cortisone, or an IV antihistamine. When respiratory difficulty occurs, a tracheostomy may need to be performed.

Nursing Alert

After administering penicillin IM in the outpatient setting, the nurse asks the client to wait in the area for at least 30 minutes. Anaphylactic reactions are most likely to occur within 30 minutes after injection.

The nurse also closely observes the patient for signs of a bacterial or fungal superinfection in the vaginal or anal area. It is important to report any signs and symptoms of a superinfection to the primary health care provider before administering the next dose of the drug. When symptoms are severe, additional treatment measures may be necessary, such as administration of an antipyretic drug for fever or an antifungal drug.

DIARRHEA. Diarrhea may be an indication of a superinfection of the gastrointestinal tract or pseudomembranous colitis. The nurse inspects all stools and notifies the primary health care provider if diarrhea occurs because it may be necessary to stop the drug. If diarrhea does occur and there appears to be blood and mucus in the stool, it is important to save a sample of the stool and test for occult blood using a test such as Hemoccult. If the stool tests positive for blood, the nurse saves the sample for possible further laboratory analysis.

IMPAIRED SKIN INTEGRITY. Dermatologic reactions such as hives, rashes, and skin lesions can occur with the administration of penicillin. In mild cases or where the benefit of the drug outweighs the discomfort of skin lesions, the nurse administers frequent skin care. Emollients, antipyretic creams, or a topical corticosteroid may be prescribed. An antihistamine may be prescribed. Harsh soaps and perfumed lotions are avoided. The nurse instructs the patient to avoid rubbing the area and not to wear rough or irritating clothing. It is important to report a rash or hives to the primary health care provider because this may be a precursor to a severe anaphylactic reaction (see Hypersensitivity Reactions). In severe cases, the primary health care provider may discontinue penicillin therapy.

IMPAIRED ORAL MUCOUS MEMBRANES. The administration of oral penicillin may result in a fungal superinfection in the oral cavity. With impaired oral mucous membranes there will be varying degrees of inflamed oral mucous membranes, swollen and red tongue, swollen gums, and pain in the mouth and throat. To detect this problem early, the nurse inspects the patient's mouth daily for evidence of glossitis, sore tongue, ulceration, or a black, furry tongue. The nurse can explain that, if the diet permits, yogurt, buttermilk, or acidophilus capsules may be taken to reduce the risk of fungal superinfection.

The nurse inspects the mouth and gums often and gives frequent mouth care with a nonirritating solution. A soft bristled toothbrush is used when brushing is needed. A nonirritating soft diet may be required. The nurse monitors the dietary intake to assure the patient is receiving adequate nutrition. Antifungal agents and/or local anesthetics are sometimes recommended to soothe the irritated membranes.

FEVER. The nurse takes vital signs every 4 hours or more often if necessary. It is important to report any increase in temperature to the primary health care provider because additional treatment measures, such as administration of an antipyretic drug or change in the drug or dosage, may be necessary. An increase in body temperature several days after the start of therapy may indicate a secondary bacterial infection or failure of the drug to control the original infection. On occasion the fever may be caused from an adverse reaction to the penicillin. In these cases the fever can usually be managed by using an antipyretic drug.

Educating the Patient and Family

Any time a drug is prescribed for a patient, the nurse is responsible for ensuring that the patient has a thorough understanding of the drug, the treatment regimen, and adverse reactions. Some patients do not adhere to the prescribed drug regimen for a variety of reasons, such as failure to comprehend the prescribed regimen or failure to understand the importance of continued and uninterrupted therapy. The nurse describes the drug regimen and stresses the importance of continued and uninterrupted therapy when teaching the patient who is prescribed an antibiotic.

The nurse teaches the following information to patients prescribed an antibiotic:

- Prophylaxis—Take the drug as prescribed until the primary health care provider discontinues therapy.
- Infection—Complete the full course of therapy. Do not stop taking the drug, even if the symptoms have disappeared, unless directed to do so by the primary health care provider.
- Take the drug at the prescribed times of day because it is important to keep an adequate amount of drug in the body throughout the entire 24 hours of each day.
- Penicillin (oral)—Take the drug on an empty stomach either 1 hour before or 2 hours after meals (exceptions: bacampicillin, penicillin V, amoxicillin).
- Take each dose with a full glass of water.
- To reduce the risk of superinfection, take yogurt, buttermilk, or acidophilus capsules.

- Notify the primary health care provider immediately if any one or more of the following should occur: skin rash; hives (urticaria); severe diarrhea; vaginal or anal itching; sore mouth; black, furry tongue; sores in the mouth; swelling around the mouth or eyes; breathing difficulty; or gastrointestinal disturbances such as nausea, vomiting, and diarrhea. Do not take the next dose of the drug until the problem is discussed with the primary health care provider.
- Oral suspensions—Keep the container refrigerated (if so labeled), shake the drug well before pouring (if so labeled), and return the drug to the refrigerator immediately after pouring the dose. Drugs that are kept refrigerated lose their potency when kept at room temperature. A small amount of the drug may be left after the last dose is taken. Discard any remaining drug because the drug (in suspension form) begins to lose its potency after a few weeks (7–14 days).
- Women prescribed ampicillin, bacampicillin, and penicillin V who take birth control pills containing estrogen should use additional contraception measures.
- Never give this drug to another individual even though the symptoms appear to be the same.
- Notify the primary health care provider if the symptoms of the infection do not improve or if the condition becomes worse.
- When a penicillin is to be taken for a long time for prophylaxis, you may feel well despite the need for long-term antibiotic therapy. There may be a tendency to omit one or more doses or even neglect to take the drug for an extended time. Never skip doses or stop therapy unless told to do so by the primary health care provider. (See Patient and Family Teaching Checklist: Preventing Antibiotic Resistance.)

EVALUATION

- The therapeutic drug effect is achieved and the infection is controlled.
- Adverse reactions are identified, reported to the primary health care provider, and managed successfully through appropriate nursing interventions.
- The patient and family demonstrate understanding of the drug regimen.

● *Critical Thinking Exercises*

1. *Ms. Barker had a bowel resection 4 days ago. After a culture and sensitivity test of her draining surgical wound, the primary health care provider orders penicillin G aqueous IV as a continuous drip. Determine what questions you would ask Ms. Barker before the penicillin is added to the IV solution.*

Patient and Family Teaching Checklist

Preventing Antibiotic Resistance

The nurse:

✓ Reviews the reason for the drug and the prescribed drug regimen, including drug name, correct dose, and frequency of administration.

✓ Stresses the importance of continued and uninterrupted therapy, even if the patient feels better after a few doses.

✓ Instructs the patient to continue taking the drug until all the drug is finished or the prescriber discontinues therapy.

✓ Urges the patient and family to discard any unused drug once therapy is discontinued or completed.

✓ Warns the patient not to use any leftover antibiotic or to take another family member's antibiotic as self-treatment for a suspected infection.

✓ Reviews the possible adverse reactions and the signs and symptoms of a new infection or of a worsening infection, both verbally and in writing.

✓ Instructs the patient and family to notify the health care provider at once should the patient experience any adverse reactions or signs and symptoms of infection.

2. *After administering penicillin to a patient in an outpatient setting, you request that the patient wait about 30 minutes before leaving. The patient is reluctant to stay, saying that she has a busy schedule. Discuss how you would handle this situation.*

3. *A 28-year-old married woman with three children is prescribed bacampicillin (Spectrobid) for an upper respiratory infection caused by Streptococcus pneumoniae. What information would be important for you to obtain from this woman? What special instructions would you give her because of her gender and age?*

● Review Questions

1. When reviewing Ms. Robertson's culture and sensitivity test results, the nurse learns that the bacteria causing Ms. Robertson's infection are sensitive to penicillin. The nurse interprets this result to mean that _____.

   A. Ms. Robertson is allergic to penicillin
   B. penicillin will be effective in treating the infection
   C. penicillin will not be effective in treating the infection
   D. the test must be repeated to obtain accurate results

2. Mr. Thomas, who is receiving oral penicillin, reports he has a sore mouth. Upon inspection the nurse notes a black, furry tongue and bright red oral mucous membranes. The primary care provider is notified immediately because these symptoms may be caused by _____.

   A. a vitamin C deficiency
   B. a superinfection
   C. dehydration
   D. poor oral hygiene

3. The nurse correctly administers penicillin V _____.

   A. 1 hour before or 2 hours after meals
   B. without regard to meals
   C. with meals to prevent gastrointestinal upset
   D. every 3 hours around the clock

4. After administering penicillin in an outpatient setting the nurse _____.

   A. asks the patient to wait 10 to 15 minutes before leaving the clinic
   B. instructs the patient to report any numbness or tingling of the extremities
   C. keeps pressure on the injection site for 10 minutes
   D. asks the patient to wait in the area for at least 30 minutes

● Medication Dosage Problems

1. A patient is prescribed amoxicillin for oral suspension. The drug is reconstituted to a solution of 250 mg/5 mL. Answer the following questions: How much amoxicillin will 1 teaspoon contain? _____ The primary care provider prescribes 500 mg. How many milliliters (mL) will the nurse administer? _____

2. The primary care provider orders 500 mg of Augmentin oral suspension. Read the label below to answer the following questions:

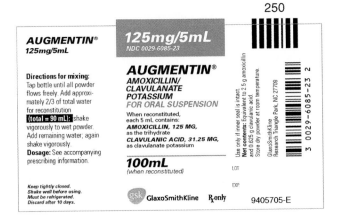

How much water will be required for reconstitution? _____ Describe the process you would go through to reconstitute this drug. _____ When reconstituted, what will be the strength of the solution? _____

Cephalosporins

Key Terms

aplastic anemia
epidermal necrolysis
nephrotoxicity

Stevens-Johnson
 syndrome

Chapter Objectives

On completion of this chapter, the student will:

- Explain the difference between the first-, second-, and third-generation cephalosporins.
- Discuss uses, general drug action, adverse reactions, contraindications, precautions, and interactions associated with the cephalosporins.
- Discuss important preadministration and ongoing assessment activities the nurse should perform on the patient taking cephalosporins.
- List some nursing diagnoses particular to a patient taking cephalosporins.
- Discuss ways to promote an optimal response to therapy, how to manage common adverse reactions, special considerations related to administration, and important points to keep in mind when educating patients about the use of the cephalosporins.

The effectiveness of penicillin in the treatment of infections prompted research directed toward finding new antibiotics with a wider range of antibacterial activity. The cephalosporins are a valuable group of drugs that are effective in the treatment of almost all of the strains of bacteria affected by the penicillins, as well as some strains of bacteria that have become resistant to penicillin. The cephalosporins are structurally and chemically related to penicillin.

The cephalosporins are divided into first-, second-, and third-generation drugs. Particular cephalosporins also may be differentiated within each group according to the microorganisms that are sensitive to them. Generally, progression from the first-generation to the second-generation and then to the third-generation drugs shows an increase in the sensitivity of gram-negative microorganisms and a decrease in the sensitivity of gram-positive microorganisms. For example, a first-generation cephalosporin would have more use against gram-positive microorganisms than would a third-generation cephalosporin. This scheme of classification is becoming less clearly defined as newer drugs are introduced. Examples of first-, second-, and third-generation cephalosporins are listed in Display 8-1. For a more complete listing see the Summary Drug Table: Cephalosporins.

ACTIONS

Cephalosporins affect the bacterial cell wall, making it defective and unstable. This action is similar to the action of penicillin. The cephalosporins are usually bactericidal (capable of destroying bacteria).

USES

The cephalosporins are used in the treatment of infections caused by susceptible microorganisms. Examples of microorganisms that may be susceptible to the cephalosporins include streptococci, staphylococci,

---

DISPLAY 8-1 ● Examples of First-, Second-, and Third-Generation Cephalosporins

First generation—cephalexin (Keflex), cefazolin (Ancef), cephapirin (Cefadyl)
Second generation—cefaclor (Ceclor), cefoxitin (Mefoxin), cefuroxime (Zinacef)
Third generation—cefoperazone (Cefobid), cefotaxime (Claforan), ceftriaxone (Rocephin)

SUMMARY DRUG TABLE CEPHALOSPORINS

GENERIC NAME	TRADE NAME*	USES	ADVERSE REACTIONS	DOSAGE RANGES
First-Generation Cephalosporins				
cefadroxil *saf-a-drox´-ill*	Duricef	Infections due to susceptible microorganisms	Nausea, vomiting, diarrhea, hypersensitivity reactions, superinfection, nephrotoxicity, headache, Stevens-Johnson syndrome, pseudomembranous colitis	1–2 g/d PO in divided doses
cefazolin sodium *sef-a´-zoe-lin*	Ancef, Kefzol, *generic*	Infections due to susceptible microorganisms; perioperative prophylaxis	Nausea, vomiting, diarrhea, hypersensitivity reactions, superinfection, nephrotoxicity, headache, Stevens-Johnson syndrome, pseudomembranous colitis	250 mg–1 g IM, IV 6–12h; perioperative, 0.5–1g IM, IV
cephalexin *sef´-a-lex-in*	Keflex, *generic*	Infections due to susceptible microorganisms	Same as cefadroxil	1–4 g/d PO in divided doses
Second-Generation Cephalosporins				
cefaclor *sef´-a-klor*	Ceclor	Treatment of infections due to susceptible organisms	Nausea, vomiting, diarrhea, hypersensitivity reactions, nephrotoxicity, headache, hematologic reactions	250 mg PO q8h
cefamandole *sef-a-man´-dole*	Mandol	Same as cefaclor	Same as cefaclor	500 mg to 1 g IM, IV q4–6h
cefotetan *sef-oh-tee´-tan*	Cefotan	Same as cefaclor; perioperative prophylaxis	Same as cefaclor	1–6 g IM, IV in equally divided doses; perioperative: 1–2 g IV
cefoxitin *sef-ox´-i-tin*	Mefoxin	Same as cefaclor; perioperative prophylaxis	Same as cefaclor	1–2 g IM q6–8h; 1–12 g/d IV in equally divided doses; perioperative, 1–2 g IV
cefpodoxime *sef-poed-ox´-eem*	Vantin	Same as cefaclor	Same as cefaclor	200–800 mg/d PO in equally divided doses
cefprozil *sef-proe´-zil*	Cefzil	Same as cefaclor	Same as cefaclor	250–500 mg PO q12h
cefuroxime *sef-yoor-ox´-eem*	Ceftin, Kefurox, Zinacef	Same as cefaclor; perioperative prophylaxis	Same as cefaclor	250 mg PO BID; 750 mg–1.5 g IM or IV q8h; perioperative, 1.5 g IV
loracarbef *lor-ah-kar´-bef*	Lorabid	Same as cefaclor	Same as cefaclor	200–400 mg PO q12h
Third-Generation Cephalosporins				
cefdinir *sef´-din-er*	Omnicef	Same as cefaclor	Same as cefaclor	300 mg PO q12h or 600 mg q24h PO
cefepime hydrochloride *sef´-ah-pime*	Maxipime	Same as cefaclor	Same as cefaclor	0.5 mg–2 g IV, IM q12h
cefixime *sef-ix´-eem*	Suprax	Same as cefaclor	Same as cefaclor	400 mg/d as a single dose or divided doses

SUMMARY DRUG TABLE CEPHALOSPORINS (*Continued*)

GENERIC NAME	TRADE NAME*	USES	ADVERSE REACTIONS	DOSAGE RANGES
cefoperazone *sef-oh-per'-a-zone*	Cefobid	Same as cefaclor	Same as cefaclor	2–4 g/d IM, IV in equally divided doses
cefotaxime *sef-oh-taks'-eem*	Claforan	Same as cefaclor; perioperative prophylaxis	Same as cefaclor	2–8 g/d IM or IV in equally divided doses q6–8h; maximum 12 g/d
ceftazidime *sef-taz'-i-deem*	Frotaz, Tazidime, Ceptaz	Same as cefaclor	Same as cefaclor	250 mg–2 g IV, IM q8-12h
ceftibuten hydrochloride *sef-ta-byoo'-ten*	Cedax	Same as cefaclor	Same as cefaclor	400 mg/d for 10 days
ceftizoxime *sef-ti-zox'-eem*	Cefizox	Same as cefaclor	Same as cefaclor	1–2 g (range, 1–4 g) IM or IV q8–12h; maximum, 12 g/d
ceftriaxone *sef-try-ax'-on*	Rocephin	Same as cefaclor; perioperative prophylaxis; gonorrhea	Same as cefaclor	1–2 g/d IM, IV QID, BID; maximum, 4 g/d; perioperative, 1 g IV; gonorrhea, 250 mg IM as a single dose

*The term *generic* indicates the drug is available in generic form.

citrobacters, gonococci, shigella, and clostridia. Culture and sensitivity tests (see Chap. 7) are performed whenever possible to determine which antibiotic, including a cephalosporin, will best control an infection caused by a specific strain of bacteria. Pharyngitis, tonsillitis, otitis media, lower respiratory infections, urinary tract infections, septicemia, and gonorrhea are examples of the types of infections that may be treated with the cephalosporins.

The cephalosporins also may be used perioperatively, that is, during the preoperative, intraoperative, and postoperative periods, to prevent infection in patients having surgery on a contaminated or potentially contaminated area, such as the gastrointestinal tract or vagina. In some instances, a specific drug may be recommended for postoperative prophylactic use only.

ADVERSE REACTIONS

The most common adverse reactions seen with administration of the cephalosporins are gastrointestinal disturbances, such as nausea, vomiting, and diarrhea.

Hypersensitivity (allergic) reactions may occur with administration of the cephalosporins and range from mild to life threatening. Mild hypersensitivity reactions include pruritus, urticaria, and skin rashes. More serious hypersensitivity reactions include **Stevens-Johnson syndrome** (fever, cough, muscular aches and pains, headache, and the appearance of lesions on the skin, mucous membranes, and eyes), hepatic and renal dysfunction, **aplastic anemia** (anemia due to deficient red blood cell production), and **epidermal necrolysis** (death of the epidermal layer of the skin).

Because of the close relation of the cephalosporins to penicillin, a patient allergic to penicillin also may be allergic to the cephalosporins.

Other adverse reactions that may be seen with administration of the cephalosporins are headache, dizziness, **nephrotoxicity** (damage to the kidneys by a toxic substance), malaise, heartburn, and fever. Intramuscular (IM) administration often results in pain, tenderness, and inflammation at the injection site. Intravenous (IV) administration has resulted in thrombophlebitis and phlebitis.

Therapy with cephalosporins may result in a bacterial or fungal superinfection. Diarrhea may be an indication of pseudomembranous colitis, which is one type of bacterial superinfection. See Chapter 7 for a discussion of bacterial and fungal superinfections and pseudomembranous colitis.

CONTRAINDICATIONS

The nurse should not administer cephalosporins if the patient has a history of allergies to cephalosporins or penicillins.

PRECAUTIONS

The nurse should use cephalosporins cautiously in patients with renal or hepatic impairment and in patients with bleeding disorders. Safety of cephalosporin administration has not been established in pregnancy or lactation; these drugs are assigned to Pregnancy Category B.

INTERACTIONS

The risk of nephrotoxicity increases when the cephalosporins are administered with the aminoglycosides (see Chap. 10). The risk for bleeding increases when the cephalosporins are taken with oral anticoagulants. A disulfiram-like reaction may occur if alcohol is consumed within 72 hours after cephalosporin administration. Symptoms of a disulfiram-like reactions include flushing, throbbing in the head and neck, respiratory difficulty, vomiting, sweating, chest pain, and hypotension. Severe reactions may cause arrhythmias and unconsciousness. When the cephalosporins are administered with the aminoglycosides, the risk for nephrotoxicity increases.

NURSING PROCESS

● The Patient Receiving a Cephalosporin

ASSESSMENT

As with most drugs, assessment depends on the drug, the patient, and the reason for administration.

Preadministration Assessment

Before the administration of the first dose of a cephalosporin, it is important to obtain a general health history. The health history includes an allergy history, a history of all medical and surgical treatments, a drug history, and the current symptoms of the infection. If the patient has a history of allergy, particularly a drug allergy, the nurse explores this area to ensure that the patient is not allergic to a cephalosporin. Patients with a history of an allergy to penicillin may also be allergic to a cephalosporin (see Chap. 7) even though they have never received one of these drugs. If an allergy to either of these drug groups is suspected, the nurse informs the primary health care provider of this before the first dose of the drug is given. Liver and kidney function tests may be ordered by the primary health care provider. The nurse should check to be sure any cultures for sensitivity testing are done before the first dose of the drug is administered.

Ongoing Assessment

An ongoing assessment is important in evaluating the patient's response to therapy, such as a decrease in temperature, the relief of symptoms caused by the infection (eg, pain or discomfort), an increase in appetite, and a change in the appearance or amount of drainage (when originally present). The nurse notifies the primary health care provider if symptoms of the infection appear to worsen. The nurse checks the patient's skin regularly for rash and is alert for any loose stools or diarrhea.

NURSING DIAGNOSES

Drug-specific nursing diagnoses are highlighted in the Nursing Diagnoses Checklist. Other, more general nursing diagnoses are discussed in Chapter 4.

PLANNING

The expected outcomes for the patient depend on the reason for administration but may include an optimal response to therapy (infectious process controlled), management of adverse drug reactions, and an understanding of and compliance with the prescribed treatment regimen.

IMPLEMENTATION

Promoting an Optimal Response to Therapy

The nurse must question the patient about allergy to cephalosporins or the penicillins before administering the first dose, even when an accurate drug history has been taken. Information regarding a drug allergy may have been forgotten at the time the initial drug history was obtained. If a patient gives a history of possible cephalosporin or penicillin allergy, the nurse withholds the drug and contacts the primary health care provider.

ORAL ADMINISTRATION. The nurse administers cephalosporins around the clock to the patient to provide adequate blood levels. Most cephalosporins may be taken with food to prevent gastric upset. Cefdinir may be taken without regard to food. The absorption of oral cefuroxime and cefpodoxime is increased when given with food. However, if the patient experiences gastrointestinal upset, the nurse can administer the drug with

---

Nursing Diagnoses Checklist

☑ **Risk for Imbalanced Body Temperature: Hyperthermia** related to infection

☑ **Diarrhea** related to superinfection secondary to cephalosporin therapy

☑ **Risk for Impaired Skin Integrity** related to adverse reactions secondary to cephalosporin therapy

food. The nurse should shake oral suspensions well before administering them.

Some cephalosporins are available as powder for a suspension and are reconstituted by a pharmacist or a nurse. It is important to keep this form of the drug refrigerated until it is used.

PARENTERAL ADMINISTRATION. The nurse should read the manufacturer's package insert for each drug for instructions regarding reconstitution of powder for injection, storage of unused portions, life of the drug after it is reconstituted, methods of IV administration, and precautions to be taken when the drug is administered.

Some cephalosporins are given by direct IV, intermittent infusion, or continuous IV infusion. When the direct IV method is used, the nurse gives the dose directly into a vein. Intermittent IV infusion is given by means of Y tubing while another solution is being given on a continuous basis. When this method is used, the nurse clamps off IV fluid given on a continuous basis while the drug is allowed to infuse. Continuous IV infusion requires that the nurse add the drug to a specified amount of an IV solution at a drip rate or volume per hour prescribed by the primary health care provider.

☀ Nursing Alert

When the drug is given IV, the nurse inspects the needle insertion site for signs of extravasation or infiltration (see Chap. 2). In addition, it is important to inspect the needle insertion site and the area above the site several times a day for signs of redness, which may indicate thrombophlebitis (inflammation of a vein with formation of a clot within the vein) or phlebitis (inflammation of a vein). If either problem occurs, the nurse contacts the primary health care provider and the IV must be discontinued and restarted in another vein, preferably in another extremity.

❄ Gerontologic Alert

When a cephalosporin is given IM, the nurse injects the drug into a large muscle mass, such as the gluteus muscle or lateral aspect of the thigh. It is important to rotate injection sites. The nurse warns the patient that at the time the drug is injected into the muscle, there may be a stinging or burning sensation and the area may be sore for a short time. The nurse informs the primary health care provider if previously used areas for injection appear red or if the patient reports continued pain in the area.

Monitoring and Managing Adverse Reactions

The nurse observes the patient closely for any adverse drug reactions, particularly signs and symptoms of a hypersensitivity reaction. It is important to report a rash or hives to the primary health care provider because this may be a precursor to a severe anaphylactic reaction (see Chap. 7). In severe cases, the primary health care provider may discontinue the cephalosporin therapy. The nurse closely observes the patient for signs and symptoms of a bacterial or fungal superinfection (see Chap. 7). If any occur, the nurse contacts the primary health care provider before the next dose of the drug is due.

Rare cases of hemolytic anemia, including fatalities, have been reported with the administration of the cephalosporins. The patient should be monitored for anemia. If a patient experiences anemia within 2 to 3 weeks after the start of cephalosporin therapy, drug-induced anemia should be considered. If hemolytic anemia is suspected, the primary health care provider will discontinue the drug therapy. The patient may require blood transfusions to correct the anemia. Frequent hematological studies may be required.

☀ Nursing Alert

Nephrotoxicity may occur with the administration of these drugs. Early signs of this adverse reaction may become apparent by a decrease in urine output. The nurse should measure and record the fluid intake and output and notify the primary health care provider if the output is less than 500 mL/d. Any changes in the fluid intake-and-output ratio or in the appearance of the urine may indicate nephrotoxicity. It is important that the nurse report these findings to the primary health care provider promptly.

❄ Gerontologic Alert

The older adult is more susceptible to the nephrotoxic effects of the cephalosporins, particularly if renal function is already diminished because of age or disease. If renal impairment is present, a lower dosage and monitoring of blood creatinine levels are indicated. Blood creatinine levels greater than 4 mg/dL indicate serious renal impairment. In elderly patients with decreased renal function, a dosage adjustment may be necessary.

FEVER. The nurse takes vital signs every 4 hours or as ordered by the primary health care provider. It is important to report any increase in temperature to the primary health care provider because additional treatment measures, such as administration of an antipyretic drug or change in the drug or dosage, may be necessary.

DIARRHEA. Frequent liquid stools may be an indication of a superinfection or pseudomembranous colitis. If pseudomembranous colitis occurs, it is usually seen 4 to 10 days after treatment is started.

The nurse inspects each bowel movement and immediately reports to the primary health care provider the occurrence of diarrhea or loose stools containing blood and mucus because it may be necessary to discontinue the drug use and institute treatment for diarrhea, a superinfection, or pseudomembranous colitis.

If there appears to be blood and mucus in the stool, the nurse saves a sample of the stool and tests for occult blood using a test such as Hemoccult. If the stool tests positive for blood, the sample is saved for possible laboratory testing for blood.

IMPAIRED SKIN INTEGRITY. The nurse inspects the skin every 4 hours for redness, rash, or lesions that appear as red wheals or blisters. When a skin rash or irritation is present, the nurse administers frequent skin care. Emollients, antipyretic creams, or a topical corticosteroid may be prescribed. An antihistamine may be prescribed. Harsh soaps and perfumed lotions are avoided. The nurse instructs the patient to avoid rubbing the area and not to wear rough or irritating clothing.

❋ Nursing Alert

The patient is at risk for Stevens-Johnson syndrome when taking the cephalosporins. Stevens-Johnson syndrome is manifested by fever, cough, muscular aches and pains, headache, and the appearance of lesions on the skin, mucous membranes, and eyes. The lesions appear as red wheals or blisters, often starting on the face, in the mouth, or on the lips, neck, and extremities. This syndrome, which also may occur with the administration of other types of drugs, can be fatal. The nurse should report any of these symptoms to the primary health care provider immediately.

Educating the Patient and Family

The nurse carefully reviews the dose regimen with the patient and family and teaches the patient the following information:

- Complete the full course of therapy. Do not stop the drug even if the symptoms have disappeared unless directed to do so by the primary health care provider.
- Take the drug at the prescribed times of day because it is important to keep an adequate amount of drug in the body throughout the entire 24 hours of each day.
- It is a good idea to take each dose with food or milk if gastrointestinal upset occurs after administration.
- Avoid drinking alcoholic beverages when taking the cephalosporins and for 3 days after completing the

course of therapy because severe reactions may occur.

- Notify the primary health care provider immediately if any one or more of the following occurs: vomiting, skin rash, hives (urticaria), severe diarrhea, vaginal or anal itching, sores in the mouth, swelling around the mouth or eyes, breathing difficulty or gastrointestinal disturbances, such as nausea, vomiting, and diarrhea. Do not take the next dose of the drug until the problem is discussed with the primary health care provider (see Home Care Teaching Checklist: Teaching About Superinfection).
- Oral suspensions—keep the container refrigerated (if so labeled), shake the drug well before pouring (if so labeled), and return the drug to the refrigerator immediately after pouring the dose. Drugs that are kept refrigerated lose their potency when kept at room temperature. If a small amount of the drug is left after the last dose is taken, discard it because the drug (in suspension form) begins to lose potency after a few weeks.
- Never give this drug to another individual even though the symptoms appear to be the same.
- Notify the primary health care provider if the symptoms of the infection do not improve or if the condition becomes worse.

EVALUATION

- Therapeutic effect is achieved; infection is controlled.
- Adverse reactions are identified, reported to the primary health care provider, and managed successfully with nursing interventions.
- Patient and family demonstrate understanding of the drug regimen.
- Patient verbalizes importance of complying with the prescribed therapeutic regimen.

● *Critical Thinking Exercises*

1. *Mr. Jonas is receiving a cephalosporin IM. He tells you that he has had to get out of bed several times this morning because he has diarrhea. Determine what questions you would ask Mr. Jonas. Analyze what steps you would take to resolve this problem.*

2. *A patient who is a recent immigrant to the United States is seen in the outpatient clinic for a severe upper respiratory infection. The primary health care provider prescribes a cephalosporin and asks you to give the patient instructions for taking the drug. You note that the patient appears to understand very little English. Discuss how you would solve this problem. Determine what information you would include in a teaching plan*

Home Care Checklist

TEACHING ABOUT SUPERINFECTION

Antibiotics are one of the most commonly administered types of drug therapy in the home. Any patient taking antibiotics, especially cephalosporins, is susceptible to superinfection. The nurse makes sure the patient knows the signs and symptoms of superinfection.

A bacterial superinfection commonly occurs in the bowel. The nurse teaches the patient to report any of the following:

✓ Diarrhea, possibly severe with visible blood and mucus

✓ Fever

✓ Abdominal cramps

✓ A fungal superinfection commonly occurs in the mouth, vagina, and anogenital areas. The nurse teaches the patient to report any of the following:

✓ Scaly, reddened, papular rash commonly in the breast folds, at the axillae, groin, or umbilicus

✓ White or yellow vaginal discharge

✓ Localized redness, inflammation, and excoriation, particularly inside the mouth, in the groin, or skin folds of the anogenital area

✓ Anal or vaginal itching

✓ Creamy white lacelike patches on the tongue, mouth, or throat

✓ Burning sensation in the mouth or throat

and how you would evaluate the effectiveness of the teaching plan for this patient.

3. *Analyze what assessments you would make if you suspect that a patient receiving a cephalosporin is experiencing Stevens-Johnson syndrome.*

● *Review Questions*

1. The nurse observes a patient taking a cephalosporin for common adverse reactions, which include_____.

   A. hypotension, dizziness, urticaria
   B. nausea, vomiting, diarrhea
   C. skin rash, constipation, headache
   D. bradycardia, pruritus, insomnia

2. When giving a cephalosporin by the intramuscular route, the nurse tells the patient that _____.

   A. a stinging or burning sensation and soreness at the site may be experienced
   B. the injection site will be red for several days
   C. all injections will be given in the same area
   D. the injection will not cause any discomfort

3. A nurse asks why it is so important to determine if the patient is allergic to penicillin before the first dose of the cephalosporin is given. The most correct answer is that persons allergic to penicillin _____.

   A. are usually allergic to most antibiotics
   B. respond poorly to antibiotic therapy
   C. require higher doses of other antibiotics
   D. have a higher incidence of allergy to the cephalosporins

4. The nurse observes a patient receiving a cephalosporin for the Stevens-Johnson syndrome. The signs and symptoms that might indicate this syndrome include _____.

   A. swelling of the extremities
   B. increased blood pressure and pulse rate
   C. lesions on the skin and/or mucous membranes
   D. pain in the joints

● *Medication Dosage Problems*

1. Ceclor 500 mg is prescribed for a patient. Use the drug label below to determine the dosage.

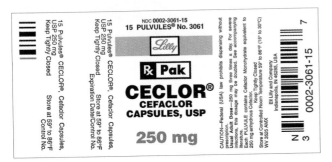

The nurse would administer _____.

2. The physician prescribes 1 g of Mefoxin (cefoxitin) for parenteral administration. Mefoxin is available in a solution of 250 mg/1 mL. What amount of Mefoxin would the nurse prepare? _____

Tetracyclines, Macrolides, and Lincosamides

Key Terms

bacteriostatic
bactericidal
myasthenia gravis

photosensitivity
reaction
prophylaxis

Chapter Objectives

On completion of this chapter, the student will:

- Discuss the uses, general drug action, adverse reactions, contraindications, precautions, and interactions of the tetracyclines, macrolides, and lincosamides.
- Discuss important preadministration and ongoing assessment activities the nurse should perform on the patient taking a tetracycline, macrolide, or lincosamide.
- List some nursing diagnoses particular to a patient taking a tetracycline, macrolide, or lincosamide.
- Discuss ways to promote an optimal response to therapy, how to manage adverse reactions, and important points to keep in mind when educating patients about the use of a tetracycline, macrolide, or lincosamide.

This chapter discusses three groups of broad-spectrum antibiotics: the tetracyclines, the macrolides, and the lincosamides. Examples of the tetracyclines include doxycycline (Vibramycin), minocycline (Minocin), and tetracycline (Sumycin). Examples of the macrolides include azithromycin (Zithromax), clarithromycin (Biaxin), and erythromycin (E-Mycin). The lincosamides include clindamycin (Cleocin) and lincomycin (Lincocin). The Summary Drug Table: Tetracyclines, Macrolides, and Lincosamides describes the types of broad-spectrum antibiotics discussed in this chapter.

TETRACYCLINES

The tetracyclines are a group of anti-infectives composed of natural and semisynthetic compounds. They are useful in select infections when the organism shows sensitivity (see Chap. 7) to the tetracyclines, such as in cholera, Rocky Mountain spotted fever, and typhus.

ACTIONS

The tetracyclines exert their effect by inhibiting bacterial protein synthesis, which is a process necessary for reproduction of the microorganism. The ultimate effect of this action is that the bacteria are either destroyed or their multiplication rate is slowed. The tetracyclines are **bacteriostatic** (capable of slowing or retarding the multiplication of bacteria), whereas the macrolides and lincosamides may be bacteriostatic or **bactericidal** (capable of destroying bacteria).

USES

These antibiotics are effective in the treatment of infections caused by a wide range of gram-negative and gram-positive microorganisms. The tetracyclines are used in infections caused by Rickettsiae (Rocky Mountain spotted fever, typhus fever, and tick fevers). Tetracyclines are also used in situations in which penicillin is contraindicated, in the treatment of intestinal amebiasis, and in some skin and soft tissue infections. Oral

83

SUMMARY DRUG TABLE TETRACYCLINES, MACROLIDES, AND LINCOSAMIDES

GENERIC NAME	TRADE NAME*	USES	ADVERSE REACTIONS	DOSAGE RANGES
Tetracyclines				
demeclocycline *deh-meh-kloe-sye´-kleen*	Declomycin	Treatment of infections due to susceptible microorganisms	Nausea, vomiting, diarrhea, hypersensitivity reactions, photosensitivity reactions, pseudomembranous colitis, hematologic changes, discoloration of teeth in fetus and young children	150 mg PO QID or 300 mg PO BID; gonorrhea: 600 mg PO initially then 300 mg PO q12h for 4 d
doxycycline *dox-i-sye´-kleen*	Doxychel Hyclate, Vibra-Tabs, Vibramycin, *generic*	Same as demeclocycline	Same as demeclocycline	100 mg PO q12h first day then 100–200 mg/d PO; gonorrhea: 200 mg PO immediately and 100 mg PO hs then 100 mg PO BID for 3 d; 200 mg IV first day then 100–200 mg/d IV
minocycline *min-oh-sye´-kleen*	Minocin, Minocin IV	Same as demeclocycline	Same as demeclocycline	200 mg PO initially then 100 mg IV q12h 100–200 mg initially then 50 mg PO QID
oxytetracycline *ox-i-tet-ra-sye´-kleen*	Terramycin, Terramycin IM, Uri-Tet	Same as demeclocycline	Nausea, vomiting, diarrhea, hypersensitivity reactions, photosensitivity reactions, pseudomembranous colitis, hematologic changes, discoloration of teeth in fetus and young children	1–2 g/d PO; 250 mg qd or 300 mg individualized doses q8–12h IM; 250–500 mg IV q12h
tetracycline *tet-ra-sye´-kleen*	Panmycin, Sumycin, Tetracap, *generic*	Same as demeclocycline	Same as demeclocycline	1–2 g/d PO in 2–4 divided doses
Macrolides				
azithromycin *ay-zi-thro-my´-cin*	Zithromax	Same as demeclocycline	Nausea, vomiting, diarrhea, abdominal pains, hypersensitivity reactions, pseudomembranous colitis	500 mg PO first day then 250 mg/d PO for 4 d
clarithromycin *klar-ith-ro-my´-cin*	Biaxin	Same as demeclocycline	Same as azithromycin	250–500 mg PO BID
dirithromycin *dir-ith-ro-my´-cin*	Dynabac	Same as demeclocycline	Nausea, vomiting, diarrhea, hypersensitivity reactions, photosensitivity reactions, pseudomembranous colitis, electrolyte imbalance	500 mg PO for 7–14 d
erythromycin base *er-ith-roe-my´-sin*	E-Mycin, Eryc, *generic*	Same as demeclocycline	Same as azithromycin	250 mg PO q6h or 333 mg q8h
erythromycin ethylsuccinate	EryPed, E.E.S., *generic*	Same as demeclocycline	Same as azithromycin	400 mg PO q6h
erythromycin estolate	Ilosone, *generic*	Same as demeclocycline	Same as azithromycin	250 mg PO q6h
erythromycin IV	Ilotycin Glucepate, *generic*	Same as demeclocycline	Same as azithromycin	Up to 4 g/d IV in divided doses
troleandomycin	Tao	Same as demeclocycline	Same as clindamycin	250–500 mg QID PO

GENERIC NAME	TRADE NAME*	USES	ADVERSE REACTIONS	DOSAGE RANGES
Lincosamides				
clindamycin *klin-da-my´-sin*	Cleocin, *generic*	Same as demeclocycline	Abdominal pain, esophagitis, nausea, vomiting, diarrhea, skin rash, blood dyscrasias, pseudomembranous colitis, hypersensitivity reactions	150–450 mg PO q6h; 600–2700 mg/d in 2–4 equal doses; up to 4.8 g/d IV, IM
lincomycin *lin-koe-my´-sin*	Lincocin, Lincorex	Same as demeclocycline	Same as clindamycin	500 mg PO q6–8h; 600 mg IM q12–24h; up to 8 g/d IV

*The term *generic* indicates the drug is available in generic form.

tetracyclines are used in the treatment of uncomplicated urethral, endocervical, or rectal infections caused by *Chlamydia trachomatis* and as adjunctive treatment in severe acne. Tetracycline in combination with metronidazole and bismuth subsalicylate is useful in treating *Helicobacter pylori* (a bacteria in the stomach that can cause peptic ulcer).

ADVERSE REACTIONS

Gastrointestinal reactions that may occur during tetracycline administration include nausea, vomiting, diarrhea, epigastric distress, stomatitis, and sore throat. Skin rashes also may be seen. A **photosensitivity** (phototoxic) **reaction** may be seen with this group of drugs, manifested by an exaggerated sunburn reaction when the skin is exposed to sunlight even for brief periods. Demeclocycline seems to cause the most serious photosensitivity reaction, whereas minocycline is least likely to cause this type of reaction.

The tetracyclines are not given to children younger than 9 years of age unless their use is absolutely necessary because these drugs may cause permanent yellow-gray-brown discoloration of the teeth. The use of the tetracyclines, especially prolonged or repeated therapy, may result in bacterial or fungal overgrowth of nonsusceptible organisms.

CONTRAINDICATIONS

The tetracyclines are contraindicated if the patient is known to be hypersensitive to any of the tetracyclines. Tetracyclines also are contraindicated during pregnancy because of the possibility of toxic effects to the developing fetus. The tetracyclines are classified Pregnancy Category D drugs. These drugs also are contraindicated

during lactation and in children younger than 9 years (may cause permanent discoloration of the teeth).

PRECAUTIONS

It is important to use the tetracyclines cautiously in patients with renal function impairment. In addition, doses greater that 2 g/d can be extremely damaging to the liver. The nurse should carefully check the expiration dates of the tetracyclines before administration because degradation of the tetracyclines can occur; after degradation, the agents are highly toxic to the kidneys.

INTERACTIONS

Antacids containing aluminum, zinc, magnesium, or bismuth salts, or foods high in calcium impair absorption of the tetracyclines. When the tetracyclines are administered with oral anticoagulants, an increase in the effects of the anticoagulant may occur. When tetracyclines are administered to women using oral contraceptives, a decrease in the effect of the oral contraceptive may be seen. This may result in breakthrough bleeding or pregnancy. When digoxin is administered with the tetracyclines there is an increased risk for digitalis toxicity (see Chapter 39). The effects of this could last for months after tetracycline administration is discontinued. Tetracyclines may reduce insulin requirements. Blood glucose levels should be monitored frequently during tetracycline therapy.

MACROLIDES

The macrolides are effective against a wide variety of pathogenic organisms, particularly infections of the respiratory and genital tract.

ACTIONS

The macrolides are bacteriostatic or bactericidal in susceptible bacteria. The drugs act by binding to cell membranes and causing changes in protein function.

USES

These antibiotics are effective in the treatment of infections caused by a wide range of gram-negative and gram-positive microorganisms. In addition, the drugs are used to treat acne vulgaris and skin infections, in conjunction with sulfonamides to treat upper respiratory infections caused by *Hemophilus influenzae,* and as prophylaxis before dental or other procedures in patients allergic to penicillin.

ADVERSE REACTIONS

Most of the adverse reactions seen with the administration of azithromycin and clarithromycin are related to the gastrointestinal tract and include nausea, vomiting, diarrhea, and abdominal pain. Abdominal cramping, nausea, vomiting, diarrhea, and allergic reactions have been reported with the administration of erythromycin. However, there appears to be a low incidence of adverse reactions associated with normal oral doses of erythromycin. As with almost all antibacterial drugs, pseudomembranous colitis may occur ranging in severity from mild to life threatening.

CONTRAINDICATIONS

These drugs are contraindicated in patients with a hypersensitivity to the macrolides and patients with pre-existing liver disease.

PRECAUTIONS

It is important to use these drugs cautiously during pregnancy and lactation. Azithromycin and erythromycin are Pregnancy Category B drugs, and clarithromycin, dirithromycin, and troleandomycin are Pregnancy Category C drugs. Because azithromycin, erythromycin, and troleandomycin are primarily eliminated from the body by the liver, these drugs should be used with great caution in patients with liver dysfunction. There is a decreased gastrointestinal absorption of the macrolides when administered with kaolin, aluminum salts, or magaldrate.

INTERACTIONS

Use of the macrolides increases serum levels of digoxin and increases the effects of anticoagulants. Use of antacids decreases the absorption of most macrolides. The macrolides should not be administered with clindamycin, lincomycin, or chloramphenicol; a decrease in the therapeutic activity of the macrolides can occur. Concurrent administration of the macrolides with theophylline may increase serum theophylline levels.

LINCOSAMIDES

The lincosamides, another group of anti-infectives, are effective against many gram-positive organisms, such as streptococci and staphylococci. However, because of their high potential for toxicity, the lincosamides are usually used only for the treatment of serious infections in which penicillin or erythromycin (a macrolide) is not effective.

ACTIONS

The lincosamides act by inhibiting protein synthesis in susceptible bacteria, causing death.

USES

These antibiotics are effective in the treatment of infections caused by a wide range of gram-negative and gram-positive microorganisms. The lincosamides are used for the more serious infections. In serious infections they may be used in conjunction with other antibiotics.

ADVERSE REACTIONS

Abdominal pain, esophagitis, nausea, vomiting, diarrhea, skin rash, and blood dyscrasias may be seen with the use of the lincosamides. These drugs also can cause pseudomembranous colitis, which may range from mild to very severe. Discontinuing the drug may relieve mild symptoms of pseudomembranous colitis.

CONTRAINDICATIONS

The lincosamides are contraindicated in patients with hypersensitivity to the lincosamides, those with minor bacterial or viral infections, and during lactation and infancy.

PRECAUTIONS

It is important to use these drugs with caution in patients with a history of gastrointestinal disorders, renal disease, or liver impairment. The neuromuscular blocking action of the lincosamides poses a danger to patients with **myasthenia gravis** (an autoimmune disease manifested by extreme weakness and exhaustion of the muscles).

INTERACTIONS

When kaolin or aluminum is administered with the lincosamides, the absorption of the lincosamide is decreased. When the lincosamides are administered with the neuromuscular blocking drugs (drugs that are used as adjuncts to anesthetic drugs that cause paralysis of the respiratory system) the action of the neuromuscular blocking drug is enhanced, possibly leading to severe and profound respiratory depression.

NURSING PROCESS

● **The Patient Receiving a Tetracycline, Macrolide, or Lincosamide**

ASSESSMENT

Preadministration Assessment

It is important to establish an accurate database before the administration of any antibiotic. The nurse should identify and record signs and symptoms of the infection. Signs and symptoms may vary and often depend on the organ or system involved and whether the infection is external or internal. Examples of some of the signs and symptoms of an infection in various areas of the body are pain, drainage, redness, changes in the appearance of sputum, general malaise, chills and fever, cough, and swelling.

The nurse obtains a thorough allergy history, especially a history of drug allergies. Some antibiotics have a higher incidence of hypersensitivity reactions in those with a history of allergy to drugs or other substances. If the patient has a history of allergies and has not told the primary health care provider, the nurse should not administer the first dose of the drug until this problem is discussed with the primary health care provider.

It also is important to take and record vital signs before the first dose of the antibiotic is given. The primary health care provider may order culture and sensitivity tests, and these should also be performed before the first dose of the drug is given. Other laboratory tests such as renal and hepatic function tests, complete blood count, and urinalysis may also be ordered by the primary health care provider.

Ongoing Assessment

An ongoing assessment is important during therapy with the tetracyclines, macrolides, and lincosamides. The nurse should take vital signs every 4 hours or as ordered by the primary health care provider. The nurse must notify the primary health care provider if there are changes in the vital signs, such as a significant drop in blood pressure, an increase in the pulse or respiratory rate, or a sudden increase in temperature.

Each day, the nurse compares current signs and symptoms of the infection against the initial signs and symptoms and records any specific findings in the patient's chart.

When an antibiotic is ordered for the prevention of a secondary infection **(prophylaxis)**, the nurse observes the patient for signs and symptoms that may indicate the beginning of an infection despite the prophylactic use of the antibiotic. If signs and symptoms of an infection occur, the nurse must report them to the primary health care provider.

NURSING DIAGNOSES

Drug-specific nursing diagnoses are highlighted in the Nursing Diagnoses Checklist. Other nursing diagnoses applicable to these drugs are discussed in Chapter 4.

PLANNING

The expected outcomes of the patient may include an optimal response to therapy, which includes control of the infectious process or prophylaxis of bacterial infection, an absence of adverse drug effects, and an understanding of and compliance with the prescribed treatment regimen.

IMPLEMENTATION

Promoting an Optimal Response to Therapy

Before therapy is begun, culture and sensitivity tests (see Chap. 7) are performed to determine which antibiotic will best control the infection. These drugs are of no value in the treatment of infections caused by a virus or fungus. There may be times when a secondary bacterial infection has occurred or potentially will occur when the patient has a fungal or viral infection. The primary health care provider may then order one of the

---

Nursing Diagnoses Checklist

☑ **Risk for Imbalanced Body Temperature: Hyperthermia** related to infection

☑ **Diarrhea** related to superinfection secondary to antibiotic therapy, adverse drug reaction

☑ **Risk for Impaired Skin Integrity** related to adverse drug reaction

broad-spectrum antibiotics, but its purpose is for the prevention (prophylaxis) or treatment of a secondary bacterial infection that could potentially develop after the primary fungal or viral infection.

ORAL ADMINISTRATION. To control the infectious process or prevent a bacterial infection, the nurse must keep several important things in mind when administering the tetracyclines, macrolides, and lincosamides.

Tetracyclines. It is important to give the tetracyclines on an empty stomach; tetracyclines are not to be taken with dairy products (milk or cheese). The exceptions are doxycycline (Vibramycin) and minocycline (Minocin), which may be taken with dairy products or food. The nurse should give clindamycin with food or a full glass of water. The nurse can give troleandomycin and clarithromycin without regard to meals. All tetracyclines should be given with a full glass of water (240 mL).

Nursing Alert

The nurse should not give tetracyclines along with dairy products (milk or cheese), antacids, laxatives, or products containing iron. When these drugs are prescribed, the nurse makes sure they are given 2 hours before or after the administration of a tetracycline. Food or drugs containing calcium, magnesium, aluminum, or iron prevent the absorption of the tetracyclines if ingested concurrently.

Macrolides. The nurse gives clarithromycin without regard to meals. Clarithromycin may be taken with milk, if desired. Azithromycin tablets may be given without regard to meals. However, azithromycin suspension is given 1 hour or more before a meal or 2 hours or more after a meal. Dirithromycin is given with food or within 1 hour of eating. Erythromycin is given on an empty stomach (1 hour before or 2 hours after meals) and with 180 to 240 mL of water.

Lincosamides. Food impairs the absorption of lincomycin. The patient should take nothing by mouth (except water) for 1 to 2 hours before and after taking lincomycin. Clindamycin may be given without regard to food.

PARENTERAL ADMINISTRATION. When these drugs are given intramuscularly, the nurse inspects previous injection sites for signs of pain or tenderness, redness, and swelling. Some antibiotics may cause temporary local reactions, but persistence of a localized reaction should be reported to the primary health care provider. It is important to rotate injection sites and record the site used for injection in the patient's chart.

When these drugs are given intravenously (IV), the nurse should inspect the needle site and area around the needle for signs of extravasation of the IV fluid or signs of tenderness, pain, and redness (which may indicate phlebitis or thrombophlebitis). If these symptoms are apparent, the nurse should restart the IV in another vein and bring the problem to the attention of the primary health care provider.

Monitoring and Managing Adverse Drug Reactions

The nurse observes the patient at frequent intervals, especially during the first 48 hours of therapy. It is important to report to the primary health care provider the occurrence of any adverse reaction before the next dose of the drug is due. The nurse should report serious adverse reactions, such as a severe hypersensitivity reaction, respiratory difficulty, severe diarrhea, or a decided drop in blood pressure, to the primary health care provider immediately because a serious adverse reaction may require emergency intervention.

The nurse observes the patient for the signs and symptoms of a bacterial or fungal superinfection, such as vaginal or anal itching, sore throat, sores in the mouth, diarrhea, fever, chills, and sore throat. It is important to report any new signs and symptoms occurring during antibiotic therapy to the primary health care provider, who must then decide if these problems are part of the original infection or if a superinfection has occurred.

HYPERTHERMIA. The nurse monitors the temperature at frequent intervals, usually every 4 hours unless the patient has an elevated temperature. When the patient has an elevated temperature the nurse checks the temperature, pulse, and respirations every hour until the temperature returns to normal and administers an antipyretic if prescribed by the primary care provider.

DIARRHEA. Diarrhea may be an indication of a superinfection or pseudomembranous colitis, both of which can be serious. The nurse should inspect all stools for the presence of blood or mucus. If diarrhea does occur and there appears to be blood and mucus in the stool, the nurse saves a sample of the stool and tests for occult blood using a test such as Hemoccult. If the stool tests positive for blood, the nurse saves the stool for possible further laboratory analysis.

The nurse should encourage the patient with diarrhea to drink fluids to replace those lost with the diarrhea. It is important to maintain an accurate intake and output record to help determine fluid balance.

Educating the Patient and Family

The patient and family must understand the prescribed therapeutic regimen. It is not uncommon for patients to stop taking a prescribed drug because they feel better. A detailed plan of teaching helps to reduce the incidence of this problem.

The nurse should explain, in easy to understand terms, the adverse reactions associated with the specific

Home Care Checklist

AVOIDING DRUG–FOOD INTERACTIONS

In some instances, drugs may be taken with food or milk to minimize the risk for gastrointestinal upset. However, most tetracyclines, when given with foods containing calcium, such as dairy products, are not absorbed as well as when they are taken on an empty stomach. So, if the patient is to receive tetracycline at home, it is important to be sure he or she knows to take the drug on an empty stomach, 1 hour before or 2 hours after a meal. In addition, the nurse teaches the patient to avoid the following foods before or after taking the drug:

✓ Milk (whole, low-fat, skim, condensed, or evaporated)

✓ Cream (half-and-half, heavy, light)

✓ Sour cream

✓ Coffee creamers

✓ Creamy salad dressings

✓ Eggnog

✓ Milkshakes

✓ Cheese (natural and processed)

✓ Yogurt (regular, low-fat, or nonfat)

✓ Cottage cheese

✓ Ice cream

✓ Frozen custard

✓ Frozen yogurt

✓ Ice milk

prescribed antibiotic. The nurse tells the patient to contact the primary health care provider if any potentially serious adverse reactions, such as hypersensitivity reactions, moderate to severe diarrhea, sudden onset of chills and fever, sore throat, or sores in the mouth, occur.

The nurse develops a teaching plan that includes the following information:

- Take the drug at the prescribed time intervals. These time intervals are important because a certain amount of the drug must be in the body at all times for the infection to be controlled.
- Do not to increase or omit the dose unless advised to do so by the primary health care provider.
- Complete the entire course of treatment. Never stop the drug, except on the advice of a primary health care provider, before the course of treatment is

completed even if symptoms improve or disappear. Failure to complete the prescribed course of treatment may result in a return of the infection.

- Take each dose with a full glass of water. Follow the directions given by the pharmacist regarding taking the drug on an empty stomach or with food (see Home Care Checklist: Avoiding Drug–Food Interactions).
- Notify the primary health care provider if symptoms of the infection become worse or there is no improvement in the original symptoms after about 5 days.
- Avoid the use of alcoholic beverages during therapy unless use has been approved by the primary health care provider.
- When a tetracycline has been prescribed, avoid exposure to the sun or any type of tanning lamp or bed. When exposure to direct sunlight is unavoidable, completely cover the arms and legs and wear a

wide-brimmed hat to protect the face and neck. Application of a sunscreen may or may not be effective. Therefore, consult the primary health care provider before using a sunscreen to prevent a photosensitivity reaction.

EVALUATION

● The therapeutic effect is achieved, and the infection is controlled or prevented.
● Adverse reactions are identified, reported to the primary health care provider, and managed successfully through appropriate nursing interventions.
● The patient and family demonstrate understanding of the drug regimen.
● The patient verbalizes the importance of complying with the prescribed therapeutic regimen.

● *Critical Thinking Exercises*

1. *Ms. Jones has been prescribed tetracycline. She works nights and is home sleeping during the day. To decrease the possibility of noncompliance with the treatment regimen, discuss how and what you would teach Ms. Jones about her drug regimen.*
2. *Mr. Park, a patient in a nursing home, has been receiving clarithromycin (Biaxin) for an upper respiratory infection for 9 days. The nurse assistant reports that he has been incontinent of feces for the past 2 days. Analyze whether this matter should be investigated.*
3. *When taking the drug history of Mr. Woods, a patient in the outpatient clinic, you note that he has been taking 0.25 mg digoxin, one baby aspirin, and the tetracycline minocycline (Minocin). Based on your knowledge of the tetracyclines, determine whether there is any reason to be concerned about the drug regimen that Mr. Woods is on. Explain your answer.*
4. *Ms. Evans, age 75 years, is to be dismissed on a regimen of doxycycline (Vibramycin). You note that she is alert and has good communication skills. Because she lives alone, she will be responsible for administering her own drug. Devise a teaching plan for Ms. Evans. You may want to use the teaching plan form in Chapter 5.*

● *Review Questions*

1. A patient asks the nurse why the primary health care provider prescribed an antibiotic when she was told that she has a viral infection. The most correct response by the nurse is that the antibiotic may be used to prevent a _____.
   A. primary fungal infection
   B. repeat viral infection
   C. secondary bacterial infection
   D. breakdown of the immune system

2. A patient is receiving erythromycin for an infection. The patient's response to therapy is best evaluated by _____.
   A. monitoring vital signs every 4 hours
   B. comparing initial and current signs and symptoms
   C. monitoring fluid intake and output
   D. asking the patient if he is feeling better

3. When asked to describe a photosensitivity reaction, the nurse correctly states that this reaction may be described as a(n) _____.
   A. tearing of the eyes on exposure to bright light
   B. aversion to bright lights and sunlight
   C. sensitivity to products in the environment
   D. exaggerated sunburn reaction when the skin is exposed to sunlight

4. When giving one of the macrolide antibiotics, the nurse assesses the patient for the most common adverse reactions, which are _____.
   A. related to the gastrointestinal tract
   B. skin rash and urinary retention
   C. sores in the mouth and hypertension
   D. related to the nervous system

● *Medication Dosage Problems*

1. Mr. Baker is prescribed azithromycin for a lower respiratory tract infection. The nurse tells Mr. Baker to take the drug on an empty stomach. Azithromycin is available in 250-mg tablets. The primary health care provider has ordered 500 mg on the first day, followed by 250 mg on days 2 to 5. How many tablets would Mr. Baker take on the first day? _____ On the last day of therapy?_____

2. A patient is prescribed 600 mg of lincomycin every 12 hours IM. The drug is available as 300 mg/mL. How many milliliters would the nurse administer?

3. A patient is prescribed 200 mg of minocycline oral suspension initially, followed by 100 mg PO every 12 hours. The minocycline is available as an oral suspension of 50 mg/5 mL. How many milliliters would the nurse administer as the initial dose? _____

Fluoroquinolones and Aminoglycosides

Chapter Objectives

On completion of this chapter, the student will:

- Discuss the uses, general drug action, contraindications, precautions, interactions, and adverse reactions of the fluoroquinolones and amino-glycosides.
- Discuss preadministration and ongoing assessment activities the nurse should perform on the patient taking the fluoroquinolones and amino-glycosides.
- List some nursing diagnoses particular to a patient receiving a fluoro-quinolone or aminoglycoside.
- Discuss ways to promote an optimal response to therapy, how to manage adverse reactions, and important points to keep in mind when educating patients about the use of a fluoroquinolone or aminoglycoside.

As antibiotics became resistant to various microorganisms, researchers sought to develop more powerful drugs that would be effective against these resistant pathogens. The fluoroquinolones and aminoglycosides are two groups of broad-spectrum antibiotics that resulted from this research. The Summary Drug Table: Fluoroquinolones and Aminoglycosides lists the fluoroquinolones and aminoglycosides discussed in this chapter.

FLUOROQUINOLONES

The fluoroquinolones include ciprofloxacin (Cipro), enoxacin (Penetrex), gatifloxacin (Tequin), lome-floxacin (Maxaquin), moxifloxacin (Avelox), ofloxacin (Floxin), and sparfloxacin (Zagam).

ACTIONS

The fluoroquinolones exert their bactericidal (bacteria-destroying) effect by interfering with an enzyme (DNA gyrase) needed by bacteria for the synthesis of DNA.

This interference prevents cell reproduction, leading to death of the bacteria.

USES

The fluoroquinolones are used in the treatment of infections caused by susceptible microorganisms. The fluoroquinolones are effective in the treatment of infections caused by gram-positive and gram-negative microorganisms. They are primarily used in the treatment of susceptible microorganisms in lower respiratory infections, infections of the skin, urinary tract infections, and sexually transmitted diseases. Ciprofloxacin, norfloxacin, and ofloxacin are available in ophthalmic forms for infections in the eyes.

ADVERSE REACTIONS

Bacterial or fungal superinfections and pseudomembranous colitis (see Chap. 7) may occur with the use of both of these drugs. The administration of any drug may result in a hypersensitivity reaction, which can

SUMMARY DRUG TABLE FLUOROQUINOLONES AND AMINOGLYCOSIDES

GENERIC NAME	TRADE NAME*	USES	ADVERSE REACTIONS	DOSAGE RANGES
Fluoroquinolones				
ciprofloxacin *si-proe-flox´-a-sin*	Cipro, Cipro IV	Treatment of infections due to susceptible microorganisms	Nausea, diarrhea, headache, abdominal discomfort, photosensitivity, superinfections, hypersensitivity reactions	250–750 mg PO q12h; 200–400 mg IV q12h
enoxacin *en-ox´-a-sin*	Penetrex	Same as ciprofloxacin	Same as ciprofloxacin	200–400 mg PO q12h
gatifloxacin *ga-tah-flox´-a-sin*	Tequin	Same as ciprofloxacin	Same as ciprofloxacin	200–400 mg qd PO or IV
levofloxacin *lee-voe-flox´-a-sin*	Levaquin	Same as ciprofloxacin	Same as ciprofloxacin	250–500 mg/d PO, IV
lomefloxacin *loh-meh-flox´-a-sin*	Maxaquin	Same as ciprofloxacin	Same as ciprofloxacin	400 mg PO once daily
moxifloxacin *mocks-ah-flox´-a-sin*	Avelox	Same as ciprofloxacin	Same as ciprofloxacin	400 mg qd PO
norfloxacin *nor- flox´-a-sin*	Noroxin	Same as ciprofloxacin, urinary tract infections, uncomplicated gonorrhea, prostatitis	Same as ciprofloxacin	400 mg PO q12h; 800 mg as single dose for gonorrhea
ofloxacin *oe-flox´-a-sin*	Floxin	Same as ciprofloxacin	Same as ciprofloxacin	200–400 mg PO, IV q12h
trovafloxacin *troh-va-flox´-a-sin* alatrofloxacin	Trovan Trovan IV	Same as ciprofloxacin	Same as ciprofloxacin, serious liver toxicity	100–200 mg/d PO, IV
Aminoglycosides				
amikacin *am-i-kay´-sin*	Amikin, Amikacin, *generic*	Treatment of serious infections caused by susceptible strains of microorganisms	Nausea, vomiting, diarrhea, rash, ototoxicity, nephrotoxicity, hypersensitivity reactions, neurotoxicity, superinfections, neuromuscular blockade	15 mg/kg IM, IV, in divided doses, not to exceed 1.5 g/d
gentamicin *jen-ta-mye´-sin*	Garamycin, *generic*	Same as amikacin	Same as amikacin	3 mg/kg/d q8h IM, IV, not to exceed 5 mg/kg/d in divided doses
kanamycin *kan-a-mye´-sin*	Kantrex, *generic*	Same as amikacin; oral use for hepatic coma and for suppression of intestinal bacteria	Same as amikacin	7.5–15 mg/kg/d in divided doses IM; 15 mg/kg/d in divided doses IV; suppression of intestinal bacteria 1 g qh for 4h then 1 g q6h for 36--72 h PO; hepatic coma 8–12 g/d in divided doses PO

SUMMARY DRUG TABLE FLUOROQUINOLONES AND AMINOGLYCOSIDES (*Continued*)

GENERIC NAME	TRADE NAME*	USES	ADVERSE REACTIONS	DOSAGE RANGES
neomycin *nee-o-mye´-sin*	Mycifradin, Neo-Tabs, *generic*	Same as amikacin, same as kanamycin	Same as amikacin	15 mg/kg/d q6h for 4 doses, then 300 mg IM bid, not to exceed 1 g/d; pre-op preparation of the bowel, see manufacturer's recommendations for complex 3-day regimen; hepatic coma 4–12 g/d
netilmicin *ne-til-mye´-sin*	Netromycin	Same as amikacin	Same as amikacin	Up to 6.5 mg/kg/d IV in divided doses
streptomycin *strep-toe-mye´-sin*	*Generic*	Same as amikacin, fourth drug in the treatment of TB	Same as amikacin	15 mg/kg/d IM or 25–30 mg/kg IM 2–3 times per week
tobramycin *toe-bra-mye´-sin*	Nebcin, *generic*	Same as amikacin	Same as amikacin	3–5 mg/kg/d IM, IV q8h

*The term *generic* indicates the drug is available in generic form.

range from mild to severe and in some cases can be life threatening. Mild hypersensitivity reactions may only require discontinuing the drug, whereas the more serious reactions require immediate treatment. (Chapters 1 and 7 contain discussions of hypersensitivity reactions.)

The more common adverse effects seen with the administration of these drugs include nausea, diarrhea, headache, abdominal pain or discomfort, and dizziness. A more serious adverse reaction seen with the administration of the fluoroquinolones, especially lomefloxacin and sparfloxacin, is a photosensitivity reaction. This is manifested by an exaggerated sunburn reaction when the skin is exposed to the ultraviolet rays of sunlight or sunlamps.

CONTRAINDICATIONS

The fluoroquinolones are contraindicated in patients with a history of hypersensitivity to the fluoroquinolones, in children younger than 18 years, and in pregnant women (Pregnancy Category C). These drugs also are contraindicated in patients whose life-styles do not allow for adherence to the precautions regarding photosensitivity.

PRECAUTIONS

The fluoroquinolones are used cautiously in patients with renal impairment or a history of seizures, in geriatric patients, and in patients on dialysis.

INTERACTIONS

Concurrent use of the fluoroquinolones with theophylline causes an increase in serum theophylline levels. When used concurrently with cimetidine, the cimetidine may interfere with the elimination of the fluoroquinolones. Use of the fluoroquinolones with an oral anticoagulant may cause an increase in the effects of the oral coagulant. Administration of the fluoroquinolones with antacids, iron salts, or zinc will decrease absorption of the fluoroquinolones. There is a risk of seizures if fluoroquinolones are given with the NSAIDs. There is a risk of severe cardiac arrhythmias when the fluoroquinolones gatifloxacin and moxifloxacin are administered with drugs that increase the QT interval (eg, quinidine, procainamide, amiodarone, and sotalol).

AMINOGLYCOSIDES

The aminoglycosides include amikacin (Amikin), gentamicin (Garamycin), kanamycin (Kantrex), neomycin (Mycifradin), netilmicin (Netromycin), streptomycin, and tobramycin (Nebcin).

ACTIONS

The aminoglycosides exert their bactericidal effect by blocking a step in protein synthesis necessary for bacterial multiplication. They disrupt the functional ability of the bacterial cell membrane causing cell death.

USES

The aminoglycosides are used in the treatment of infections caused by susceptible microorganisms. The aminoglycosides are used primarily in the treatment of infections caused by gram-negative microorganisms.

Because the oral aminoglycosides are poorly absorbed, they are useful to suppressing gastrointestinal bacteria. The oral aminoglycosides kanamycin (Kantrex) and neomycin (Mycifradin) are used preoperatively to reduce the number of bacteria normally present in the intestine (**bowel prep**). A reduction in intestinal bacteria is thought to lessen the possibility of abdominal infection that may occur after surgery on the bowel.

Kanamycin, neomycin, and paromomycin are used orally in the management of **hepatic coma**. In this disorder, liver failure results in an elevation of blood ammonia levels. By reducing the number of ammonia-forming bacteria in the intestines, blood ammonia levels may be lowered, thereby temporarily reducing some of the symptoms associated with this disorder.

ADVERSE REACTIONS

The aminoglycosides are capable of causing nephrotoxicity (damage to the kidneys by a toxic substance) and **ototoxicity** (damage to the organs of hearing by a toxic substance). Signs and symptoms of nephrotoxicity may include protein in the urine (**proteinuria**), **hematuria** (blood in the urine), increase in the blood urea nitrogen level, decrease in urine output, and an increase in the serum creatinine concentration. Nephrotoxicity is usually reversible once the drug is discontinued. Signs and symptoms of ototoxicity include tinnitus, dizziness, roaring in the ears, vertigo, and a mild to severe loss of hearing. If hearing loss occurs, it is most often permanent. Ototoxicity may occur during drug therapy or even after the drug is discontinued. The short-term administration of kanamycin and neomycin as a preparation for bowel surgery rarely causes these two adverse reactions.

Neurotoxicity (damage to the nervous system by a toxic substance) may also be seen with the administration of the aminoglycosides. Signs and symptoms of neurotoxicity include numbness, skin tingling, circumoral (around the mouth) paresthesia, peripheral paresthesia, tremors, muscle twitching, convulsions, muscle weakness, and **neuromuscular blockade** (acute muscular paralysis and apnea).

Additional adverse reactions seen with administration of the aminoglycosides may include nausea, vomiting, anorexia, rash, and urticaria. When these drugs are given, individual drug references, such as the package insert, should be consulted for more specific adverse reactions.

Like the other anti-infectives, bacterial or fungal superinfections and pseudomembranous colitis (see Chap. 7) may occur with the use of these drugs. The administration of the aminoglycosides may result in a hypersensitivity reaction, which can range from mild to severe and in some cases can be life threatening. Mild hypersensitivity reactions may only require discontinuing the drug, whereas the more serious reactions require immediate treatment.

CONTRAINDICATIONS

The aminoglycosides are contraindicated in patients with hypersensitivity to aminoglycosides. The aminoglycosides should not be given to patients requiring long-term therapy because of the potential for ototoxicity and nephrotoxicity. One exception is the use of streptomycin for long-term management of tuberculosis. These drugs are contraindicated in patients with preexisting hearing loss, myasthenia gravis, parkinsonism, and during lactation or pregnancy. Neomycin, amikacin, gentamicin, kanamycin, netilmicin, and tobramycin are Pregnancy Category D drugs; the remainder are Category C.

PRECAUTIONS

The aminoglycosides are used cautiously in patients with renal failure (dosage adjustments may be necessary), in the elderly, and in patients with neuromuscular disorders.

INTERACTIONS

Administration of the aminoglycosides with the cephalosporins may increase the risks of nephrotoxicity. When the aminoglycosides are administered with loop diuretics there is an increased risk of ototoxicity (irreversible hearing loss). There is an increased risk of neuromuscular blockage (paralysis of the respiratory muscles) if the aminoglycosides are given shortly after general anesthetics (neuromuscular junction blockers).

● The Patient Receiving a Fluoroquinolone or Aminoglycoside

ASSESSMENT

Preadministration Assessment

Before administering a fluoroquinolone or an aminoglycoside, the nurse identifies and records the signs and symptoms of the infection. It is particularly important for the nurse to obtain a thorough allergy history, especially a history of drug allergies. The nurse should take and record vital signs as well.

The primary health care provider may order culture and sensitivity tests, and the culture is obtained before the first dose of the drug is given. When an aminoglycoside is to be given, laboratory tests such as renal and hepatic function tests, complete blood count, and urinalysis also may be ordered.

When kanamycin or neomycin is given for hepatic coma, the nurse must evaluate the patient's level of consciousness and ability to swallow.

Ongoing Assessment

During drug therapy with the aminoglycosides or the fluoroquinolones, it is important for the nurse to perform an ongoing assessment. In general, the nurse compares the initial signs and symptoms of the infection, which were recorded during the initial assessment, to the current signs and symptoms. The nurse then records these findings in the patient's chart. When kanamycin or neomycin is given for hepatic coma, the nurse evaluates and records the patient's general condition daily.

The nurse monitors the patient's vital signs every 4 hours or as ordered by the primary health care provider. The nurse should notify the primary health care provider if there are changes in the vital signs, such as a significant drop in blood pressure, an increase in the pulse or respiratory rate, or a sudden increase in temperature.

When an aminoglycoside is being administered, it is important to monitor the patient's respiratory rate because neuromuscular blockade has been reported with the administration of these drugs. The nurse reports any changes in the respiratory rate or rhythm to the primary health care provider because immediate treatment may be necessary.

NURSING DIAGNOSES

Drug-specific nursing diagnoses are highlighted in the Nursing Diagnoses Checklist. Other nursing diagnoses applicable to these drugs are discussed in Chapter 4.

Nursing Diagnoses Checklist

☑ **Risk for Imbalanced Body Temperature: Hyperthermia** related to infectious process

☑ **Diarrhea** related to superinfection secondary to antibiotic therapy, adverse drug reaction

☑ **Disturbed Sensory Perception: Auditory** related to adverse drug reactions of the aminoglycosides

☑ **Ineffective Tissue Perfusion: Renal** related to adverse drug reactions of the aminoglycosides

---

PLANNING

The expected outcomes for the patient may include an optimal response to therapy, which includes control of the infectious process, an absence of adverse drug effects, and an understanding of and compliance with the prescribed treatment regimen.

IMPLEMENTATION

Promoting an Optimal Response to Therapy: Fluoroquinolones

The nurse encourages patients who receive the fluoroquinolones to increase their fluid intake. Norfloxacin and enoxacin are given on an empty stomach (eg, 1 hour before or 2 hours after meals). Ciprofloxacin and lomefloxacin can be given without regard to meals. However, the manufacturer recommends that the drug be given 2 hours after a meal. Moxifloxacin is given once a day for the period prescribed. If the patient is taking an antacid, moxifloxacin should be administered 4 hours before or 8 hours after the antacid.

Ciprofloxacin, gatifloxacin, and ofloxacin are the only fluoroquinolones given intravenously (IV). None of the fluoroquinolones are given intramuscularly (IM).

MONITORING FOR HYPERTHERMIA. The infectious process is accompanied by an elevation in temperature. When the patient is being treated for the infection the nurse must monitor the vital signs, particularly the body temperature. As the anti-infective works to rid the body of the infectious organism, the body temperature should return to normal. The nurse monitors the vital signs (temperature, pulse, and respiration) frequently to monitor the drug's effectiveness in eradicating the infectious process. The nurse checks the vital signs every 4 hours or more frequently if the temperature is elevated. The primary health care provider is notified if a temperature is greater than 101° Fahrenheit.

Promoting an Optimal Response to Therapy: Aminoglycosides

The oral aminoglycosides may be given without regard to meals. If there is any doubt about administration of these drugs with or without food, consult the hospital pharmacist.

With the exception of paromomycin, all of the aminoglycoside drugs can be given intramuscularly (IM). For optimal results, the nurse should inspect previous injection sites for signs of pain or tenderness, redness, and swelling. The nurse informs the primary health care provider of any persistence in a localized reaction of pain, redness, or extreme tenderness. It is important to rotate injection sites and record the site used on the patient's chart. With the exception of paromomycin and streptomycin, all of the aminoglycoside drugs can be given intravenously (IV).

SUPPRESSION OF INTESTINAL BACTERIA. When kanamycin or neomycin is given for suppression of intestinal bacteria before surgery, the primary health care provider's orders regarding the timing of the administration of the drug are extremely important. Omission of a dosage or failure to give the drug at the specified time may result in inadequate suppression of intestinal bacteria. When neomycin is given, enteric-coated erythromycin (see Chap. 9) may be given at the same time as part of the bowel preparation.

HEPATIC COMA. When the aminoglycosides kanamycin or neomycin are given orally as treatment for hepatic coma, the nurse exercises care when giving the drug. During the early stages of this disorder, various changes in the level of consciousness may be seen. At times, the patient may appear lethargic and respond poorly to commands. Because of these changes in the level of consciousness, the patient may have difficulty swallowing, and a danger of aspiration is present. If the patient appears to have difficulty taking an oral drug, the nurse withholds the drug and contacts the primary health care provider.

Monitoring and Managing Adverse Drug Reactions

A variety of adverse reactions can be seen with the administration of the fluoroquinolones or aminoglycosides. The nurse observes the patient, especially during the first 48 hours of therapy. It is important to report the occurrence of any adverse reaction to the primary health care provider before the next dose of the drug is due. If a serious adverse reaction such as a hypersensitivity reaction, respiratory difficulty, severe diarrhea, or a decided drop in blood pressure occurs, the nurse contacts the primary health care provider immediately.

The nurse always listens, evaluates, and reports any complaints the patient may have; certain complaints may be an early sign of an adverse drug reaction. The nurse should report all changes in the patient's condition and any new problems that occur (eg, nausea or diarrhea) as soon as possible. It is then up to the primary health care provider to decide if these changes or problems are a part of the patient's infectious process or the result of an adverse drug reaction.

MONITORING FOR DIARRHEA. Because superinfections and pseudomembranous colitis can occur during therapy with these drugs, the nurse checks the patient's stools and reports any incidence of diarrhea immediately because this may indicate a superinfection or pseudomembranous colitis. If diarrhea does occur and blood and mucus appear in the stool, the nurse should save a sample of the stool and test it for occult blood using a test such as Hemoccult. If the stool tests positive for blood, it is important to save the sample for possible additional laboratory tests.

MONITORING DRUGS GIVEN INTRAVENOUSLY. For optimal results, the nurse inspects the needle site and the area around the needle every hour for signs of extravasation of the IV fluid. The nurse performs these assessments more frequently if the patient is restless or uncooperative. It is important to check the rate of infusion every 15 minutes and adjust it as needed. The nurse should inspect the vein used for the IV infusion every 4 hours for signs of tenderness, pain, and redness (which may indicate phlebitis or thrombophlebitis). If these are apparent, the nurse must restart the IV in another vein and bring the problem to the attention of the primary health care provider.

Monitoring and Managing Adverse Drug Reactions: Fluoroquinolones

All fluoroquinolone drugs can cause pain, inflammation, or rupture of a tendon. The Achilles tendon is particularly vulnerable. This problem can be so severe that prolonged disability results, and, at times, surgical intervention may be necessary to correct the problem. In addition, the fluoroquinolone drugs, particularly sparfloxacin and lomefloxacin, cause dangerous photosensitivity reactions. Patients have experienced severe reactions even when sunscreens or sunblocks were used.

Monitoring and Managing Adverse Drug Reactions: Aminoglycosides

The aminoglycosides are potentially neurotoxic, nephrotoxic, and ototoxic and are capable of causing permanent damage to these organs and structures. The nurse notifies the primary health care provider immediately when one or more signs and symptoms of these adverse reactions is suspected.

MONITORING FOR NEUROTOXICITY. The nurse should be alert for symptoms such as numbness or tingling of the skin, circumoral paresthesia, peripheral paresthesia (numbness or tingling in the extremities), tremors, and muscle twitching or weakness. The nurse reports any symptom of neurotoxicity immediately to the primary health care provider. Convulsions can occur if the drug is not discontinued.

Nursing Alert

Neuromuscular blockade or respiratory paralysis may occur after administration of the aminoglycosides. Therefore, it is extremely important that any symptoms of respiratory difficulty be reported immediately. If neuromuscular blockade occurs, it may be reversed by the administration of calcium salts, but mechanical ventilation may be required.

INEFFECTIVE TISSUE PERFUSION: RENAL. The patient taking an aminoglycoside is at risk for nephrotoxicity. The nurse measures and records the intake and output and notifies the primary health care provider if the output is less than 750 mL/day. It is important to keep a record of the fluid intake and output as well as a daily weight to assess hydration and renal function. The nurse encourages fluid intake to 2000 mL/day (if the patient's condition permits). Any changes in the intake and output ratio or in the appearance of the urine may indicate nephrotoxicity. The nurse reports these types of changes to the primary health care provider promptly. The primary health care provider may order daily laboratory tests (ie, serum creatinine and blood urea nitrogen [BUN]) to monitor renal function. The nurse reports any elevation in the creatinine or BUN level to the primary health care provider because an elevation may indicate renal dysfunction.

DISTURBED SENSORY PERCEPTION: AUDITORY. The patient taking aminoglycosides is at risk for ototoxicity. Auditory changes are irreversible, usually bilateral, and may be partial or total. The risk is greater in patients with renal impairment or those with preexisting hearing loss. It is important for the nurse to detect any problems with hearing and report them to the primary health care provider because continued administration could lead to permanent hearing loss.

Nursing Alert

To detect ototoxicity, the nurse carefully evaluates the patient's complaints or comments related to hearing, such as a ringing or buzzing in the ears or difficulty hearing. If hearing problems do occur, the nurse reports this problem to the primary health care provider immediately. To monitor for damage to the eighth cranial nerve, an evaluation of hearing may be done by audiometry before and throughout the course of therapy.

Educating the Patient and Family

Carefully planned patient and family education is important to foster compliance, relieve anxiety, and promote therapeutic effect. The nurse explains all adverse reactions associated with the specific prescribed antibiotic to the patient. The nurse advises the patient of the signs and symptoms of potentially serious adverse reactions, such as hypersensitivity reactions, moderate to severe diarrhea, sudden onset of chills and fever, sore throat, sores in the mouth, or extreme fatigue. The nurse should explain to the patient the necessity of contacting the primary health care provider immediately if such symptoms occur. The nurse cautions the patient against the use of alcoholic beverages during therapy unless approved by the primary health care provider. To reduce the incidence of noncompliance to the treatment regimen, a teaching plan is developed to include the following information:

- Take the drug at the prescribed time intervals. These time intervals are important because a certain amount of the drug must be in the body at all times for the infection to be controlled.
- Drink six to eight large glasses of fluids while taking these drugs and take each dose with a full glass of water.
- Do not increase or omit the dose unless advised to do so by the primary health care provider.
- Complete the entire course of treatment. Do not stop the drug, except on the advice of a primary health care provider, before the course of treatment is completed even if symptoms improve or disappear. Failure to complete the prescribed course of treatment may result in a return of the infection.
- Follow the directions supplied with the prescription regarding taking the drugs with meals or on an empty stomach. For drugs that must be taken on an empty stomach, take them 1 hour before or 2 hours after a meal.
- Notify the primary health care provider if symptoms of the infection become worse or there is no improvement in the original symptoms after 5 to 7 days of drug therapy.
- Avoid any exposure to sunlight or ultraviolet light (tanning beds, sunlamps) while taking these drugs and for several weeks after completing the course of therapy. Wear sunblock, sunglasses, and protective clothing when exposed to sunlight.
- Avoid tasks requiring mental alertness until response to the drug is known.

SPECIFIC INSTRUCTIONS REGARDING FLUOROQUINOLONE THERAPY

- When taking the fluoroquinolones, report any signs of tendinitis, such as pain or soreness in the leg, shoulder, or back of the heel. Periodic applications of ice may help relieve the pain. Until tendinitis or tendon rupture can be excluded, rest the involved area and avoid exercise.

● Do not take antacids or drugs containing iron or zinc because these drugs will decrease absorption of the fluoroquinolone.

SPECIFIC INSTRUCTIONS REGARDING AMINOGLYCOSIDE THERAPY

● Notify the primary health care provider of any ringing in the ears or difficulty hearing, numbness or tingling around the mouth or in the extremities, and of any change in urinary patterns.

SPECIFIC INSTRUCTIONS FOR A PREOPERATIVE PREPARATION OF THE BOWEL

● When taking an aminoglycoside for preparation of the bowel before surgery, take the prescribed drug at the exact times indicated on the prescription container. Some bowel prep regimens are complex. For example, when kanamycin is prescribed for suppression of intestinal bacteria in preparation for bowel surgery, the drug is given orally every hour for 4 hours followed by 1 g every 6 hours for 36 to 72 hours.

EVALUATION

● The therapeutic effect is achieved, the infection is controlled, and the bowel is cleansed sufficiently.
● Adverse reactions are identified, reported to the primary health care provider, and managed successfully through nursing interventions.
● The patient and family demonstrate understanding of the drug regimen.
● The patient verbalizes the importance of complying with the prescribed therapeutic regimen.

● *Critical Thinking Exercises*

1. *Mr. Baker is receiving amikacin (Amikin) IV as treatment for a bacterial septicemia. When checking a drug reference you note that this drug is an aminoglycoside. Considering the most serious toxic effects associated with this group of drugs, determine what daily assessments you would perform to detect early signs and symptoms of these adverse drug effects.*

2. *Ms. Carson is seen in the outpatient clinic for a severe respiratory infection and is prescribed ciprofloxacin. Discuss what you would include in the teaching plan for this patient.*

3. *A patient is prescribed ciprofloxacin for a severe respiratory infection. What serious adverse reaction(s)*

should the nurse warn the patient to be especially observant for? What common adverse reactions should the patient be aware of? What important information should the nurse include in the teaching plan concerning adverse reactions?

● *Review Questions*

1. Mr. Allison is taking gentamicin for a severe gram-negative infection. The nurse observes him for signs of neurotoxicity, which include _____.
   A. anorexia and abdominal pain
   B. decreased urinary output and dark, concentrated urine
   C. muscle twitching and numbness
   D. headache and agitation

2. Patients taking a fluoroquinolone are encouraged to _____.
   A. nap 1 to 2 hours daily while taking the drug
   B. eat a high-protein diet
   C. increase their fluid intake
   D. avoid foods high in carbohydrate

3. Which of the following complaints by a patient taking tobramycin would be most indicative the patient is experiencing ototoxicity?
   A. tingling of the extremities
   B. complaints that he is unable to hear the television
   C. changes in mental status
   D. short periods of dizziness

4. A patient is prescribed moxifloxacin. The nurse notes that the patient is also taking an antacid. The nurse correctly administers moxifloxacin _____.
   A. once daily PO, 4 hours before the antacid
   B. twice daily PO, immediately following the antacid
   C. once daily IM without regard to the administration of the antacid
   D. every 12 hours IV without regard to the administration of the antacid

5. The nurse is asked why kanamycin is given as a "bowel prep" before gastrointestinal surgery. The nurse correctly replies _____.
   A. abdominal surgery requires starting antibiotic therapy 4 days before surgery
   B. the bacteria found in the bowel cannot be destroyed after surgery
   C. a reduction of intestinal bacteria lessens the possibility of postoperative infection
   D. anesthesia makes the bowel resistant to an antibiotic after surgery

● *Medication Dosage Problems*

1. A patient is prescribed 40 mg of tobramycin IM. Use the drug label shown below to determine the amount of drug to administer. The nurse would administer _____ .

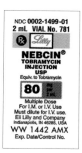

NDC 0002-1499-01
2 mL VIAL No. 781
℞ *Lilly*
NEBCIN®
TOBRAMYCIN
INJECTION
USP
Equiv. to Tobramycin
80 mg per 2 mL
Multiple Dose
For I.M. or I.V. Use
Must dilute for I.V. use.
Eli Lilly and Company
Indianapolis, IN 46285, USA
WW 1442 AMX
Exp. Date/Control No.

2. The primary health care provider prescribed 400 mg gatifloxacin PO daily for 7 days. The drug is available in 200-mg tablets. How many tablets would the nurse administer each day?

photosensitivity. Pseudomembranous colitis and thrombocytopenia are the more serious adverse reactions caused by linezolid.

CONTRAINDICATIONS, PRECAUTIONS, AND INTERACTIONS

The drug is contraindicated in the presence of an allergy to the drug, pregnancy (Category C), lactation, and phenylketonuria (oral form only). Linezolid is used cautiously in patients with bone marrow depression, hepatic dysfunction, renal impairment, hypertension, and hyperthyroidism.

When linezolid is used with antiplatelet drugs such as aspirin or the NSAIDs (see Chap. 18) there is an increased risk of bleeding and thrombocytopenia. When administered with the MAOIs (see Chap. 31) the effects of the MAOIs are decreased. There is a risk of severe hypertension if linezolid is combined with large amounts of food containing tyramine (eg, aged cheese, caffeinated beverages, yogurt, chocolate, red wine, beer, pepperoni).

MEROPENEM

ACTION AND USES

Meropenem (Merrem IV) inhibits synthesis of the bacterial cell wall and causes the death of susceptible cells. This drug is used for intra-abdominal infections caused by *Pseudomonas aeruginosa, Escherichia coli, Klebsiella pneumoniae,* and other susceptible organisms. Meropenem also is effective against bacterial meningitis caused by *Neisseria meningitidis, Streptococcus pneumoniae,* and *Hemophilus influenzae.*

ADVERSE REACTIONS

The most common adverse reactions with meropenem include headache, nausea, vomiting, diarrhea, anorexia, abdominal pain, generalized pain, flatulence, rash, and superinfections. This drug also can cause an abscess or phlebitis at the injection site. An abscess is suspected if the injection site appears red or is tender and warm to the touch. Tissue sloughing at the injection site also may occur.

CONTRAINDICATIONS, PRECAUTIONS, AND INTERACTIONS

Meropenem is contraindicated in patients who are allergic to cephalosporins and penicillins and in patients with renal failure. This drug is not recommended in children younger than 3 months or for women during pregnancy (Category B) or lactation. Meropenem is used cautiously in patients with central nervous system (CNS) disorders, seizure disorders, and in patients with renal or hepatic failure. When administered with probenecid, the excretion of meropenem is inhibited.

METRONIDAZOLE

ACTIONS AND USES

The mode of action of metronidazole (Flagyl) is not well understood, but it is thought to disrupt DNA and protein synthesis in susceptible organisms. This drug may be used in the treatment of serious infections, such as intra-abdominal, bone, soft tissue, lower respiratory, gynecologic, and CNS infections caused by susceptible **anaerobic** (able to live without oxygen) microorganisms.

ADVERSE REACTIONS

The most common adverse reactions seen with this drug are related to the gastrointestinal tract and may include nausea, anorexia, and occasionally vomiting and diarrhea. The most serious adverse reactions are associated with the CNS and include seizures and numbness of the extremities. Hypersensitivity reactions also may be seen. Thrombophlebitis may occur with intravenous (IV) use of the drug.

CONTRAINDICATIONS, PRECAUTIONS, AND INTERACTIONS

This drug is contraindicated in patients with known hypersensitivity to the drug and during the first trimester of pregnancy (Category B). This drug is used cautiously in patients with blood dyscrasias, seizure disorders, and hepatic dysfunction. Safety in children (other than orally for amebiasis) has not been established.

The metabolism of metronidazole may decrease when administered with cimetidine. When administered with phenobarbital, the effectiveness of metronidazole may decrease. When metronidazole is administered with warfarin, the effectiveness of the warfarin is increased.

PENTAMIDINE ISETHIONATE

ACTIONS AND USES

Pentamidine isethionate (Pentam 300, the parenteral form; NebuPent, the aerosol form) is used in the treatment (parenteral form) or prevention (aerosol form) of

Pneumocystis carinii pneumonia, a pneumonia seen in those with acquired immunodeficiency syndrome. The mode of action of this drug is not fully understood.

ADVERSE REACTIONS

More than half of the patients receiving this drug by the parenteral route experience some adverse reaction. Severe and sometimes life-threatening reactions include leukopenia (low white blood cell count), **hypoglycemia** (low blood sugar), thrombocytopenia (low platelet count), and **hypotension** (low blood pressure). Moderate or less severe reactions include changes in some laboratory tests, such as the serum creatinine and liver function tests. Other adverse reactions include anxiety, headache, hypotension, chills, nausea, and anorexia. Aerosol administration may result in fatigue, a metallic taste in the mouth, shortness of breath, and anorexia.

CONTRAINDICATIONS, PRECAUTIONS, AND INTERACTIONS

This drug is contraindicated in individuals who have had previous hypersensitivity reactions to pentamidine isethionate. Pentamidine isethionate is used cautiously in patients with hypertension, hypotension, hyperglycemia, renal impairment, diabetes mellitus, liver impairment, bone marrow depression, pregnancy (Category C), or lactation.

An additive nephrotoxicity develops when pentamidine isethionate is administered with other nephrotoxic drugs (eg, aminoglycosides, vancomycin, or amphotericin B). An additive bone marrow depression occurs when the drug is administered with antineoplastic drugs or when the patient has received radiation therapy recently.

SPECTINOMYCIN

ACTIONS AND USES

Spectinomycin (Trobicin) is chemically related to but different from the aminoglycosides (see Chap. 10). This drug exerts its action by interfering with bacterial protein synthesis. Spectinomycin is used for the treatment of gonorrhea.

ADVERSE REACTIONS

Soreness at the injection site, urticaria, dizziness, rash, chills, fever, and hypersensitivity reactions may be seen with the administration of this drug.

CONTRAINDICATIONS, PRECAUTIONS, AND INTERACTIONS

This drug is contraindicated in known cases of hypersensitivity to spectinomycin. In addition, the drug should not be given to infants. If another sexually transmitted disease is present with gonorrhea, additional anti-infectives may be needed to eradicate the infectious processes. Safe use during pregnancy (Category B) or lactation or in children has not been established.

No known significant drug or food interactions for spectinomycin are known.

VANCOMYCIN

ACTIONS AND USES

Vancomycin (Vancocin) acts against susceptible gram-positive bacteria by inhibiting bacterial cell wall synthesis and increasing cell wall permeability. This drug is used in the treatment of serious gram-positive infections that do not respond to treatment with other anti-infectives. It also may be used in treating anti-infective–associated pseudomembranous colitis caused by *Clostridium difficile*.

ADVERSE REACTIONS

Nephrotoxicity (damage to the kidneys) and ototoxicity (damage to the organs of hearing) may be seen with the administration of this drug. Additional adverse reactions include nausea, chills, fever, urticaria, sudden fall in blood pressure with parenteral administration, and skin rashes.

CONTRAINDICATIONS, PRECAUTIONS, AND INTERACTIONS

This drug is contraindicated in patients with known hypersensitivity to vancomycin. Vancomycin is used cautiously in patients with renal or hearing impairment and during pregnancy (Category C) and lactation.

When administered with other ototoxic and nephrotoxic drugs, additive effects may be seen.

NURSING PROCESS

● **The Patient Receiving a Miscellaneous Anti-infective**

ASSESSMENT

Preadministration Assessment

Before administering these drugs, the nurse takes and records the patient's vital signs and identifies and records the symptoms of the infection. It is very important to take a thorough allergy history, especially a history of drug allergies. When culture and sensitivity tests are ordered, these procedures must be performed before the first dose of the drug is given. Other laboratory tests such as renal and hepatic function tests, complete blood count, and urinalysis also may be ordered before and during drug therapy for early detection of toxic reactions.

Ongoing Assessment

The nurse should monitor the patient's vital signs every 4 hours or as ordered by the primary health care provider. It is important to notify the primary health care provider if there are changes in the vital signs, such as a significant drop in blood pressure, an increase in the pulse or respiratory rate, or a sudden increase in temperature.

The nurse observes the patient at frequent intervals, especially during the first 48 hours of therapy. It is important to report any adverse reaction to the primary health care provider before the next dose of the drug is due.

NURSING DIAGNOSES

Drug-specific nursing diagnoses are highlighted in the Nursing Diagnoses Checklist. Other nursing diagnoses applicable to these drugs are discussed in Chapter 4.

PLANNING

The expected outcomes for the patient depend on the reason for administration of the anti-infective but may include an optimal response to drug therapy, management of adverse drug reactions, a decrease in anxiety, and an understanding of and compliance with the prescribed drug regimen.

IMPLEMENTATION

Promoting an Optimal Response to Therapy

Monitoring each patient for response to drug therapy and for the appearance of adverse reactions is an integral part of promoting an optimal response to therapy. The nurse immediately reports serious adverse reactions, such as signs and symptoms of a hypersensitivity reaction or superinfection, respiratory difficulty, or a marked drop in blood pressure.

Nursing Diagnoses Checklist

- ☑ **Anxiety** related to infection, seriousness of illness, route of administration, other factors (specify)
- ☑ **Diarrhea** related to adverse drug reaction, superinfection
- ☑ **Pain** related to intramuscular injection
- ☑ **Risk for Disturbed Sensory Perception: Auditory** related to adverse drug effects (ototoxicity)
- ☑ **Risk for Impaired Urinary Elimination** related to adverse drug effects (nephrotoxicity)

INTRAMUSCULAR ADMINISTRATION. To promote an optimal response to therapy when giving these drugs intramuscularly (IM), the nurse inspects previous injection sites for signs of pain or tenderness, redness, and swelling. In addition, the nurse reports any persistent local reaction to the primary health care provider. It also is important to develop a plan for rotation of injection sites and to record the site used after each injection.

INTRAVENOUS ADMINISTRATION. When giving these drugs IV, the nurse inspects the needle site and area around the needle at frequent intervals for signs of extravasation of the IV fluid. More frequent assessments are performed if the patient is restless or uncooperative.

The rate of infusion is checked every 15 minutes and adjusted as needed. This is especially important when administering vancomycin because rapid infusion of the drug can result in severe hypotension and shock. The nurse inspects the vein used for the IV infusion every 4 to 8 hours for signs of tenderness, pain, and redness (which may indicate phlebitis or thrombophlebitis). If these symptoms are apparent, the nurse restarts the IV in another vein and brings the problem to the attention of the primary health care provider.

SPECIAL CONSIDERATIONS FOR SPECIFIC DRUGS. To promote an optimal response to therapy, the nurse should know the following special considerations for specific drugs.

Chloramphenicol. When the drug is given orally, the nurse gives it to the patient whose stomach is empty, 1 hour before or 2 hours after meals. If gastrointestinal distress occurs, it is acceptable to give the drug with food. Chloramphenicol is also given IV. The drug should be administered around the clock to maintain therapeutic blood levels of the drug.

⁂ Nursing Alert

The blood dyscrasias may occur with the administration of chloramphenicol during either short- or long-term therapy. The nurse observes patients closely for signs and symptoms that may indicate a blood dyscrasia—fever, sore throat, sores in the mouth, easy bruising or bleeding (even several weeks after the drug regimen is completed) and extreme fatigue.

It is important to monitor closely serum blood levels of chloramphenicol, particularly in patients with impaired liver or kidney function or when administering chloramphenicol with other drugs metabolized by the liver. Blood concentration levels exceeding 25 mcg/mL increase the risk of the patient developing bone marrow depression.

Linezolid. The drug is given orally or intravenously (IV). When the drug is taken orally, it is administered every 12 hours and may be taken with or without food. If nausea develops, the drug may be taken with food. Foods high in tyramine (see Chap. 31) are avoided because of the risk of hypertension. When given IV, the drug is infused during a period of 30 to 120 minutes. The nurse protects the drug from light by leaving the overwrap in place until ready to administer. It is important to monitor the patient's platelet count regularly, particularly if the drug is used for longer than 2 weeks.

Meropenem. This drug is administered only by the IV route. The nurse gives meropenem every 8 hours over a period of 15 to 30 minutes if the drug is diluted or over a period of 3 to 5 minutes as a bolus injection (5–20 mL).

Metronidazole. When the nurse prepares the drug, the package insert should be consulted for reconstitution of the powder form because the directions for the order of preparation for IV administration must be followed. After reconstitution, the solution should be clear to pale yellow to pale green; do not use if the solution is cloudy or contains particulates. The drug should be used within 24 hours. When given orally, it is important to give the drug with meals to avoid gastrointestinal upset. The nurse informs the patient that an unpleasant metallic taste may be noted during therapy. When the drug is given on an outpatient basis, it is a good idea to advise the patient to avoid drinking alcoholic beverages during and for at least 1 day after treatment. When metronidazole is mixed with alcohol, the patient may experience flushing, nausea, vomiting, headache, and abdominal cramping.

The nurse informs patients being treated for gynecologic infections, such as trichomoniasis, that sexual contact with infected partners may lead to reinfection, so sexual partners must be treated concurrently.

Pentamidine Isethionate. When the drug is given IM or IV, the nurse prepares the drug according to the manufacturer's directions. When the drug is given by the IV route, it is important to infuse the drug over 1 hour. When the drug is given by aerosol, the nurse uses a special nebulizer (Respirgard II) and delivers the drug until the chamber is empty. It also is a good idea to explain or demonstrate the use of the nebulizer to the patient. The nurse monitors blood pressure frequently during administration because sudden, severe hypotension may occur after administration. Because hypotension can occur after a single dose, the nurse should always have the patient lying down when the drug is administered. The nurse assesses the patient for signs of hypoglycemia (weakness, diaphoresis, cool skin, shakiness) and hyperglycemia (flushed dry skin, fruity breath odor, increased thirst, and increased urination).

Spectinomycin. Spectinomycin may be given as a single dose, but multiple doses may be prescribed for complicated, widespread gonorrhea. The nurse warns the patient that the IM injection may be uncomfortable and that soreness at the injection site may be noted for a brief time. The nurse emphasizes the importance of following the primary health care provider's recommendations regarding a follow-up examination to determine if the infection has been eliminated. In addition, the nurse explains to the patient that all sexual contacts need to receive treatment.

Vancomycin. The nurse can administer vancomycin orally or by intermittent IV infusion. This drug is not administered IM. Unused portions of reconstituted oral suspensions and parenteral solutions are stable for 14 days when refrigerated after reconstitution.

☀ Nursing Alert

The nurse should administer each IV dose of vancomycin over 60 minutes. Too rapid an infusion may result in a sudden and profound fall in blood pressure and shock. When giving the drug IV, the nurse closely monitors the infusion rate and the patient's blood pressure. The nurse reports any decrease in blood pressure or reports of throbbing neck or back pain. These symptoms could indicate a severe adverse reaction referred to as "red neck" or "red man" syndrome. Symptoms of this syndrome include a sudden and profound fall in blood pressure, fever, chills, paresthesias, and erythema (redness) of the neck and back.

The nurse reports patient complaints of difficulty hearing or tinnitus (ringing in the ears) to the primary health care provider before the next dose is due. In addition, the nurse monitors the fluid intake and output and brings any decrease in the urinary output to the attention of the primary health care provider.

Monitoring and Managing Adverse Reactions

MANAGING ANXIETY. Patients may exhibit varying degrees of anxiety related to their illness and infection and the necessary drug therapy. When these drugs are given by the parenteral route, patients may experience anxiety because of the discomfort or pain that accompanies an IM injection or IV administration. The nurse reassures the patient that every effort will be made to reduce pain and discomfort although complete pain relief may not always be possible.

MANAGING DIARRHEA. Diarrhea may be a sign of a superinfection or pseudomembranous colitis, both of which are adverse reactions that may be seen with the administration of any anti-infective. The nurse checks each stool and reports any changes in color or consistency. When vancomycin is given as part of the treatment for pseudomembranous colitis, it is important to record the color and consistency of each stool to determine the effectiveness of therapy.

MANAGING PAIN. Pain at the injection site may occur when these drugs are given IM. The nurse warns the patient that discomfort may be felt when it is injected and that additional discomfort may be experienced for a brief time afterward. The nurse places a warm moist compress over the injection site to help alleviate the discomfort.

Home Care Checklist

ADMINISTERING PENTAMIDINE AT HOME

The patient may be required to receive aerosol pentamidine at home. Before discharge, the nurse checks to make sure that arrangements have been made to deliver the specialized equipment and supplies, such as a Respirgard II nebulizer and diluent, to the home. The nurse also instructs the patient and caregiver on how to administer the drug:

✓ Prepare the solution immediately before its use.

✓ Dissolve the contents of one vial in 6 mL sterile water and protect the solution from light.

✓ Place the entire solution in the reservoir. Do not put any other drugs into the reservoir.

✓ Attach the tubing to the nebulizer and reservoir.

✓ Place the mouthpiece in your mouth and turn on the nebulizer.

✓ Breathe in and out deeply and slowly. The entire treatment should last 30 to 45 minutes.

✓ Tap the reservoir periodically to ensure that all of the drug is aerosolized.

✓ When the treatment is finished, turn off the nebulizer.

✓ Clean the equipment according to the manufacturer's instructions.

✓ Allow tubing, reservoir, and mouthpiece to air dry.

✓ Store the equipment in a clean plastic bag and put it away for the next dose.

✓ Use a calendar to mark the days you are to receive the drug and check off each time you've done the treatment.

MONITORING FOR NEPHROTOXICITY AND OTOTOXICITY. It is important for the nurse to monitor for nephrotoxicity. The nurse measures and records intake and output during the time the patient is receiving these drugs. Any changes in the intake and output ratio or in the appearance of the urine must be reported immediately because these may indicate nephrotoxicity.

The nurse also closely monitors for ototoxicity in all patients receiving an anti-infective. It is important to report any ringing in the ears, difficulty hearing, or dizziness to the primary health care provider. Changes in hearing may not be noticed initially by the patient, but when changes occur they usually progress from difficulty in hearing high-pitched sounds to problems hearing low-pitched sounds.

Educating the Patient and Family

Anytime a drug is prescribed for a patient, the nurse is responsible to ensure that the patient has a thorough understanding of the drug, the treatment regimen, and the potential adverse reactions. Not all of the miscellaneous anti-infectives are prescribed for use within the clinical setting. Chloramphenicol, metronidazole, and

vancomycin can be given orally and prescribed for outpatient use. However, patients requiring oral chloramphenicol are usually hospitalized so that blood studies can be done during treatment.

When pentamidine is prescribed for aerosol use at home, the nurse reviews the use of the special nebulizer, as well as directions for cleaning and maintaining the nebulizer equipment (see Home Care Checklist: Administering Pentamidine at Home).

When metronidazole is prescribed, the nurse warns the patient to avoid the use of alcoholic beverages because a severe reaction may occur.

To decrease the chance of noncompliance, the nurse emphasizes the following points when any of these drugs are prescribed on an outpatient basis:

● Take the drug at the prescribed time intervals. These time intervals are important because a certain amount of the drug must be in the body at all times for the infection to be controlled.
● Take the drug with food or on an empty stomach as directed on the prescription container.

- Do not increase or omit the dose unless advised to do so by the primary health care provider.
- Complete the entire course of treatment. Do not stop the drug, except on the advice of a primary health care provider, before the course of treatment is completed even if symptoms have improved or have disappeared. Failure to complete the prescribed course of treatment may result in a return of the infection.
- Notify the primary health care provider if symptoms of the infection become worse or there is no improvement in the original symptoms after about 5 to 7 days.
- Contact the primary health care provider as soon as possible if a rash, fever, sore throat, diarrhea, chills, extreme fatigue, easy bruising, ringing in the ears, difficulty hearing, or other problems occur.
- Avoid drinking alcoholic beverages unless use has been approved by the primary health care provider.

EVALUATION

- The therapeutic drug effect is achieved and the infection is controlled.
- Adverse reactions are identified, reported to the primary health care provider, and managed successfully.
- Pain or discomfort following IM or IV administration is relieved or eliminated.
- Anxiety is reduced.
- The patient and family demonstrate understanding of the drug regimen.

● *Critical Thinking Exercises*

1. *The charge nurse asks you to discuss the drug metronidazole (Flagyl) at a team conference. Determine what specific points regarding administration and patient and family teaching you would discuss at the conference.*
2. *Mr. Stone is receiving vancomycin. One adverse reaction that may be seen with the administration of this drug is ototoxicity. Rather than ask Mr. Stone directly whether he is having any problem with his hearing, discuss how you might determine if ototoxicity might be occurring.*
3. *Mr. Reeves has a severe infection and is receiving chloramphenicol IV. The nurse notes several bruises on Mr. Reeves arm after 2 days of therapy. What action (if any) should the nurse take. Give a rationale for your answer.*

● *Review Questions*

1. When educating a patient about the drug linezolid the nurse instructs the patient _____.
   - **A.** to take the drug without food to enhance absorption
   - **B.** to avoid foods high in tyramine such as chocolate, coffee, tea, and red wine
   - **C.** to avoid alcohol for at least 10 days after taking the drug
   - **D.** that frequent liver function tests will be necessary while taking the drug

2. When giving a drug that is potentially neurotoxic, the nurse reports which of the patient's complaints related to neurotoxicity?
   - **A.** light-headedness and abdominal pain
   - **B.** severe headache and feeling chilly
   - **C.** numbness of the extremities and dizziness
   - **D.** blurred vision and tinnitus

3. When giving spectinomycin to Mr. Jackson for gonorrhea, the nurse advises him to _____.
   - **A.** return for a follow-up examination
   - **B.** limit his fluid intake to 1200 mL per day while taking the drug
   - **C.** return the next day for a second injection
   - **D.** avoid drinking alcohol for the next 10 days

4. When monitoring the IV infusion of vancomycin, the nurse makes sure the drug infuses over a period of 60 minutes because rapid infusion can result in a _____.
   - **A.** fluid overload and respiratory distress
   - **B.** sudden and profound fall in blood pressure
   - **C.** fluid deficit and dehydration
   - **D.** sudden and severe rise in blood pressure

● *Medication Dosage Problems*

1. A patient is prescribed 500 mg of vancomycin PO every 6 hours. The drug is available in 500-mg tablets. The nurse administers _____.

2. Metronidazole 250 mg IV is ordered. The drug is available in a vial with 500 mg/2 mL. The nurse administers _____.

3. The primary health care provider prescribes linezolid 400 mg PO. The drug is available as an oral suspension in a strength of 100 mg/5 mL. The nurse administers _____.

chapter 12

Antitubercular Drugs

Key Terms

anaphylactoid
  reactions
antitubercular drugs
bacteriostatic
circumoral
extrapulmonary
gout
Mycobacterium
  tuberculosis

nephrotoxicity
optic neuritis
ototoxicity
peripheral neuropathy
prophylactic
tinnitus
tuberculosis
vertigo

Chapter Objectives

On completion of this chapter, the student will:

- Discuss the drugs used in the treatment of tuberculosis.
- Discuss the uses, general drug action, contraindications, precautions, interactions, and general adverse reactions associated with the administration of the antitubercular drugs.
- Discuss important preadministration and ongoing assessment activities the nurse should perform on the patient taking an antitubercular drug.
- List some nursing diagnoses particular to a patient taking an antitubercular drug.
- Explain directly observed therapy (DOT).
- Discuss ways to promote an optimal response to therapy, how to manage adverse reactions, and important points to keep in mind when educating patients about the use of the antitubercular drugs.

Tuberculosis is a major health problem throughout the world, infecting more than 8 million individuals each year. It is the world's leading cause of death from infectious disease. Individuals living in crowded conditions, those with compromised immune systems, and individuals with debilitative conditions are especially susceptible to tuberculosis.

Tuberculosis is an infectious disease caused by the ***Mycobacterium tuberculosis*** bacillus. The pathogen is also referred to as the tubercle bacillus. The disease is transmitted from one person to another by droplets dispersed in the air when an infected person coughs or sneezes. These droplet nuclei are released into the air and inhaled by noninfected persons. Although tuberculosis primarily affects the lungs, other organs may also be affected. For example, if the immune system is poor, the infection can spread from the lungs to other organs of the body. **Extrapulmonary** (outside of the lungs) tuberculosis is the term used to distinguish tuberculosis affecting the lungs from infection with the *M. tuberculosis* bacillus in other organs of the body. Organs that can be affected include the liver, kidneys, spleen, and uterus. People with acquired immunodeficiency syndrome (AIDS) are at risk for tuberculosis because of

their compromised immune systems. Tuberculosis responds well to long-term treatment with a combination of three or more antitubercular drugs.

Antitubercular drugs are used to treat active cases of tuberculosis and as a **prophylactic** to prevent the spread of tuberculosis. The drugs used to treat tuberculosis do not "cure" the disease, but they render the patient noninfectious to others. Antitubercular drugs are classified as primary and second-line drugs. Primary (first-line) drugs provide the foundation for treatment. Second-line or secondary drugs are less effective and more toxic than primary drugs. These drugs are used in various combinations to treat tuberculosis. Sensitivity testing may be done to determine the most effective combination treatment, especially in areas of the country showing resistance. Second-line drugs are used to treat extrapulmonary tuberculosis or drug-resistant organisms. The primary antitubercular drugs are discussed in this chapter. Both primary and second-line antitubercular drugs are listed in the Summary Drug Table: Antitubercular Drugs. Certain fluoroquinolones such as ciprofloxacin, ofloxacin, levofloxacin, and sparfloxacin have proven effective against tuberculosis and are considered second-line drugs. See Chapter 10 for a discussion of the fluoroquinolones.

SUMMARY DRUG TABLE ANTITUBERCULAR DRUGS

GENERIC NAME	TRADE NAME*	USES	ADVERSE REACTIONS	DOSAGE RANGES
Primary Drugs				
ethambutol *eth-am´-byoo-tole*	Myambutol	Pulmonary tuberculosis (TB)	Optic neuritis, fever, pruritis, headache, nausea, anorexia, dermatitis, hypersensitivity, psychic disturbances	15–25 mg/kg/d PO
isoniazid *eye-soe-nye´-a-zid*	INH, Laniazid, Nydrazid, *generic*	Active TB; prophylaxis for TB	Peripheral neuropathy, nausea, vomiting, epigastric distress, jaundice, hepatitis, pyridoxine deficiency, skin eruptions, hypersensitivity	Active TB: up to 300 mg/d PO or up to 300 mg/d IM, to 900 mg IM 2–3 times/wk First-line treatment: 300 mg INH and 600 mg rifampin PO in single dose TB prophylaxis: 30 mg/d PO
pyrazinamide *peer-a-zin´-a-mide*	*generic*	Active TB	Hepatotoxicity, nausea, vomiting, diarrhea, myalgia, rashes	15–30 mg/kg/d maximum, 3 g/d PO; 50–70 mg/kg twice weekly PO
rifabutin *rif-ah-byou´-tin*	Mycobutin	Active TB	Nausea, vomiting, diarrhea, rash, discolored urine	300 mg PO as a single dose or BID
rifampin *rif-am´-pin*	Rifadin, Rimactane, *generic*	Active TB	Heartburn, drowsiness, fatigue, dizziness, epigastric distress, hematologic changes, renal insufficiency, rash	600 mg PO, IV
streptomycin *strep-toe-mye´-sin*	*generic*	TB; infections due to susceptible microorganisms	Nephrotoxicity, ototoxicity, numbness, tingling, paresthesia of the face, nausea, dizziness	Up to 1 g/d IM
isoniazid (150 mg) and rifampin 300 mg	Rifamate	TB	See individual drugs	1–2 tablets daily PO
Second-line Drugs				
aminosalicylate *a-meen-oh-sal´-sa-late* (p-aminosalicylic acid; 4-aminosalicylic acid)	Paser	TB	Nausea, vomiting, diarrhea, abdominal pain, hypersensitivity reactions	4 g (1 packet) PO TID
capreomycin sulfate *kap-ree-oh-mye´-sin*	Capastat Sulfate	TB	Hypersensitivity reactions, nephrotoxicity, hepatic impairment, pain and induration at injection site, ototoxicity	I g/d (maximum, 20 mg/kg/d) IM
cycloserine *sye-kloe-ser´-een*	Seromycin Pulvules	TB	Convulsions, somnolence, confusion, renal impairment, sudden development of congestive heart failure, psychoses	500 mg to 1 g PO in divided doses

*The term *generic* indicates the drug is available in generic form.

ACTIONS

Most antitubercular drugs are **bacteriostatic** (slow or retard the growth of bacteria) against the *M. tuberculosis* bacillus. These drugs usually act to inhibit bacterial cell wall synthesis, which slows the multiplication rate of the bacteria. Only isoniazid is bactericidal, with rifampin and streptomycin having some bactericidal activity.

USES

Antitubercular drugs are used in combination with other antitubercular drugs to treat active tuberculosis. Isoniazid (INH) is the only antitubercular drug used alone. While isoniazid is used in combination with other drugs for the treatment of primary tuberculosis, a primary use is in preventive therapy (prophylaxis) against tuberculosis. For example, when a diagnosis of tuberculosis is present, family members of the infected individual must be given prophylactic treatment with isoniazid for 6 months to 1 year. Display 12-1 identifies prophylactic uses for isoniazid.

RESISTANCE TO THE ANTITUBERCULAR DRUGS

Of increasing concern is the development of mutant strains of tuberculosis that are resistant to many of the antitubercular drugs currently in use. Bacterial resistance develops, sometimes rapidly, with the use of antitubercular drugs. Treatment is individualized and based on laboratory studies identifying the drugs to which the organism is susceptible. To slow the development of bacterial resistance, the Centers for Disease Control (CDC) recommends the use of three or more drugs with initial therapy, as well as in retreatment. Using a combination of drugs slows the development of bacterial resistance.

Tuberculosis caused by drug-resistant organisms should be considered in patients who have no response to therapy and in patients who have been treated in the past.

STANDARD TREATMENT

Standard treatment for tuberculosis is divided into two phases: the initial phase followed by a continuing phase. During the initial phase, drugs are used to kill the rapidly multiplying *M. tuberculosis* and to prevent drug resistance. The initial phase lasts approximately 2 months and the continuing phase approximately 4 months, with the total treatment regimen lasting for 6 to 9 months, depending on the patient's response to therapy.

The initial phase must contain three or more of the following drugs: isoniazid, rifampin, and pyrazinamide, along with either ethambutol or streptomycin. The CDC recommends treatment to begin as soon as possible after the diagnosis of tuberculosis. The treatment recommendation regimen is for the administration of rifampin, isoniazid, and pyrazinamide for a minimum of 2 months (8 weeks), followed by rifampin and isoniazid for 4 months (16 weeks) in areas with a low incidence of tuberculosis. In areas of high incidence of tuberculosis, the CDC recommends the addition of streptomycin or ethambutol for the first 2 months.

RETREATMENT

At times treatment fails due to noncompliance with the drug regimen or to inadequate initial drug treatment. When treatment fails, retreatment is necessary. Retreatment generally includes the use of four or more antitubercular drugs. Retreatment drug regimens most often consist of the secondary drugs ethionamide, aminosalicylic acid, cycloserine, and capreomycin. Ofloxacin and ciprofloxacin may also be used in retreatment. At times during retreatment, as many as seven or more drugs may be used, with the ineffective drugs discontinued when susceptibility test results are available.

This chapter will discuss the following primary antitubercular drugs: ethambutol, isoniazid, pyrazinamide, rifampin, and streptomycin. Other primary and secondary drugs are listed in the Summary Drug Table: Antitubercular Drugs.

DISPLAY 12-1 Prophylactic Uses for Isoniazid

Isoniazid may be used in the following situations:
- Household members and other close associates of those recently diagnosed as having tuberculosis
- Those whose tuberculin skin test has become positive in the last 2 years
- Those with positive skin tests whose radiographic findings indicate nonprogressive, healed, or quiescent (causing no symptoms) tubercular lesions
- Those at risk of developing tuberculosis (eg, those with Hodgkin's disease, severe diabetes mellitus, leukemia, and other serious illnesses and those receiving corticosteroids or drug therapy for a malignancy)
- All patients younger than 35 years (primarily children to age 7) who have a positive skin test
- Persons with acquired immunodeficiency syndrome or those who are positive for the human immunodeficiency virus and have a positive tuberculosis skin test or a negative tuberculosis skin test but a history of a prior significant reaction to purified protein derivative (a skin test for tuberculosis)

ETHAMBUTOL

ADVERSE REACTIONS

Optic neuritis (a decrease in visual acuity and changes in color perception), which appears to be related to the dose given and the duration of treatment, has occurred in some patients receiving ethambutol. Usually, this adverse reaction disappears when the drug is discontinued. Other adverse reactions are dermatitis, pruritus, **anaphylactoid reactions** (unusual or exaggerated allergic reactions), joint pain, anorexia, nausea, and vomiting.

CONTRAINDICATIONS, PRECAUTIONS, AND INTERACTIONS

Ethambutol is contraindicated in patients with a history of hypersensitivity to the drug. Ethambutol is not recommended for children younger than 13 years. The drug is used with caution during lactation, in patients with hepatic and renal impairment, and during pregnancy (Category B). Because of the danger of optic neuritis, the drug is used cautiously in patients with diabetic retinopathy or cataracts.

ISONIAZID

ADVERSE REACTIONS

The incidence of adverse reactions appears to be higher when larger doses of isoniazid are prescribed. Adverse reactions include hypersensitivity reactions, hematologic changes, jaundice, fever, skin eruptions, nausea, vomiting, and epigastric distress. Severe, and sometimes fatal, hepatitis has been associated with isoniazid therapy and may appear after many months of treatment. **Peripheral neuropathy** (numbness and tingling of the extremities) is the most common symptom of toxicity.

CONTRAINDICATIONS, PRECAUTIONS, AND INTERACTIONS

Isoniazid is contraindicated in patients with a history of hypersensitivity to the drug. The drug is used with caution during lactation, in patients with hepatic and renal impairment, and during pregnancy (Category C). Daily consumption of alcohol when taking isoniazid may result in a higher incidence of drug-related

hepatitis. Aluminum salts may reduce the oral absorption of isoniazid. The action of the anticoagulants may be enhanced when taken with isoniazid. There is a possibility of increased serum levels of phenytoin with concurrent use of isoniazid. When isoniazid is taken with foods containing tyramine, such as aged cheese and meats, bananas, yeast products, and alcohol, an exaggerated sympathetic-type response can occur (eg, hypertension, increased heart rate, palpitations).

PYRAZINAMIDE

ADVERSE REACTIONS

Hepatotoxicity is the principal adverse reaction seen with pyrazinamide use. Symptoms of hepatotoxicity may range from none (except for slightly abnormal hepatic function tests) to a more severe reaction such as jaundice. Nausea, vomiting, diarrhea, myalgia, and rashes also may be seen.

CONTRAINDICATIONS, PRECAUTIONS, AND INTERACTIONS

Pyrazinamide is contraindicated in patients with a history of hypersensitivity to the drug. The drug is also contraindicated in patients with acute **gout** (a metabolic disorder resulting in increased levels of uric acid) and in patients with severe hepatic damage. The drug is used with caution during lactation, in patients with hepatic and renal impairment, and during pregnancy (Category C). Pyrazinamide is used cautiously in patients infected with human immunodeficiency virus, who may require longer treatment, and in patients with diabetes mellitus, in whom management is more difficult. Pyrazinamide decreases the effects of allopurinol, colchicines, and probenecid.

RIFAMPIN

ADVERSE REACTIONS

Nausea, vomiting, epigastric distress, heartburn, fatigue, dizziness, rash, hematologic changes, and renal insufficiency may be seen with administration of rifampin. Rifampin may also cause a reddish-orange discoloration of body fluids, including urine, tears, saliva, sweat, and sputum.

CONTRAINDICATIONS, PRECAUTIONS, AND INTERACTIONS

Rifampin is contraindicated in patients with a history of hypersensitivity to the drug. The drug is used with caution during lactation, in patients with hepatic and renal impairment, and during pregnancy. Serum concentrations of digoxin may be decreased by rifampin. Isoniazid and rifampin administered concurrently may result in a higher risk of hepatotoxicity than when either drug is used alone. The use of rifampin with the oral anticoagulants or oral hypoglycemics may decrease the effects of the anticoagulant or hypoglycemic drug. There is a decrease in the effect of the oral contraceptives, chloramphenicol, phenytoin, and verapamil when these agents are administered concurrently with rifampin.

STREPTOMYCIN

ADVERSE REACTIONS

Nephrotoxicity (damage to the kidneys), **ototoxicity** (damage to the organs of hearing by a toxic substance), numbness, tingling, **tinnitus** (ringing in the ears), nausea, vomiting, **vertigo** (dizziness), and **circumoral** (around the mouth) paresthesia may be noted with the administration of streptomycin. Soreness at the injection site may also be noted, especially when the drug is given for a long time.

CONTRAINDICATIONS, PRECAUTIONS, AND INTERACTIONS

Streptomycin is contraindicated in patients with a history of hypersensitivity to the drug or any other aminoglycoside. Streptomycin is a Pregnancy Category D drug and can cause fetal harm when administered to a pregnant woman. This drug is used cautiously in patients with preexisting hearing difficulty or tinnitus and in patients with renal insufficiency. The ototoxic effects of streptomycin are potentiated when administered with ethacrynic acid, furosemide, and mannitol. (See Chapter 10 for additional information about streptomycin.)

NURSING PROCESS

● **The Patient Receiving an Antitubercular Drug**

ASSESSMENT

Preadministration Assessment

Once the diagnosis of tuberculosis is confirmed, the primary health care provider selects the drug that will best control the spread of the disease and make the patient noninfectious to others. Many laboratory and diagnostic tests may be necessary before starting antitubercular therapy, including radiographic studies, culture and sensitivity tests, and various types of laboratory tests, such as a complete blood count. It also is important to include a family history and a history of contacts, if the patient has active tuberculosis, as part of the assessment.

Depending on the severity of the disease, patients may be treated initially in the hospital and then discharged to their home for supervised follow-up care, or they may have all treatment instituted on an outpatient basis.

Ongoing Assessment

When performing the ongoing assessment, the nurse observes the patient daily for the appearance of adverse reactions. These observations are especially important when a drug is known to be nephrotoxic or ototoxic. It is important to report any adverse reactions to the primary health care provider. In addition, the nurse carefully monitors vital signs daily or as frequently as every 4 hours when the patient is hospitalized.

NURSING DIAGNOSES

Drug-specific nursing diagnoses are highlighted in the Nursing Diagnoses Checklist. The nursing diagnoses Noncompliance and Ineffective Management of Therapeutic Regimen also are discussed in Chapter 4.

PLANNING

The expected outcomes for the patient may include an optimal response to antitubercular therapy, management of common adverse reactions, and an understanding of and compliance with the prescribed treatment regimen.

IMPLEMENTATION

Promoting an Optimal Response to Therapy

The diagnosis, as well as the necessity of long-term treatment and follow-up, is often distressing to the

---

Nursing Diagnoses Checklist

☑ **Disturbed Sensory Perception: Tactile, Auditory, Visual** related to adverse reactions of antitubercular drugs

☑ **Risk for Impaired Skin Integrity** related to adverse reactions of the antitubercular drugs

☑ **Noncompliance** related to indifference, lack of knowledge, other factors

☑ **Risk of Ineffective Therapeutic Regimen Management** related to indifference, lack of knowledge, long-term treatment regimen, other factors

patient. Patients with a diagnosis of tuberculosis may have many questions about the disease and its treatment. The nurse allows time for the patient and family members to ask questions. In some instances, it may be necessary to refer the patient to other health care workers, such as a social service worker or a dietitian.

When administering the antitubercular drug by the parenteral route, the nurse is careful to rotate the injection sites. At the time of each injection, the nurse inspects previous injection sites for signs of swelling, redness, and tenderness. If a localized reaction persists or if the area appears to be infected, it is important to notify the primary health care provider.

The nurse should give antitubercular drugs by the oral route and on an empty stomach, unless gastric upset occurs. If gastric upset occurs, it is important to notify the primary health care provider before the next dose is given.

DIRECTLY OBSERVED THERAPY (DOT). Because the antitubercular drugs must be taken for prolonged periods, compliance with the treatment regimen becomes a problem and increases the risk of the development of resistant strains of tuberculosis. To help prevent the problem of noncompliance, directly observed therapy (DOT) is used to administer these drugs. When using DOT, the patient makes periodic visits to the office of the primary care provider or the health clinic, where the drug is taken in the presence of the nurse. The nurse watches the patient swallow each dose of the medication regimen. In some cases, the nurse uses the direct observation method to administer the antitubercular drug in the patient's home, place of employment, or school. DOT may occur daily or two to three times weekly, depending on the patient's health care regimen. Studies indicate that taking the antitubercular drugs intermittently does not cause a drop in the therapeutic blood levels of antitubercular drugs, even if the drugs were given only two or three times a week.

MANAGING VARIOUS TREATMENT REGIMENS. The nurse uses the following interventions in the management of patients receiving antitubercular drugs to promote an optimal response to therapy.

Ethambutol. The nurse administers ethambutol once every 24 hours at the same time each day. It is a good idea to give the drug with food to prevent gastric upset. If a dose is missed, the nurse should tell the patient not to double the dose the next day. The nurse should explain to the patient that the urine, feces, saliva, sputum, sweat, and tears may be colored reddish-orange or brownish-orange and that this is normal.

Isoniazid. The nurse gives isoniazid to the patient whose stomach is empty, at least 1 hour before or 2 hours after

meals. If gastrointestinal upset occurs, the patient can take the drug with food. The nurse teaches the patient to minimize alcohol consumption because of the increased risk of hepatitis. To prevent pyridoxine (vitamin B_6) deficiency, 6 to 50 mg pyridoxine daily may be prescribed.

Pyrazinamide. This drug is given once a day with food to prevent gastric upset. An alternative dosing regimen of twice weekly dosing has been developed to promote patient compliance on an outpatient basis. When administered on an outpatient basis, this drug, as well as the other antitubercular drugs, is administered using DOT.

Rifampin. The nurse administers rifampin once daily to the patient with an empty stomach, at least 1 hour before or 2 hours after meals. It is a good idea to explain to patients that their urine, feces, saliva, sputum, sweat, and tears may be colored reddish-orange and that this is normal.

Streptomycin. Streptomycin is usually administered daily as a single IM injection. The preferred site is the upper outer quadrant of the buttock or the midlateral thigh. The deltoid area is used only if the area is well developed. In patients 60 years of age or older, the dosage is reduced because of the risk of increased toxicity.

Monitoring and Managing Adverse Reactions

Managing adverse reactions in patients taking antitubercular drugs is an important responsibility of the nurse. The nurse must continuously observe for signs of adverse reactions and immediately report them to the primary health care provider. Some information specific to the different antitubercular drugs is provided below.

ETHAMBUTOL. The nurse monitors for any changes in visual acuity and promptly reports any visual changes to the primary health care provider. Vision changes are usually reversible if the drug is discontinued as soon as symptoms appear. The patient may need assistance with ambulation if visual disturbances occur. Psychic disturbances may occur. If the patient appears depressed, withdrawn, noncommunicative, or has other personality changes, the nurse must report the problem to the primary health care provider.

ISONIAZID. Severe and sometimes fatal hepatitis may occur with isoniazid therapy. The nurse must carefully monitor all patients at least monthly for any evidence of liver dysfunction. It is important to instruct patients to report any of the following symptoms: anorexia, nausea, vomiting, fatigue, weakness, yellowing of the skin or eyes, darkening of the urine, or numbness in the hands and feet.

❄ Gerontologic Alert

Older adults are particularly susceptible to a potentially fatal hepatitis when taking isoniazid, especially if they consume alcohol on a regular basis. Two other antitubercular drugs, rifampin and pyrazinamide, can cause liver dysfunction in the older adult. Careful observation and monitoring for signs of liver impairment are necessary (eg, increased serum aspartate transaminase, increased serum alanine transferase, increased serum bilirubin, and jaundice).

PYRAZINAMIDE. Patients should have baseline liver functions tests to use as a comparison when monitoring liver function during pyrazinamide therapy. The nurse should monitor the patient closely for symptoms of a decline in hepatic functioning (ie, yellowing of the skin, malaise, liver tenderness, anorexia, or nausea). The primary health care provider may order periodic liver function tests. Hepatotoxicity appears to be dose related and may appear at any time during therapy.

RIFAMPIN. The patient is informed about the reddish-orange or reddish-brown discoloration of body fluids (eg, tears, sweat, sputum, saliva). Advise the patient not to wear soft contact lenses during therapy because they may be permanently stained.

STREPTOMYCIN. This drug may cause ototoxicity, resulting in hearing loss. The nurse should monitor for any signs of hearing loss, including tinnitus, and vertigo. The patient may have hearing checked by audiometry before beginning therapy and periodically during therapy. Tinnitus, roaring noises, or a sense of fullness in the ears indicates the need for audiometric examination or termination of the drug. Hearing loss occurs most often for high-frequency sounds. These drugs must be discontinued if the patient reports any hearing loss or if tinnitus occurs. Prompt action by the nurse is critical in preventing permanent hearing loss.

Educating the Patient and Family

Antitubercular drugs are given for a long time, and careful patient and family education and close medical supervision are necessary. Noncompliance can be a problem whenever a disease or disorder requires long-term treatment. For this reason, the DOT method of administration is preferred. The patient and family must understand that short-term therapy is of no value in treating this disease. The nurse remains alert for statements made by the patient or family that may indicate future noncompliance with the drug regimen necessary in controlling the disease. (See Patient and Family Teaching Checklist: Increasing Compliance in Tubercular Drug Treatment Programs.)

Patient and Family Teaching Checklist

Increasing Compliance in Tubercular Drug Treatment Program

The nurse:

☑ Discusses tuberculosis, its causes and communicability, and the need for long-term therapy for disease control.

☑ Reinforces that short-term treatment is ineffective.

☑ Reviews the drug therapy regimen, including the prescribed drugs, doses, and frequency of administration.

☑ Reassures the patient that various combinations of drugs are effective in treating tuberculosis.

☑ Urges the patient to take the drugs exactly as prescribed and not to omit, increase, or decrease the dosage unless directed to do so by the health care provider.

☑ Instructs the patient about possible adverse reactions and the need to notify prescriber should any occur.

☑ Arranges for direct observation therapy with the patient and family.

☑ Instructs the patient in measures to minimize gastrointestinal upset.

☑ Advises the patient to avoid alcohol and the use of nonprescription drugs, especially those containing aspirin, unless use is approved by the health care provider.

☑ Reassures the patient and family that the results of therapy will be monitored by periodic laboratory and diagnostic tests and follow-up visits with the health care provider.

The nurse reviews the dosage schedule and adverse effects associated with the prescribed antitubercular drug with the patient and family. Information that applies to all patients taking these drugs includes:

- The results of antitubercular therapy will be monitored at periodic intervals. Laboratory and diagnostic tests and visits to the primary health care provider's office or clinic are necessary.
- Take these drugs exactly as directed on the prescription container. Do not omit, increase, or decrease a dose unless advised to do so by the primary health care provider.
- Avoid the use of nonprescription drugs, especially those containing aspirin, unless use has been approved by the primary health care provider.
- Discuss the drinking of alcoholic beverages with the primary health care provider. A limited amount of alcohol may be allowed, but excessive intake should usually be avoided.

The nurse includes the following information in the teaching plan when a specific antitubercular drug is prescribed:

Ethambutol: Take this drug once a day at the same time each day. If a dose is missed, do not double the dose the next day. Notify the primary health care provider of any changes in vision or the occurrence of a skin rash.

Isoniazid: Take this drug 1 hour before or 2 hours after meals. However, if gastric upset occurs, take isoniazid with food. Notify the primary health care provider of weakness, yellowing of the skin, loss of appetite, darkening of the urine, skin rashes, or numbness or tingling of the hands or feet. Avoid tyramine-containing foods (see Chap. 31). To prevent pyridoxine (vitamin B_6) deficiency, 6 to 50 mg of pyridoxine daily may be prescribed.

Pyrazinamide: Notify the primary health care provider if any of the following occurs: nausea, vomiting, loss of appetite, fever, malaise, visual changes, yellow discoloration of the skin, or severe pain in the knees, feet, or wrists. (Note: Pain in these areas may be a sign of active gout.)

Rifampin: Take the drug once daily on an empty stomach (1 hour before or 2 hours after meals). A reddish-brown or reddish-orange discoloration of tears, sputum, urine, or sweat may occur. Soft contact lenses may be permanently stained if worn while the patient is taking the drug. Notify the primary health care provider of any yellow discoloration of the skin, fever, chills, unusual bleeding or bruising, and skin rash or itching. If taking an oral contraceptive, check with primary health care provider because reliability of the contraceptive may be affected.

EVALUATION

- The therapeutic effect is achieved.
- Adverse reactions are identified, reported to the primary health care provider, and managed successfully.
- The patient verbalizes an understanding of treatment modalities and the importance of continued follow-up care.
- The patient and family demonstrate understanding of the drug regimen.
- The patient complies with the prescribed drug regimen.

● *Critical Thinking Exercises*

1. *Ms. Burns has received a diagnosis of tuberculosis. She is concerned because her primary health care provider has informed her that the treatment regimen consists of three drugs, isoniazid, rifampin, and pyrazinamide, taken for the next 2 months, followed by a 4-month treatment regimen with two of the drugs.*

Determine what rationales the nurse can give Ms. Burns for the use of multiple drugs and the need for long-term therapy.

2. *While Mr. Johnson is taking isoniazid, explain what instructions the nurse should give him concerning side effects.*

● *Review Questions*

1. The nurse explains to the patient that to slow bacterial resistance to an antitubercular drug the primary health care provider may prescribe _____.
   A. at least three antitubercular drugs
   B. an antibiotic to be given with the drug
   C. vitamin B_6
   D. that the drug be given only once a week

2. Which of the following drugs is the only antitubercular drug to be prescribed alone?
   A. rifampin
   B. pyrazinamide
   C. streptomycin
   D. isoniazid

3. The nurse monitors the patient taking isoniazid for toxicity. The most common symptom of toxicity is _____.
   A. peripheral edema
   B. circumoral edema
   C. peripheral neuropathy
   D. jaundice

4. Which of the following is a dose-related adverse reaction to ethambutol?
   A. peripheral neuropathy
   B. optic neuritis
   C. hyperglycemia
   D. fatal hepatitis

5. Which of the following antitubercular drugs is contraindicated in patients with gout?
   A. rifampin
   B. streptomycin
   C. isoniazid
   D. pyrazinamide

● *Medication Dosage Problems*

1. A patient is prescribed isoniazid syrup 300 mg. The isoniazid is available as 50 mg/mL. The nurse should administer _____.

2. Rifampin 600 mg PO is prescribed. The drug is available in 150-mg tablets. The nurse should administer _____.

Leprostatic Drugs

Key Terms

hemolysis
leprosy

Mycobacterium
leprae

Chapter Objectives

On completion of this chapter, the student will:

- Discuss the drugs used in the treatment of leprosy.
- Discuss the uses, general drug action, contraindications, precautions, interactions, and general adverse reactions associated with the administration of the leprostatic drugs.
- Discuss important preadministration and ongoing assessment activities the nurse should perform on the patient taking a leprostatic drug.
- List some nursing diagnoses particular to a patient taking a leprostatic drug.
- Discuss the ways to promote an optimal response to therapy, how to manage adverse reactions, and important points to keep in mind when educating patients about the use of the leprostatic drugs.

Leprosy is a chronic, communicable disease spread by prolonged, intimate contact with an infected person. Peripheral nerves are affected, and skin involvement is present. Lesions may be confined to a few isolated areas or may be fairly widespread over the entire body. Treatment with the leprostatic drugs provides a good prospect for controlling the disease and preventing complications.

Leprosy, also referred to as Hansen's disease, is caused by the bacterium *Mycobacterium leprae.* Although rare in colder climates, this disease may be seen in tropical and subtropical zones. Dapsone and clofazimine (Lamprene) are the two drugs currently used to treat leprosy. The leprostatic drugs are listed in the Summary Drug Table: Leprostatic Drugs.

CLOFAZIMINE

ACTIONS AND USES

Clofazimine is primarily bactericidal against *M. leprae.* The exact mode of action of this drug is unknown. Clofazimine is used to treat leprosy.

ADVERSE REACTIONS

Clofazimine may cause pigmentation of the skin, abdominal pain, diarrhea, nausea, and vomiting.

CONTRAINDICATIONS, PRECAUTIONS, AND INTERACTIONS

Clofazimine is used cautiously in patients with gastrointestinal disorders, diarrhea, and during pregnancy (Pregnancy Category C) and lactation. If clofazimine is used during pregnancy, the infant may be born with pigmented skin. No significant drug–drug interactions are associated with the use of clofazimine.

DAPSONE

ACTIONS AND USES

Dapsone is bactericidal and bacteriostatic against *M. leprae.* The drug is used to treat leprosy. Dapsone

SUMMARY DRUG TABLE LEPROSTATIC DRUGS

GENERIC NAME	TRADE NAME*	USES	ADVERSE REACTIONS	DOSAGE RANGES
clofazimine *kloe-fazz-ih-meen*	Lamprene	Leprosy	Skin pigmentation (pink to brownish-black), skin dryness, rash, abdominal/epigastric pain, nausea, dryness, burning, or itching of the eyes	100–200 mg/d PO
dapsone *dap´-sone*	generic	Leprosy; dermatitis herpetiformis	Blood cell hemolysis, anemia, peripheral neuropathy, headache, insomnia, phototoxicity, nausea, vomiting, anorexia, blurred vision	50–300 mg/d PO

*The term *generic* indicates the drug is available in generic form.

may also be used in the treatment of dermatitis herpetiformis, a chronic, inflammatory skin disease.

ADVERSE REACTIONS

Administration of dapsone may result in **hemolysis** (destruction of red blood cells), nausea, vomiting, anorexia, and blurred vision.

CONTRAINDICATIONS, PRECAUTIONS, AND INTERACTIONS

Dapsone is used with caution in patients with anemia, severe cardiopulmonary disease, hepatic dysfunction, and during pregnancy (Pregnancy Category C). Dapsone is contraindicated during lactation. Substantial amounts of dapsone are excreted in breast milk and can cause hemolytic reactions in neonates. No significant drug–drug interactions are associated with the use of dapsone.

NURSING PROCESS

● **The Patient Receiving a Leprostatic Drug**

ASSESSMENT

Preadministration Assessment

It is important to perform a complete physical examination and history before the institution of therapy. The nurse examines the involved areas and describes them in detail on the patient's record to provide a database for comparison during therapy.

ONGOING ASSESSMENT

These drugs are often given on an outpatient basis. Each time the patient is seen in the clinic or primary health care provider's office, the nurse performs a general physical examination, with particular attention given to the affected areas.

NURSING DIAGNOSES

Drug-specific nursing diagnoses are highlighted in the Nursing Diagnoses Checklist. More general nursing diagnoses applicable to these drugs are discussed in depth in Chapter 4.

PLANNING

The expected outcomes for the patient may include an optimal response to drug therapy and an understanding of and compliance with the prescribed treatment regimen.

IMPLEMENTATION

Promoting an Optimal Response to Therapy

Treatment with a leprostatic drug may require many years. These patients are faced with long-term medical and drug therapy and possibly severe disfigurement. The nurse must spend time with these patients, allowing them to verbalize their anxieties, problems, and fears.

It is important to give the leprostatic drugs orally and with food to minimize gastric upset. The nurse can give antitubercular drugs, such as rifampin, concurrently

Nursing Diagnoses Checklist

☑ **Impaired Skin Integrity** related to adverse reactions of the leprostatic drugs

during initial therapy to minimize bacterial resistance to the leprostatic drug.

Educating the Patient and Family

The nurse is alert to patient statements regarding compliance with the long-term treatment regimen. It is important to note factors, such as depression or indifference, that may be indicative of treatment noncompliance. The nurse uses a positive approach when doing patient and family teaching. The nurse informs the patient that changes in skin pigmentation may occur, ranging from red to brownish-black. Skin discoloration may take months to years to reverse after use of the drug is discontinued.

To ensure compliance with the treatment regimen, the nurse explains the dosage schedule, possible adverse effects, and the importance of scheduled follow-up visits to the patient and family members. In particular, the nurse emphasizes the importance of adhering to the prescribed dosage schedule.

EVALUATION

- The therapeutic drug effect is achieved.
- The patient verbalizes an understanding of treatment modalities and the importance of continued follow-up care.
- The patient and family demonstrate understanding of the drug regimen.
- The patient complies with the prescribed drug regimen.

● Critical Thinking Exercises

1. *Mr. Winters is very anxious about his newly diagnosed leprosy and his treatment regimen with dapsone. Discuss what you could do to decrease his anxiety. Determine what information you would include when educating Mr. Winters about the treatment regimen.*
2. *Mr. York has been prescribed clofazimine daily to manage his leprosy. Discuss what preadministration assessments the nurse should make. Explain what information you would include in a teaching plan for Mr. York.*

● Review Questions

1. Before administration of the initial dose of a leprostatic drug, it is most important for the nurse to assess _____.
   - **A.** range of motion
   - **B.** mental ability
   - **C.** vital signs
   - **D.** affected areas on the patient's body

2. Which of the following adverse reactions would the nurse expect with the administration of clofazimine?
   - **A.** hypotension
   - **B.** blurred vision
   - **C.** pigmentation of the skin
   - **D.** jaundice

3. Which of the following hematologic changes may result from the administration of dapsone?
   - **A.** hemolysis
   - **B.** leukopenia
   - **C.** decreased platelets
   - **D.** increase in the hematocrit

4. When educating the patient about taking a leprostatic drug, the nurse would include which of the following information?
   - **A.** This drug regimen will require that you take the drug faithfully for at least 3 months.
   - **B.** Take the drug with food to minimize gastric upset.
   - **C.** Skin lesions should clear within 3 days.
   - **D.** The drug should be taken on an empty stomach at bedtime to minimize gastric upset.

● Medication Dosage Problems

1. The patient is prescribed 150 mg of dapsone. On hand are 50-mg tablets. The nurse administers _____.

2. A patient with leprosy is prescribed clofazimine 100 mg daily PO. The drug is available in 200-mg tablets. The nurse administers _____.

c h a p t e r **14**

Antiviral Drugs

Key Terms

anticholinergic effects
exacerbations
granulocytopenia
remissions
retinitis

Chapter Objectives

On completion of this chapter, the student will:

- Discuss the uses, general drug action, adverse reactions, contraindications, precautions, and interactions of antiviral drugs.
- Discuss important preadministration and ongoing assessment activities the nurse should perform on the patient receiving an antiviral drug.
- List some nursing diagnoses particular to a patient taking an antiviral drug.
- List possible goals for a patient taking an antiviral drug.
- Discuss ways to promote an optimal response to therapy, how to manage adverse reactions, and special considerations to keep in mind when educating the patient and the family about the antiviral drugs.

More than 200 viruses have been identified as capable of producing disease. Acute viruses, such as the common cold, have a rapid onset and quick recovery. Chronic viral infections, such as acquired immunodeficiency syndrome (AIDS), have recurrent episodes of **exacerbations** (increases in severity of symptoms of the disease) and **remissions** (periods of partial or complete disappearance of the signs and symptoms). Display 14-1 describes the viruses discussed in this chapter.

Although viral infections are common, for many years only a limited number of drugs were available for their treatment. Over the past several years, the number of antiviral drugs has increased significantly. Several of the antiviral drugs will be discussed in greater detail than others. These include acyclovir (Zovirax), amantadine (Symmetrel), didanosine (Videx), ribavirin (Virazole), zanamivir (Relenza), and zidovudine (AZT, Retrovir). The Summary Drug Table: Antiviral Drugs presents a more complete listing of the antiviral drugs currently in use.

ACTIONS

Viruses can reproduce only within a living cell. A virus consists of either DNA or RNA surrounded by a protein shell. The virus is capable of reproducing only when it

Herbal Alert: Lemon Balm

Lemon balm is a perennial herb with heart-shaped leaves that has been used for hundreds of years. Its scientific name is Melissa officinalis. Traditionally the herb has been used for Graves' disease (see Chap. 51), as a sedative, antispasmodic, and an antiviral agent. When used topically, lemon balm has antiviral activity against herpes simplex virus (HSV). No adverse reactions have been reported when lemon balm is used topically.

uses the body's cellular material (Fig. 14-1). Most antiviral drugs act by inhibiting viral DNA or RNA replication in the virus, causing viral death.

USES

Although infections caused by a virus are common, antiviral drugs have limited use because they are effective against only a small number of specific viral infections.

General uses of the antiviral drugs include the treatment of:

- Initial and recurrent mucosal and cutaneous herpes simplex virus (HSV) 1 and 2 infections in

Other contraindications and precautions are listed below, according to the specific drug. Numerous interactions are possible with the antiviral drugs. Only the most significant interactions are listed for selected drugs. The nurse should consult an appropriate source for a more extensive listing of interactions.

Acyclovir

This drug is used cautiously in patients with pre-existing neurologic, renal, hepatic, respiratory, or fluid and electrolyte abnormalities. The nurse gives the drug with caution to patients with a history of seizures. Acyclovir is a Pregnancy Category C drug and is used cautiously during pregnancy and lactation. Incidences of extreme drowsiness have occurred when acyclovir is given with zidovudine. There is an increased risk of nephrotoxicity when acyclovir is administered with other nephrotoxic drugs. When administered with amphotericin B, the risk of nephrotoxicity is increased. Administration with probenecid causes a decrease in the renal excretion of acyclovir, prolonging the effects of acyclovir and increasing the risk of drug toxicity.

Amantadine

Amantadine is used cautiously in patients with seizure disorders, psychiatric problems, renal impairment, and cardiac disease. Amantadine is a Pregnancy Category B drug and is used cautiously during pregnancy and lactation. Concurrent use of antihistamines, phenothiazines, tricyclic antidepressants, disopyramide, and quinidine may increase the **anticholinergic effects** (dry mouth, blurred vision, constipation) of amantadine.

Didanosine

This drug is used cautiously in patients with peripheral vascular disease, neuropathy, chronic pancreatitis, or impaired liver function. Didanosine is a Pregnancy Category B drug and is used cautiously during pregnancy and lactation. There may be a decrease in the effectiveness of dapsone in preventing *Pneumocystis carinii* pneumonia when didanosine is administered with dapsone. Use of didanosine with zalcitabine may cause additive neuropathy. Absorption of didanosine is decreased when it is administered with food.

Ribavirin

Ribavirin may be teratogenic and embryotoxic (Pregnancy Category X) and is contraindicated during pregnancy, in patients with chronic obstructive pulmonary disease (COPD), and during lactation. Ribavirin is used cautiously at all times during administration of the drug. Ribavirin may antagonize the antiviral action of zidovudine and potentiate the hematologic toxic effects of zidovudine. When ribavirin is used concurrently with digitalis, the risk of digitalis toxicity increases.

Zanamivir

Zanamivir is used cautiously with pregnancy (Category C), lactation, asthma, COPD, or other underlying respiratory diseases. No significant drug interactions have been reported with the use of zanamivir.

Zidovudine

This drug is used cautiously in patients with bone marrow depression or severe hepatic or renal impairment. Zidovudine is a Pregnancy Category C drug and is used cautiously during pregnancy and lactation. There is an increased risk of bone marrow depression when zidovudine is administered with antineoplastic drugs, other drugs causing bone marrow depression, and in patients having or recently taking radiation therapy. An additive neurotoxicity may occur when zidovudine is administered with acyclovir. Clarithromycin decreases blood levels of zidovudine. The blood levels of zidovudine are increased when it is given with lamivudine.

N U R S I N G   P R O C E S S

● **The Patient Receiving an Antiviral Drug**

ASSESSMENT

Preadministration Assessment

Preadministration assessment of the patient receiving an antiviral drug depends on the patient's symptoms or diagnosis. These patients may have a serious infection that causes a decrease in their natural defenses against disease. Before administering the antiviral drug, the nurse determines the patient's general state of health and resistance to infection. The nurse then records the patient's symptoms and complaints. In addition, the nurse takes and records the patient's vital signs. Additional assessments may be necessary in certain types of viral infections or in patients who are acutely ill. For example, in patients with HSV 1 or 2 the nurse inspects the areas of the body affected with the lesions (eg, the mouth, face, eyes, or genitalia) before treatment for comparison during treatment.

Ongoing Assessment

The ongoing assessment depends on the reason for giving the antiviral drug. It is important to make a daily assessment for improvement of the signs and symptoms

Nursing Diagnoses Checklist

✓ **Risk for Imbalanced Nutrition: Less than Body Requirements** related to adverse reaction of antiviral drugs

✓ **Risk for Impaired Skin Integrity** related to initial infection, adverse drug reactions, IV administration of the antiviral drug

✓ **Risk for Injury** related to adverse reactions of the drug

✓ **Risk for Infection** related to inadequate defense mechanisms (immunosuppression)

identified in the initial assessment. The nurse monitors for and reports any adverse reactions from the antiviral drug. It also is important to inspect the IV site several times a day for redness, inflammation, or pain. The nurse should report any signs of phlebitis (inflammation of the vein).

NURSING DIAGNOSES

Drug-specific nursing diagnoses are highlighted in the Nursing Diagnoses Checklist. Other, more general nursing diagnoses applicable to the antiviral drugs are discussed in Chapter 4.

PLANNING

The expected outcomes for the patient depend on the reason for administration of the antiviral drug but may include an optimal response to therapy, management of adverse reactions, and an understanding of and compliance with the prescribed treatment regimen.

IMPLEMENTATION

Promoting an Optimal Response to Therapy

Because these drugs may be used in the treatment of certain types of severe and sometimes life-threatening viral infections, the patient may be concerned about the diagnosis and prognosis. The nurse should allow the patient time to talk and ask questions about methods of treatment, especially when the drug is given IV. It is important to explain the treatment methods to the patient and family members.

The antiviral drugs are not given intramuscularly or subcutaneously. It is important to prepare the antiviral drugs according to the manufacturer's directions. The administration rate is ordered by the primary health care provider. The nurse takes care to prevent trauma because even slight trauma can result in bruising if the platelet count is low. If injections are given, pressure is applied at the injection site to prevent bleeding. Occasionally, headache or a slight fever may occur in patients taking antiviral drugs. An analgesic may be prescribed to manage these effects.

ACYCLOVIR. Treatment with acyclovir is begun as soon as symptoms of herpes simplex appear. The drug may be given topically, orally, or intravenously. When the drug is given orally, the nurse may give the drug without regard to food. However, if GI upset occurs, acyclovir is administered with food. Patients with a history of congestive heart failure may not be able to tolerate an increase in fluids, so it is important to monitor them closely to prevent fluid overload. Neurologic symptoms such as seizures may occur with the administration of acyclovir. When the drug is administered topically, the nurse should use a finger cot or glove to prevent spread of infection.

AMANTADINE. The nurse administers this drug for the prevention or treatment of respiratory tract illness caused by influenza A virus. Some patients are prescribed this drug to manage extrapyramidal effects caused by drugs used to treat Parkinsonism (See Chaps. 29 and 32). The nurse should protect the capsules from moisture to prevent deterioration. When the drug is administered for symptoms of influenza, it is important to start therapy within 24 to 48 hours after symptoms begin.

DIDANOSINE. For patients with HIV infection who cannot tolerate zidovudine or who have exhibited decreased therapeutic effect with zidovudine, the nurse should administer this drug to the patient with an empty stomach (at least 1 hour before or 2 hours after meals). The tablets are not swallowed whole; the patient should chew them or crush and mix them thoroughly with at least 1 oz of water. The nurse mixes buffered powder with 4 oz of water (not juice), stirs until dissolved, and gives it to the patient to drink immediately. The nurse avoids generating dust when preparing the medication. When cleaning up powdered products, a wet mop or damp sponge is used. The surface is cleaned with soap and water.

RIBAVIRIN. The nurse gives ribavirin by inhalation using a small particle aerosol generator (SPAG-2 aerosol generator). It is important to discard and replace the solution every 24 hours. Treatment with ribavirin lasts for at least 3 days, but not more than 7, for 12 to 18 h/d. Women of childbearing age should not take this drug because evidence links it to birth defects.

ZANAMIVIR. This drug is available as a powder blister for inhalation. The usual dose is 2 inhalations (one 5-mg blister per inhalation) administered with a Diskhaler device. The drug should be started within 2 days' onset of flu symptoms. The drug is taken every 12 hours.

ZIDOVUDINE. The nurse assesses the patient for an increase in severity of symptoms of HIV and for symptoms of opportunistic infections. Capsules and syrup should be protected from light.

Monitoring and Managing Adverse Reactions

Serious adverse reactions can occur in patients taking antiviral drugs. The nurse must notify the primary health care provider of any adverse reactions to these drugs.

ACYCLOVIR. When given IV, acyclovir can cause crystalluria (presence of crystals in the urine) and mental confusion. The nurse helps the patient maintain adequate hydration to prevent crystalluria by encouraging the patient to drink 2000 to 3000 mL of fluid each day (if the disease condition permits). In addition, the nurse should give careful attention to assessing the mental status of the patient.

AMANTADINE. The nurse should monitor the patient for the occurrence of drowsiness, dizziness, light-headedness, or mood changes (irritability or mood change).

DIDANOSINE. Although rare, pancreatitis and peripheral neuropathy are possible adverse reactions seen with didanosine. The nurse must be alert for symptoms of pancreatitis (nausea, vomiting, abdominal pain, jaundice, elevated enzymes) and for signs of peripheral neuropathy (numbness, tingling, or pain in the feet or hands). It is important to immediately report these signs to the primary health care provider.

RIBAVIRIN. This drug can cause worsening of the respiratory status. Sudden deterioration of respiratory status can occur in infants receiving ribavirin. It is important to monitor respiratory function closely throughout therapy. The nurse should immediately report any worsening of respiratory function to the primary health care provider.

ZANAMIVIR. There is a risk for bronchospasm in patients with asthma or COPD. A fast-acting bronchodilator should be on hand in case bronchospasm occurs. Zanamivir use should be discontinued and the primary health care provider notified promptly if respiratory symptoms worsen.

ZIDOVUDINE. With zidovudine, bone marrow depression may occur, making the patient susceptible to infection and easy bruising. The patient is protected against individuals with upper respiratory infection. All caregivers are reminded to use good handwashing technique. The nurse takes care to prevent trauma because even slight trauma can result in bruising if the platelet count is low. If injections are given, pressure is applied at the injection site to prevent bleeding.

NUTRITIONAL IMBALANCE. The antiviral drugs may cause anorexia, nausea, or vomiting. These effects range from mild to severe. The patient may be able to tolerate small, frequent meals with soft, nonirritating foods if nausea is mild. Frequent sips of carbonated beverages or hot tea may be helpful for others. It is important to keep the atmosphere clean and free of odors. The nurse provides good oral care before and after meals. If nausea is severe or the patient is vomiting, the nurse notifies the primary health care provider.

IMPAIRED SKIN INTEGRITY. The nurse monitors the skin lesions carefully for worsening or improvement. Should the lesions not improve, the nurse informs the primary health care provider. Accurate observation and documentation is essential. If an antiviral drug is administered topically, the nurse uses gloves when applying to avoid spreading the infection. These drugs may also cause a rash as an adverse reaction. The nurse notes and reports any rash to the primary health care provider. When administering the drug by the IV route, the nurse must closely observe the injection site for signs of phlebitis, and depending on the patient's symptoms, the nurse monitors vital signs every 4 hours or as ordered by the primary health care provider.

RISK FOR INJURY. Some patients with a viral infection are acutely ill. Others may experience fatigue, lethargy, dizziness, or weakness as an adverse reaction to the antiviral agent. The nurse monitors these patients carefully. Call lights are placed in a convenient place for the patient and are answered promptly by the nurse. If fatigue, dizziness, or weakness is present, the patient may require assistance with ambulation or activities of daily living. The nurse plans activities so as to provide adequate rest periods.

RISK FOR INFECTION IN IMMUNOSUPPRESSED PATIENTS. When patients are immunosuppressed, they are at increased risk for bacterial or other infection. The patient is protected against individuals with upper respiratory infection. All caregivers are reminded to use good handwashing technique.

✳ Nursing Alert

Patients receiving antiviral drugs for HIV infections may continue to develop opportunistic infections and other complications of HIV. The nurse monitors all patients closely for signs of infection such as fever (even low-grade fever), malaise, sore throat, or lethargy.

Educating the Patient and Family

When an antiviral drug is given orally, the nurse explains the dosage regimen to the patient and family.

The nurse instructs the patient to take the drug exactly as directed and for the full course of therapy. If a dose is missed, the patient should take it as soon as remembered but should not double the dose at the next dosage time. Any adverse reactions should be reported to the primary health care provider or the nurse. The patient must understand that these drugs do not cure viral infections but should decrease symptoms and increase feelings of well-being.

The nurse instructs patients to report any symptoms of infection such as an elevated temperature (even a slight elevation), sore throat, difficulty breathing, weakness, or lethargy. The patient must be aware of possible signs of pancreatitis (nausea, vomiting, abdominal pain, jaundice [yellow discoloration of the skin or eyes]) and peripheral neuritis (tingling, burning, numbness, or pain in the hands or feet). Any indication of pancreatitis or peripheral neuritis must be reported at once.

The nurse includes the following information in the teaching plan for specific antiviral drugs:

- Acyclovir: This drug is not a cure for herpes simplex, but it will shorten the course of the disease and promote healing of the lesions. The drug will not prevent the spread of the disease to others. Topical application should not exceed the frequency prescribed. Apply this drug with a finger cot or gloves and cover all lesions. Do not have sexual contact while lesions are present. Notify the primary health care provider if burning, stinging, itching, or rash worsens or becomes pronounced.
- Amantadine: Do not drive a car or do work for which mental alertness is necessary until the effect of the drug is apparent because vision and coordination can be affected. Rise slowly from a prone to a sitting position to decrease the possibility of light-headedness caused by orthostatic hypotension. Report changes such as nervousness, tremors, slurred speech, or depression. Some patients are on an alternate dosage schedule. If this is the situation, it is important to mark the calendar to designate the days the drug is to be taken.
- Didanosine: Take this drug on an empty stomach because food decreases absorption. Follow the instructions for administration carefully. Crush the drug and mix it with water. Discontinue use of the drug and notify the primary health care provider if any numbness or tingling of the extremities is experienced. Report any signs of abdominal pain, nausea, or vomiting. Didanosine is not a cure for AIDS and does not prevent the spread of the disease, but it may decrease the symptoms of AIDS.
- Ribavirin: The patient is told that this drug is given with a small-particle aerosol generator. Any worsening of respiratory function, dizziness, confusion, or

shortness of breath should be reported. If a child is taking this drug it is important for any female caregivers to know that the drug is a Pregnancy Category X drug and women of childbearing age should take care not to inhale the drug. It may be necessary for the mother or other females of childbearing age who have direct contact with the child to observe respiratory precautions while the child is taking the drug.
- Zanamivir: This drug is taken every 12 hours for 5 days using a Diskhaler delivery system. If a bronchodilator is also prescribed, the bronchodilator is used before the zanamivir if both are prescribed at the same time. The drug may cause dizziness. The patient should use caution if driving an automobile or operating dangerous machinery. Treatment with this drug does not decrease the risk of transmission of the "flu" to others.
- Zidovudine: This drug may cause dizziness. Avoid activities requiring alertness until the drug response is known. This drug does not cure AIDS and does not prevent transmission to others. Notify the primary health care provider if fever, sore throat, or signs of infection occur. The primary health care provider may prescribe frequent blood tests to monitor for a decrease in the immune response indicating the need to decrease the dosage or to discontinue use of the drug for a period of time.

EVALUATION

- The therapeutic effect is achieved and symptoms of disease process subside or diminish.
- Adverse reactions are identified, reported to the primary health care provider, and managed successfully through nursing interventions.
- The patient and family demonstrate an understanding of the drug regimen.
- The patient verbalizes the importance of complying with the prescribed treatment regimen.

● *Critical Thinking Exercises*

1. *A young mother is concerned because her 2-month-old daughter has received a diagnosis of RSV. The infant is receiving inhalation treatments with ribavirin. The mother questions this treatment. Describe how the nurse could explain treatment with ribavirin to the mother. Discuss what possible effects the drug could have on the infant and on the mother.*
2. *Ms. Jenkins, age 77 years, has herpes zoster. The primary health care provider prescribes acyclovir 200 mg every 4 hours while awake. Discuss what information you would give Ms. Jenkins concerning herpes zoster, the drug regimen, and the possible adverse reactions.*

3. *Jim, age 25 years, has recently received a diagnosis of HIV infection and is placed on a treatment regimen of zidovudine and lamivudine. Determine what information you would give him concerning the drugs he will be taking. What adverse reactions would you discuss with Jim?*

● Review Questions

1. Which of the following adverse reactions would the nurse expect in a patient receiving acyclovir by the oral route?

A. nausea and vomiting
B. constipation and urinary frequency
C. conjunctivitis and blurred vision
D. nephrotoxicity

2. Which of the following would the nurse report immediately in a 3-month-old patient receiving ribavirin?

A. any worsening of the respiratory status
B. refusal to take foods or fluids
C. drowsiness
D. constipation

3. The nurse is administering didanosine properly when _____.

A. tablets are crushed and mixed thoroughly with 1 oz of water
B. the drug is prepared for subcutaneous injection
C. the drug is given with meals
D. the drug is given mixed with orange juice or apple juice

4. Intravenous administration of acyclovir can result in _____.

A. shock
B. crystalluria
C. cardiac arrest
D. hypertensive crisis

● Medication Dosage Problems

1. The patient is prescribed amantadine 200 mg. The drug is available in 100-mg tablets. The nurse administers _____.

2. A patient is prescribed 2 inhalations of zanamivir. The drug is available as one 5-mg blister per inhalation and is to be given with a Diskhaler device. How many milligrams will the nurse administer with 2 inhalations?

3. The nurse is to administer 100 mg of zidovudine PO. The drug is available as syrup 50 mg/5 mL. The nurse administers _____.

chapter 15

Antifungal Drugs

Key Terms

fungicidal
fungistatic
fungus
mycotic infections

onychomycosis
tinea corporis
tinea cruris
tinea pedi

Chapter Objectives

On completion of this chapter, the student will:

- Distinguish between superficial and systemic fungal infections
- Discuss the uses, general drug action, adverse reactions, contraindications, precautions, and interactions of antifungal drugs.
- Discuss important preadministration and ongoing assessment activities the nurse should perform on the patient receiving an antifungal drug.
- List some nursing diagnoses particular to a patient taking an antifungal drug.
- List possible goals for a patient taking an antifungal drug.
- Discuss ways to promote an optimal response to therapy, how to manage adverse reactions, and important points to keep in mind when educating the patient and the family about the antifungal drugs.

Fungal infections range from superficial skin infections to life-threatening systemic infections. Systemic fungal infections are serious infections that occur when fungi gain entrance into the interior of the body.

A **fungus** is a colorless plant that lacks chlorophyll. Fungi that cause disease in humans may be yeastlike or moldlike; the resulting infections are called **mycotic infections** or fungal infections.

Mycotic (fungal) infections may be one of two types:

1. Superficial mycotic infections
2. Deep (systemic) mycotic infections

The superficial mycotic infections occur on the surface of, or just below, the skin or nails. Superficial infections include **tinea pedis** (athlete's foot), **tinea cruris** (jock itch), **tinea corporis** (ringworm), **onychomycosis** (nail fungus), and yeast infections, such as those caused by *Candida albicans*. Yeast infections or those caused by *C. albicans* affect women in the vulvovaginal area and can be difficult to control. Women who are at increased risk for vulvovaginal yeast infections are those who have diabetes, are pregnant, or are taking oral contraceptives, antibiotics, or corticosteroids.

Deep mycotic infections develop inside the body, such as in the lungs. Treatment for deep mycotic infections is often difficult and prolonged. The Summary Drug Table: Antifungal Drugs identifies drugs that are used to combat fungal infections.

ACTIONS

Antifungal drugs may be **fungicidal** (able to destroy fungi) or **fungistatic** (able to slow or retard the multiplication of fungi). Amphotericin B (Fungizone IV), miconazole (Monistat), nystatin (Mycostatin), and ketoconazole (Nizoral) are thought to have an effect on the cell membrane of the fungus, resulting in a fungicidal or fungistatic effect. The fungicidal or fungistatic effect of these drugs appears to be related to their concentration in body tissues. Fluconazole (Diflucan) has fungistatic activity that appears to result from the depletion of sterols (a group of substances related to fats) in the fungus cells.

Griseofulvin (Grisactin) exerts its effect by being deposited in keratin precursor cells, which are then gradually lost (due to the constant shedding of top skin cells), and replaced by new, noninfected cells. The mode of action of flucytosine (Ancobon) is not clearly understood. Clotrimazole (Lotrimin, Mycelex) binds with phospholipids in the fungal cell membrane,

TABLE 15-2	Vaginal Antifungal Drugs
GENERIC NAME	**SELECT TRADE NAME(S)**
butoconazole nitrate *byoo-toe-koe'-nuh-zole*	Femstat 3, Gynazole-1, Mycelex-3
clotrimazole *kloe-trye'-ma-zole*	Lotrimin 3, Mycelex-7, *generic*
miconazole nitrate *mi-kon'-a-zole*	Monistat 3, Monistat 7, Monistat Dual Pak, M-Zole 3 Combination Pack, *generic*
nystatin *nye-stat'-in*	*generic*
terconazole *ter-kon'-a-zole*	Terazol 7, Terazol 3
tioconazole *tee-o-kon'-a-zole*	Monistat 1, Vagistat-1

including fever, shaking, chills, headache, malaise, anorexia, joint and muscle pain, abnormal renal function, nausea, vomiting, and anemia. This drug is given parenterally, usually for a period of several months. Its use is reserved for serious and potentially life-threatening fungal infections. Some of these adverse reactions may be lessened by use of aspirin, antihistamines, or antiemetics.

Fluconazole

Administration may result in nausea, vomiting, headache, diarrhea, abdominal pain, and skin rash. Abnormal liver function tests may be seen and may require follow-up tests to determine if liver function has been affected.

Flucytosine

Administration may result in nausea, vomiting, diarrhea, rash, anemia, leukopenia, and thrombocytopenia. Signs of renal impairment include elevated blood urea nitrogen (BUN) and serum creatinine levels. Periodic renal function tests are usually performed during therapy.

Griseofulvin

Administration may result in a hypersensitivity-type reaction that includes rash and urticaria. Nausea, vomiting, oral thrush, diarrhea, and headache also may be seen.

Itraconazole

The most common adverse reactions are nausea, vomiting, and diarrhea. On occasion, severe hypokalemia (low potassium level) has occurred in patients receiving 600 mg or more of the drug on a daily basis. Hepatotoxicity is a possibility with itraconazole administration.

Ketoconazole

This drug is usually well tolerated, but nausea, vomiting, headache, dizziness, abdominal pain, and pruritus may be seen. Most adverse reactions are mild and transient. On rare occasions, hepatic toxicity may be seen, and use of the drug must be discontinued immediately. Periodic hepatic function tests are recommended to monitor for hepatic toxicity.

Miconazole

Administration of miconazole for a vulvovaginal fungal infection may cause irritation, sensitization, or vulvovaginal burning. Skin irritation may result in redness, itching, burning, or skin fissures. Other adverse reactions with miconazole include cramping, nausea, and headache. Adverse reactions associated with topical use are usually not severe.

CONTRAINDICATIONS, PRECAUTIONS, AND INTERACTIONS

Amphotericin B

Amphotericin B is contraindicated in patients with a history of allergy to the drug and during lactation. It is used cautiously in patients with renal dysfunction, electrolyte imbalances, and in combination with antineoplastic drugs (because it can cause severe bone marrow suppression). This drug is a Pregnancy Category B drug and is used during pregnancy only when the situation is life threatening. When given with the corticosteroids, severe hypokalemia may occur. There may be an increased risk of digitalis toxicity if digoxin is administered concurrently with amphotericin B. Administration with nephrotoxic drugs (eg, aminoglycosides or cyclosporine) may increase the risk of nephrotoxicity in patients also taking amphotericin B. Amphotericin B decreases the effects of miconazole. Amphotericin B is given only under close supervision in the hospital setting.

Fluconazole

Fluconazole is contraindicated in patients with known hypersensitivity to the drug. The drug is used cautiously in patients with renal impairment and during pregnancy (Category C) and lactation. The drug is given during pregnancy only if the benefit of the drug clearly outweighs any possible risk to the infant. When fluconazole is administered with oral hypoglycemics, there is an increased effect of the oral hypoglycemics.

Fluconazole may decrease the metabolism of phenytoin and warfarin.

Flucytosine

Flucytosine is contraindicated in patients with known hypersensitivity to the drug. Flucytosine is used cautiously in patients with bone marrow depression and with extreme caution in those with renal impairment. The drug is also used cautiously during pregnancy (Category C) and lactation. When flucytosine and amphotericin B are administered concurrently, the risk of flucytosine toxicity is increased.

Griseofulvin

Griseofulvin is contraindicated in patients with known hypersensitivity to the drug and in those with severe liver disease. This drug is used cautiously during pregnancy (Category C) and lactation. It is important to use caution when administering concurrently with penicillin because there is a possibility of cross-sensitivity. When griseofulvin is administered with warfarin, the anticoagulant effect may be decreased. When administered with the barbiturates the effect of griseofulvin may be decreased. A decrease in the effects of oral contraceptives may occur with griseofulvin therapy, causing breakthrough bleeding, pregnancy, or amenorrhea. Blood salicylate concentrations may be decreased when the salicylates are administered with griseofulvin.

Itraconazole

Itraconazole is contraindicated in patients with a known hypersensitivity to the drug. The drug is used cautiously in patients with hepatitis, those with human immunodeficiency virus, impaired liver function, and in pregnant women (Pregnancy Category C). In patients with hypochlorhydria, the absorption of itraconazole is decreased. Multiple drug interactions occur with itraconazole. Itraconazole elevates blood concentrations of digoxin and cyclosporine. Phenytoin decreases blood levels of itraconazole and alters the metabolism of phenytoin. Histamine antagonists, isoniazid, and rifampin decrease plasma levels of itraconazole. There is an increased anticoagulant effect when warfarin is administered concurrently with itraconazole.

Ketoconazole

Ketoconazole is contraindicated in patients with known hypersensitivity to the drug. Ketoconazole is used cautiously in patients with hepatic impairment, those who are pregnant (Category C), and during lactation. The absorption of ketoconazole is impaired when the drug is taken with histamine antagonists and antacids. Ketoconazole enhances the anticoagulant effect of warfarin and causes an additive hepatotoxicity when given with other hepatotoxic drugs and alcohol. Administration of ketoconazole with rifampin or isoniazid may decrease the blood levels of ketoconazole.

Miconazole

Miconazole is contraindicated in patients with known hypersensitivity to the drug. The drug is given cautiously in cases of chronic or recurrent candidiasis. With recurrent or chronic candidiasis the patient may have underlying diabetes. Recurrent or chronic candidiasis requires an evaluation for diabetes. The drug is used cautiously during pregnancy (Category C). If used during pregnancy, a vaginal applicator may be contraindicated. Manual insertion of the vaginal tablets may be preferred. Because small amounts of these drugs may be absorbed from the vagina, the drug is used during the first trimester only when essential.

NURSING PROCESS

● **The Patient Receiving an Antifungal Drug**

ASSESSMENT

Preadministration Assessment

Information gathered before the administration of the first dose establishes a database for comparison during therapy. In performing the preadministration assessment before giving the first dose of an antifungal drug, the nurse assesses the patient for signs of the infection. The nurse inspects for superficial fungal infections of the skin or skin structures (eg, hair, nails) and describes them on the patient's record. The nurse carefully documents any skin lesions, such as rough itchy patches, cracks between the toes, and sore and reddened areas, to obtain an accurate database. It also is important to describe any vaginal discharge or white plaques or sore areas of the mucous membranes. The nurse takes and records vital signs. The nurse weighs the patient scheduled to receive amphotericin or flucytosine because the dosage of the drug is determined according to the patient's weight.

Ongoing Assessment

The ongoing assessment involves careful observation of the patient every 2 to 4 hours for adverse drug reactions when the antifungal drug is given by the oral or parenteral route. When these drugs are applied topically to the skin, the nurse inspects the area at the time of each application for localized skin reactions. When these drugs are administered vaginally, the nurse questions the patient regarding any discomfort or other sensations experienced after insertion of the antifungal preparation. The nurse notes improvement or deterioration of lesions of the skin, mucous membranes, or vaginal secretions in the chart. It is important for the nurse to evaluate and chart the patient's response to therapy daily.

NURSING DIAGNOSES

Drug-specific nursing diagnoses are highlighted in the Nursing Diagnoses Checklist. More general nursing diagnoses applicable to these drugs are discussed in depth in Chapter 4.

PLANNING

The expected outcomes for the patient depend on the reason for administration of the antifungal drug but may include a therapeutic response to the antifungal drug, management of adverse reactions, and an understanding of and compliance with the prescribed treatment regimen.

IMPLEMENTATION

Promoting an Optimal Response to Therapy

Superficial and deep fungal infections respond slowly to antifungal therapy. Many patients experience anxiety and depression over the fact that therapy must continue for a prolonged time. Depending on the method of treatment, patients may be faced with many problems during therapy and therefore need time to talk about problems as they arise. Examples of problems are the cost of treatment, hospitalization (when required), the failure of treatment to adequately control the infection, and loss of income. The nurse must help the patient and the family to understand that therapy must be continued until the infection is under control. In some cases, therapy may take weeks or months.

DISTURBED BODY IMAGE. The lesions caused by the fungal infections may cause the patient to feel negatively about the body or a body part. It is important for the nurse to develop a therapeutic nurse–patient relationship that conveys an attitude of caring and develops a sense of trust. The nurse listens to the patient's concerns and assists the patient in accepting the situation as temporary. The nurse encourages the patient to verbalize any feelings or anxiety about the effect of the disorder on body image. The nurse explains the disorder and the treatment regimen in terms the patient can understand and discusses the need at times for long-term treatment to eradicate the infection.

RISK FOR INEFFECTIVE TISSUE PERFUSION: RENAL. When the patient is taking a drug that is potentially toxic to the kidneys, the nurse must carefully monitor fluid intake and output. In some instances, the nurse may need to perform hourly measurements of the urinary output. Periodic laboratory tests are usually ordered to monitor the patient's response to therapy and to detect toxic drug reactions. Serum creatinine levels and BUN levels are checked frequently during the course of therapy to monitor kidney function. If the BUN exceeds 40 mg/dL or if the serum creatinine level exceeds 3 mg/dL, the primary health care provider may discontinue the drug therapy or reduce the dosage until renal function improves.

IMPAIRED SKIN INTEGRITY AND RISK FOR INFECTION. Many fungal infections are associated with lesions that are at risk for infection. The nurse monitors the patient's temperature, pulse, respirations, and blood pressure every 4 hours or more often if needed. The nurse inspects for superficial fungal infections of the skin or skin structures (eg, hair, nails) and describes them on the patient's record. The nurse carefully documents any skin lesions, such as rough itchy patches, cracks between the toes, and sore and reddened areas. The nurse checks the skin for localized signs of infection (ie, increased redness or swelling). The nurse monitors the skin lesions daily, describing lesions and any changes observed. It is important that the nurse note any improvement or healing of the lesions. Gloves are used when caring for open lesions to minimize autoinoculation or transmission of the disease.

Administering Specific Antifungal Drugs

AMPHOTERICIN B. The nurse administers this drug daily or every other day over several months. The patient is often acutely ill with a life-threatening deep fungal infection. The nurse should reconstitute the drug according to the manufacturer's instructions. Sterile water is used for reconstitution because any other diluent may cause precipitation. Immediately after the drug is reconstituted, the nurse administers the IV infusion over a period of 6 hours or more.

The manufacturer recommends that the IV solution be protected from exposure to light. It is a good idea to wrap a brown paper bag or aluminum foil around the

---

Nursing Diagnoses Checklist

Drug-specific nursing diagnoses are listed below. Depending on the drug, dose, and reason for administration, one or more of the following nursing diagnoses may apply to a person receiving an antifungal drug:

☑ **Disturbed Body Image** related to changes in skin and mucous membranes

☑ **Risk for Ineffective Tissue Perfusion: Renal** related to adverse reactions of the antifungal drug

☑ **Risk for Infection** related to the presence of skin lesions

☑ **Impaired Skin Integrity** related to the presence of skin lesions

infusion bottle after reconstitution of the powder and during administration of the solution. Although solutions of amphotericin B are light sensitive, research indicates that if used within 8 hours, there is negligible loss of drug activity. Because the solution decomposes slowly, it is probably not necessary to protect the container from light if the drug is used within 8 hours of reconstitution. The nurse should consult the primary health care provider or hospital pharmacist regarding whether or not to use a protective covering for the infusion container.

The nurse checks the IV infusion rate and the infusion site frequently during administration of the drug. This is especially important if the patient is restless or confused.

On occasion amphotericin B may be administered as an oral solution for oral candidiasis. The patient is instructed to swish and hold the solution in the mouth for several minutes (or as long as possible) before swallowing. The oral solution may be used for as long as 2 weeks.

FLUCONAZOLE. The drug may be administered orally or intravenously. Initially the patient receives 200 to 400 mg, followed by 100 to 200 mg per day for at least 14 days. When given as a continuous infusion, the drug is infused at a maximum rate of 200 mg per hour. When administering IV do not remove the overwrap until ready to use. The nurse tears the overwrap down the side at the slit and removes the solution container. When administering IV, the nurse must follow the manufacturer's directions regarding removal of the wrapping around the container. It is important not to administer solution that is cloudy or contains precipitate. The nurse then checks the bag for minute leaks by squeezing firmly. The solution is discarded if any leaks are found.

FLUCYTOSINE. The nurse gives flucytosine orally. The prescribed dose may range from 2 to 6 capsules/dose. To decrease or avoid nausea and vomiting, the capsules may be taken a few at a time during a 15-minute period.

GRISEOFULVIN. This drug is given orally as a single dose or in two to four divided doses. Prolonged therapy is usually needed to eradicate the fungus.

KETOCONAZOLE. This drug is given with food to minimize gastrointestinal irritation. Tablets may be crushed. Ketoconazole is absorbed best in an acid environment. Do not administer antacids, anticholinergics, or histamine blockers until at least 2 hours after ketoconazole is given.

ITRACONAZOLE. Give the drug orally with food to increase absorption. When administering IV, use only components provided by the manufacturer for reconstitution. Do not dilute with any other diluent. The drug

is infused during a period of 60 minutes. Doses greater than 200 mg are given in 2 divided dosages.

MICONAZOLE. This drug is self-administered on an outpatient basis. See Patient and Family Education for information to give to the patient concerning this drug.

Monitoring and Managing Adverse Reactions

AMPHOTERICIN B. Fever (sometimes with shaking chills) may occur within 15 to 20 minutes of initiation of the treatment regimen. It is important to monitor the patient's temperature, pulse, respirations, and blood pressure carefully during the first 30 minutes to 1 hour of treatment. The nurse should monitor vital signs every 2 to 4 hours during therapy, depending on the patient's condition.

The nurse must carefully monitor fluid intake and output because this drug may be nephrotoxic (harmful to the kidneys). In some instances, the nurse may need to perform hourly measurements of the urinary output. Periodic laboratory tests are usually ordered to monitor the patient's response to therapy and detect toxic drug reactions.

Nursing Alert

Renal damage is the most serious adverse reaction with the use of amphotericin B. Renal impairment usually improves with modification of dosage regimen (reduction of dosage or increasing time between dosages). Serum creatinine levels and BUN levels are checked frequently during the course of therapy to monitor kidney function. If the BUN exceeds 40 mg/dL or if the serum creatinine level exceeds 3 mg/dL, the primary health care provider may discontinue the drug or reduce the dosage until renal function improves.

FLUCONAZOLE. Because older adults are more likely to have decreased renal function, they are at increased risk for further renal impairment or renal failure.

Gerontological Alert

Before administering this drug to an elderly patient or one that has renal impairment, the primary health care provider may order a creatinine clearance. The initial dose is 50 to 100 mg PO or IV, depending on the results of the creatinine clearance. The nurse reports the laboratory results to the primary health care provider because dosage adjustments may be made on the results of the creatinine clearance.

FLUCYTOSINE. To reduce the incidence of gastrointestinal distress, the nurse may give the capsules one or two at a time during a 15-minute period. If gastrointestinal distress still occurs, the nurse should notify the primary health care provider. Before therapy is begun, electrolytes, hematological status, and renal status are

Home Care Checklist

USING TOPICAL ANTIFUNGAL AGENTS

Often patients are required to apply topical drugs for fungal infections of the skin. A majority of the adverse effects that occur with topical drugs are a result of applying the drug improperly. Typically, if applied correctly, the drug usually is not systemically absorbed. However, many times, patients think that if a little or some is good, then "more is better." Applying more than the amount necessary increases the patient's risk for systemic absorption. To ensure that the patient applies the topical antifungal drug properly, the nurse includes the following points in the teaching plan:

✓ Gather all necessary supplies and wash hands before starting.

✓ Wash the area first to remove any debris and old drug.

✓ Pat the area dry with a clean cloth.

✓ Open the container (or tube) and place the lid or cap upside down on the counter or surface.

✓ Use a tongue blade, gloved finger (either with a nonsterile gloved hand or finger cot), cotton swab, or gauze pad to remove the drug, then apply it to the skin.

✓ Wipe the drug onto the affected area using long smooth strokes in the direction of hair growth.

✓ Apply a thin layer of drug to the area (more is *not* better).

✓ Use a new tongue blade, applicator, or clean gloved finger to remove additional drug from the container (if necessary).

✓ Apply a clean, dry dressing (if appropriate) over the area.

---

determined. Renal impairment can cause accumulation of the drug.

ITRACONAZOLE. Although rare, the patient may develop hepatitis during itraconazole administration. The nurse closely monitors the patient for signs of hepatitis, including anorexia, abdominal pain, unusual tiredness, jaundice, and dark urine. The primary health care provider may order periodic liver function tests.

Educating the Patient and Family

If the patient is being treated with topical antifungal drugs, the nurse includes the following points in the teaching plan (see Home Care Checklist: Using Topical Antifungal Drugs):

- Clean the involved area and apply the ointment or cream to the skin as directed by the primary health care provider.
- Do not increase or decrease the amount used or the number of times the ointment or cream should be applied unless directed to do so by the primary health care provider.
- During treatment for a ringworm infection, keep towels and facecloths used for bathing separate from those of other family members to avoid the spread of the infection. It is important to keep the affected area clean and dry.

Drug-specific teaching points include:

- Flucytosine: Nausea and vomiting may occur with this drug. Reduce or eliminate these effects by taking a few capsules at a time during a 15-minute period. If nausea, vomiting, or diarrhea persists, notify the primary health care provider as soon as possible.
- Griseofulvin: Beneficial effects may not be noticed for some time; therefore, take the drug for the full course of therapy. Avoid exposure to sunlight and sunlamps because an exaggerated skin reaction (which is similar to a severe sunburn) may occur even after a brief exposure to ultraviolet light. Notify the primary health care provider if fever, soar throat, or skin rash occurs.
- Ketoconazole: Complete the full course of therapy as prescribed by the primary health care provider. Do not take this drug with an antacid. In addition, avoid the use of nonprescription drugs unless use of a specific drug is approved by the primary health care provider. This drug may produce headache,

dizziness, and drowsiness. If drowsiness or dizziness should occur, observe caution while driving or performing other hazardous tasks. Notify the primary health care provider if abdominal pain, fever, or diarrhea becomes pronounced.

● Itraconazole: The drug is taken with food. Therapy will continue for at least 3 months until infection is controlled. Report unusual fatigue, yellow skin, darkened urine, anorexia, nausea, and vomiting.

● Miconazole: If the drug (cream or tablet) is administered vaginally, insert the drug high in the vagina using the applicator provided with the product. Wear a sanitary napkin after insertion of the drug to prevent staining of the clothing and bed linen. Continue taking the drug during the menstrual period if vaginal route is being used. Do not have intercourse while taking this drug, or advise the partner to use a condom to avoid reinfection. To prevent recurrent infections, avoid nylon and tight-fitting garments. If there is no improvement in 5 to 7 days, stop using the drug and consult a primary care provider because a more serious infection may be present. If abdominal pain, pelvic pain, rash, fever, or offensive-smelling vaginal discharge is present, do not use the drug, but notify the primary health care provider.

EVALUATION

● The therapeutic effect occurs and signs and symptoms of infection improve.
● Optimal skin integrity is maintained.
● Adverse reactions are identified, reported to the primary health care provider, and managed through appropriate nursing interventions.
● The patient and family demonstrate an understanding of the drug regimen.
● The patient verbalizes the importance of complying with the prescribed treatment regimen.

● *Critical Thinking Exercises*

1. *A nurse is preparing to administer amphotericin B to a patient with a systemic mycotic infection. This is the first time the nurse has administered amphotericin B. Determine what information the nurse should be aware of concerning the administration of this drug. Explain your answer.*

2. *Mr. Harding, age 35 years, has received a diagnosis of a fungal infection. The primary health care provider has prescribed a topical antifungal drug. Develop a teaching plan concerning the application of a topical antifungal drug.*

● *Review Questions*

1. Mr. Carr is receiving amphotericin B for a systemic fungal infection. Which of the following would most likely indicate to the nurse that Mr. Carr is experiencing an adverse reaction to amphotericin B?
   A. fever and chills
   B. abdominal pain
   C. drowsiness
   D. flushing of the skin

2. Which of the following laboratory tests would the nurse monitor in patients receiving flucytosine?
   A. liver function tests
   B. complete blood count
   C. renal functions tests
   D. prothrombin levels

3. The nurse monitors a patient taking itraconazole for the most common adverse reaction, which is _____.
   A. nausea
   B. hypokalemia
   C. irregular pulse
   D. confusion

4. The nurse would withhold griseofulvin if the patient has _____.
   A. anemia
   B. respiratory disease
   C. had a recent myocardial infarction
   D. severe liver disease

● *Medication Dosage Problems*

1. A patient weighs 140 pounds. If amphotericin B 1.5 mg/kg per day is prescribed, what is the total daily dosage of amphotericin B for this patient?

2. The primary care provider has prescribed fluconazole 200 mg PO initially, followed by 100 mg PO daily. On hand are fluconazole 100-mg tablets. What would the nurse administer as the initial dose?

Antiparasitic Drugs

Key Terms

amebiasis
anthelmintic
cinchonism
gametocytes
helminthiasis

helminths
merozoites
parasite
sporozoites

Chapter Objectives

On completion of this chapter, the student will:

- Discuss the uses, general drug action, adverse effects, contraindications, precautions, and interactions of the drugs used in the treatment of helminth infections, malaria, and amebiasis.
- Discuss important preadministration and ongoing assessment activities the nurse should perform on the patient taking an anthelmintic, antimalarial, or amebicide drug.
- List some nursing diagnoses particular to a patient taking an anthelmintic, antimalarial, or amebicide drug.
- Discuss ways to promote an optimal response to therapy, how to manage adverse reactions, and important points to keep in mind when educating patients about the use of the anthelmintics, antimalarials, and amebicides.

A **parasite** is an organism that lives in or on another organism (the host) without contributing to the survival or well-being of the host. **Helminthiasis** (invasion of the body by helminths [worms]), malaria (an infectious disease caused by a protozoan and transmitted to humans through a bite from an infected mosquito), and **amebiasis** (invasion of the body by the ameba *Entamoeba histolytica*) are worldwide health problems caused by parasites.

Pinworm is a helminth infection that is universally common; most other helminth infections are predominantly found in countries or areas of the world that lack proper sanitary facilities. Malaria is rare in the United States, but it is sometimes seen in individuals who have traveled to or lived in areas where this disease is a health problem. The first antimalarial drug, quinine, is derived from the bark of the cinchona tree. Amebiasis is seen throughout the world, but it is less common in developed countries where sanitary facilities prevent the spread of the causative organism.

ANTHELMINTIC DRUGS

Anthelmintic (against helminths) drugs are used to treat helminthiasis. Roundworms, pinworms, whipworms,

hookworms, and tapeworms are examples of helminths. Table 16-1 lists the organisms that cause helminth infections. The anthelmintic drugs are listed in the Summary Drug Table: Anthelmintic Drugs.

ACTION, USES, AND ADVERSE REACTIONS

Although the actions of anthelmintic drugs vary, their prime purpose is to kill the parasite. Adverse reactions associated with the anthelmintic drugs, if they do occur, are usually mild when the drug is used in the recommended dosage.

Albendazole

Albendazole (Albenza) interferes with the synthesis of the parasite's microtubules, resulting in death of susceptible larva. This drug is used to treat larval forms of pork tapeworm and to treat liver, lung, and peritoneum disease caused by the dog tapeworm.

Mebendazole

Mebendazole (Vermox) blocks the uptake of glucose by the helminth, resulting in a depletion of the helminth's

TABLE 16-1	Common Names and Causative Organisms of Parasitic Infections

COMMON NAME	CAUSATIVE ORGANISM
Roundworm	*Ascaris lumbricoides*
Pinworm	*Enterobius vermicularis*
Whipworm	*Trichuris trichiura*
Threadworm	*Strongyloides stercoralis*
Hookworm	*Ancylostoma duodenale, Necator americanus*
Beef tapeworm	*Taenia saginata*
Pork tapeworm	*Taenia solium*
Fish tapeworm	*Diphyllobothrium latum*

own glycogen. Glycogen depletion results in a decreased formation of adenosine triphosphate, which is required by the helminth for reproduction and survival. This drug is used to treat whipworm, pinworm, roundworm, American hookworm, and the common hookworm. Treatment with mebendazole may cause transient abdominal pain and diarrhea.

Pyrantel

The activity of pyrantel (Antiminth) is probably due to its ability to paralyze the helminth. Paralysis causes the helminth to release its grip on the intestinal wall; it is then excreted in the feces. Pyrantel is used to treat roundworm and pinworm. Some patients receiving pyrantel may experience gastrointestinal side effects, such as nausea, vomiting, abdominal cramps, or diarrhea.

Thiabendazole

The exact mechanism of action of thiabendazole (Mintezol) is unknown. This drug appears to suppress egg or larval production and therefore may interrupt the life cycle of the helminth. Thiabendazole is used to treat threadworm. Thiabendazole may cause hypersensitivity reactions, drowsiness, and dizziness.

CONTRAINDICATIONS, PRECAUTIONS, AND INTERACTIONS

Albendazole

Albendazole is contraindicated in patients with known hypersensitivity to the drug and during pregnancy (Category C). The drug has exhibited embryotoxic and teratogenic effects in experimental animals. Albendazole is used cautiously in patients with hepatic impairment and during lactation. The effects of albendazole are increased with dexamethasone and cimetidine.

Mebendazole

Mebendazole is contraindicated in patients with known hypersensitivity. Mebendazole is also contraindicated during pregnancy (Category C). The drug, like albendazole, has exhibited embryotoxic and teratogenic effects in experimental animals. Administration of mebendazole with the hydantoins and carbamazepine may reduce plasma levels of mebendazole.

SUMMARY DRUG TABLE ANTHELMINTIC DRUGS

GENERIC NAME	TRADE NAME*	USES	ADVERSE REACTIONS	DOSAGE RANGES
albendazole *al-ben'-dah-zohl*	Albenza	Parenchymal neurocysticerosis due to pork tapeworms, hydatid disease (caused by the larval form of the dog tapeworm)	Abnormal liver function tests, abdominal pain, nausea, vomiting, headache, dizziness	≥60 kg: 400 mg BID: <60 kg: 15 mg/kg/d
mebendazole *me-ben'-dah-zole*	Vermox, *generic*	Treatment of whipworm, pinworm, roundworm, common and American hookworm	Transient abdominal pain, diarrhea	100 mg PO morning and evening for 3 consecutive d; pinworm: 100 mg PO as a single dose
pyrantel *pi-ran'-tel*	Antiminth, Reese's Pinworm	Treatment of pinworm and roundworm	Anorexia, nausea, vomiting, abdominal cramps, diarrhea, rash	11 mg/kg PO as a single dose
thiabendazole *thye-a-ben'-da-zole*	Mintezol	Treatment of threadworm	Hypersensitivity reactions, drowsiness, dizziness	<150 lb: 10 mg/lb per dose PO >150 lb: 1.5 g/dose PO Maximum daily dose, 3g

*The term *generic* indicates the drug is available in generic form.

Pyrantel

Pyrantel is contraindicated in patients with known hypersensitivity. Pyrantel is used with caution in individuals with liver dysfunction, malnutrition, or anemia. Pyrantel is a Pregnancy Category C drug and is used during pregnancy only if the potential benefit outweighs the risk to the fetus. Pyrantel and piperazine are antagonists and should not be given together.

Thiabendazole

Thiabendazole is contraindicated in patients with known hypersensitivity. Thiabendazole is used with caution in patients with hepatic or renal disease. Thiabendazole is a Pregnancy Category C drug and is used during pregnancy only if the potential benefit outweighs the risk to the fetus. When thiabendazole is administered with the xanthine derivatives, the plasma level of the xanthine may increase to toxic levels. It is important to monitor xanthine plasma levels closely in case a dosage reduction is necessary.

NURSING PROCESS

● The Patient Receiving an Anthelmintic Drug

ASSESSMENT

Preadministration Assessment

During the preadministration assessment, the nurse obtains vital signs before the first dose of the anthelmintic drug is given. The nurse also may need to weigh the patient if the drug's dosage is determined by weight or if the patient is acutely ill.

Ongoing Assessment

Unless ordered otherwise, the nurse should save all stools that are passed after the drug is given. It is important to visually inspect each stool for passage of the helminth. If stool specimens are to be saved for laboratory examination, the nurse follows hospital procedure for saving the stool and transporting it to the laboratory. If the patient is acutely ill or has a massive infection, it is important to monitor vital signs every 4 hours and measure and record fluid intake and output. The nurse observes the patient for adverse drug reactions, as well as severe episodes of diarrhea. It is important to notify the primary health care provider if these occur.

NURSING DIAGNOSES

The nursing diagnoses depend on the patient and the type of helminth infection. Drug-specific nursing diagnoses are highlighted in the Nursing Diagnoses Checklist. Other nursing diagnoses are discussed in depth in Chapter 4.

Nursing Diagnoses Checklist

☑ **Imbalanced Nutrition: Less Than Body Requirements** related to infestation with helminths or anthelmintic adverse drug reactions

PLANNING

The expected outcomes for the patient may include a reduction in anxiety, an optimal response to therapy, management of adverse reactions, and an understanding of and compliance with the prescribed therapeutic regimen.

IMPLEMENTATION

Promoting an Optimal Response to Therapy

The diagnosis of a helminth infection is made by examination of the stool for ova and all or part of the helminth. Several stool specimens may be necessary before the helminth is seen and identified. The patient history also may lead to a suspicion of a helminth infection, but some patients have no symptoms.

When a pinworm infection is suspected, the nurse takes a specimen from the anal area, preferably early in the morning before the patient gets out of bed. Specimens are taken by swabbing the perianal area with a cellophane tape swab.

Patients with massive helminth infections may or may not be acutely ill. The acutely ill patient requires hospitalization, but many individuals with helminth infections can be treated on an outpatient basis.

The diagnosis of a helminth infection is often distressing to patients and their family. The nurse should allow time to explain the treatment and future preventive measures, as well as to allow the patient or family members to discuss their concerns or ask questions.

Depending on hospital policy, as well as the type of helminth infection, linen precautions may be necessary. The nurse wears gloves when changing bed linens, emptying bedpans, or obtaining or handling stool specimens. It is important to wash hands thoroughly after removing the gloves. The nurse instructs the patient to wash the hands thoroughly after personal care and use of the bedpan.

ADMINISTERING AN ANTHELMINTIC DRUG. The method of administration of an anthelmintic drug may vary somewhat from the administration of other drugs. To achieve an optimal response to therapy, it is most important that the drug be given as directed by the primary health care provider, drug label, or package insert. Display 16-1 provides specific instructions for administering anthelmintic drugs.

Monitoring and Managing Adverse Reactions

The nurse monitors the patient taking an anthelmintic drug closely for adverse reactions.

RISK FOR IMBALANCED NUTRITION. Gastrointestinal upset may occur, causing nausea, vomiting, abdominal pain, and diarrhea. Taking the drug with food often helps to alleviate the nausea. The patient may require frequent, small meals of easily digested food. The nurse considers the patient's food preferences and encourages the patient to eat nutritious, balanced meals. If vomiting is present, the primary health care provider may prescribe an antiemetic or a different anthelmintic agent. If diarrhea is present, the nurse notifies the primary health care provider because a change in the drug regimen may be needed. The nurse keeps a record of the number, consistency, color, and frequency of stools. The nurse monitors the fluid intake and output. It is important to keep the patient clean and the room free of odor.

Educating the Patient and Family

When an anthelmintic is prescribed on an outpatient basis, the nurse gives the patient or a family member complete instructions about taking the drug, as well as household precautions that should be followed until the helminth is eliminated from the intestine. The nurse develops a patient education plan to include the following:

- Report any symptoms of infection (low-grade fever or sore throat) or thrombocytopenia (easy bruising or bleeding).
- Follow the dosage schedule exactly as printed on the prescription container. (See Administering an Anthelmintic Drug for the directions specific for each drug.) It is absolutely necessary to follow the directions for taking the drug to eradicate the helminth.
- Follow-up stool specimens will be necessary because this is the only way to determine the success of drug therapy.
- To prevent reinfection and the infection of others in the household, change and launder bed linens and undergarments daily, separately from those of other members of the family.
- Daily bathing (showering is best) is recommended. Disinfect toilet facilities daily, and disinfect the bathtub or shower stall immediately after bathing. Use the disinfectant recommended by the primary health care provider or use chlorine bleach. Scrub the surfaces thoroughly and allow the disinfectant to remain in contact with the surfaces for several minutes.
- Wash the hands thoroughly after urinating or defecating and before preparing and eating food. Clean under the fingernails daily and avoid putting fingers in the mouth or biting the nails.
- Albendazole can cause serious harm to a developing fetus. Use a barrier contraceptive during the course of therapy and for 1 month after discontinuing the therapy.

EVALUATION

- The therapeutic effect is achieved.
- Adverse reactions are identified, reported to the primary health care provider, and managed successfully using appropriate nursing interventions.
- The infection is resolved.
- Stool specimens or perineal swabs are negative for parasites.
- The patient verbalizes an understanding of the therapeutic regimen modalities and the importance of continued follow-up testing.
- The patient describes or lists measures used to prevent the spread of infection to others.
- The patient verbalizes the importance of complying with the prescribed treatment regimen and preventive measures.

ANTIMALARIAL DRUGS

Malaria is transmitted from person to person by a certain species of the *Anopheles* mosquito. The four different protozoans causing malaria are *Plasmodium falciparum*, *P. malariae*, *P. ovale*, and *P. vivax*. Drugs used to treat or prevent malaria are called antimalarial drugs. Three antimalarial drugs are discussed in the chapter: chloroquine, doxycycline, and quinine sulfate. Other examples of antimalarial drugs in use today are listed in the Summary Drug Table: Antimalarial Drugs.

ACTIONS

The plasmodium causing malaria must enter the mosquito to develop, reproduce, and be transmitted. When the mosquito bites a person infected with malaria, it ingests the male and female forms (**gametocytes**) of the plasmodium. The gametocytes mate in the mosquito's

SUMMARY DRUG TABLE ANTIMALARIAL DRUGS

GENERIC NAME	TRADE NAME*	USES	ADVERSE REACTIONS	DOSAGE RANGES
atovaquone and proquanil HCl *uh-toe'-vuh-kwone*	Malarone	Prevention and treatment of malaria	Headache, fever, myalgia, abdominal pain, diarrhea	Prevention: 1–2 d before travel 1 tablet PO per day during period of exposure and for 7 days after exposure. Treatment: 4 tablets PO daily for 3 d
chloroquine *klor'-oh-kwin*	Aralen	Treatment and prevention of malaria	Hypotension, electrocardiographic changes, headache, nausea, vomiting, anorexia, diarrhea, abdominal cramps, visual disturbances	Treatment: *Dose expressed as base.* 160–200 mg (4–5 mL) IM and repeat in 6 h if necessary. Prevention: 300 mg PO weekly; treatment: initially 600 mg PO and 300 mg PO 6 h later, then 300 mg/d PO for 2 d
doxycycline *dox-i-sye'-kleen*	Monodox, Vibramycin, Vibra-Tabs, *generic*	Short-term prevention of malaria	Photosensitivity, anorexia, nausea, vomiting, diarrhea, superinfection, rash	100 mg PO QD
halofantrine *hay'-low-fan-trin*	Halfan	Treatment of malaria	Abdominal pain, nausea, vomiting, anorexia, diarrhea, dizziness	500 mg PO q6h for 3 doses, repeat dose regimen in 7 days
hydroxychloroquine sulfate *hye-drox-ee-klor'-oh-kwin*	Plaquenil Sulfate	Prevention and treatment of malaria	Same as chloroquine	*Dose expressed as base.* Prevention: 310 mg PO weekly; treatment: initially 620 mg PO, and 310 mg 6 h later, then 310 mg/d PO for 2 d
mefloquine hydrochloride *me'-flow-kwin*	Lariam	Prevention and treatment of malaria	Vomiting, dizziness, disturbed sense of balance, nausea, fever, headache, visual disturbances	Prevention: 250 mg/wk PO for 4 wk, then 250 mg PO every other week; treatment: 5 tablets PO as a single dose
primaquine phosphate *prim'-a-kween*	*generic*	Treatment of malaria	Nausea, vomiting, epigastric distress, abdominal cramps	*Dose expressed as base.* 15 mg/d PO for 14 d
pyrimethamine *peer-i-meth'-a-mine*	Daraprim	Prevention and treatment of malaria	Nausea, vomiting, hematologic changes, anorexia	Prevention: 25 mg PO once weekly; treatment: 50 mg/d for 2 days
quinine sulfate *kwi'-nine*	*generic*	Treatment of malaria	Cinchonism, vertigo, hematologic changes, skin rash, visual disturbances	260–650 mg TID for 6–12 days
sulfadoxine and pyrimethamine *sul-fa-dox'-een peer-i-meth'-a-meen*	Fansidar	Prevention and treatment of malaria	Hematologic changes, nausea, emesis, headache, hypersensitivity reactions, Stevens-Johnson syndrome	Prevention: 1 tablet PO weekly or 2 tablets every 2 wk; treatment: 2–3 tablets PO as a single dose

*The term *generic* indicates the drug is available in generic form.

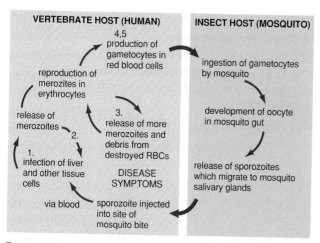

FIGURE 16-1. Life cycle of the malarial parasite. Points numbered on the illustration indicate the location in the malarial life cycle where specific drugs might be effective. (**1**) Chlorguanide, pyrimethamine, and primaquine used for causal prophylaxis. (**2**) Primaquine used to prevent relapses. (**3**) Drugs against the erythrocytic phase: potent action—chloroquine, amodiaquine, quinine; limited action—primaquine and chlorguanide. (**4**) Gametocidal drugs: primaquine. (**5**) Gametocyte-sterilizing drugs: chlorguanide, pyrimethamine.

stomach and ultimately form **sporozoites** (an animal reproductive cell) that make their way to the salivary glands of the mosquito. When the mosquito bites a non-infected person, the sporozoites enter the person's bloodstream and lodge in the liver and other tissues. The sporozoites then undergo asexual cell division and reproduction and form **merozoites** (cells formed as a result of asexual reproduction). The merozoites then divide asexually and enter the red blood cells of the person, where they form the male and female forms of the plasmodium. The symptoms of malaria (shaking, chills, and fever) appear when the merozoites enter the individual's red blood cells.

Antimalarial drugs interfere with, or are active against, the life cycle of the plasmodium, primarily when it is present in the red blood cells. Destruction at this stage of the plasmodium life cycle prevents the development of the male and female forms of the plasmodium. This in turn keeps the mosquito (when the mosquito bites an infected individual) from ingesting the male and female forms of the plasmodium, thus effectively ending the plasmodium life cycle (Fig. 16-1).

USES

Two terms are used when discussing the uses of antimalarial drugs:

1. Suppression—the prevention of malaria
2. Treatment—the management of a malarial attack

Not all antimalarial drugs are effective in suppressing or treating all four of the Plasmodium species that cause

malaria. In addition, resistant strains have developed, and some antimalarial drugs are no longer effective against some of these strains. The primary health care provider must select the antimalarial drug that reportedly is effective, at present, for the type of malaria the individual either has (treatment) or could be exposed to (prevention) in a specific area of the world.

Chloroquine (Aralen) is also used in the treatment of extraintestinal amebiasis (see section on Amebicides). Doxycycline is also used to treat infections caused by *Neisseria gonorrhoeae*, *Treponema pallidum*, *Listeria monocytogenes*, *Clostridium*, and *Bacillus anthracis* when penicillin is contraindicated. Quinine also may be used for the prevention and treatment of nocturnal leg cramps.

ADVERSE REACTIONS

Chloroquine

The adverse reactions associated with the administration of chloroquine (Aralen HCl and phosphate) and hydroxychloroquine include hypotension, electrocardiographic changes, visual disturbances, headache, nausea, vomiting, anorexia, diarrhea, and abdominal cramps.

Doxycycline

Doxycycline (Vibramycin) is an antibiotic belonging to the tetracycline group of antibiotics. The adverse reactions associated with this drug are discussed in Chapter 9 and include photosensitivity, anorexia, nausea, and vomiting.

Quinine

The use of quinine can cause cinchonism at full therapeutic doses. **Cinchonism** is a group of symptoms associated with quinine, including tinnitus, dizziness, headache, gastrointestinal disturbances, and visual disturbances. These symptoms usually disappear when the dosage is reduced. Other adverse reactions include hematologic changes, vertigo, and skin rash.

CONTRAINDICATIONS, PRECAUTIONS, AND INTERACTIONS

Chloroquine

Chloroquine is contraindicated in patients with known hypersensitivity. It is a good idea to use chloroquine cautiously in patients with hepatic disease or bone marrow depression and during pregnancy. Children are very sensitive to chloroquine, and the drug should be used with extreme caution in children.

Because the effects of chloroquine during pregnancy (Pregnancy Category C) are unknown, this drug is given only when clearly needed and the potential benefits outweigh potential hazards to the fetus. There is an increased risk of hepatotoxicity when chloroquine is administered with other hepatotoxic drugs.

Foods that acidify the urine (cranberries, plums, prunes, meats, cheeses, eggs, fish, and grains) may increase excretion and decrease the effectiveness of chloroquine.

Doxycycline

Doxycycline is contraindicated in patients with known hypersensitivity. Because the effects of doxycycline during pregnancy (Category D) are unknown, this drug is contraindicated during pregnancy. The drug is used cautiously in patients with renal or hepatic impairment and during lactation. There is a decreased absorption of the drug when administered with antacids or iron. There is a decrease of the therapeutic effects of doxycycline when the drug is administered with barbiturates, phenytoins, and carbamazepine. There is an increased risk of digoxin toxicity when digoxin is administered with doxycycline.

Quinine

Quinine is contraindicated in patients with known hypersensitivity. The drug is also contraindicated in pregnant women (Pregnancy Category X) and in patients with myasthenia gravis (may cause respiratory distress and dysphagia). Quinine absorption is delayed when administered with antacids containing aluminum. Plasma digitalis levels may increase when digitalis preparations and quinine are given concurrently. Plasma levels of warfarin are increased when administered with quinine.

NURSING PROCESS

● **The Patient Receiving an Antimalarial Drug**

ASSESSMENT

Preadministration Assessment

When an antimalarial drug is given to a hospitalized patient for treatment of malaria, the preadministration assessment includes vital signs and a summary of the nature and duration of the symptoms. Laboratory tests may be ordered for the diagnosis of malaria. Additional laboratory tests, such as a complete blood count, may be ordered to determine the patient's general health status.

Ongoing Assessment

If the patient is hospitalized with malaria, the nurse takes the vital signs every 4 hours or as ordered by the

---

Nursing Diagnoses Checklist

☑ **Risk for Injury** related to adverse reactions

☑ **Risk for Imbalanced Nutrition: Less Than Body Requirements** related to adverse drug reactions or disease process (malaria)

☑ **Disturbed Sensory Perception: Visual** related to adverse drug reactions

---

primary health care provider. The nurse observes the patient every 1 to 2 hours for the symptoms of malaria (headache, nausea, muscle aching, and high fever). Improvement or exacerbation of signs and symptoms of malaria is documented and reported to the primary health care provider. Antipyretics may be ordered for fever. If the patient is acutely ill, the nurse carefully measures and records the fluid intake and output. In some instances, intravenous fluids may be required.

NURSING DIAGNOSES

The specific nursing diagnoses for a patient receiving an antimalarial depend on the reason for administration (prevention or treatment) of the antimalarial drug. Drug-specific nursing diagnoses are highlighted in the Nursing Diagnoses Checklist.

PLANNING

The expected outcomes for the patient may include an optimal response to therapy, maintenance of adequate nutrition, management of common adverse reactions, and an understanding of and compliance with the prescribed therapeutic or prevention regimen.

IMPLEMENTATION

Promoting an Optimal Therapeutic Response

When administering an antimalarial drug such as chloroquine for prophylaxis (prevention), therapy should begin 2 weeks before exposure and continue for 6 to 8 weeks after the client leaves the area where malaria is prevalent. Initial treatment with quinine may be given parenterally. When administered intravenously (IV), quinine should be well diluted and administered slowly. The nurse must frequently examine the injection site and areas along the vein because quinine is irritating to the vein. Parenteral injection of chloroquine is avoided because the drug can cause respiratory distress, shock, and cardiovascular collapse when given intramuscularly or IV. If chloroquine must be given parenterally, the route should be changed to oral as soon as possible.

RISK FOR IMBALANCED NUTRITION. Patients receiving an antimalarial drug may experience nausea. Good nutrition is essential in the healing process. The nurse assists patients to identify food preferences and aversions and helps them in planning a nutritious diet. The nurse can consult a registered dietitian if necessary. If the patient is hospitalized with an active case of malaria, the nurse keeps the room environment clean and pleasant during mealtime. Meals should be nutritious and attractively served. Several small meals may be preferable to three large meals.

Monitoring and Managing Adverse Reactions

The nurse monitors for adverse reactions associated with the antimalarial drugs, such as dizziness, hypotension, and visual disturbances. Other adverse reactions are listed in the Summary Drug Table: Antimalarial Drugs.

RISK FOR INJURY. Some patients experience dizziness and hypotensive episodes when taking antimalarial drugs. The nurse should frequently monitor blood pressure if the patient is hospitalized. If dizziness occurs, the nurse may need to assist the patient with ambulation. The nurse instructs the patient to rise slowly from a reclining position, sit a few minutes before standing, and stand a few minutes before beginning to walk. When the patient is taking these drugs on an outpatient basis, the nurse instructs the patient to avoid driving or performing hazardous tasks if dizziness occurs.

DISTURBED SENSORY PERCEPTION: VISUAL. The patient taking chloroquine may experience a number of visual disturbances, such as disturbed color vision, blurred vision, night blindness, diminished visual fields, or optic atrophy. The nurse questions the patient about visual disturbances.

> ### ✳ Nursing Alert
>
> *The nurse reports any visual disturbance in patients taking chloroquine to the primary health care provider. Irreversible retinal damage has occurred in patients on long-term therapy with these drugs.*

Frequent ophthalmic examinations are necessary for patients receiving long-term or high-dose regimens of chloroquine. When vision is affected, the patient is assessed for the extent of visual impairment. If treated outside the hospital, it is important to instruct the patient not to drive until assessed by an ophthalmologist. Environmental safety is accomplished by measures such as positioning doors and furniture so they are out of walkways, removing scatter rugs, placing items frequently used in convenient places, and strategically placing grab bars to aid in maintaining balance. Assistance with ambulation may be necessary.

Educating the Patient and Family

When an antimalarial drug is prescribed for the prevention (suppression) of malaria, the nurse thoroughly reviews the drug regimen with the patient. When the drug is to be taken once a week, the nurse advises patients to select a day of the week that will best remind them to take the drug. The nurse emphasizes the importance of taking the drug exactly as prescribed because failure to take the drug on an exact schedule will not give protection against malaria.

The patient must have a complete understanding of the therapeutic regimen. The nurse reviews the drug dosage schedule with the patient and stresses the importance of adhering to the prescribed dosage schedule.

When an antimalarial drug is used for prevention of malaria and taken once a week, the patient must take the drug on the same day each week. The program of prevention is usually started 1 week before departure to an area where malaria is prevalent.

The following additional information is relevant to specific antimalarial drugs:

Chloroquine: Take this drug with food or milk. Avoid foods that acidify the urine (cranberries, plums, prunes, meats, cheeses, eggs, fish, and grains). This drug may cause diarrhea, loss of appetite, nausea, stomach pain, or vomiting. Notify the primary health care provider if these symptoms become pronounced. Chloroquine may cause a yellow or brownish discoloration to the urine; this is normal and will go away when the drug therapy is discontinued. Notify the primary health care provider if any of the following occur:

- Visual changes
- Ringing in the ears
- Difficulty in hearing
- Fever
- Sore throat
- Unusual bleeding or bruising
- Unusual color (blue-black) of the skin
- Skin rash
- Unusual muscle weakness

Doxycycline: This drug can cause photosensitivity. Even relatively brief exposure to sunlight may cause sunburn. Avoid exposure to the sun by wearing protective clothing (eg, long-sleeved shirts and wide-brimmed hats) and by using a sunscreen.

Quinine: Take this drug with food or immediately after a meal. Do not drive or perform other hazardous tasks requiring alertness if blurred vision or dizziness occurs. If the tablet or capsule is difficult to swallow, do not chew the tablet or open the capsule because the drug is irritating to the stomach. If itching, rash, fever, difficult breathing, or vision problems occur, stop taking the drug and notify the primary health care provider.

EVALUATION

- The therapeutic effect is achieved.
- Adverse reactions are identified, reported to the health care provider, and managed using appropriate nursing interventions.
- The patient verbalizes the importance of complying with the prescribed therapeutic or prophylactic regimen.
- The patient verbalizes an understanding of the prophylaxis or treatment schedule.

AMEBICIDES

Amebicides (drugs that kill amebas) are used to treat amebiasis caused by the parasite *E. histolytica*. An ameba is a one-celled organism found in soil and water. Examples of amebicides are listed in the Summary Drug Table: Amebicides.

ACTIONS AND USES

These drugs are amebicidal (ie, they kill amebas). There are two types of amebiasis: intestinal and extraintestinal.

In the intestinal form, the ameba is confined to the intestine. In the extraintestinal form, the ameba is found outside of the intestine, such as in the liver. The extraintestinal form of amebiasis is more difficult to treat.

Iodoquinol (Yodoxin) and metronidazole (Flagyl) are used to treat intestinal amebiasis. Metronidazole is also used to treat infections caused by susceptible microorganisms and is discussed in Chapter 11. Paromomycin is an aminoglycoside with amebicidal activity and is used to treat intestinal amebiasis. Chloroquine hydrochloride (Aralen) is used to treat extraintestinal amebiasis.

ADVERSE REACTIONS

Chloroquine

Hypotension, electrocardiographic changes, headache, nausea, vomiting, anorexia, diarrhea, abdominal cramps, and psychic stimulation can occur with the use of chloroquine hydrochloride or phosphate.

Iodoquinol

Various types of skin eruptions, nausea, vomiting, fever, chills, abdominal cramps, vertigo, and diarrhea can occur with administration of iodoquinol.

SUMMARY DRUG TABLE AMEBICIDES

GENERIC NAME	TRADE NAME*	USES	ADVERSE REACTIONS	DOSAGE RANGES
chloroquine hydrochloride *klor´-oh-kwin*	Aralen	Extraintestinal amebiasis when oral therapy not feasible	Hypotension, electrocardiographic (ECG) changes, headache, nausea, vomiting, anorexia, diarrhea, abdominal cramps, psychic stimulation, visual disturbances	*Dose expressed as base.* 160–200 mg/d IM for 10–12 d
chloroquine phosphate *klor´-oh-kwin*	Aralen Phosphate, *generic*	Extraintestinal amebiasis when oral therapy not feasible	Hypotension, ECG changes, headache, nausea, vomiting, anorexia, diarrhea, abdominal cramps, psychic stimulation	1 g (600 mg base)/d for 2 d, then 500 mg (300 mg base)/d for 2–3 wk
iodoquinol *eye-oh-doe-kwin´-ole*	Yodoxin	Treatment of intestinal amebiasis	Skin eruptions, nausea, vomiting, fever, chills, abdominal cramps, vertigo, diarrhea	650 mg PO TID after meals for 20 d
metronidazole *me-troe-ni´-da-zole*	Flagyl, *generic*	Treatment of intestinal amebiasis	Headache, nausea, peripheral neuropathy, disulfiram-like interaction with alcohol	750 mg PO TID for 5–10 d
paromomycin *par-oh-moe-mye´-sin*	Humatin	Treatment of intestinal amebiasis	Nausea, vomiting, diarrhea	25–35 mg/kg/d in 3 divided doses with meals for 5–10 d

*The term *generic* indicates the drug is available in generic form.

Metronidazole

Convulsive seizures, headache, nausea, and peripheral neuropathy (numbness and tingling of the extremities) have been reported with the use of metronidazole.

Paromomycin

This drug has relatively few adverse reactions. The most common include nausea, vomiting, and diarrhea. The more serious adverse reactions, although rare, are nephrotoxicity and ototoxicity.

CONTRAINDICATIONS, PRECAUTIONS, AND INTERACTIONS

Chloroquine

Chloroquine is contraindicated in patients with known hypersensitivity. Precautions and interactions for chloroquine are provided in the discussion of the drug in the Antimalarial Drugs section.

Iodoquinol

Iodoquinol is contraindicated in patients with known hypersensitivity. Iodoquinol is used with caution in patients with thyroid disease and during pregnancy and lactation. Iodoquinol may interfere with the results of thyroid function tests. This interference not only occurs during therapy, but may last as long as 6 months after iodoquinol therapy is discontinued.

Metronidazole

Metronidazole is contraindicated in patients with known hypersensitivity. Metronidazole is contraindicated during the first trimester of pregnancy (Category B). Metronidazole is given during the second and third trimesters of pregnancy. Metronidazole is used cautiously in patients with blood dyscrasias, seizure disorders, and severe hepatic impairment. The patient must avoid alcohol while taking metronidazole.

When metronidazole is administered with cimetidine, the metabolism of metronidazole is decreased; when it is administered with phenobarbital, the metabolism is increased, possibly causing a decrease in the effectiveness of metronidazole. Metronidazole increases the effects of warfarin.

Paromomycin

Paromomycin is contraindicated in patients with known hypersensitivity. Paromomycin is given with caution during pregnancy. Paromomycin is used with caution in patients with bowel disease. High doses and prolonged therapy are avoided because the drug may be absorbed in large amounts by patients with bowel disease, causing ototoxicity and renal impairment.

NURSING PROCESS

● The Patient Receiving an Amebicide

ASSESSMENT

Preadministration Assessment

Diagnosis of amebiasis is made by examining the stool, as well as by considering the patient's symptoms. Once the patient has received a diagnosis of amebiasis, local health department regulations often require investigation into the source of infection. A thorough history of foreign travel is necessary. If the patient has not traveled to a foreign country, further investigation of the patient's lifestyle, such as local travel, use of restaurants, and the local water supply (especially well water) may be necessary to identify the source of the infection. In addition, it is common practice to test immediate family members for amebiasis.

Before the first dose of an amebicide is given, the nurse records the patient's vital signs and weight. The nurse evaluates the general physical status of the patient and looks for evidence of dehydration, especially if severe vomiting and diarrhea have occurred.

Ongoing Assessment

If the patient is acutely ill or has vomiting and diarrhea, the nurse measures the fluid intake and output and observes the patient closely for signs of dehydration. If dehydration is apparent, the nurse notifies the primary health care provider. If the patient is or becomes dehydrated, oral or IV fluid and electrolyte replacement may be necessary. The nurse takes vital signs every 4 hours or as ordered by the primary health care provider.

NURSING DIAGNOSES

The specific nursing diagnoses used depend on the type of amebiasis and the condition of the patient. Drug-specific nursing diagnoses are highlighted in the Nursing Diagnoses Checklist. More general nursing diagnoses are discussed in greater depth in Chapter 4.

Nursing Diagnoses Checklist

☑ **Diarrhea** related to amebiasis

☑ **Risk for Deficient Fluid Volume** related to amebiasis

☑ **Imbalanced Nutrition: Less Than Body Requirements** related to adverse effects of drug therapy

PLANNING

The expected outcomes for the patient may include an optimal response to therapy, management of common adverse reactions, an absence of diarrhea, maintenance of an adequate intake of fluids, maintenance of adequate nutrition, an understanding of the therapeutic regimen (hospitalized patients), and an understanding of and compliance with the prescribed therapeutic regimen (outpatients).

IMPLEMENTATION

Promoting an Optimal Response to Therapy

The patient with amebiasis may or may not be acutely ill. Nursing management depends on the condition of the patient and the information obtained during the initial assessment.

Isolation is usually not necessary, but hospital policy may require isolation procedures. Stool precautions are usually necessary. The nurse washes the hands thoroughly after all patient care and the handling of stool specimens.

Monitoring and Managing Adverse Reactions

The nurse monitors the patient for adverse reactions associated with the amebicides such as diarrhea and gastrointestinal upsets. Other adverse reactions are listed on the Summary Drug Table: Amebicides.

DIARRHEA AND DEFICIENT FLUID VOLUME. The nurse records the number, character, and color of stools passed. Daily stool specimens may be ordered to be sent to the laboratory for examination. The nurse immediately delivers all stool specimens saved for examination to the laboratory because the organisms die (and therefore cannot be seen microscopically) when the specimen cools. The nurse should inform laboratory personnel that the patient has amebiasis because the specimen must be kept at or near body temperature until examined under a microscope.

The nurse observes the patient with severe or frequent episodes of diarrhea for symptoms of a fluid volume deficit. The primary health care provider is notified if signs of dehydration become apparent because IV fluids may be necessary.

IMBALANCED NUTRITION. Because most amebicides cause gastrointestinal upsets, particularly nausea, the maintenance of adequate nutrition is important. A discussion of eating habits, food preferences, and food aversions will assist in meal planning. The nurse monitors body weight daily to identify any changes (increase or decrease). The nurse should make sure that meals are well balanced nutritionally, appetizing, and attractively served. Small frequent meals (five to six daily) may be more appealing than three large meals. The nurse may consult the dietitian if necessary.

Educating the Patient and Family

The nurse stresses the importance of completing the full course of treatment. The nurse should provide the following information to patients receiving an amebicide on an outpatient basis:

- Follow directions: Take the drug exactly as prescribed. Complete the full course of therapy to eradicate the ameba. Failure to complete treatment may result in a return of the infection.
- Prevention: Follow measures to control the spread of infection. Wash hands immediately before eating or preparing food and after defecation.
- Chef/waitstaff: Food handlers should not resume work until a full course of treatment is completed and stools do not contain the ameba.
- Chloroquine: Notify the primary health care provider if any of the following occurs: ringing in the ears, difficulty hearing, visual changes, fever, sore throat, or unusual bleeding or bruising.
- Iodoquinol: Notify the primary health care provider if nausea, vomiting, or other gastrointestinal distress becomes severe.
- Metronidazole: This drug may cause gastric upset. Take this drug with food or meals. Avoid the use of alcohol, in any form, until the course of treatment is completed. The ingestion of alcohol may cause a mild to severe reaction, with symptoms of severe vomiting, headache, nausea, abdominal cramps, flushing, and sweating. These symptoms may be so severe that hospitalization may be required.
- Paromomycin: Take this drug three times a day with meals. Report any ringing in the ears, dizziness, severe gastrointestinal upset, decrease in urinary output, or other urinary difficulties.

EVALUATION

- The therapeutic effect is achieved.
- Adverse reactions are identified, reported to the primary health care provider, and managed successfully through nursing interventions.
- Bowel elimination is normal.
- The patient verbalizes an understanding of the therapeutic modalities and importance of continued follow-up care.
- The patient verbalizes the importance of complying with the prescribed therapeutic regimen.

● Critical Thinking Excercises

1. *While he was living outside the country for 3 years, Mr. Evans became infected with a helminth. The parasite has been identified and the appropriate drug prescribed. Discuss the points you would include in a teaching plan for this patient.*

2. *A child in a family of four children is found to have pinworms. Determine what you would include in a teaching plan to prevent the spread of pinworms to other family members.*

3. *Explain what precautions should be taken when administering paromomycin.*

4. *Mr. Adkins, age 68 years, is being treated with metronidazole for intestinal amebiasis. He tells you that he lives alone, eats out for most of his meals, and likes to have a glass of wine before retiring. Analyze what information would be most important for you to give Mr. Adkins before he begins taking metronidazole.*

● Review Questions

1. When discussing the adverse reactions of the anthelmintic, the nurse correctly states that _____.
   A. patients must be closely observed for 2 hours after the drug is given
   B. adverse reactions are usually mild when recommended doses are used
   C. most patients experience severe adverse reaction and must be monitored closely
   D. there are no adverse reactions associated with these drugs

2. A patient asks how antimalarial drugs prevent or treat malaria. The nurse correctly responds that this group of drugs _____.
   A. kills the mosquito that carries the protozoa
   B. interferes with the life cycle of the protozoa causing malaria
   C. ruptures the red blood cells that contain merozoites
   D. increases the body's natural immune response to the protozoa

3. When explaining the drug regimen to a patient who will be taking chloroquine for the prevention of malaria the nurse instructs the patient _____.
   A. to take the drug on an empty stomach
   B. to protect the skin from the sun because the drug can cause a severe sunburn
   C. therapy should begin 2 weeks before exposure
   D. to take the drug with a citrus drink to enhance absorption

4. While administering paromomycin, the nurse monitors the patient for which of the following adverse reactions?
   A. ototoxicity
   B. cinchonism
   C. convulsions
   D. hypertension

● Medication Dosage Problems

1. Pyrantel 360 mg is prescribed. The drug is available in 180-mg capsules. The nurse administers _____.

2. Hydroxychloroquine 0.4 g is ordered. The drug is available in 200-mg tablets. The nurse administers _____.

c h a p t e r **17**

Nonnarcotic Analgesics: Salicylates and Nonsalicylates

Key Terms

acute pain
aggregation
analgesic
antipyretic
chronic pain
jaundice
pain

pancytopenia
prostaglandin
Reye's syndrome
salicylate
salicylism
tinnitus

Chapter Objectives

On completion of this chapter, the student will:

● Discuss the types, uses, general drug actions, common adverse reactions, contraindications, precautions, and interactions of the salicylates and acetaminophen.
● Discuss important preadministration and ongoing assessment activities the nurse should perform on the patient taking salicylates or acetaminophen.
● List some nursing diagnoses particular to a patient taking the salicylates or acetaminophen.
● Discuss the ways to promote an optimal response to therapy, how to manage common adverse reactions, and important points to keep in mind when educating patients about the use of the salicylates or acetaminophen.

Pain can be defined as an unpleasant sensory and emotional experience that is associated with actual or potential tissue damage. Pain is subjective, and the patient's report of pain should always be taken seriously. Pain management in acute and chronic illness is an important responsibility of the nurse. Many nurses consider pain as the fifth vital sign and assessment of pain just as important as the assessment of temperature, pulse, respirations, and blood pressure. Accurate assessment of pain is necessary if pain management is to be effective. Patients with pain are often undertreated.

Basically there are three types of pain: acute pain, chronic pain associated with malignant disease, and chronic pain not associated with malignant disease. **Acute pain** is of short duration and lasts less than 3 to 6 months. Intensity of acute pain is from mild to severe. Causes of acute pain include postoperative pain, procedural pain, and traumatic pain. Acute pain usually subsides when the injury heals.

Chronic pain lasts longer than 6 months and ranges in intensity from mild to severe. Chronic pain associated with malignancy includes the pain of cancer, acquired

immunodeficiency syndrome (AIDS), multiple sclerosis, sickle cell disease, and end-stage organ system failure.

The exact cause of chronic pain of a nonmalignant nature may or may not be known. This type of pain includes the pain associated with various neuropathic and musculoskeletal disorders such as headaches, fibromyalgia, rheumatoid arthritis, and osteoarthritis.

The next three chapters deal with drugs used in the management of pain: the nonnarcotic **analgesics** (salicylates, nonsalicylates [acetaminophen], and the nonsteroidal anti-inflammatory drugs) and the narcotic analgesics.

The nonnarcotic analgesics are a group of drugs used to relieve pain without the possibility of causing physical dependency, which can occur with the use of the narcotic analgesics. The nonnarcotic analgesics can be divided into the salicylates, nonsalicylates (acetaminophen), and the nonsteroidal anti-inflammatory drugs (NSAIDs). There are a number of combination nonnarcotic analgesics that are available over the counter and by prescription. The NSAIDs have emerged as important drugs in the treatment of the chronic pain and inflammation associated with disorders such as rheumatoid arthritis or osteoarthritis. Examples of NSAIDs include celecoxib (Celebrex) and rofecoxib (Vioxx). This chapter deals with the nonnarcotic analgesics: the salicylates and acetaminophen. Subsequent chapters cover the NSAIDs and the narcotic analgesics.

SALICYLATES

The **salicylates** include aspirin (acetylsalicylic acid) and **related** drugs, such as magnesium salicylate and sodium salicylate. The salicylates have analgesic (relieves pain), **antipyretic** (reduces elevated body temperature), and anti-inflammatory effects. All the salicylates are similar in pharmacologic activity; however, aspirin has a greater anti-inflammatory effect than the other salicylates. Specific salicylates are listed in the Summary Drug Table: Nonnarcotic Analgesics: Salicylates and Nonsalicylates.

✿ Herbal Alert: Willow Bark

Willow bark has a long history of use as an analgesic. Willows are small trees or shrubs that grow in moist places, often along riverbanks in temperate or cold climates. When used as a medicinal herb, willow bark is collected in early spring from young branches. In addition to its use as a pain reliever, various species of willow bark and leaf have been used to lower fever and as an anti-inflammatory. The salicylates were isolated from willow bark and identified as the most like source of the bark's anti-inflammatory effects. The chemical structure was replicated in the lab and mass produced as synthetic salicylic acid. Years later, a modified version (acetylsalicylic acid) was first sold as aspirin. Aspirin became the most widely used pain reliever, fever reducer, and anti-inflammatory agent, leaving willow bark to be cast aside. The synthetic anti-inflammatory drugs work quickly and have a higher potency than willow bark. Willow bark takes longer to work and may need fairly high doses to achieve a noticeable effect. However, fewer adverse reactions are associated with willow bark than with the salicylates. Although adverse reactions are rare with willow bark, it should be used with caution in patients with peptic ulcers and medical conditions in which aspirin is contraindicated.

ACTIONS

The manner in which salicylates relieve pain and reduce inflammation is not fully understood. It is thought that the analgesic action of the salicylates is due to the inhibition of prostaglandins. **Prostaglandins** are fatty acid derivatives found in almost every tissue of the body and body fluid. Release of prostaglandin is thought to increase the sensitivity of peripheral pain receptors. The inhibitory action of the salicylates on the prostaglandins is also thought to account for the anti-inflammatory activity. Salicylates lower an elevated body temperature by dilating peripheral blood vessels, which in turn cools the body.

Aspirin more potently inhibits prostaglandin synthesis and has greater anti-inflammatory effects that the other salicylates. In addition, aspirin also prolongs the bleeding time by inhibiting the **aggregation** (clumping) of platelets. When the bleeding time is prolonged, it takes a longer time for the blood to clot after a cut, surgery, or other injury to the skin or mucous membranes. The other salicylates do not have as great an effect on platelets as does aspirin. This effect of aspirin on the platelets is irreversible and lasts for the life of the platelet (7–10 days).

USES

The salicylate nonnarcotic analgesics are used for the following reasons:

- Relief of mild to moderate pain;
- Reduction of elevated body temperature (except for diflunisal which is not used as an antipyretic);
- Treatment of inflammatory conditions, such as rheumatoid arthritis, osteoarthritis, and rheumatic fever;
- Reduction of the risk of myocardial infarction in those with unstable angina or previous myocardial infarction (aspirin only); and
- Reduction of the risk of transient ischemic attacks or strokes in men who have had transient ischemia of the brain due to fibrin platelet emboli (aspirin only). This use has been found to be effective only in men (not women).

ADVERSE REACTIONS

Gastric upset, heartburn, nausea, vomiting, anorexia, and gastrointestinal bleeding may occur with salicylate use. Although these drugs are relatively safe when taken as recommended on the label or by the primary health care provider, their use can occasionally result in more serious reactions. Some individuals are allergic to aspirin and the other salicylates. Allergy to the salicylates may be manifested by hives, rash, angioedema, bronchospasm with asthma-like symptoms, and anaphylactoid reactions.

Loss of blood through the gastrointestinal tract occurs with salicylate use. The amount of blood lost is

Patients receiving long-term opioid therapy rarely have problems with respiratory depression. In instances where respiratory depression occurs, administration of a narcotic antagonist (see Chap. 20) may be ordered by the primary health care provider if the respiratory rate continues to fall.

> ### ❄ Gerontologic Alert
>
> *The older adult is especially prone to adverse reactions of the narcotic analgesics, particularly respiratory depression, somnolence (sedation), and confusion. The primary health care provider may order a lower dosage of the narcotic for the older adult.*

Narcotics may depress the cough reflex. The nurse should encourage patients receiving a narcotic on a regular basis, even for a few days, to cough and breathe deeply every 2 hours. This task prevents the pooling of secretions in the lungs, which can lead to hypostatic pneumonia and other lung problems. If the patient experiences nausea and vomiting, the nurse should notify the primary health care provider. A different analgesic or an antiemetic may be necessary.

RISK FOR INJURY. Narcotics may produce orthostatic hypotension, which in turn results in dizziness. The nurse should assist the patient with ambulatory activities and with rising slowly from a sitting or lying position. **Miosis** (pinpoint pupils) may occur with the administration of some narcotics and is most pronounced with morphine, hydromorphone, and hydrochlorides of opium alkaloids. Miosis decreases the ability to see in dim light. The nurse keeps the room well lit during daytime hours and advises the patient to seek assistance when getting out of bed at night.

CONSTIPATION. The nurse checks the bowel elimination pattern daily because constipation can occur with repeated doses of a narcotic. The nurse keeps a daily record of bowel movements and informs the primary health care provider if constipation appears to be a problem. Most patients should begin taking a stool softener or laxative with the initial dose of a narcotic analgesic. Many patients need to continue taking a laxative as long as the narcotic analgesic is taken. If the patient is constipated despite the use of a stool softener, the primary health care provider may prescribe an enema or another means of relieving constipation.

IMBALANCED NUTRITION. When a narcotic is prescribed for a prolonged time, anorexia (loss of appetite) may occur. Those receiving a narcotic for the relief of pain caused by terminal cancer often have severe anorexia from the disease and the narcotic. The nurse assesses food intake after each meal. When anorexia is prolonged, the nurse weighs the patient weekly or as ordered by the primary health care provider. It is important for the nurse to notify the primary health care provider of continued weight loss and anorexia.

NARCOTIC DRUG DEPENDENCE. Most patients receiving the narcotic analgesics for medical purposes do not develop dependence. However, drug dependence can occur when a narcotic is administered over a long period. For some patients, such as those who are terminally ill and in severe pain, drug dependence is not considered a problem because the most important task is to keep the patient as comfortable as possible for the time he or she has remaining (see "Relieving Chronic Severe Pain").

When a patient does not have a painful terminal illness, drug dependence must be avoided. Signs of drug dependence include occurrence of withdrawal symptoms (acute abstinence syndrome) when the narcotic is discontinued, requests for the narcotic at frequent intervals around the clock, personality changes if the narcotic is not given immediately, and constant complaints of pain and failure of the narcotic to relieve pain. Although these behaviors can have other causes, the nurse should consider drug dependence and discuss the problem with the primary health care provider. Specific symptoms of the abstinence syndrome are listed in Display 19-3.

Drug dependence can also occur in a newborn whose mother was dependent on opiates during pregnancy. Withdrawal symptoms in the newborn usually appear during the first few days of life. Symptoms include irritability, excessive crying, yawning, sneezing, increased respiratory rate, tremors, fever, vomiting, and diarrhea.

Educating the Patient and Family

The nurse informs the patient that the drug he or she is receiving is for pain. It also is a good idea to include additional information, such as how often the drug can be given and the name of the drug being given. If a patient is receiving drugs through a PCA infusion pump, the nurse discusses the following points:

● The location of the control button that activates the administration of the drug;

> ### DISPLAY 19-3 ● Symptoms of the Abstinence Syndrome
>
> **EARLY SYMPTOMS**
> Yawning, lacrimation, rhinorrhea, sweating
>
> **INTERMEDIATE SYMPTOMS**
> Mydriasis, tachycardia, twitching, tremor, restlessness, irritability, anxiety, anorexia
>
> **LATE SYMPTOMS**
> Muscle spasm, fever, nausea, vomiting, kicking movements, weakness, depression, body aches, weight loss, severe backache, abdominal and leg pains, hot and cold flashes, insomnia, repetitive sneezing, increased blood pressure, respiratory rate, and heart rate

Home Care Checklist

USING A PATIENT-CONTROLLED ANALGESIA PUMP

In some situations, narcotic analgesics may be ordered for pain relief using patient-controlled analgesia (PCA). If the patient will be receiving PCA at home, the nurse makes sure to review the following steps with the patient and the caregiver:

✓ How the pump works

✓ What drug is being given

✓ When to administer a dose

✓ What the power source is (battery or electricity)

✓ What to do if the battery fails or a power failure occurs

✓ How to check the insertion site

✓ How to change the cartridge or syringe

If the patient or caregiver will be responsible for changing the drug cartridge or syringe, the nurse teaches the following steps:

✓ Gather new syringe with drug (if refrigerated, remove it at least 30 minutes before using).

✓ Attach pump specific tubing to the drug.

✓ Prime the tubing.

✓ Turn off the pump and clamp the infusion tubing.

✓ Remove the tubing from the infusion site.

✓ Flush the site (if ordered).

✓ Remove used cartridge or syringe from the pump.

✓ Insert the new cartridge or syringe into the pump.

✓ Connect the new infusion tubing to the infusion site.

✓ Turn on the pump and have the patient provide a drug dose when needed.

- The difference between the control button and the button to call the nurse (when both are similar in appearance and feel);
- The machine regulates the dose of the drug as well as the time interval between doses;
- If the control button is used too soon after the last dose, the machine will not deliver the drug until the correct time;
- Pain relief should occur shortly after pushing the button;
- Call the nurse if pain relief does not occur after two successive doses.

Narcotics for outpatient use may be prescribed in the oral form or as a timed-release transdermal patch. In certain cases, such as when terminally ill patients are being cared for at home, the nurse may give the family instruction in the parenteral administration of the drug or use of PCA (see Home Care Checklist: Using a Patient Controlled Analgesia Pump). When a narcotic has been prescribed, the nurse includes the following points in the teaching plan:

- This drug may cause drowsiness, dizziness, and blurring of vision. Use caution when driving or performing tasks requiring alertness.
- Avoid the use of alcoholic beverages unless use has been approved by the primary health care provider. Alcohol may intensify the action of the drug and cause extreme drowsiness or dizziness.

In some instances, the use of alcohol and a narcotic can have extremely serious and even life-threatening consequences that may require emergency medical treatment.

- Take the drug as directed on the container label and do not exceed the prescribed dose. Contact the primary health care provider if the drug is not effective.
- If gastrointestinal upset occurs, take the drug with food.
- Notify the primary health care provider if nausea, vomiting, and constipation become severe.
- To administer the transdermal system, remove the system from the package and immediately apply it to the skin of the upper torso. To ensure complete contact with the skin surface, press for 10 to 20 seconds with the palm of the hand. After 72 hours, remove the system and, if continuous therapy is prescribed, apply a new system. Use only water to cleanse the site before application because soaps, oils, and other substances may irritate the skin. Rotate site of application. The used patch should be folded carefully so the system adheres to itself.

EVALUATION

- The therapeutic effect occurs and pain is relieved.
- The patient demonstrates the ability to effectively use PCA.
- Adverse reactions are identified, reported to the primary health care provider, and managed through appropriate nursing interventions.
- No evidence of injury is seen.
- Body weight is maintained.
- Diet is adequate.
- The patient is free of drug dependence.
- The patient and family demonstrate understanding of the drug regimen.

● *Critical Thinking Exercises*

1. *Ms. Taylor is receiving meperidine for postoperative pain management. In assessing Ms. Taylor approximately 20 minutes after receiving an injection of meperidine, the nurse discovers Ms. Taylor's vital signs are blood pressure 100/50 mm Hg, pulse rate 100 bpm, and respiratory rate 10/min. Determine what action, if any, the nurse should take.*

2. *Mr. Talley, a 64-year-old retired schoolteacher, has cancer and is to receive morphine through a PCA infusion pump. His wife is eager to help, but Mr. Talley is very independent and refuses any assistance from her. Formulate a teaching plan for Mr. Talley that includes the use of PCA, adverse reactions to expect, and what adverse reactions to report. Discuss what methods the nurse might use to include Mrs. Talley in the care of her husband.*

3. *Roger Baccus, age 23 years, is prescribed Demerol for postoperative pain. You discover in his health history on the chart that he has a history of alcohol and drug use. Determine what further assessments you would need to make. Explain how Roger's answers would influence the actions that you as a nurse would take.*

4. *Discuss the important preadministration assessments that must be made on the patient receiving a narcotic analgesic.*

5. *Joe Thompson, age 48 years, is taking morphine to manage severe pain occurring as the result of cancer. The primary health care provider has prescribed an around-the-clock dosage regimen. Joe is asking for the pain drug 1 to 2 hours before the next dose is due. One of your co-workers feels that Joe is becoming addicted to the narcotic analgesic. Analyze this situation. What signs and symptoms would you look for in Joe? What information (if any) would you discuss with your co-worker. Discuss the actions you would take in providing the best possible care for this patient.*

● *Review Questions*

1. The nurse explains to the patient that some narcotics may be used as part of the preoperative medication regimen to _____.
   - A. increase intestinal motility
   - B. facilitate passage of an endotracheal tube
   - C. enhance the effects of the skeletal muscle relaxant
   - D. lessen anxiety and sedate the patient

2. Each time the patient requests a narcotic analgesic, the nurse must _____.
   - A. check the patient's diagnosis
   - B. talk to the patient to be sure he or she is not becoming addicted to the narcotic
   - C. determine the exact location of the pain, a description of the pain, and when the pain began
   - D. administer the narcotic with food to prevent gastric upset

3. Which of the following findings requires that the nurse withhold a narcotic and immediately contact the health care provider?
   - A. a pulse rate of 80 bpm
   - B. a significant decrease in blood pressure or a systolic pressure below 100 mm Hg
   - C. a respiratory rate of 20/min
   - D. blood pressure with a systolic pressure of 140 mm Hg

4. When administering narcotic analgesics to an elderly patient, the nurse monitors the patient closely for _____.
   - A. an increased heart rate
   - B. euphoria

C. confusion

D. a synergistic reaction

5. When monitoring a patient receiving a narcotic agonist-antagonist, the nurse must be aware that _____.

  A. symptoms of narcotic withdrawal may occur in those addicted to narcotics
  B. severe respiratory depression may occur
  C. serious cardiac arrhythmias may develop
  D. CNS stimulation is possible

● *Medications Dosage Problems*

1. A patient is prescribed oral morphine 12 mg. The dosage available is 10 mg/mL. The nurse administers _____.

2. A patient is prescribed fentanyl (Sublimaze) 50 mcg IM 30 minutes before surgery. The nurse has available a vial with a dosage strength of 0.05 mg/1 mL. The nurse calculates the dosage and administers _____.

Narcotic Antagonists

Chapter Objectives

On completion of this chapter, the student will:

- Discuss the uses, general drug action, general adverse reactions, contraindications, precautions, and interactions of the narcotic antagonists.
- Discuss important preadministration and ongoing assessment activities the nurse should perform on the patient taking the narcotic antagonists.
- List some nursing diagnoses particular to a patient taking a narcotic antagonist.
- Discuss ways to promote optimal response to therapy, how to manage adverse reactions, and important points to keep in mind when educating patients about the use of narcotic antagonists.

An **antagonist** is a substance that counteracts the action of something else. A drug that is an antagonist has an affinity for a cell receptor, and by binding to it, prevents the cell from responding. Thus, a narcotic antagonist reverses the actions of a narcotic. Specific antagonists have been developed to reverse the respiratory depression associated with the opiates. The two narcotic antagonists in use today are naloxone (Narcan) and naltrexone (ReVia; see the Summary Drug Table: Narcotic Antagonists). Naloxone is capable of restoring respiratory function within 1 to 2 minutes after administration. Naltrexone is used primarily for the treatment of narcotic dependence to block the effects of the opiates, especially the euphoric effects experienced in opiate dependence.

NALOXONE

ACTIONS

Administration of naloxone prevents or reverses the effects of the opiates. The exact mechanism of action is not fully understood, but it is believed that naloxone reverses opioid effects by competing for opiate receptor sites (see Chap. 19). If the individual has taken or received an opiate, the effects of the opiate are reversed.

If the individual has not taken or received an opiate, naloxone has no drug activity.

USES

This drug is used for complete or partial reversal of narcotic depression, including respiratory depression. Narcotic depression may be due to intentional or accidental overdose (self-administration by an individual), accidental overdose by medical personnel, and drug idiosyncrasy. Naloxone also may be used for diagnosis of a suspected acute opioid overdosage.

ADVERSE REACTIONS

Although not a true adverse reaction, abrupt reversal of narcotic depression may result in nausea, vomiting, sweating, tachycardia, increased blood pressure, and tremors.

CONTRAINDICATIONS, PRECAUTIONS, AND INTERACTIONS

Naloxone is contraindicated in those with a hypersensitivity to the narcotic antagonists. Naloxone is used cautiously in those with a narcotic addiction. Naloxone

SUMMARY DRUG TABLE NARCOTIC ANTAGONISTS

GENERIC NAME	TRADE NAME*	USES	ADVERSE REACTIONS	DOSAGE RANGES
nalmefene *nal'-me-feen*	Revex	Complete or partial reversal of opioid effects	Nausea, vomiting, tachycardia, hypertension, return of postoperative pain, fever, dizziness	Initial dose: 0.5 mg/70 kg IV PRN, second dose of 1 mg/70 kg 2–5 min later; maximum dose, 1.5 mg/70 kg
naloxone hydrochloride *nal-ox'-ohn*	Narcan	Narcotic overdose, postoperative narcotic depression	Abrupt reversal of narcotic depression may result in nausea, vomiting, sweating, increased blood pressure, tachycardia	0.4–2 mg IV initially with additional doses repeated at 2–3 min intervals; smaller doses used for postoperative narcotic depression
naltrexone hydrochloride *nal-trex'-ohn*	ReVia, Depade	Narcotic addiction, alcohol dependence	Anxiety, difficulty sleeping, abdominal cramps, nasal congestion, joint and muscle pain, nausea, vomiting, dizziness, irritability	Maintenance treatment: 50 mg PO daily or 100 mg every other day, or 150 mg PO every third day; 2 mL IV, SC

*The term *generic* indicates the drug is available in generic form.

is used cautiously in patients with cardiovascular disease; those who are pregnant (Pregnancy Category B); and in infants of opioid-dependent mothers.

These drugs may produce withdrawal symptoms in those physically dependent on the narcotics. The patient must not have taken any opiate for the last 7 to 10 days. Naloxone may prevent the action of opioid antidiarrheals, antitussives, and analgesics. This drug is used cautiously during lactation.

NALTREXONE

ACTIONS

Naltrexone completely blocks the effects of IV opiates, as well as drugs with agonist-antagonist actions (butorphanol, nalbuphine, and pentazocine). The mechanism of action appears to be the same as that for naloxone.

USES

Naltrexone is used to treat persons dependent on opioids. Patients receiving naltrexone have been detoxified and are enrolled in a program for treatment of narcotic addiction. Naltrexone, along with other methods of treatment (counseling, psychotherapy), is used to maintain an opioid-free state. Patients taking naltrexone on a

scheduled basis will not experience any narcotic effects if they use an opioid.

ADVERSE REACTIONS

Administration of naltrexone may result in anxiety, difficulty sleeping, abdominal cramps, nasal congestion, joint and muscle pain, nausea, vomiting, dizziness, irritability, depression, fatigue, and drowsiness.

CONTRAINDICATIONS, PRECAUTIONS, AND INTERACTIONS

Naltrexone is contraindicated in those with a hypersensitivity to the narcotic antagonists. Naltrexone is contraindicated during pregnancy (Category C). Naltrexone is used cautiously in those with a narcotic addiction; in patients with cardiovascular disease, acute hepatitis, liver failure, or depression; and in patients who are suicidal. Naltrexone is used cautiously during lactation.

Naltrexone may produce withdrawal symptoms in those physically dependent on narcotics. The patient must not have taken any opiate for the last 7 to 10 days. Concurrent use of naltrexone with thioridazine may cause increased drowsiness and lethargy. Naltrexone may prevent the action of opioid antidiarrheals, antitussives, and analgesics.

● **The Patient Receiving a Narcotic Antagonist for Respiratory Depression**

ASSESSMENT

Preadministration Assessment

Before the administration of naloxone, the nurse obtains the blood pressure, pulse, and respiratory rate and reviews the record for the drug suspected of causing the overdosage. If there is sufficient time, the nurse also should review the initial health history, allergy history, and current treatment modalities.

Ongoing Assessment

As part of the ongoing assessment during the administration of naloxone, the nurse monitors the blood pressure, pulse, and respiratory rate at frequent intervals, usually every 5 minutes, until the patient responds. After the patient has shown response to the drug, the nurse monitors vital signs every 5 to 15 minutes. The nurse should notify the primary health care provider if any adverse drug reactions occur because additional medical treatment may be needed. The nurse monitors the respiratory rate, rhythm, and depth; pulse; blood pressure; and level of consciousness until the effects of the narcotics wear off.

> **Nursing Alert**
>
> *The effects of some narcotics may last longer than the effects of naloxone. A repeat dose of naloxone may be ordered by the primary health care provider if results obtained from the initial dose are unsatisfactory. The duration of close patient observation depends on the patient's response to the administration of the narcotic antagonist.*

NURSING DIAGNOSIS

Drug-specific nursing diagnoses are highlighted in the Nursing Diagnoses Checklist. Other nursing diagnoses applicable to these drugs are discussed in depth in Chapter 4.

> **Nursing Diagnoses Checklist**
>
> ☑ **Ineffective Airway Clearance** related to administration of a narcotic (specify overdose, drug idiosyncrasy, or other cause)
>
> ☑ **Risk for Impaired Gas Exchange** related to decreased respiratory rate

PLANNING

The expected outcome for the patient with respiratory depression is an optimal response to therapy, which essentially is a return to normal respiratory rate, rhythm, and depth.

IMPLEMENTATION

Promoting an Optimal Response to Therapy

Depending on the patient's condition, the nurse may use cardiac monitoring, artificial ventilation (respirator), and other drugs during and after the administration of naloxone. It is important to keep suction equipment readily available because abrupt reversal of narcotic depression may cause vomiting. The nurse must maintain a patent airway and should suction the patient as needed.

If naloxone is given by IV infusion, the primary health care provider orders the IV fluid and amount, the drug dosage, and the infusion rate. Giving the drug by IV infusion requires use of a secondary line or IV piggyback.

> **Nursing Alert**
>
> *When naloxone is used to reverse respiratory depression and the resulting somnolence, the drug is given slow IV push until the respiratory rate begins to increase and somnolence abates. Giving a rapid bolus will cause withdrawal and return of intense pain.*

The nurse monitors fluid intake and output and notifies the primary health care provider of any change in the fluid intake-output ratio. The nurse should notify the primary health care provider if there is any sudden change in the patient's condition.

EVALUATION

● The therapeutic effect is achieved.
● The patient's respiratory rate, rhythm, and depth are normal.
● A clear airway is maintained.

● **The Patient Receiving a Narcotic Antagonist for Treatment of Opioid Dependency**

ASSESSMENT

Preadministration Assessment

During the preadministration assessment, the nurse obtains a complete drug history. In addition, the nurse performs a complete physical examination and psychological evaluation before initiating therapy. The extent of the pretreatment assessment is usually based on the guidelines set up by the clinic or agency dispensing the drug.

Ongoing Assessment

Each time the patient visits the outpatient clinic, the nurse evaluates the patient's response to therapy and looks for any signs that drug dependency might again be a problem.

NURSING DIAGNOSES

Drug-specific nursing diagnoses are highlighted in the Nursing Diagnoses Checklist. Other nursing diagnoses applicable to these drugs are discussed in depth in Chapter 4.

Nursing Diagnoses Checklist

✓ **Ineffective Coping** related to difficulty staying drug free

✓ **Noncompliance** related to anxiety, difficulty in staying drug free, other factors (specify)

✓ **Risk of Ineffective Therapeutic Regimen Management** related to indifference, requirements of treatment program, other factors (specify)

PLANNING

The expected outcomes of the person formerly dependent on opioids may include an optimal response to therapy, which includes compliance with the treatment program, remaining drug free, and an understanding of the drug rehabilitation program.

IMPLEMENTATION

Promoting an Optimal Response to Drug Therapy

Entering a program for drug dependency may cause great anxiety due to many factors. Examples of possible causes of anxiety include the socioeconomic impact of drug dependency, the effectiveness of the treatment program, and concern over remaining drug free. Individuals vary in their ability to communicate their fears and concerns. At times, the nurse may be able to identify those situations causing anxiety and explore possible solutions to the many problems faced by these patients.

One of the greatest problems associated with former drug dependency is remaining drug free. The nurse must follow precisely the administration techniques of the drug treatment program. Some people find it difficult to break away from situations, individuals, or pressures that promote drug use. Because of this, some opioid users entering a drug rehabilitation program may, in time, not report to the program or agency to receive

their drug and thus are more apt to return to the use of an opiate.

All staff members of the rehabilitation program should work to encourage adherence to the regimen and attempt to identify situations that may encourage a return to drug use.

Educating the Patient and Family

The nurse instructs patients under treatment for narcotic addiction to wear or carry identification indicating that they are receiving naltrexone. If the patient is taking naltrexone and requires hospitalization, it is important that all medical personnel be aware of therapy with this drug. Narcotics administered to these patients have no effect and therefore do not relieve pain. Patients receiving naltrexone may pose a problem if they experience acute pain. The primary health care provider must decide what methods must be used to control pain in these patients.

The nurse should teach the patient taking naltrexone the impact of therapy. While taking the drug, any use of heroin or other opiate by the patient results in no effect. In fact, large doses of heroin or other opiates can overcome the drug's effect and result in coma or death.

EVALUATION

- The therapeutic effect is achieved, and the patient remains drug free.
- The patient complies with the prescribed treatment regimen.
- The patient demonstrates an understanding of the therapeutic regimen and requirements of the rehabilitation program.

● *Critical Thinking Exercises*

1. *Jerry Jones is to begin receiving methadone for the treatment of heroin dependency. Jerry asks why methadone, a narcotic, is effective in the treatment of narcotic dependency. How would you explain this to the patient? What information would be important to give this patient while he is in the methadone program?*

2. *Discuss important preadministration and ongoing nursing assessments you would make when giving a patient naloxone for severe respiratory depression caused by morphine.*

● *Review Questions*

1. Which narcotic antagonist would most likely be prescribed for treatment of a patient who is experiencing an overdose of a narcotic?

   A. naltrexone

   B. naloxone

C. naproxen

D. nifedipine

2. When given a narcotic analgesic for acute pain, a patient taking naltrexone for narcotic addiction _____.

   A. may have an acute hypersensitivity reaction
   B. is at increased risk for respiratory arrest
   C. will not have pain relief
   D. will have additive effects of the narcotic

3. When naltrexone is administered with thioridazine, the nurse monitors the patient for

   A. elevated temperature
   B. severe occipital headache

C. increased blood pressure

D. increased drowsiness

● Medications Dosage Problems

1. A patient is prescribed 0.8 mg naloxone IM for an overdose of morphine. Available is a vial with 1 mg/mL. The nurse administers _____.

2. The physician prescribes naltrexone (ReVia) 25 mg PO initially. The nurse is to observe the patient carefully and if no withdrawal signs appear, 100 mg PO of the drug is prescribed every other day. On hand is naltrexone 50-mg tablets. The nurse administers _____ as the initial dose.

chapter **21**

Drugs Used to Treat Disorders of the Musculoskeletal System

Key Terms

chrysiasis
corticosteroids
dermatitis
gout

musculoskeletal
osteoarthritis
rheumatoid arthritis
stomatitis

Chapter Objectives

On completion of this chapter, the student will:

- List the types of drugs used to treat musculoskeletal disorders.
- Discuss the uses, general drug actions, adverse reactions, contraindications, precautions, and interactions of the drugs used to treat musculoskeletal disorders.
- Discuss important preadministration and ongoing assessment activities the nurse should perform on the patient taking drugs used to treat musculoskeletal disorders.
- List some nursing diagnoses particular to a patient taking a drug for the treatment of musculoskeletal disorders.
- Discuss ways to promote an optimal response to therapy, management of adverse reactions, and important points to keep in mind when educating the patient about drugs used to treat musculoskeletal disorders.

A variety of drugs are used in the treatment of **musculoskeletal** (bone and muscle) disorders. Examples of the musculoskeletal disorders discussed in this chapter include osteoarthritis, rheumatoid arthritis, gout, and Paget's disease. A description of these and other musculoskeletal disorders is given in Table 21-1. The drug selected is based on the musculoskeletal disorder being treated, the severity of the disorder, and the patient's positive or negative response to past therapy. For example, early cases of rheumatoid arthritis may respond well to the salicylates, whereas advanced rheumatoid arthritis not responding to other drug therapies may require the use of one of the gold compounds.

The salicylates and nonsteroidal anti-inflammatory drugs (NSAIDs) are important in the treatment of arthritic conditions. For example, the salicylates and NSAIDs are used in the treatment of **rheumatoid arthritis** (a chronic disease characterized by inflammatory changes within the body's connective tissue) and **osteoarthritis** (a noninflammatory joint disease resulting in degeneration of the articular cartilage and

changes in the synovial membrane), as well as relief of pain or discomfort resulting from musculoskeletal injuries such as sprains. The reader is referred to Chapters 17 and 18, where these drugs are discussed in detail.

GOLD COMPOUNDS

Gold suppresses or prevents but, but does not cure, arthritis and synovitis. The therapeutic effects from gold compounds occur slowly. Early improvement is often limited to reduction in morning stiffness. The full effects of gold therapy are not known for 6 to 8 weeks or in some cases after 6 months of therapy.

ACTIONS

The exact mechanism of action of the gold compounds (for example, gold sodium thiomalate, aurothioglucose, and auranofin) in the suppression or prevention of

185

TABLE 21-1	Selected Musculoskeletal Disorders

DISORDER	DESCRIPTION
Synovitis	Synovitis is an inflammation of the synovial membrane of a joint resulting in pain, swelling, and inflammation. It occurs in disorders such as rheumatic fever, rheumatoid arthritis, and gout.
Arthritis	Arthritis is the inflammation of a joint. The term is frequently used to refer to any disease involving pain or stiffness of the musculoskeletal system.
Osteoarthritis or degenerative joint disease (DJD)	Osteoarthritis is a noninflammatory degenerative joint disease marked by degeneration of the articular cartilage, changes in the synovial membrane, and hypertrophy of the bone at the margins.
Rheumatoid arthritis (RA)	RA is a chronic systemic disease that produces inflammatory changes throughout the connective tissue in the body. It affects joints and other organ systems of the body. Destruction of articular cartilage occurs, affecting joint structure and mobility. RA primarily affects individuals between 20 and 40 years of age.
Gout	Gout is a form of arthritis in which uric acid accumulates in increased amounts in the blood and often is deposited in the joints. The deposit or collection of urate crystals in the joints causes the symptoms (pain, redness, swelling, joint deformity).
Osteoporosis	Osteoporosis is a loss of bone density occurring when the loss of bone substance exceeds the rate of bone formation. Bones become porous, brittle, and fragile. Compression fractures of the vertebrae are common. This disorder occurs most often in postmenopausal women, but can occur in men as well.
Paget's disease (osteitis deformans)	Paget's disease is a chronic bone disorder characterized by abnormal bone remodeling. The disease disrupts the growth of new bone tissue causing the bone to thicken and become soft. This weakens the bone, which increases susceptibility of fracture even with slight trauma or collapse of the bone (eg, the vertebrae).

inflammation is unknown. Gold compounds decrease synovial inflammation and retard cartilage and bone destruction. Gold decreases the concentration of rheumatoid factor and immunoglobulins.

USES

Gold compounds are used to treat active juvenile and adult rheumatoid arthritis not controlled by other anti-inflammatory drugs. It is important to note that when cartilage and bone damage has already occurred, gold cannot reverse structural changes to the joints. The greatest benefit appears to occur in patients in the early stages of disease.

ADVERSE REACTIONS

Adverse reactions to the gold compounds may occur any time during therapy, as well as many months after therapy has been discontinued. **Dermatitis** (inflammation of the skin) and **stomatitis** (inflammation of mucosa of the mouth, gums, and possibly the tongue) are the most common adverse reactions seen. Pruritus (itching) often occurs before the skin eruption becomes apparent. Photosensitivity reactions (exaggerated sunburn

reaction when the skin is exposed to sunlight or ultraviolet light) may also occur. **Chrysiasis** (grey to blue pigmentation of the skin) may occur and is caused by gold deposits in tissues. Gold dermatitis is exacerbated by exposure to sunlight.

CONTRAINDICATIONS

The gold compounds are contraindicated in patients with known hypersensitivity to any component of the drug. Parenteral administration is contraindicated in patients with uncontrolled diabetes, hepatic disease, uncontrolled hypertension, uncontrolled congestive heart failure, systemic lupus erythematosus, and blood dyscrasias and in those with recent radiotherapy. Oral administration is contraindicated in patients with necrotizing enterocolitis, pulmonary fibrosis, and hematologic disorders and during pregnancy (Category C) and lactation.

PRECAUTIONS

The gold compounds are used cautiously in patients with a history of hypersensitivity to other drugs, previous kidney or liver disease, diabetes, or hypertension.

Nursing Alert

Tolerance to gold usually decreases with age. The older adult must be carefully monitored when receiving gold therapy.

INTERACTIONS

Concurrent administration of auranofin with phenytoin may increase phenytoin blood levels.

DRUGS USED IN THE TREATMENT OF GOUT

Gout is a form of arthritis in which uric acid accumulates in increased amounts in the blood and often is deposited in the joints. The deposit or collection of urate crystals in the joints causes the symptoms (pain, redness, swelling, joint deformity) of gout.

ACTIONS

Allopurinol (Zyloprim) reduces the production of uric acid, thus decreasing serum uric acid levels and the deposit of urate crystals in joints. The exact mechanism of action of colchicine is unknown, but it does reduce the inflammation associated with the deposit of urate crystals in the joints. This probably accounts for its ability to relieve the severe pain of acute gout. Colchicine has no effect on uric acid metabolism.

In those with gout, the serum uric acid level is usually elevated. Sulfinpyrazone increases the excretion of uric acid by the kidneys, which lowers serum uric acid levels and consequently retards the deposit of urate crystals in the joints. Probenecid (Benemid) works in the same manner and may be given alone or with colchicine as combination therapy when there are frequent, recurrent attacks of gout. Probenecid also has been used to prolong the plasma levels of the penicillins and cephalosporins.

USES

Drugs indicated for treatment of gout may be used to manage acute attacks of gout or in preventing acute attacks of gout (prophylaxis).

ADVERSE REACTIONS

One adverse reaction associated with allopurinol is skin rash, which in some cases has been followed by serious hypersensitivity reactions such as exfoliative dermatitis

and Stevens-Johnson syndrome (see Chap. 6 for a description of this syndrome). Other adverse reactions include nausea, vomiting, diarrhea, abdominal pain, and hematologic changes.

Colchicine administration may result in nausea, vomiting, diarrhea, abdominal pain, and bone marrow depression. When this drug is given to patients with an acute attack of gout, the primary health care provider may order the drug given at frequent intervals until gastrointestinal symptoms occur. Probenecid administration may cause headache, gastrointestinal symptoms, urinary frequency, and hypersensitivity reactions. Upper gastrointestinal disturbances may be seen with the administration of sulfinpyrazone. Even when the drug is given with food, milk, or antacids, gastrointestinal distress may persist and the drug therapy may need to be discontinued. The adverse reactions seen with other agents used in the treatment of gout are listed in the Summary Drug Table: Drugs Used to Treat Musculoskeletal Disorders.

CONTRAINDICATIONS

The drugs used for gout are contraindicated in patients with known hypersensitivity. Probenecid is contraindicated in patients with blood dyscrasias or uric acid kidney stones and in children younger than 2 years. Sulfinpyrazone is contraindicated in patients with peptic ulcer disease and gastrointestinal inflammation. Colchicine is contraindicated in patients with serious gastrointestinal, renal, hepatic, or cardiac disorders and those with blood dyscrasias.

PRECAUTIONS

Allopurinol is used cautiously in patients with liver and renal impairment and during pregnancy (Pregnancy Category C) and lactation. Probenecid is used cautiously in patients with renal impairment, previous hypersensitivity to sulfa drugs, peptic ulcer disease, and those who are pregnant (Pregnancy Category B). Sulfinpyrazone is used cautiously in patients with renal function impairment and those who are pregnant (category unknown). Colchicine is used with caution in older adults and during pregnancy (Pregnancy Category C) and lactation.

INTERACTIONS

There is an increased incidence of skin rash when allopurinol and ampicillin are administered concurrently. Concurrent administration of allopurinol and theophylline

ACTIONS

Alendronate, etidronate, and risedronate act primarily on the bone by inhibiting normal and abnormal bone resorption. This results in increased bone mineral density, reversing the progression of osteoporosis.

USES

The bisphosphonates are used to treat osteoporosis in postmenopausal women, Paget's disease of the bone, and postoperative treatment after total hip replacement (etidronate).

ADVERSE REACTIONS

Adverse reactions with the bisphosphonates include nausea, diarrhea, increased or recurrent bone pain, headache, dyspepsia, acid regurgitation, dysphagia, and abdominal pain.

CONTRAINDICATIONS

These drugs are contraindicated in patients who are hypersensitive to the bisphosphonates. Alendronate and risedronate are contraindicated in patients with hypocalcemia. Alendronate is a pregnancy Category C drug and is contraindicated during pregnancy. These drugs are contraindicated in patients with renal impairment with serum creatinine less than 5 mg/dL. Concurrent use of these drugs with hormone replacement therapy is not recommended.

PRECAUTIONS

These drugs are used cautiously in patients with gastrointestinal disorders, renal function impairment and those who are pregnant or lactating.

INTERACTIONS

When administered with ranitidine, alendronate bioavailability is increased. When calcium supplements or antacids are administered with risedronate or alendronate, absorption of the bisphosphonates is decreased. In addition, risedronate absorption is inhibited when the drug is administered with magnesium and aluminum. There is an increased risk of gastrointestinal effects when the bisphosphonates are administered with aspirin.

CORTICOSTEROIDS

ACTIONS

Corticosteroids are hormones secreted from the adrenal cortex. These hormones arise from the cortex of the adrenal gland and are made from the crystalline steroid alcohol cholesterol. Synthetic forms of the natural adrenal cortical hormones are available. The potent anti-inflammatory action of the corticosteroids makes these drugs useful in the treatment of many types of musculoskeletal disorders. The corticosteroids are discussed in Chapter 50.

USES

The corticosteroids may be used to treat rheumatic disorders such as ankylosing spondylitis, rheumatoid arthritis, gout, bursitis (inflammation of the bursa, usually the bursa of the shoulder), and osteoarthritis.

ADVERSE REACTIONS

Corticosteroids may be given in high doses for some arthritic disorders. Many adverse reactions are associated with high-dose and long-term corticosteroid therapy. Chapter 50 discusses some of the adverse reactions associated with corticosteroid therapy. A comprehensive list of adverse reactions is provided in Display 50-2. Contraindications, precautions, and interactions of the corticosteroids are discussed in Chapter 50.

MISCELLANEOUS DRUGS

The miscellaneous drugs are used to treat a variety of musculoskeletal disorders. Penicillamine, methotrexate (MTX), and hydroxychloroquine are used to treat rheumatoid arthritis in patients who have had an insufficient therapeutic response to or are intolerant of other antirheumatic drugs such as the sailcylates and NSAIDs. The Summary Drug Table: Drugs Used to Tream Musculoskeletal Disorders provides additional information about these and other drugs. One compound, hylan G-F 20, listed in the Summary Drug Table is not used for rheumatoid arthritis, but rather, for osteoarthritis knee pain. It is a viscous, elastic sterile mixture made of hylan A fluid, hylan B gel, and salt water that is administered directly into the knee.

ACTIONS

The mechanism of action of penicillamine, MTX, and hydroxychloroquine in the treatment of rheumatoid arthritis is unknown.

USES

Penicillamine, MTX, and hydroxychloroquine are used in the treatment of rheumatoid arthritis. The administration of MTX is reserved for severe, disabling disease that is not responsive to other treatment.

ADVERSE REACTIONS

Hydroxychloroquine administration may result in irritability, nervousness, anorexia, nausea, vomiting, and diarrhea. This drug also may have adverse effects on the eye, including blurred vision, corneal edema, halos around lights, and retinal damage. Hematologic effects, such as aplastic anemia and leukopenia, may also be seen.

The adverse reactions seen with penicillamine include pruritus, rash, anorexia, nausea, vomiting, epigastric pain, bone marrow depression, proteinuria, hematuria, increased skin friability, and tinnitus. Penicillamine is capable of causing severe toxic reactions.

MTX is a potentially toxic drug that is also used in the treatment of malignancies and psoriasis. Nausea, vomiting, a decreased platelet count, leukopenia (decreased white blood cell count), stomatitis (inflammation of the oral cavity), rash, pruritus, dermatitis, diarrhea, alopecia (loss of hair), and diarrhea may be seen with the administration of this drug.

CONTRAINDICATIONS

These drugs are contraindicated in patients with known hypersensitivity. Hydroxychloroquine is contraindicated in patients with porphyria (a group of serious inherited disorders affecting the bone marrow or the liver), psoriasis (chronic skin disorder), and retinal disease (may cause irreversible retinal damage). MTX is contraindicated during pregnancy because it is a Pregnancy Category X drug and may cause birth defects in the developing fetus. Penicillamine is contraindicated in patients with a history of allergy to penicillin.

PRECAUTIONS

Hydroxychloroquine is used cautiously in patients with hepatic disease or alcoholism and during pregnancy (Pregnancy Category C) and lactation. MTX is used cautiously in patients with renal impairment, women of childbearing age, and older adults or individuals who are chronically ill or debilitated. Penicillamine is used with extreme caution during pregnancy (Pregnancy Category C) and lactation.

INTERACTIONS

There is an increased risk of toxicity of MTX when administered with the NSAIDs, salicylates, oral antidiabetic drugs, phenytoin, tetracycline, and probenecid. There is an additive bone marrow depressant effect when administered with other drugs known to depress the bone marrow or with radiation therapy. There is an increased risk for nephrotoxicity when MTX is administered with other drugs that cause nephrotoxicity. When penicillamine is administered with digoxin, decreased blood levels of digoxin may occur. There is a decreased absorption of penicillamine when the drug is administered with food, iron preparations, and antacids.

> ### ❀ Health Supplement Alert: Glucosamine and Chondroitin
>
> *Both glucosamine and chondroitin are used, in combination or alone, to treat arthritis, particularly osteoarthritis. Chondroitin acts as the flexible connecting matrix between the protein filaments in cartilage. Chondroitin can be produced in the laboratory or can come from natural sources (eg, shark cartilage). Some studies suggest that if chondroitin sulfate is available to the cell matrix, synthesis of the matrix can occur. For this reason it is used to treat arthritis. Although there is not much information on chrondroitin's long-term effects, it is generally not considered to be harmful.*
>
> *Glucosamine is found in mucopolysaccharides, mucoproteins, and chitin. Chitin is found in various marine invertebrates and other lower animals and members of the plant family. In osteoarthritis there is a progressive degeneration of cartilage glycosaminoglycans. Oral glucosamine theoretically provides a building block for regeneration of damaged cartilage. The absorption of oral glucosamine is 90% to 98%, making it widely accepted for use. However, chondroitin molecules are very large (50–300 times larger than glucosamine), and only 0% to 13% of chondroitin is absorbed. There is speculation that these larger molecules are undeliverable to cartilage cells. Glucosamine is generally well tolerated, and no adverse reactions have been reported with its use.*

NURSING PROCESS

● **The Patient Receiving a Drug for a Musculoskeletal Disorder**

ASSESSMENT

Preadministration Assessment

The nurse obtains the patient's history, that is, a summary of the disorder, including onset, symptoms, and current treatment or therapy. In some instances, it may be necessary to question patients regarding their ability to carry out activities of daily living, including employment when applicable.

For the physical assessment, the nurse generally appraises the patient's physical condition and limitations. If the patient has arthritis (any type), the nurse examines the affected joints in the extremities for appearance of the skin over the joint, evidence of joint deformity, and mobility of the affected joint. Patients with osteoporosis are assessed for pain particularly in the upper and lower back or hip. Vital signs and weight are taken to provide a baseline for comparison during therapy. If the patient has gout, the nurse examines the affected joints and notes the appearance of the skin over the joints and any joint enlargement.

Ongoing Assessment

Periodic evaluation is an important part of therapy for musculoskeletal disorders. With some disorders such as acute gout, the patient can be expected to respond to therapy in hours. Therefore, it is important for the nurse to inspect the joints involved every 1 to 2 hours to identify immediately a response or nonresponse to therapy. At this time, the nurse questions the patient regarding the relief of pain, as well as adverse drug reactions. In other disorders, response is gradual and may take days, weeks, and even months of treatment. Depending on the drug administered and the disorder being treated, the evaluation of therapy may be daily or weekly. These recorded evaluations help the primary health care provider plan current and future therapy, including dosage changes, changes in the drug administered, and institution of physical therapy.

Some of these drugs are toxic. The nurse closely observes the patient for the development of adverse reactions. Should any one or more adverse reactions occur, the nurse notifies the primary health care provider before the next dose is due.

NURSING DIAGNOSES

Drug-specific nursing diagnoses are highlighted in the Nursing Diagnoses Checklist. Other nursing diagnoses applicable to these drugs are discussed in depth in Chapter 4.

Nursing Diagnoses Checklist

✓ **Risk for Injury** related to adverse drug reactions (dizziness, drowsiness)

✓ **Risk for Impaired Skin Integrity** related to adverse drug reactions (dermatitis, rash)

✓ **Altered Oral Mucous Membranes** related to adverse reactions (stomatitis)

✓ **Diarrhea** related to adverse drug reaction

✓ **Constipation** related to adverse drug reaction

PLANNING

The expected outcomes for the patient depend on the reason for administration but may include an optimal response to therapy, management of common adverse drug reactions, and an understanding of and compliance with the prescribed therapeutic regimen.

IMPLEMENTATION

Promoting an Optimal Response to Therapy

The patient with a musculoskeletal disorder may be in acute pain or have longstanding mild to moderate pain, which can be just as difficult to tolerate as severe pain. Along with pain, there may be skeletal deformities, such as the joint deformities seen with advanced rheumatoid arthritis. For many musculoskeletal conditions, drug therapy is a major treatment modality. Therapy with these drugs may keep the disorder under control (eg, therapy for gout), improve the patient's ability to carry out the activities of daily living, or make the pain and discomfort tolerable.

Patients on bed rest require position changes and good skin care every 2 hours. The patient with an arthritis disorder may experience much pain or discomfort and may require assistance with activities, such as ambulating, eating, and grooming. Patients with osteoporosis may require a brace or corset when out of bed.

Patients with a musculoskeletal disorder often have anxiety related to the symptoms and the chronicity of their disorder. In addition to physical care, these patients often require emotional support, especially when a disorder is disabling and chronic. The nurse explains to the patient that therapy may take weeks or longer before any benefit is noted. When this is explained before therapy is started, the patient is less likely to become discouraged over the slow results of drug therapy.

GOLD COMPOUNDS. Aurothioglucose and gold sodium thiomalate are given intramuscularly, preferably in the upper outer quadrant of the gluteus muscle. The nurse gives auranofin orally.

DRUGS USED FOR GOUT. The nurse gives allopurinol, probenecid, and sulfinpyrazone with, or immediately after, meals to minimize gastric distress. Colchicine usually can be given with food or milk. When this drug is used for the treatment of an acute gout attack, the nurse may give it every 1 to 2 hours until the pain is relieved. The primary health care provider writes specific orders for administration of the drug and when the drug is to be stopped. The nurse evaluates the patient carefully for relief of pain or the occurrence of nausea, vomiting, or diarrhea. After this evaluation, the nurse decides whether to administer or withhold the drug. Colchicine may be given intravenously for severe gout.

SKELETAL MUSCLE RELAXANTS. The nurse gives these drugs with food to minimize gastrointestinal distress. In addition to drug therapy, rest, physical therapy, and other measures may be part of treatment.

BISPHOSPHONATES. When administering alendronate or risedronate the nurse gives the drug orally in the morning before the first food or drink of the day. Risedronate and etidronate are administered once daily. Etidronate is not administered within 2 hours of food, vitamin and mineral supplements, or antacids.

> ### ☀ Nursing Alert
>
> *Alendronate is administered orally each day or as a once-a-week dose. The nurse should check the physician's order to be certain of the dosage and the times of administration. When administering the drug for treatment of osteoporosis in postmenopausal women, the dosage is 70 mg once weekly or 10 mg daily. When administering the drug for prevention of osteoporosis, 5 mg of the drug is given daily or 35 mg once a week.*

When alendronate and risedronate are administered, serum calcium levels are monitored before, during, and after therapy.

To facilitate delivery of the drug to the stomach and minimize adverse gastrointestinal effects, the nurse administers the drug with 6 to 8 oz of water while the patient is in an upright position. The patient is instructed to remain upright (avoid lying down) for at least 30 minutes after taking the drug.

CORTICOSTEROIDS. When the patient is receiving one of these drugs on alternate days (alternate-day therapy), the drug must be given before 9 AM. It is extremely important that these drugs not be omitted or discontinued suddenly.

MISCELLANEOUS DRUGS. The nurse administers hydroxychloroquine with food or milk to help prevent

> ### ☀ Nursing Alert
>
> *When corticosteroid use is discontinued, the dosage must be tapered gradually over several days. If high dosages have been given, it may take a week or more to taper the dosage.*

gastrointestinal upset. The nurse administers MTX orally. A therapeutic response usually begins within 3 to 6 weeks of therapy, and improvement may continue for another 12 weeks. Treatment with this drug may continue for as long as 2 years. Penicillamine must be given to a patient with an empty stomach, 1 hour before or 2 hours after a meal.

Monitoring and Managing Adverse Drug Reactions

GOLD COMPOUNDS. The nurse observes the patient closely for evidence of dermatitis. Itching may occur before a skin reaction and should be reported to the primary health care provider immediately. If itching occurs, the nurse may apply a soothing lotion or an antiseptic cream. The nurse also keeps the environment free of irritants that aggravate itching, such as rough fabrics, excessive warmth, or excessive dryness.

The nurse inspects the patient's mouth daily for ulceration of the mucous membranes. A metallic taste may be noted before stomatitis becomes evident. The nurse advises the patient to inform the primary health care provider or nurse if a metallic taste occurs. Good oral care is necessary. The teeth should be brushed after each meal and the mouth rinsed with plain water to remove food particles. Mouthwash may also be used, but excessive use may result in oral infections due to the destruction of the normal bacteria present in the mouth.

> ### ❄ Gerontologic Alert
>
> *Gold compounds are given cautiously to older adults. Tolerance for gold therapy decreases with advancing age.*

While taking gold compounds the patient is monitored closely for thrombocytopenia (abnormally low numbers of platelets in the blood). The primary health care provider orders frequent blood studies (usually once a month or more frequently).

> ### ☀ Nursing Alert
>
> *If the platelet count falls below 100,000/mm³ or if the patient experiences signs and symptoms of thrombocytopenia (eg, easy bruising, bleeding gums, epistaxis, melena), the nurse notifies the physician immediately.*

DRUGS USED FOR GOUT. The nurse encourages a liberal fluid intake and measures the intake and output. The daily urine output should be at least 2 liters. An increase in urinary output is necessary to excrete the urates (uric acid) and prevent urate acid stone formation in the genitourinary tract.

The nurse provides adequate fluids and reminds the patient frequently of the importance of increasing fluid intake. If the patient fails to increase the oral intake, the nurse informs the primary health care provider. In some instances, it may be necessary to administer intravenous fluids to supplement the oral intake when the patient fails to drink about 3000 mL of fluid per day.

Administration of allopurinol may result in skin rash. This rash may precede a serious adverse reaction, Stevens-Johnson syndrome (see Chaps. 6 and 8). The nurse immediately reports to the primary health care provider the presence of any rash.

SKELETAL MUSCLE RELAXANTS. These drugs may cause drowsiness. Because of the risk of injury, the nurse evaluates the patient carefully before allowing the patient to ambulate alone. If drowsiness does occur, assistance with ambulatory activities is necessary. If drowsiness is severe, the nurse notifies the primary health care provider before the next dose is due.

BISPHOSPHONATES. The nurse monitors the patient taking the bisphosphonates for any adverse reactions such as nausea, diarrhea, increased or recurrent bone pain, headache, dyspepsia, acid regurgitation, dysphagia, and abdominal pain. Analgesic may be administered for headache. Notify the primary health care provider of adverse reactions such as the return of bone pain or severe diarrhea.

MISCELLANEOUS DRUGS. The nurse closely observes the patient taking hydroxychloroquine for adverse reactions. It is important for the nurse to be alert to skin rash, fever, cough, easy bruising, or unusual bleeding, or the patient's complaints of sore throat, visual changes, mood changes, loss of hair, tinnitus, or hearing loss. The nurse immediately reports adverse reactions. Particular attention is paid to visual changes because irreversible retinal damage may occur. The nurse observes the patient for signs of easy bruising and infection, which may indicate bone marrow depression, an adverse reaction related to the platelets and white blood cells. A decreased platelet count may cause the patient to bleed easily. The nurse applies pressure to all venipuncture puncture sites for at least 10 minutes and avoids intramuscular injections. The mouth is inspected daily for signs of inflammation or ulceration. The nurse also inspects each stool for diarrhea or signs of gastrointestinal bleeding.

Administration of penicillamine has been associated with many adverse reactions, some of which are potentially serious and even fatal. The nurse carefully evaluates any complaint or comment made by the patient and reports it to the primary health care provider. Increased skin friability may occur, which may result in easy breakdown of the skin at pressure sites, such as the hips, elbows, and shoulders. If the patient is unable to ambulate, the nurse changes the patient's position and inspects pressure sites for skin breakdown every 2 hours.

MTX is potentially toxic. Therefore, the nurse observes closely for development of adverse reactions, such as thrombocytopenia (see Nursing Alert in Gold Compounds section) and leukopenia (see discussion of adverse reactions associated with hydroxychloroquine). Hematology, liver, and renal function studies are monitored every 1 to 3 months with MTX therapy. The primary care provider is notified of abnormal hematology, liver function, or kidney function findings. The nurse immediately brings all adverse reactions or suspected adverse reactions to the attention of the primary health care provider.

Educating the Patient and Family

To ensure compliance with the treatment regimen, the patient must understand the importance of complying with the prescribed treatment regimen and taking the drug exactly as directed to obtain the best results from therapy. To meet this goal, the nurse develops an effective plan of patient and family teaching.

The points included in a patient and family teaching plan depend on the type and severity of the musculoskeletal disorder being treated. The nurse must carefully explain that treatment for the disorder includes drug therapy, as well as other medical management, such as diet, exercise, limitations or nonlimitations of activity, and periodic physical therapy treatments. The nurse emphasizes the importance of not taking any nonprescription drugs unless their use has been approved by the primary health care provider. The following points for specific drugs are included in the teaching plan. Information included for the patient taking a corticosteroid is explained in Chapter 50.

GOLD COMPOUNDS

- Toxic reactions are possible when taking gold compounds. Report adverse reactions to the primary health care provider as soon as possible.
- Contact the primary health care provider if a metallic taste is noted.
- Arthralgia (pain in the joints) may be noted for 1 or 2 days after the parenteral form is given.
- Chrysiasis may occur, especially on areas exposed to sunlight. Avoid exposure to sunlight or ultraviolet light.

DRUGS USED FOR GOUT

- Drink at least 10 glasses of water a day until the acute attack has subsided.
- Take this drug with food to minimize gastrointestinal upset.
- If drowsiness occurs, avoid driving or performing other hazardous tasks.
- Acute gout—Notify the primary health care provider if pain is not relieved in a few days.
- Colchicine for acute gout—Take this drug at the intervals prescribed by the primary health care provider and stop taking the drug when the pain is relieved or when diarrhea or vomiting occurs. If the pain is not relieved in about 12 hours, notify the primary health care provider.
- Allopurinol—Notify the primary health care provider if a skin rash occurs.
- Colchicine—Notify the primary health care provider if skin rash, sore throat, fever, unusual bleeding or bruising, unusual fatigue, or weakness occurs.

SKELETAL MUSCLE RELAXANTS

- This drug may cause drowsiness. Do not drive or perform other hazardous tasks if drowsiness occurs.
- This drug is for short-term use. Do not use the drug for longer than 2 to 3 weeks.
- Avoid alcohol or other depressants while taking this drug.

BISPHOSPHONATES

Alendronate and risedronate. These drugs are taken with 6 to 8 oz of water first thing in the morning. Do not lie down for at least 30 minutes after taking the drug and wait at least 30 minutes before taking any other food or drink. The drugs are taken exactly as prescribed. The primary care provider may prescribe alendronate as a once weekly dose or to be taken daily. Risedronate is taken daily. Take supplemental calcium and vitamin D if dietary intake is inadequate. Take all medication, including vitamin and mineral supplements, at a different time of the day to prevent interference with absorption of the drug.

MISCELLANEOUS DRUGS

Penicillamine. The primary health care provider will explain the treatment regimen and adverse reactions before therapy is started. You must know which toxic reactions require contacting the primary health care provider immediately. Take penicillamine on an empty stomach, 1 hour before or 2 hours after a meal. If other drugs are prescribed, penicillamine is taken 1 hour apart from any other drug. Observe skin areas over the elbows, shoulders, and buttocks for evidence of bruising, bleeding, or break in the skin (delayed wound healing may occur). If these occur, do not self-treat the problem, but notify the primary health care provider immediately. An alteration in taste perception may occur. Taste perception should return to normal within 2 to 3 months.

Methotrexate. Take MTX exactly as directed. If a weekly dose is prescribed, use a calendar or some other method to take the drug on the same day each week. Never increase the prescribed dose of this drug. Mistaken daily use has led to fatal toxicity. Notify the primary health care provider immediately if any of the following occur: sore mouth, sores in the mouth, diarrhea, fever, sore throat, easy bruising, rash, itching, or nausea and vomiting. Women of childbearing age should use an effective contraceptive during therapy with MTX and for 8 weeks after therapy.

Hydroxychloroquine. Take hydroxychloroquine with food or milk. Contact the primary health care provider immediately if any of the following occur: hearing or visual changes, skin rash or severe itching, hair loss, change in the color of the hair (bleaching), changes in the color of the skin, easy bruising or bleeding, fever, sore throat, muscle weakness, or mood changes. It may be several weeks before symptoms are relieved.

EVALUATION

- The therapeutic drug effect is achieved.
- Adverse reactions are identified, reported to the primary health care provider, and managed using appropriate nursing interventions.
- The patient verbalizes the importance of complying with the prescribed therapeutic regimen.
- The patient and family demonstrate an understanding of the drug regimen.

● *Critical Thinking Exercises*

1. *Mary is a nurse who has returned to nursing after 15 years absence to raise a family. Mary asks you what should be included in a teaching plan for a patient with rheumatoid arthritis now taking high doses of salicylates. Discuss what information you would suggest Mary emphasize in a teaching plan.*

2. *Ms. Leeds is prescribed methotrexate for rheumatoid arthritis not responding to other therapies. She is nervous about starting the drug after she was told that the drug can cause many serious adverse reactions. Discuss what you could say to Ms. Leeds to relieve her anxiety. Identify specific instructions you would give her before she begins therapy with this drug.*

3. *Discuss important points the nurse should consider when administering colchicine to a patient with an acute attack of diarrhea.*

4. *Discuss the important points to include when educating a patient prescribed alendronate 35 mg once weekly.*

What suggestions could you give the patient to help him remember when to take the drug?

● Review Questions

1. When a patient is taking gold compound therapy on an outpatient basis, the nurse advises the patient to inform the primary care provider if _____.

   A. the appetite decreases
   B. a severe headache occurs
   C. a metallic taste is noted
   D. hair loss occurs

2. When administering a skeletal muscle relaxant the nurse observes the patient for the most common adverse reaction, which is _____.

   A. drowsiness
   B. gastrointestinal bleeding
   C. vomiting
   D. constipation

3. When a patient is prescribed a corticosteroid for arthritis and alternate-day therapy is used, the nurse administers the drug _____.

   A. with food or milk
   B. on an empty stomach
   C. before 9:00 AM
   D. at bedtime

4. When allopurinol (Zyloprim) is used for the treatment of gout, the nurse _____.

   A. administers the drug with juice or milk
   B. administers the drug after the evening meal
   C. restricts fluids during evening hours
   D. encourages a liberal fluid intake

5. What teaching points would the nurse include when educating the patient prescribed risedronate?

   A. The drug is administered once weekly.
   B. Take a daily laxative because the drug will likely cause constipation.
   C. Take the drug in the morning before breakfast and immediately lie down for 30 minutes to facilitate absorption.
   D. After taking the drug, remain upright for at least 30 minutes.

● Medication Dosage Problems

1. A patient is to receive allopurinol 300 mg PO for gout. The nurse has 100-mg tablets available. How many tablets would the nurse administer?

2. The physician prescribes 1.5 g methocarbamol (Robaxin) PO for a musculoskeletal disorder. Available for administration are 500-mg tablets. The nurse administers _____.

Adrenergic Drugs

Chapter Objectives

On completion of this chapter, the student will:

- Discuss the activity of the central nervous system and the peripheral nervous system.
- Discuss the types of shock, physiologic responses of shock, and the use of adrenergic drugs in the treatment of shock.
- Discuss the uses, general drug actions, contraindications, precautions, interactions, and adverse reactions associated with the administration of adrenergic drugs.
- Discuss important preadministration and ongoing assessment activities the nurse should perform on the patient taking adrenergic drugs.
- List some nursing diagnoses particular to a patient taking the adrenergic drugs.
- Discuss ways to promote an optimal response to therapy, how to manage common adverse reactions, and important points to keep in mind when educating patients about the use of adrenergic drugs.

The adrenergic drugs produce pharmacologic effects similar to the effects that occur in the body when the adrenergic nerves and the medulla are stimulated. The primary effects of these drugs occur on the heart, the blood vessels, and the smooth muscles, such as the bronchi. A basic knowledge of the nervous system is necessary to understand these drugs and how they work in the body.

THE NERVOUS SYSTEM

The nervous system is a complex part of the human body concerned with the regulation and coordination of body activities such as movement, digestion of food, sleep, and elimination of waste products. The nervous system has two main divisions: the central nervous system (CNS) and the peripheral nervous system (PNS). Figure 22-1 illustrates the divisions of the nervous system.

    The **CNS** consists of the brain and the spinal cord and receives, integrates, and interprets nerve impulses.

The PNS is the term used to describe all nerves outside of the brain and spinal cord. The PNS connects all parts of the body with the CNS.

Peripheral Nervous System

The **PNS** is further divided into the somatic nervous system and the autonomic nervous system. The somatic branch of the PNS is concerned with sensation and voluntary movement. The sensory part of the **somatic nervous system** sends messages to the brain concerning the internal and external environment, such as sensations of heat, pain, cold, and pressure. The voluntary part of the somatic nervous system is concerned with the voluntary movement of skeletal muscles, such as walking, chewing food, or writing a letter.

Autonomic Branch of the Peripheral Nervous System

The autonomic branch of the PNS is concerned with functions essential to the survival of the organism. Functional activity of the **autonomic nervous system**

TABLE 22-3	Types of Shock
TYPE*	**DESCRIPTION**
Hypovolemic	Occurs when the volume of extracellular fluid is significantly diminished. Examples include hemorrhage, fluid loss caused by burns, diarrhea, vomiting, or excess diuresis
Cardiogenic	Occurs when the heart is unable to deliver an adequate cardiac output to maintain perfusion to the vital organs. Examples include: as the result of an acute myocardial infarction, ventricular arrhythmias, congestive heart failure (CHF), or severe cardiomyopathy.
Septic	Occurs as a result of circulatory insufficiency associated with overwhelming infection
Obstructive	Occurs when obstruction of blood flow results in inadequate tissue perfusion. Examples include a severe reduction of blood flow as the result of massive pulmonary embolism, pericardial tamponade, restrictive pericarditis, and severe cardiac valve dysfunction
Neurogenic	Occurs as a result of blockade of neurohumoral outflow. Examples include: from a pharmacological source (ie, spinal anesthesia) or direct injury to the spinal cord. This type of shock is rare.

*Other causes of shock include anaphylaxis, hypoglycemia, hypothyroidism, or Addison's disease.

"cool" or "cold" shock. Regardless of the type, shock results in a decrease in cardiac output, decrease in arterial blood pressure (hypotension), reabsorption of water by the kidneys (causing a decrease in urinary output), decrease in the exchange of oxygen and carbon dioxide in the lungs, increase in carbon dioxide in the blood and decrease in oxygen in the blood, hypoxia (decreased oxygen reaching the cells), and increased concentration of intravascular fluid. This scenario compromises the functioning of vital organs such as the heart, brain, and kidneys. The various physiologic responses caused by shock within the body are listed in Table 22-4.

The adrenergic drugs are useful in improving hemodynamic status by improving myocardial contractility and increasing heart rate, which results in increased cardiac output. Peripheral resistance is increased by vasoconstriction. In cardiogenic shock or advanced shock associated with low cardiac output, the adrenergic drug may be used with a vasodilating drug. A vasodilator such as nitroprusside (Chap. 42) or nitroglycerin (Chap. 41) improves myocardial performance as the adrenergic drug maintains blood pressure.

ADVERSE REACTIONS

The adverse reactions associated with the administration of adrenergic drugs depend on the drug used, the dose administered, and individualized patient response. Some of the more common adverse reactions include cardiac arrhythmias, such as bradycardia and tachycardia, headache, insomnia, nervousness, anorexia, and an increase in blood pressure (which may reach dangerously high levels). Additional adverse reactions for specific adrenergic drugs are listed in the Summary Drug Table: Adrenergic Drugs.

CONTRAINDICATIONS

Adrenergic drugs are contraindicated in patients with known hypersensitivity. Isoproterenol is contraindicated in patients with tachyarrhythmias, tachycardia or heart block caused by digitalis toxicity, ventricular arrhythmias, and angina pectoris. Dopamine is contraindicated in those with pheochromocytoma (tumor of adrenal gland), unmanaged arrhythmias, and ventricular fibrillation. Epinephrine is contraindicated in patients with narrow-angle glaucoma, cerebral arteriosclerosis, and cardiac insufficiency. Norepinephrine and ephedrine are contraindicated in patients who are hypotensive from blood volume deficits. Midodrine is contraindicated in those with severe organic heart disease, acute renal disease, pheochromocytoma, and supine hypertension.

TABLE 22-4	Physiologic Manifestations of Shock
BODY SYSTEM	**POSSIBLE SIGNS AND SYMPTOMS**
Integumentary (skin)	Pallor, cyanosis, cold and clammy, sweating
Central nervous system	Agitation, confusion, disorientation, coma
Cardiovascular	Hypotension, tachycardia, arrhythmias, wide pulse pressure, gallop rhythm
Respiratory	Tachypnea, pulmonary edema
Renal	Urinary output < 20 mL/h
Metabolic	Acidosis

PRECAUTIONS

These drugs are used cautiously in patients with coronary insufficiency, cardiac arrhythmias, angina pectoris, diabetes, hyperthyroidism, occlusive vascular disease, or prostatic hypertrophy, and in those taking digoxin. Patients with diabetes may require an increased dosage of insulin. Epinephrine is used cautiously in patients with Parkinson's disease (may temporarily increase rigidity and tremor) or ventricular fibrillation and in the elderly. Ephedrine is used cautiously in patients with acute-closure glaucoma. Midodrine is used cautiously in patients with urinary problems or hepatic disease and during lactation. Adrenergic drugs are classified as Pregnancy Category C and are used with extreme caution during pregnancy.

INTERACTIONS

There is an increased risk of hypertension when dobutamine is administered with the β-adrenergic blocking drugs. When dopamine is administered with the monoamine oxidase inhibitors (see Chap. 31) or the tricyclic antidepressants (see Chap. 31), there is a risk for increased effects of dopamine. There is an increased risk of seizures, hypotension, and bradycardia when dopamine is administered with phenytoin. When epinephrine is administered with the tricyclic antidepressants, there is an increased risk of sympathomimetic effects. Excessive hypertension can occur when epinephrine is administered with propranolol. A decreased bronchodilating effect occurs when epinephrine is administered with the β-adrenergic drugs. Metaraminol is used cautiously in patients taking digoxin because of an increased risk for cardiac arrhythmias. When midodrine is administered with cardiac glycosides, psychotropic drugs, or β blockers, bradycardia, heart block, or arrhythmias can occur.

NURSING PROCESS

● **The Patient Receiving an Adrenergic Drug**

ASSESSMENT

Assessment of the patient receiving an adrenergic drug differs depending on the drug, the patient, and the reason for administration. For example, assessment of the patient in shock who is to be treated with norepinephrine is different from that for the patient receiving nose drops containing phenylephrine. Both are receiving adrenergic drugs, but the circumstances are much different.

✿ Herbal Alert: Ephedra

Many members of the Ephedra family have been used medicinally (ie, E. sinica and E. intermedia). Ephedra preparations have traditionally been used to relieve cold symptoms, improve respiratory function, as an adjunct in weight loss, and to treat a variety of conditions from headaches to sexually transmitted disease. Large doses may cause a variety of adverse reactions, such as hypertension, irregular heart rate, tremors, epigastric pain, nausea, vomiting, sweating, weakness, and possible dependence. Ephedra is contraindicated in patients with hypertension, glaucoma, hypertrophy of the prostate, urinary tract problems, clotting disorders, anxiety, anorexia, colitis, thyroid disease, or diabetes. Ephedra should not be used with the cardiac glycosides, halothane, guanethidine, MAOIs, oxytocin, and in patients taking St. John's wort. Weight loss preparations containing ephedra should be avoided.

Before taking this herb the patient should consult the primary care provider. When taking a standardized extract, 12 to 25 mg total alkaloids (calculated as ephedrine) two to three times daily is the normal dosage. When taking the capsules or tablets, the normal dosage is 500 to 1000 mg two to three times daily.

The FDA warns the public not to take ephedrine-containing dietary supplements with labels that portray the products as an alternative to illegal street drugs such as Ecstasy because these products may pose serious health risks to consumers.

Preadministration Assessment

When a patient is to receive an adrenergic agent for shock, the nurse obtains the blood pressure, pulse rate and quality, and respiratory rate and rhythm. The nurse assesses the patient's symptoms, problems, or needs before administering the drug and records any subjective or objective data on the patient's chart. In emergencies, the nurse must make assessments quickly and accurately. This information provides an important database that is used during treatment.

A general survey of the patient also is necessary. It is important to look for additional symptoms of shock, such as cool skin, cyanosis, diaphoresis, and a change in the level of consciousness. Other assessments may be necessary if the hypotensive episode is due to trauma, severe infection, or blood loss.

In patients taking midodrine for orthostatic hypotension, the nurse checks the blood pressure with the patient supine and sitting before therapy is begun. This is important because midodrine is contraindicated in patients with supine hypertension.

When a patient is to have nose drops instilled for nasal congestion, the nurse examines the nasal passages and describes the type of secretions present in the nose. The nurse also should obtain the blood pressure because nose drops that contain adrenergic drugs are not given to those with high blood pressure.

Nursing Diagnoses Checklist

✓ **Ineffective Tissue Perfusion** related to hypovolemia, blood loss, impaired distribution of fluid, impaired circulation, impaired transport of oxygen across alveolar and capillary bed, other (specify)

✓ **Decreased Cardiac Output** related to altered heart rate and/or rhythm

✓ **Imbalanced Nutrition: Less Than Body Requirements** related to adverse reaction (anorexia) to the drug

✓ **Disturbed Sleep Pattern** related to adverse reactions (insomnia, nervousness) to the drug

Ongoing Assessment

During the ongoing assessment, the nurse observes the patient for the effect of the drug, such as improved breathing of the patient with asthma, response of the blood pressure to the administration of the vasopressor, or controlled orthostatic hypotension. During therapy, the nurse evaluates and documents the drug effect. The nurse also takes and documents the vital signs. Comparison of assessments made before and after administration may help the primary health care provider determine future use of the drug for this patient. It is important to report adverse drug reactions to the primary health care provider as soon as possible.

NURSING DIAGNOSES

Drug-specific nursing diagnoses are highlighted in the Nursing Diagnoses Checklist. Other nursing diagnoses applicable to these drugs are discussed in depth in Chapter 4.

PLANNING

The expected outcomes of the patient will depend on the reason for administration of an adrenergic agent but may include an optimal response to drug therapy, management of common adverse reactions, an absence of infection, and an understanding of the reason the drug is being given.

IMPLEMENTATION

Promoting an Optimal Response to Therapy

Management of the patient receiving an adrenergic agent varies and depends on the drug used, the reason for administration, and the patient's response to the drug. In most instances, adrenergic drugs are potent and potentially dangerous. The nurse must exercise great care in the calculation and preparation of these drugs for administration. Although adrenergic drugs are potentially dangerous, proper supervision and management before, during, and after administration will minimize the occurrence of any serious problems. Management of shock is aimed at providing basic life support (airway, breathing, and circulation) while attempting to correct the underlying cause. Antibiotics, inotropes, hormones (eg, insulin, thyroid), and other drugs may be used to treat the underlying disease. However, the initial pharmacologic intervention is aimed at supporting the circulation with vasopressors.

MAINTAINING ADEQUATE TISSUE PERFUSION. When a patient is in shock and experiencing ineffective tissue perfusion there is a decrease in oxygen resulting in an inability of the body to nourish its cells at the capillary level. If the patient has marked hypotension the administration of a **vasopressor** (a drug that raises the blood pressure because of its ability to constrict blood vessels) is required. The primary health care provider determines the cause of the hypotension and then selects the best method of treatment. Some hypotensive episodes require the use of a less potent vasopressor, such as metaraminol, whereas at other times a more potent vasopressor, such as dobutamine (Dobutrex), dopamine (Intropin), or norepinephrine (Levophed) is necessary.

The nurse considers the following points when administering the potent vasopressors dopamine and norepinephrine:

- Use an electronic infusion pump to administer these drugs.
- Do not mix dopamine with other drugs, especially sodium bicarbonate or other alkaline intravenous (IV) solutions. Check with the hospital pharmacist before adding a second drug to an IV solution containing this drug.
- Administer norepinephrine and dopamine only via the IV route. Do not dilute these drugs in an IV solution before administration. The primary health care provider orders the IV solution, the amount of drug added to the solution, and the initial rate of infusion.
- Monitor blood pressure every 2 minutes from the beginning of therapy until the desired blood pressure is achieved, then monitor the blood pressure and pulse rate at frequent intervals, usually every 5 to 15 minutes, during the administration of these drugs.
- Adjust the rate of administration according to the patient's blood pressure. The rate of administration of the IV solution is increased or decreased to maintain the patient's blood pressure at the systolic level ordered by the primary health care provider.
- Readjustment of the rate of flow of the IV solution is often necessary. The frequency of adjustment will depend on the patient's response to the vasopressor.
- Inspect the needle site and surrounding tissues at frequent intervals for leakage (extravasation, infiltration) of the solution into the subcutaneous tissues surrounding the needle site. If either situation occurs, establish another IV line immediately, discontinue the IV containing the vasopressor, and

notify the primary health care provider. These drugs are particularly damaging to the tissues if leakage into the surrounding tissue occurs. The nurse should keep phentolamine nearby to use when extravasation occurs. The affected area is infiltrated with 5 to 10 mg of phentolamine in 10 to 15 mL of saline.

● Never leave the patient receiving these drugs unattended.

Monitoring the patient in shock requires vigilance on the part of the nurse. The patient's heart rate, blood pressure, and ECG are monitored continuously. The urinary output is measured often (usually hourly), and an accurate intake and output is taken. Monitoring of central venous pressure via a central venous catheter will provide an estimation of the patient's fluid status. Sometimes additional hemodynamic monitoring is necessary with a pulmonary artery catheter. The use of a pulmonary artery catheter allows the nurse to monitor a number of parameters, such as cardiac output and peripheral vascular resistance. The nurse adjusts therapy according to the primary health care provider's instructions.

The less potent vasopressors, such as metaraminol, also require close patient supervision during administration. The nurse follows the same procedure as that for norepinephrine and dopamine but may take blood pressure and pulse determinations at less frequent intervals, usually every 15 to 30 minutes. The nurse needs sound clinical judgment to determine the frequency because there is no absolute minimum or maximum time limit between determinations.

MAINTAINING CARDIAC OUTPUT. The heart rate and stroke volume determine cardiac output. The stroke volume is determined in part by the contractile state of the heart and the amount of blood in the ventricle available to be pumped out. The interventions listed above help to support the cardiac output of the patient in shock.

It is important for the nurse to monitor vital signs carefully when the patient is in shock. The nurse monitors the vital signs (heart rate and rhythm, respiratory rate, and blood pressure) often (every 15 to 30 minutes) to determine the severity of shock. For example, as cardiac output decreases, compensatory tachycardia develops to increase cardiac output. As shock deepens, the pulse volume becomes progressively weaker and assumes a "thready" feel. The heart rate increases and the heart rhythm may become irregular. Initially the respiratory rate is rapid as the patient experiences air hunger, but in profound shock the respiratory rate decreases. Blood pressure decreases as shock progresses.

CARING FOR THE PATIENT TAKING MIDODRINE. This drug is administered only when the patient is out of bed. Bedridden patients should not receive the drug. The patient taking midodrine will need frequent moni-

> ### ☀ Nursing Alert
>
> *Regardless of the actual numerical reading of the blood pressure, a progressive fall of the blood pressure is serious. The nurse reports to the primary health care provider any progressive fall of the blood pressure, a fall in systolic blood pressure below 100 mm Hg, or any fall of 20 mm Hg or more of the patient's normal blood pressure.*

toring of blood pressure and heart rate. Bradycardia is common at the beginning of therapy. Persistent bradycardia should be reported to the primary health care provider for evaluation. Because the drug can cause dysuria, the patient is asked to void before administration of the drug.

Monitoring and Managing Adverse Reactions

The nurse reports and documents any complaint the patient may have while taking the adrenergic drugs. However, nursing judgment is necessary when reporting adverse reactions. The nurse must report some adverse effects, such as the development of cardiac arrhythmias immediately, regardless of the time of day or night. The nurse should report other adverse effects, such as anorexia, but this is usually not an emergency.

> ### ☀ Nursing Alert
>
> *Supine hypertension is a potentially dangerous adverse reaction when taking midodrine. The nurse can minimize this reaction by administering the medication during the day while the patient is in an upright position. Keeping the patient in an upright position can sometimes control supine hypertension. This requires that the patient sleep with the head of the bed elevated.*
>
> *The following is a suggested dosing schedule for the administration of midodrine: shortly before arising in the morning, midday, and late afternoon (not after 6:00 PM). The nurse should continue drug therapy only in the patient whose orthostatic hypotension improves during the initial treatment.*

> ### ❄ Gerontologic Alert
>
> *The older adult is particularly vulnerable to adverse reactions of the adrenergic drugs, particularly epinephrine. In addition, older adults are more likely to have preexisting cardiovascular disease that predisposes them to potentially serious cardiac arrhythmias. The nurse closely monitors all elderly patients taking an adrenergic drug. It is important to report any changes in the pulse rate or rhythm immediately. In addition, epinephrine may temporarily increase tremor and rigidity in older adults with Parkinson's disease.*

MAINTAINING ADEQUATE TISSUE PERFUSION AND CARDIAC OUTPUT. Administration of an adrenergic drug may cause hypertension or tachycardia. These adverse reactions may cause a decrease in oxygenation at the cellular level. It is important for the nurse to monitor the pulse and blood pressure during the administration of an adrenergic drug. If the patient is being given the adrenergic drug for hypotension, there is already a potential problem with tissue perfusion. Administration of the adrenergic drug may correct the problem or, if the blood pressure becomes too high, tissue perfusion may again be a problem. Maintaining the blood pressure at the systolic rate prescribed by the primary health care provider will maintain tissue perfusion. If the pulse rate increases to a rate of 100 bpm or more or a change in rhythm occurs, the primary health care provider is notified.

> ### ✳ Nursing Alert
>
> *Prolonged high-dose therapy of the adrenergic drugs can produce cyanosis and tissue necrosis of distal extremities. It is important to remember to use the lowest possible dose that produces an adequate response for the shortest period of time. The nurse monitors the patient's extremities closely for any signs of cyanosis.*

MANAGING ANOREXIA. Administration of an adrenergic drug may cause anorexia in the patient. Management of this adverse reaction requires diligence on the part of the nurse. The nurse discusses food preferences and aversions with the patient and makes modifications in the diet when possible. An easily digested diet high in carbohydrate and protein and low in fat is usually well tolerated. Several small meals may be better tolerated than three large meals. The nurse weighs the patient daily or weekly and keeps an accurate dietary record. Foods that cause increased gastric motility, such as gas-forming foods, spicy foods, and caffeinated beverages, are avoided. Good oral care is provided. The dietitian may be consulted if necessary. The nurse provides a pleasant, odor-free, relaxing environment for eating.

MANAGING SLEEP DISTURBANCES. The patient taking an adrenergic drug may experience insomnia and nervousness. This can cause a great deal of stress in the patient. It is important to inform the patient that this is an effect of the drug. It is helpful to identify circumstances that disturb sleep, such as the nurse taking vital signs during the night or turning the overhead light on during the night. The nurse plans care with as few interruptions as possible or makes modifications. For example, instead of turning the overhead light on during the night, a night light may be used. However, monitoring vital signs is an important nursing intervention when administering the adrenergic drugs. A thorough explanation of the reason for close monitoring of the vital signs by the nurse is necessary. In addition, caffeinated beverages are avoided, especially after 5:00 PM. Other sleep aids may be used (eg, warm milk, back rub, progressive relaxation, or bedtime snack). The patient is assured that sleeplessness and nervousness will pass when the drug therapy is discontinued.

Educating the Patient and Family

Only medical personnel give some adrenergic drugs, such as the vasopressors. The nurse's responsibility for teaching involves explaining the drug to the patient or family. Depending on the situation, the nurse may include facts such as how the drug will be given (eg, the route of administration) and what results are expected. The nurse must use judgment regarding some of the information given to the patient or family regarding administration of an adrenergic drug in life-threatening situations because certain facts, such as the seriousness of the patient's condition, are usually best given by the primary health care provider.

EDUCATING THE PATIENT USING A NASAL DECONGESTANT. When a nasal decongestant (drops or spray) containing an adrenergic drug has been recommended or prescribed, the nurse shows the patient or family member the correct method of instillation. The nurse explains possible adverse effects and the importance of adherence to the dose regimen prescribed by the primary health care provider. Because many nasal decongestants are over-the-counter (OTC) drugs, the nurse advises patients using them that these drugs are contraindicated in those with high blood pressure and that overuse can increase nasal congestion (rebound congestion).

EDUCATING THE PATIENT PRESCRIBED A BRONCHODILATOR. If an adrenergic drug, such as ephedrine or isoproterenol, has been prescribed as a bronchodilator, the nurse explains the drug regimen to the patient (see Chap. 37 for additional information). It is important to stress the importance of reporting adverse reactions to the primary health care provider as soon as possible. If the drug is prescribed in sublingual form, the nurse demonstrates the technique of placing the drug under the tongue. The nurse warns the patient not to use any OTC drug unless use has been approved by the primary health care provider. The nurse encourages patients receiving a bronchodilator to contact their primary health care provider if the drug fails to produce at least partial relief of their symptoms.

EDUCATING THE PATIENT PRESCRIBED MIDODRINE. When midodrine is given to patients with severe orthostatic hypotension, the nurse explains the importance of taking the drug during daytime hours when the patient is upright. The patient can take doses in 3-hour intervals, if needed to control symptoms. The drug should not be taken within 4 hours of bedtime. In addition, to control supine hypertension, a potentially fatal adverse reaction, the patient should not become fully supine. The nurse explains that it may be necessary to sleep with the head of the bed elevated. If urinary retention is a problem, the patient is instructed to urinate before taking the drug. The nurse stresses the importance of returning for regular medical evaluation. The patient is instructed to report any changes in vision, pounding in the head when lying down, slow heart rate, or difficulty urinating.

EVALUATION

- The therapeutic effect is achieved.
- Adverse reactions are identified, reported to the primary health care provider, and managed successfully.
- The patient verbalizes an understanding of treatment modalities and the importance of continued follow-up care.

● Critical Thinking Exercises

1. *Mr. Cole is receiving dopamine for the treatment of severe hypotension. In planning the care for Mr. Cole, determine what would be the most important aspects of nursing management. Explain your answers.*
2. *Plan a teaching program to explain the nervous system to a group of nurses at a staff education meeting.*
3. *Discuss the preadministration assessment for a patient requiring an adrenergic drug for hypotension.*
4. *Describe what information is important to include in an education session for a patient taking an adrenergic drug for nasal congestion.*

● Review Questions

1. The physician prescribes norepinephrine, a potent vasopressor, to be administered to a patient in shock.

The rate of the administration of the IV fluid containing the norepinephrine is
   A. maintained at a set rate of infusion
   B. adjusted accordingly to maintain the patient's blood pressure
   C. given at a rate not to exceed 5 mg/min
   D. discontinued when the blood pressure is 100 mm Hg systolic

2. At what intervals would the nurse monitor the blood pressure of a patient taking norepinephrine?
   A. every 5 to 15 minutes
   B. every 30 minute
   C. every hour
   D. every 4 hours

3. Which of the following are the common adverse reactions the nurse would expect with the administration of the adrenergic drugs?
   A. bradycardia, lethargy, bronchial constriction
   B. increase in appetite, nervousness, drowsiness
   C. nausea, vomiting, hypotension
   D. insomnia, nervousness, anorexia

4. When dobutamine is administered with the β-adrenergic blocking drugs the nurse is aware of an increased risk for _____.
   A. seizures
   A. arrhythmias
   C. hypotension
   D. hypertension

5. Epinephrine is administered cautiously in patients with Parkinson's disease because the drug may _____.
   A. precipitate congestive heart failure
   B. temporarily increase rigidity and tremor
   C. decrease the response to antiparkinsonism drugs
   D. cause confusion

● Medication Dosage Problems

1. Midodrine 2.5 mg is prescribed. The drug is available in 5-mg tablets. The nurse would administer _____.

2. The physician orders 0.5 mg of 1:1000 epinephrine solution IV. The drug is available in 1:1000 solution 1 mg/mL. The nurse administers _____.

chapter 23

Adrenergic Blocking Drugs

Key Terms

α-adrenergic blocking
  drugs
α/β-adrenergic
  blocking drugs
β-adrenergic blocking
  drugs
antiadrenergic drugs

cardiac arrhythmia
first dose effect
glaucoma
orthostatic
  hypotension
pheochromocytoma
postural hypotension

Chapter Objectives

On completion of this chapter, the student will:

- List the four types of adrenergic blocking drugs.
- Discuss the uses, general drug actions, general adverse reactions, contraindications, precautions, and interactions of the adrenergic blocking drugs.
- Discuss important preadministration and ongoing assessment activities the nurse should perform on the patient taking adrenergic blocking drugs.
- List some nursing diagnoses particular to a patient taking adrenergic blocking drugs.
- Discuss ways to promote an optimal response to therapy, how to manage common adverse reactions, nursing actions that may be taken to minimize orthostatic or postural hypotension, and important points to keep in mind when educating patients about the use of adrenergic blocking drugs.

Adrenergic blocking drugs, also called sympathomimetic blocking drugs, may be divided into four groups:

- **Alpha (α)-adrenergic blocking drugs**—drugs that block α-adrenergic receptors. These drugs produce their greatest effect on α receptors of adrenergic receptors of adrenergic nerves that control the vascular system.
- **Beta (β)-adrenergic blocking drugs**—drugs that block β-adrenergic receptors. These drugs produce their greatest effect on β receptors of adrenergic nerves, primarily the β receptors of the heart.
- **Antiadrenergic drugs**—drugs that block adrenergic nerve fibers. These drugs block the adrenergic nerve fibers within the central nervous system (CNS) or within the peripheral nervous system.
- **α/β-Adrenergic blocking drugs**—drugs that block both α- and β-adrenergic receptors. These drugs act on both α and β nerve fibers.

Each of these groups will be discussed individually followed by information concerning the use of the nursing process for the group as a whole. See the Summary Drug Table: the Adrenergic Blocking Drugs for a more complete listing of these drugs.

α-ADRENERGIC BLOCKING DRUGS

ACTIONS

Stimulation of α-adrenergic fibers results in vasoconstriction (see Table 22-1 in Chap. 22). If stimulation of these α-adrenergic fibers is interrupted or blocked, the result will be vasodilation. This is the direct opposite of the effect of an adrenergic drug having mainly α activity. Phentolamine (Regitine) is an example of an α-adrenergic blocking drug.

USES

Phentolamine (Regitine) is used for its vasodilating effect on peripheral blood vessels and therefore may be beneficial in the treatment of hypertension caused by

SUMMARY DRUG TABLE   ADRENERGIC BLOCKING DRUGS

GENERIC NAME	TRADE NAME*	USES	ADVERSE REACTIONS	DOSAGE RANGES
α-Adrenergic Blocking Agents				
phentolamine *fen-tole-a-meen*	Regitine	Diagnosis of pheochromocytoma, hypertensive episodes before and during surgery, prevention/treatment of dermal necrosis after IV administration of norepinephrine or dopamine	Weakness, dizziness, flushing, nausea, vomiting, orthostatic hypotension	5 mg IV, IM for tissue necrosis: 5–10 mg in 10 mL saline infiltrated into affected area
β-Adrenergic Blocking Drugs				
acebutolol HCl *a-se-byoo´-toe-lol*	Sectral, *generic*	Hypertension, ventricular arrhythmias	Bradycardia, dizziness, weakness, hypotension, nausea, vomiting, diarrhea, nervousness	Hypertension: 400 mg PO in 1–2 doses; arrhythmias: 400–1200 mg/d PO in divided doses
atenolol *a-ten´-oh-lol*	Tenormin, *generic*	Hypertension, angina, acute MI	Bradycardia, dizziness, fatigue, weakness, hypotension, nausea, vomiting, diarrhea, nervousness	50–200 mg/d PO; 5 mg IV
betaxolol HCL *beh-tax´-oh-lol*	Kerlone	Hypertension	Bradycardia, dizziness, hypotension, bronchospasm, nausea, vomiting, diarrhea, nervousness	5–20 mg/d PO
betaxolol HCL *beh-tax´-oh-lol* (ophthalmic)	Betoptic	Glaucoma	Brief ocular discomfort, tearing	I gtt BID
bisoprolol *bye-sew´-proe-lol*	Zebeta	Hypertension	Bradycardia, dizziness, weakness, hypotension, nausea, vomiting, diarrhea, nervousness	5 mg PO QD; maximum dose, 20 mg PO QD
carteolol *kar´-tee-oh-lol*	Cartrol	Hypertension	Bradycardia, dizziness, weakness, hypotension, nausea, vomiting, diarrhea, nervousness	2.5 mg–10 mg/d PO
esmolol HCL *ess´-moe-lol*	Brevibloc	Supraventricular tachycardia, noncompensatory tachycardia	Hypotension, weakness, light-headedness, urinary retention	25–500 mcg/kg/min IV
metoprolol *me-toe´-proe-lol*	Lopressor, Toprol-XL, *generic*	Hypertension, angina, MI	Dizziness, hypotension, CHF, arrhythmia, nausea, vomiting, diarrhea	100–450 mg/d PO; 5 mg IV; extended release: 50–100 mg/d PO
nadolol *nay-doe´-lol*	Corgard, *generic*	Angina, hypertension	Dizziness, hypotension, nausea, vomiting, diarrhea, CHF, cardiac arrhythmias	40–320 mg/d PO
penbutolol *pen-byoo´-toe-lol*	Levatol	Hypertension	Bradycardia, dizziness, hypotension, nausea, vomiting, diarrhea	20 mg PO QD
pindolol *pen´-doe-lol*	Visken, *generic*	Hypertension	Bradycardia, dizziness, hypotension, nausea, vomiting, diarrhea	5–60 mg/d PO in divided doses

(continued)

SUMMARY DRUG TABLE   ADRENERGIC BLOCKING DRUGS *(Continued)*

GENERIC NAME	TRADE NAME*	USES	ADVERSE REACTIONS	DOSAGE RANGES
propranolol *pro-pran´-oh-lol*	Inderal, *generic*	Cardiac arrhythmias, MI, angina, hypertension, migraine prophylaxis	Bradycardia, dizziness, hypotension, nausea, vomiting, diarrhea, bronchospasm, hyperglycemia, pulmonary edena	Arrhythmias: 10–30 mg PO TID, QID; hypertension: 40–640 mg/d PO in divided doses; angina: 10–320 mg/d PO in divided doses; life-threatening arrhythmias: up to 1–3 mg IV; migraine: 80–240 mg/d PO in divided doses
sotalol HCl *soh´-tal-lole*	Betapace, *generic*	Ventricular arrhythmias	Dizziness, hypotension, nausea, vomiting, diarrhea, respiratory distress	80–320 mg/d PO in divided doses
timolol maleate *tye-moe´-lole*	Blocadren, *generic*	Hypertension, MI, migraine prophylaxis	Dizziness, hypotension, nausea, vomiting, diarrhea, pulmonary edena	Hypertension: 10–60 mg/d PO in divided doses; MI: 10 mg PO BID; migraine: 10–30 mg/d PO
timolol maleate (ophthalmic) *tye-moe'-lole*	Timoptic	Glaucoma	Ocular irritation, tearing	1 gtt BID

α/β-*Adrenergic Blocking Agents*

carvedilol *car-veh´-dih-lol*	Coreg	Hypertension, CHF	Bradycardia, hypotension, cardiac insufficiency, fatigue, dizziness, diarrhea	Hypertension: 6.25–50 mg PO BID; CHF: dose individualized based on patient response; initial dose 3.125 mg PO BID, increased gradually to a maximum dose of 50 mg PO BID
labetalol *lah-bet´-ah-lol*	Normodyne, Trandate, *generic*	Hypertension	Fatigue, drowsiness, insomnia, hypotension, impotence, diarrhea	100–400 mg/d PO in divided doses; 20–300 mg IV

Antiadrenergic Drugs: Centrally Acting

clonidine HCl *kloe´-ni-deen*	Catapres, Catapres-TTS, *generic*	Severe pain in patients with cancer, hypertension	Drowsiness, dizziness, sedation, dry mouth, constipation, syncope, dreams, rash	100–2400 mg/d PO; transdermal: 0.1–0.3 mg/24h
guanabenz acetate *gwan´-ah-benz*	Wytensin, *generic*	Hypertension	Dry mouth, sedation, dizziness, headache, weakness, arrhythmias	4–32 mg BID
guanfacine HCL *gwan´-fa-sine*	Tenex	Hypertension	Dry mouth, somnolence, asthenia, dizziness, headache, constipation, fatigue	1–3 mg/d PO at hs
methyldopa OR methylodopate HCL *meth´-ill-doe-pa-* *meth´-ill-doe-* *pate*	Aldomet, *generic*	Hypertension, hypertensive crisis	Bradycardia, aggravation of angina pectoris, heart failure, sedation, headache, rash, nausea, vomiting, nasal stuffiness	250 mg PO BID–TID; maintenance dose, 3 g/d; 250–500 mg q6h IV

SUMMARY DRUG TABLE ADRENERGIC BLOCKING DRUGS (*Continued*)

GENERIC NAME	TRADE NAME*	USES	ADVERSE REACTIONS	DOSAGE RANGES
Antiadrenergic Drugs: Peripherally Acting				
guanadrel *gwan´-ah-drel*	Hylorel	Hypertension	Palpitation, chest pain, fatigue, gas, headache, faintness, drowsiness, nocturia, shortness of breath on exertion, weight gain or loss, aching limbs, urination urgency	5–75 mg PO BID
guanethidine monosulfate *gwahn-eth´i-deen*	Ismelin	Hypertension, renal hypertension	Bradycardia, fluid retention, dizziness, weakness, diarrhea, nausea, dry mouth	10–50 mg/d PO
prazosin *pray-zoe´-sin*	Minipress, *generic*	Hypertension	Dizziness, postural hypotension, drowsiness, headache, loss of strength, palpitation, nausea	1–20 mg/d PO in divided doses
terazosin *tear-aye´-zoe-sin*	Hytrin	Hypertension, benign prostatic hyperplasia (BPH)	Dizziness, postural hypotension, headache, dyspnea, nasal congestion	1–20 mg/d PO

*The term *generic* indicates the drug is available in generic form.

pheochromocytoma, a tumor of the adrenal gland that produces excessive amounts of epinephrine and norepinephrine. The drug is used to control hypertension during preoperative preparation and surgical excision of pheochromocytoma.

Some drugs such as norepinephrine or dopamine are particularly damaging to the surrounding tissues if extravasation (infiltration) occurs during intravenous administration. Phentolamine is used to prevent or treat tissue damage caused by extravasation of these drugs.

ADVERSE REACTIONS

Administration of an α-adrenergic blocking drug may result in weakness, orthostatic hypotension, cardiac arrhythmias, hypotension, and tachycardia.

CONTRAINDICATIONS, PRECAUTIONS, AND INTERACTIONS

α-Adrenergic blocking drugs are contraindicated in patients who are hypersensitive to the drugs and in patients with coronary artery disease. These drugs are used cautiously during pregnancy (Pregnancy Category C)

and lactation, after a recent myocardial infarction, and in patients with renal failure or Raynaud's disease. When phentolamine is administered with epinephrine or ephedrine there is a decreased vasoconstrictor and hypertensive effects.

β-ADRENERGIC BLOCKING DRUGS

ACTIONS

β-Adrenergic blocking drugs, also called β blockers, decrease the activity of the sympathetic nervous system on certain tissues. β-Adrenergic receptors are found mainly in the heart. Stimulation of β receptors of the heart results in an increase in the heart rate. If stimulation of these β-adrenergic fibers is interrupted or blocked, the heart rate decreases and the vessels dilate (Fig. 23-1). These drugs decrease the excitability of the heart, decrease cardiac workload and oxygen consumption, and provide membrane-stabilizing effects that contribute to the antiarrhythmic activity of the β-adrenergic blocking drugs. Examples of β-adrenergic blocking drugs are esmolol (Brevibloc), metoprolol (Lopressor), nadolol (Corgard), and propranolol (Inderal).

β-Adrenergic blocking drugs, such as betaxolol (Betoptic) and timolol (Timoptic), when used topically

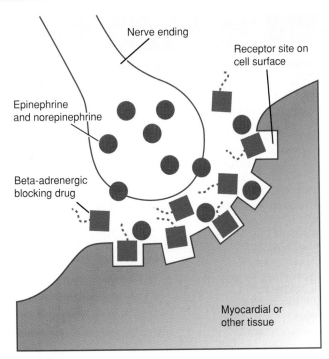

Figure 23-1. Beta-adrenergic blocking drugs prevent epinephrine and norepinephrine from occupying receptor sites on cell membranes. This action alters cell functions normally stimulated by epinephrine and norepinephrine, according to the number of receptor sites occupied by the beta-blocking drugs. (Adapted by J. Harley from *Encyclopedia Britannica Medical and Health Annual*. Chicago: Encyclopedia Britannica, 1983.)

as ophthalmic drops, appear to reduce the production of aqueous humor in the anterior chamber of the eye.

USES

These drugs are primarily used in the treatment of hypertension (see the Summary Drug Table: Adrenergic Blocking Drugs; also see Chap. 39) and certain **cardiac arrhythmia**s (abnormal rhythm of the heart), such as ventricular arrhythmias or supraventricular tachycardia. They are used to prevent reinfarction in patients with a recent myocardial infarction (1–4 weeks after MI). Some of these drugs have additional uses, such as the use of propranolol for migraine headaches and nadolol for angina pectoris.

β-Adrenergic blocking drugs also can be used topically as ophthalmic eye drops. For example, betaxolol (Betoptic) and timolol (Timoptic) are used in the treatment of glaucoma. **Glaucoma** is a narrowing or blockage of the drainage channels (canals of Schlemm) between the anterior and posterior chambers of the eye. This results in a build-up of pressure (increased intraocular pressure) in the eye. Blindness may occur if glaucoma is left untreated.

ADVERSE REACTIONS

Some of the adverse reactions observed with the administration of β-adrenergic blocking drugs include orthostatic hypotension, bradycardia, dizziness, vertigo, bronchospasm (especially in those with a history of asthma), hyperglycemia, nausea, vomiting, and diarrhea. Many of these reactions are mild and may disappear with therapy. More serious adverse reactions include symptoms of congestive heart failure (dyspnea, weight gain, peripheral edema). Examples of adverse reactions associated with the use of β-adrenergic ophthalmic preparations include headache, depression, cardiac arrhythmias, and bronchospasm.

> ❄ **Gerontologic Alert**
>
> *Older adults are at increased risk for adverse reactions when taking the β-adrenergic blocking drugs. The nurse should monitor the older adult closely for confusion, heart failure, worsening of angina, shortness of breath, and peripheral vascular insufficiency (eg, cold extremities, paresthesia of the hands, weak peripheral pulses).*

CONTRAINDICATIONS, PRECAUTIONS, AND INTERACTIONS

These drugs are contraindicated in patients with an allergy to the β blockers, in patients with sinus bradycardia, second- or third-degree heart block, heart failure, and those with asthma, emphysema, or hypotension. The drugs are used cautiously in patients with diabetes, thyrotoxicosis, and peptic ulcer.

When used with verapamil, the effects of the β blockers are increased. When the β blockers are used with indomethacin, ibuprofen, sulindac, or barbiturates, a decrease in the effects of the β blockers may occur. Diuretics may increase the hypotensive effects of the β-adrenergic blocking drugs. There is a paradoxical hypertensive effect when clonidine is given with the β-adrenergic blocking drugs. There is a risk of increased serum levels and toxic effects of the β-adrenergic blocking drugs when given with lidocaine and cimetidine.

ANTIADRENERGIC DRUGS

ACTIONS

One group of antiadrenergic drugs inhibits the release of norepinephrine (a neurohormone of the sympathetic nervous system, see Chap. 22) from certain adrenergic nerve endings in the peripheral nervous system. This group is composed of peripherally acting (ie, acting on peripheral structures) antiadrenergic drugs. An example of a peripherally acting antiadrenergic drug is guanethidine (Ismelin). The other antiadrenergic drugs are called centrally acting antiadrenergic drugs because they act on the CNS, rather than on the peripheral nervous system. This group affects specific CNS centers, thereby decreasing some of the activity of the sympathetic nervous system. Although the action of both types of antiadrenergic drugs is somewhat different, the results are basically the same. An example of a centrally acting antiadrenergic drug is clonidine (Catapres-TTS).

USES

Antiadrenergic drugs are used mainly for the treatment of certain cardiac arrhythmias and hypertension (see the Summary Drug Table: Adrenergic Blocking Drugs).

ADVERSE REACTIONS

Some of the adverse reactions associated with the administration of centrally acting antiadrenergic drugs include dry mouth, drowsiness, sedation, anorexia, rash, malaise, and weakness. Adverse reactions associated with the administration of the peripherally acting antiadrenergic drugs include hypotension, weakness, light-headedness, and bradycardia.

CONTRAINDICATIONS, PRECAUTIONS, AND INTERACTIONS

The centrally acting antiadrenergic drugs are contraindicated in active hepatic disease such as acute hepatitis or active cirrhosis and in patients with a history of hypersensitivity to these drugs. The centrally acting antiadrenergic drugs are used cautiously in patients with a history of liver disease, renal function impairment, and during pregnancy and lactation. If methyldopa is administered with anesthetics, there is an increased effect of the anesthetic. The centrally acting antiadrenergic drugs increase the activity of sympathomimetics, possibly causing hypertension. Clonidine decreases the effectiveness of levodopa. When clonidine is administered with β-adrenergic blocking drugs, a potentially life-threatening hypertensive episode may occur.

The peripherally acting antiadrenergic drugs are contraindicated in patients with a hypersensitivity to any of the drugs. Reserpine is contraindicated in patients who have an active peptic ulcer or ulcerative colitis and in

patients who are mentally depressed. Reserpine is used cautiously in patients with a history of depression, in patients with renal impairment or cardiovascular disease, and during pregnancy and lactation. Guanethidine, another peripherally acting antiadrenergic drug, is contraindicated in patients with pheochromocytoma and congestive heart failure. The drug is used cautiously in patients with bronchial asthma and renal impairment and during pregnancy and lactation. Anorexiants, haloperidol, the monoamine oxidase inhibitors, tricyclic antidepressants, and phenothiazines decrease the hypotensive effects of guanethidine.

α/β-ADRENERGIC BLOCKING DRUGS

ACTIONS

α/β-Adrenergic blocking drugs block the stimulation of α- and β-adrenergic receptors, resulting in peripheral vasodilation. The two drugs in this category are carvedilol (Coreg) and labetalol (Normodyne).

USES

Labetalol is used in the treatment of hypertension, either alone or in combination with another drug such as a diuretic. Carvedilol is used to treat essential hypertension and in congestive heart failure to reduce progression of the disease.

ADVERSE REACTIONS

Most adverse effects of labetalol are mild and do not require discontinuation of therapy. Examples of the adverse reactions include fatigue, drowsiness, insomnia, weakness, hypotension, diarrhea, dyspnea, and skin rash. Adverse reactions of carvedilol include fatigue, hypotension, cardiac insufficiency, chest pain, bradycardia, dizziness, diarrhea, hypotension, and fatigue.

CONTRAINDICATIONS, PRECAUTIONS, AND INTERACTIONS

Both carvedilol and labetalol are contraindicated in patients with hypersensitivity to the drug, bronchial asthma, decompensated heart failure, and severe bradycardia. The drugs are used cautiously in patients with drug-controlled congestive heart failure, chronic bronchitis, impaired hepatic or cardiac function, in those with diabetes, and during pregnancy (Category C) and lactation.

When either drug is administered with diuretics and other hypotensives, an increased hypotensive effect may occur. When labetalol is administered with cimetidine, the effects of labetalol are increased. Halothane increases the effects of labetalol. When carvedilol is administered with the antidiabetic drugs, there is an increased effectiveness of the antidiabetic drugs. There is an increased effectiveness of clonidine when carvedilol is administered with clonidine. There is an increased serum level of digoxin when digoxin is administered with carvedilol.

NURSING PROCESS

● The Patient Receiving an Adrenergic Blocking Drug

ASSESSMENT

Assessment depends on the drug, the patient, and the reason for administration.

Preadministration Assessment

The nurse establishes an accurate database before any adrenergic blocking drug is administered for the first time. If, for example, the patient has a peripheral vascular disease, the nurse notes the subjective and objective symptoms of the disorder during the initial assessment. If the drug is given for anginal pain, the nurse records the onset, type (eg, sharp, dull, squeezing), radiation, location, intensity, and duration of anginal pain. The nurse also questions the patient regarding any precipitating factors of the anginal pains, such as exertion or emotional stress. Once drug therapy is started, evaluation of the effects of therapy can be made by comparing the patient's current symptoms with the symptoms experienced before therapy was initiated.

Patients with hypertension must have their blood pressure and pulse taken on both arms in sitting, standing, and supine positions before therapy is begun. If the patient has a cardiac arrhythmia, the initial assessment includes taking the pulse rate, determining the pulse rhythm, and noting the patient's general appearance.

Subjective data (ie, the patient's complaints or description of symptoms) also are obtained at this time. The primary health care provider usually orders an electrocardiogram. Additional diagnostic studies and laboratory tests also may be ordered.

If the drug is given is given to treat congestive heart failure (ie, carvedilol), the patient is assessed for evidence of the disease, such as dyspnea (especially on exertion), peripheral edema, distended neck veins, and cough.

Ongoing Assessment

It is important for the nurse to perform ongoing assessment of the patient receiving adrenergic drug therapy. This assessment often depends on the reason the drug is administered. For all adrenergic blocking drugs, it is important for the nurse to continually observe these patients for the appearance of adverse reactions. Some adverse reactions are mild, whereas others, such as diarrhea, may cause a problem, especially if the patient is elderly or debilitated.

During therapy with an adrenergic blocking drug for hypertension, the nurse should take the patient's blood pressure before each dose is given. Some patients have an unusual response to the drugs. In addition, some drugs may, in some individuals, decrease the blood pressure at a more rapid rate than other drugs. It is important to monitor the patient's blood pressure on both arms and in the sitting, standing, and supine position for the first week or more of therapy. Once the patient's blood pressure has stabilized, the nurse should take the blood pressure before each drug administration using the same arm and position for each reading. It is a good idea to make a notation on the medication administration record or care plan about the position and arm used for blood pressure determinations. Measuring the blood pressure near the end of the dosing interval or near the end of the day after the last dose of the day helps to determine if the blood pressure is controlled throughout the day.

Ongoing assessment of patients receiving adrenergic blocking drugs for cardiac arrhythmias depends on the type of arrhythmia and the method of treatment. Some cardiac arrhythmias, such as ventricular fibrillation, are life threatening and require immediate attention. Other arrhythmias are serious and require treatment but are not life threatening. The patient with a life-threatening arrhythmia may receive an adrenergic blocking drug, such as propranolol, by the intravenous (IV) route. When these drugs are administered IV, cardiac monitoring is necessary. Patients not in a specialized unit, such as a coronary care unit, are usually transferred to one as soon as possible. When administering these drugs for a life-threatening arrhythmia, it is important for the nurse to continually supervise the patient, frequently monitor the blood pressure and respiratory rate, and perform cardiac monitoring.

When propranolol is administered orally for a less serious cardiac arrhythmia, cardiac monitoring is usually not necessary. The nurse should monitor the patient's blood pressure and pulse rate and rhythm at varying intervals, depending on the length of treatment and the patient's response to the drug.

✳ Nursing Alert

When administering a β-adrenergic blocking drug, such as propranolol (Inderal), the nurse should take an apical pulse rate and blood pressure before giving the drug. If pulse is below 60 bpm or if systolic blood pressure is less than 90 mm Hg, the nurse should withhold the drug and contact the primary health care provider.

If propranolol is given for angina, the nurse should ask the patient about the relief of symptoms and should record responses on the patient's chart.

NURSING DIAGNOSES

Drug-specific nursing diagnoses are highlighted in the Nursing Diagnoses Checklist. Other nursing diagnoses applicable to these drugs are discussed in depth in Chapter 4.

PLANNING

The expected outcomes for the patient depend on the reason for administration of an adrenergic blocking drug but may include an optimal response to drug therapy, management of common adverse drug reactions (diarrhea, constipation, anorexia, fatigue, ineffective tissue perfusion), decreased risk for injury, and an understanding of and compliance with the prescribed drug regimen.

IMPLEMENTATION

Promoting an Optimal Response to Therapy

Most adrenergic blocking drugs may be given without regard to food. However, the nurse should administer propranolol and metoprolol at the same time each day because food may enhance bioavailability. Sotalol is given on an empty stomach because food may reduce absorption of the drug.

> ✳ **Nursing Alert**
>
> *The nurse should withhold the administration of a β-adrenergic drug, such as propranolol (Inderal), and contact the primary health care provider if the patient has a heart rate of less than 60 bpm or if there is any irregularity in the patient's heart rate or rhythm.*

When adrenergic blocking drugs are given to patients to control hypertension, angina, or cardiac arrhythmias, it is important to communicate with the primary care provider about the patient's response to therapy. When given for a cardiac arrhythmia, these drugs can provoke new or worsen existing ventricular arrhythmias. If angina worsens or does not appear to be controlled by the drug, the nurse should contact the

primary care provider immediately. When the drug is administered for hypertension, the nurse monitors the patient for a decrease in the blood pressure. If there is a significant rise in the blood pressure, the nurse administers the dose and notifies the primary care provider immediately because additional drug therapy may be necessary.

When a β-adrenergic blocking ophthalmic preparation, such as timolol, is administered to patients with glaucoma, it is important to insist that they have periodic follow-up examinations by an ophthalmologist. At these examinations, the intraocular pressure should be measured to determine the effectiveness of drug therapy.

Monitoring and Managing Common Adverse Reactions

Some patients may experience one or more adverse drug reactions during treatment with adrenergic blocking drugs. As with any drug, the nurse must report adverse reactions to the primary care provider and record the reactions on the patient's chart. Nursing judgment in this matter is necessary because some adverse reactions are serious or potentially serious in nature. In these cases, the nurse should withhold the next dose of the drug and contact the primary care provider immediately. The nurse also reports to the primary care provider any adverse reactions that pose no serious threat. Adverse reactions that pose no serious threat to the patient's well-being, such as dry mouth or mild constipation, may have to be tolerated by the patient. It is important to assure the patient that, in some instances, these less serious reactions disappear or lessen in intensity after a time.

However, even minor adverse drug reactions can be distressing to the patient, especially when they persist for a long time. Therefore, when possible, the nurse should relieve minor adverse reactions with simple nursing measures. For example, the nurse can assist the patient with dry mouth by giving frequent sips of water or by allowing the patient to suck on a piece of hard candy (provided that the patient does not have diabetes or is not on a special diet that limits sugar intake) to relieve a dry mouth. The nurse can help relieve a patient's constipation by encouraging increased fluid intake, unless extra fluids are contraindicated. The primary care provider also may order a laxative or stool softener. It is important for the nurse to maintain a daily record of bowel elimination. The nurse can help the patient minimize certain gastrointestinal side effects, such as anorexia, diarrhea, and constipation by administering drugs at a specific time in relation to meals, with food, or with antacids.

MANAGING HYPOTENSION. Administration of the adrenergic blocking drugs may cause hypotension. If the drug is administered for hypertension, then a decrease is expected.

> ### ☀ Nursing Alert
>
> *If a significant decrease in the blood pressure (a drop of 20 mm Hg systolic or a systolic below 90 mm Hg) occurs after a dose of an adrenergic blocking drug, the nurse should withhold the drug and notify the primary care provider immediately. A dosage reduction or discontinuation of the drug may be necessary. Some adrenergic blocking drugs (eg, prazosin or terazosin) may cause a "first dose" effect. A **first dose effect** occurs when the patient experiences marked hypotension (or postural hypotension) and syncope with sudden loss of consciousness with the first few doses of the drug.*

The first dose effect may be minimized by decreasing the initial dose and administering the dose at bedtime. The dosage can then be slowly increased every 2 weeks until a full therapeutic effect is achieved. If the patient experiences syncope, the nurse places the patient in a recumbent position and treats supportively. This effect is self-limiting and in most cases does not recur after the initial period of therapy. Light-headedness and dizziness are more common than loss of consciousness. The section below discusses these effects and provides interventions for management.

DECREASING THE PATIENT'S RISK FOR INJURY. On occasion, patients receiving an adrenergic blocking drug may experience postural or orthostatic hypotension. **Postural hypotension** is characterized by a feeling of light-headedness and dizziness when the patient suddenly changes from a lying to a sitting or standing position, or from a sitting to a standing position. **Orthostatic hypotension** is characterized by similar symptoms as postural hypotension and occurs when the patient changes or shifts position after standing in one place for a long period. The nurse can help to minimize these adverse reactions as follows:

- Instruct patients to rise slowly from a sitting or lying position.
- Provide assistance for the patient getting out of a bed or a chair if symptoms of postural hypotension are severe. Place the call light nearby and instruct patients to ask for assistance each time they get in and out of a bed or a chair.
- Assist the patient in bed to a sitting position and have the patient sit on the edge of the bed for about 1 minute before ambulating.
- Help seated patients to a standing position and instruct them to stand in one place for about 1 minute before ambulating.
- Remain with the patient while he or she is standing in one place, as well as during ambulation.

- Instruct the patient to avoid standing in one place for prolonged periods. This is rarely a problem in the hospital but should be included in the patient and family discharge teaching plan.
- Teach the patient to avoid taking hot showers or baths, which tend to increase vasodilation.

Symptoms of postural or orthostatic hypotension often lessen with time, and the patient may be allowed to get out of bed or chair slowly without assistance. The nurse must exercise good judgment in this matter. Allowing the patient to rise from a lying or sitting position without help is done only when the determination has been made that the symptoms have lessened and ambulation poses no danger of falling.

Educating the Patient and Family

Some patients do not adhere to the prescribed drug regimen for a variety of reasons, such as failure to comprehend the prescribed regimen, the cost of drug therapy, and failure to understand the importance of continued and uninterrupted therapy. If the nurse detects failure to adhere to the prescribed drug regimen, he or she should investigate the possible cause of the problem. In some instances, financial assistance may be necessary; in other instances, patients need to know why they are taking a drug and why therapy must be continuous to attain and maintain an optimal state of health and well-being.

The nurse should describe the drug regimen and stress the importance of continued and uninterrupted therapy when teaching the patient who is prescribed an adrenergic blocking drug. Patient education will differ according to the reason the adrenergic blocking drug is prescribed.

EDUCATING THE PATIENT WITH HYPERTENSION, CARDIAC ARRHYTHMIA, OR ANGINA. If a β-adrenergic blocking drug has been prescribed for hypertension, cardiac arrhythmia, angina, or other cardiac disorders, the patient must have a full understanding of the treatment regimen. In some instances, the primary care provider may advise the hypertensive patient to lose weight or eat a special diet, such as a low-salt diet. A special diet also may be recommended for the patient with angina or a cardiac arrhythmia. When appropriate, the nurse should stress the importance of diet and weight loss in the therapy of hypertension.

It is important to include the following additional points in the teaching plan for the patient with hypertension, angina, or a cardiac arrhythmia:

- Do not stop taking the drug abruptly, except on the advice of the primary care provider. Most of these drugs require that the dosage be gradually decreased to prevent precipitation or worsening of adverse effects.

- Notify the primary health care provider promptly if adverse drug reactions occur.
- Observe caution while driving or performing other hazardous tasks because these drugs (β-adrenergic blockers) may cause drowsiness, dizziness, or light-headedness.
- Immediately report any signs of congestive heart failure (weight gain, difficulty breathing, or edema of the extremities).
- Do not use any nonprescription drug (eg, cold or flu preparations or nasal decongestants) unless use of a specific drug has been approved by the primary care provider.
- Inform dentists and other primary care providers of therapy with this drug.
- Keep all primary care provider appointments because close monitoring of therapy is essential.
- Check with a primary health care provider or pharmacist to determine if the drug is to be taken with food or on an empty stomach.

In addition, when an adrenergic blocking drug is prescribed for hypertension, the primary care provider may want the patient to monitor his or her own blood pressure between office visits. This may enable the number of visits to the primary care provider office to be reduced and will help the patient learn to manage his or her own health (see Patient and Family Teaching Checklist: Monitoring Blood Pressure).

Patient and Family Teaching Checklist

Monitoring Blood Pressure

The nurse:

✓ Teaches the patient and a family member how to take an accurate blood pressure reading. This involves choosing the correct instrument and teaching the patient the steps to taking a blood pressure reading.

✓ Supervises the patient and a family member during several trial blood pressure readings to ensure accuracy of the measurements.

✓ Suggests to the patient that the same arm and body position be used each time the blood pressure is taken.

✓ Explains that the blood pressure can vary slightly with emotion, the time of day, and the position of the body.

✓ Explains that a slight change in readings is normal, but if a drastic change in either or both the systolic or diastolic readings occurs, the patient should contact the primary health care provider as soon as possible.

EDUCATING THE PATIENT WITH GLAUCOMA. When an adrenergic blocking drug has been prescribed for glaucoma, the nurse demonstrates the technique of eye drop instillation and explains the prescribed treatment regimen to the patient. Adherence to the instillation schedule is stressed because omitting or discontinuing the drug without approval of the primary care provider may result in a marked increase in intraocular pressure, which can lead to blindness. The nurse should tell patients with glaucoma who are using adrenergic blocking eye drops to contact their primary health care provider if eye pain, excessive tearing, or any change in vision occurs.

EVALUATION

- The therapeutic effect is achieved and hypertension, cardiac arrhythmia, or glaucoma is controlled.
- Adverse reactions are identified, reported to the primary health care provider, and managed successfully through appropriate nursing interventions.
- No evidence of injury related to orthostatic or postural hypotension is seen.
- The patient and family demonstrate an understanding of the drug regimen.

● *Critical Thinking Exercises*

1. *Ms. Martin has been prescribed propranolol (Inderal) for hypertension. She arrives at the outpatient clinic and tells you that she is having episodes of dizziness and at times feels as if she is going to faint. Discuss how you would investigate this problem and what information you could give Ms. Martin that might help her.*
2. *Mr. Garcia was prescribed labetalol (Normodyne) 100 mg orally twice daily for hypertension. The health care provider wants him to monitor his blood pressure once daily. Determine what assessments you would make. Develop a teaching plan for Mr. Garcia that would help him in monitoring his blood pressure and taking labetalol.*
3. *A new nurse says that she is unsure about how the adrenergic blocking drugs work. Discuss the four types of adrenergic blocking drugs and how each one works within the body.*

● *Review Questions*

1. A patient is to receive a β-adrenergic drug for hypertension. Before the drug is administered the most important assessment the nurse performs is _____.
   - **A.** weighing the patient
   - **B.** obtaining blood for laboratory tests
   - **C.** taking a past medical history
   - **D.** taking the blood pressure on both arms

2. When an adrenergic blocking drug is given for a life-threatening cardiac arrhythmia, which of the following activities would the nurse expect to be a part of patient care?

   A. daily ECGs
   B. fluid restriction of 1000 mL per day
   C. daily weights
   D. cardiac monitoring

3. To prevent complications when administering a β-adrenergic blocking drug to an elderly patient, the nurse would be particularly alert for _____.

   A. vascular insufficiency (eg, weak peripheral pulses and cold extremities)
   B. complaints of an occipital headache
   C. insomnia
   D. hypoglycemia

4. The patient with glaucoma will likely receive a(n) _____.

   A. α/β-adrenergic blocking drug
   B. α-adrenergic blocking drug
   C. β-adrenergic blocking drug
   D. antiadrenergic drug

● **Medication Dosage Problems**

1. The primary health care provider prescribes 60 mg propranolol oral solution. The drug is available in an oral solution with a strength of 4 mg/mL. The nurse administers _____.

2. A patient is prescribed 12.5 mg of carvedilol. The drug on hand is 3.125-mg tablets. The nurse administers _____.

Cholinergic Drugs

Key Terms

acetylcholine
acetylcholinesterase
cholinergic crisis
glaucoma

micturition
myasthenia gravis
parasympathomimetic
   drugs

Chapter Objectives

On completion of this chapter, the student will:

● Discuss important aspects of the parasympathetic nervous system.
● Discuss the uses, drug actions, general adverse reactions, contraindications, precautions, and interactions of the cholinergic drugs.
● Identify important preadministration and ongoing assessment activities the nurse should perform on the patient taking cholinergic drugs.
● List some nursing diagnoses particular to a patient taking cholinergic drugs.
● Discuss ways to promote an optimal response to therapy, how to manage common adverse reactions, and important points to keep in mind when educating the patient about the use of cholinergic drugs.

Cholinergic drugs mimic the activity of the parasympathetic nervous system (PNS). They also are called **parasympathomimetic drugs.** An understanding of the PNS is useful in understanding the cholinergic drugs.

PARASYMPATHETIC NERVOUS SYSTEM

The PNS is a part of the autonomic nervous system (see Chap. 22). It helps conserve body energy and is partly responsible for activities such as slowing the heart rate, digesting food, and eliminating body wastes.

Electron microscopic study reveals an incalculably small space between nerve endings and the effector organ (eg, the muscle, cell, or gland) that is innervated (or controlled) by a nerve fiber. For a nerve impulse to be transmitted from the nerve ending (motor end plate) across the space to the effector organ, a neurohormone is needed.

The PNS has two neurohormones (neurotransmitters): **acetylcholine** (ACh) and **acetylcholinesterase** (AChE). ACh is a neurotransmitter responsible for the transmission of nerve impulses to effector cells of the parasympathetic nervous system. ACh plays an important role in the transmission of nerve impulses at synapses and myoneural junctions. ACh is quickly destroyed by the enzyme AChE, thereby allowing the nerve impulse to pass, but not remain in an excited state.

These two neurohormones are released at nerve endings of parasympathetic nerve fibers, at some nerve endings in the sympathetic nervous system, and at nerve endings of skeletal muscles. These parasympathetic neurohormones are believed to be manufactured by special cells located in the nerve ending. When a parasympathetic nerve fiber is stimulated, the nerve fiber releases ACh, and the nerve impulses pass (travel) from the nerve fiber to the effector organ or structure. After the impulse has crossed over to the effector organ or structure, ACh is inactivated (destroyed) by the neurohormone AChE. When the next nerve impulse is ready to travel along the nerve fiber, ACh is again released and then inactivated by AChE.

CHOLINERGIC DRUGS

Cholinergic drugs have limited usefulness in medicine, partly because of the adverse reactions that may occur during administration. However, in some diseases or conditions cholinergic drugs are either definitely indicated or may be of value.

town, returning to school, jet lag, pain from arthritis or headaches, stress, or anxiety. The sedatives and hypnotics are primarily used to treat insomnia.

During hospitalization, helping the patient sleep is an important part of the management of illness. Hospitalized patients are in unfamiliar surroundings that are unlike the home situation. There are noises and lights at night, which often interfere with or interrupt sleep. Sleep deprivation may interfere with the healing process; therefore, a hypnotic may be given. These drugs also may be prescribed for short-term use as hypnotics after discharge from the hospital.

Zaleplon, a miscellaneous sedative, is the first prescription sleep preparation that the patient can take, later in the night, if you have at least 4 hours in bed before you become active again. With zaleplon the patient will fall asleep quickly and wake up with little or no aftereffects of the drug.

A hypnotic may be given the night before the operation to prepare the patient for surgery. On the day of surgery, a barbiturate or miscellaneous sedative and hypnotic may be used either alone or with other drugs as part of the preoperative regimen. The anesthesiologist or surgeon selects a drug that is tailored to the patient's needs. When a barbiturate or miscellaneous sedative and hypnotic is used as a hypnotic, a dose larger than that required to produce sedation is given.

❄ Gerontologic Alert

Elderly patients may require a smaller hypnotic dose, and, in some instances, a sedative dose produces sleep.

Although the use of barbiturates and miscellaneous sedatives and hypnotics for sedation has largely been replaced by the antianxiety drugs (see Chap. 30), they occasionally may be used to provide sedation before certain types of procedures, such as cardiac catheterization or the administration of a local or general anesthesia. Sedative doses, usually given during daytime hours, may be used to treat anxiety and apprehension. Patients with chronic disease may require sedation, not only to reduce anxiety, but also as an adjunct in the treatment of their disease.

Paraldehyde, a miscellaneous sedative and hypnotic, may be used to treat delirium tremens and other psychiatric conditions. In addition, some barbiturates are used as anticonvulsants (see Chap. 28).

ADVERSE REACTIONS

Barbiturates

Adverse reactions associated with barbiturate administration include:

- CNS—somnolence, agitation, confusion, CNS depression, ataxia, nightmares, lethargy, residual sedation (drug hangover), hallucinations, paradoxical excitement
- Respiratory—hypoventilation, apnea, respiratory depression, bronchospasm, laryngospasm
- Gastrointestinal—nausea, vomiting, constipation, diarrhea, epigastric pain
- Cardiovascular—bradycardia, hypotension, syncope
- Hypersensitivity—rash, angioneurotic edema, fever, urticaria
- Other—headache and liver damage.

Miscellaneous Sedatives and Hypnotics

Adverse reactions associated with administration of the miscellaneous sedatives and hypnotics vary depending on the drug used. Common adverse reactions include dizziness, drowsiness, headache, and nausea. Other adverse reactions that may be seen with the administration of miscellaneous sedatives and hypnotics are listed in the Summary Drug Table: Miscellaneous Sedatives and Hypnotics.

CONTRAINDICATIONS

These drugs are contraindicated in patients with known hypersensitivity to the sedatives or hypnotics. The nurse should not administer these drugs to comatose patients, those with severe respiratory problems, those with a history of drug and alcohol abuse, or to pregnant or lactating women. The barbiturates (eg, amobarbital, butabarbital, secobarbital) are classified as Pregnancy Category D drugs. Most miscellaneous sedatives and hypnotics (eg, zolpidem, chloral hydrate, zaleplon) are Pregnancy Category C drugs. Some benzodiazepines (eg, estazolam, quazepam, temazepam, triazolam) are classified as Pregnancy Category X drugs and can cause damage to the developing fetus if administered during pregnancy.

☀ Nursing Alert

Women taking the barbiturates or the benzodiazepines should be warned of the potential risk to the fetus so that contraceptive methods may be instituted, if necessary. A child born to a mother taking benzodiazepines may develop withdrawal symptoms during the postnatal period.

PRECAUTIONS

All drugs entering the body ultimately leave the body. Some leave virtually unchanged, whereas others are transformed into other, less-potent chemicals or compounds **detoxified** (to make nontoxic or not harmful) before they are eliminated. Barbiturates and miscellaneous sedatives and hypnotics are detoxified by the liver and ultimately excreted by the kidney. These drugs are given with great caution to patients with liver or kidney disease because their diseased organs will not be able to detoxify or eliminate the drug, and a drug build-up will occur. The barbiturates should be administered with extreme caution to patients with a history of drug abuse (eg, alcoholics and opiate abusers) or mental illness. If the drugs are prescribed on an outpatient basis, the amount dispensed is limited to the amount needed until the next appointment. These drugs should be used with great caution during lactation. Drowsiness in infants of breastfeeding mothers who have taken the barbiturates has been reported.

Gerontologic Alert

The nurse uses these drugs cautiously in older adults or in those who are debilitated because these patients are more sensitive to the effects of the sedatives or hypnotics.

INTERACTIONS

The sedatives and hypnotics have an additive effect when administered with alcohol, antidepressants, narcotic analgesics, antihistamines, or phenothiazines.

Nursing Alert

Because narcotic analgesics depress the CNS (see Chap. 19), the nurse should not administer a barbiturate or miscellaneous sedatives and hypnotics approximately 2 hours before or after administration of a narcotic analgesic or other CNS depressant. If the time interval between administration of a narcotic analgesic and a sedative or hypnotic is less than 2 hours, the patient may experience severe respiratory depression, bradycardia, and unresponsiveness.

Health Supplement Alert: Melatonin

Melatonin is a hormone produced by the pineal gland in the brain. The use of melatonin obtained from animal pineal tissue is not recommended because of the risk of contamination. The synthetic form of melatonin does not carry this risk. However, melatonin is an over-the-counter dietary supplement and has not been evaluated for safety, effectiveness, and purity by the FDA. All of the potential risks and benefits may not be known. Supplements should be purchased from a reliable source to minimize the risk of contamination. Melatonin has been used in treating insomnia, overcoming jet lag, improving the effectiveness of the immune system, and as an antioxidant. The most significant use is for the short-term treatment of insomnia at low doses. Individuals wishing to use melatonin should consult with their primary health care provider or a pharmacist before using the supplement. Possible adverse reactions include headache and depression. Drowsiness may occur within 30 minutes after taking the herb. The drowsiness may persist for an hour or

more, affecting any activity that requires mental alertness, such as driving. Although uncommon, allergic reactions to melatonin have been reported. The supplement should be stopped and emergency care sought if symptoms of an allergic reaction (eg, difficulty breathing, hives, or swelling of lips, tongue, or face) occur.

Herbal Alert: Valerian

Valerian was originally used in Europe and was brought on the Mayflower to North America. The herb is widely used for its sedative effects in conditions of mild anxiety or restlessness. It is particularly useful in individuals with insomnia. Valerian improves overall sleep quality by shortening the length of time it takes to go to sleep and decreasing the number of nighttime awakenings. It does not cause the adverse reactions common with sedative drugs, such as addiction and "drug hangovers" the morning after taking the herb. Valerian is classified as generally recognized as safe (GRAS) for use in the United States. Valerian is used as a tea, tablet, capsule, or tincture. When valerian is used as an aid to sleep, the herb is taken approximately 1 hour before bedtime. The dose is less if used for anxiety, and the herb can be used in combination with other calming herbs, such as lemon balm or chamomile. It may take 2 to 4 weeks before the full therapeutic effect (ie, improvement of mood and sleep patterns) of the herb occurs. Dosages include the following:

Tea: 1 to 2 cups/day
Capsules/tablets: 300 to 500 mg daily
Tincture: ½ to 1 teaspoon daily
Standardized extract: 300 to 400 mg daily

NURSING PROCESS

● The Patient Receiving a Sedative or Hypnotic

ASSESSMENT

Assessment of the patient receiving a sedative or hypnotic drug depends on the reason for administration and whether the drug is given routinely or as needed.

Preadministration Assessment

Before administering a barbiturate or miscellaneous sedative and hypnotic, the nurse takes and records the patient's blood pressure, pulse, and respiratory rate. In addition to the vital signs, the nurse assesses the following patient needs.

● Is the patient uncomfortable? If the reason for discomfort is pain, an analgesic, rather than a hypnotic, may be required.
● Is it too early for the patient to receive the drug? Is a later hour preferred?
● Does the patient receive a narcotic analgesic every 4 to 6 hours? A hypnotic may not be necessary because a narcotic analgesic is also capable of causing drowsiness and sleep.

● Are there disturbances in the environment that may keep the patient awake and decrease the effectiveness of the drug?

Barbiturates have little or no analgesic action, so the nurse does not give these drugs if the patient has pain and cannot sleep. Barbiturates, when given in the presence of pain, may cause restlessness, excitement, and delirium.

If the patient is receiving one of these drugs for daytime sedation, the nurse assesses the patient's general mental state and level of consciousness. If the patient appears sedated and difficult to awaken, the nurse withholds the drug and contacts the primary health care provider as soon as possible.

Ongoing Assessment

Before administering the drug each time, the nurse should perform an assessment to include the patient's vital signs (temperature, pulse, respirations, and blood pressure) and level of consciousness (is the patient alert, confused, or lethargic). This is especially important when the drug is ordered to be given as needed. After assessing the patient, the nurse makes a decision regarding administration of the drug.

The nurse checks to see if the drug helped the patient sleep on previous nights. If not, a different drug or dose may be needed, and the nurse should consult the primary health care provider regarding the drug's ineffectiveness.

If the patient has an order for a PRN narcotic analgesic or other CNS depressant and a hypnotic, the nurse should consult the primary health care provider regarding the time interval between administration of these drugs. Usually at least 2 hours should elapse between administration of a hypnotic and any other CNS depressant, but this interval may vary, depending on factors such as the patient's age and diagnosis.

☀ Nursing Alert

The nurse withholds the drug and notifies the primary health care provider if any one or more vital signs significantly varies from the database, if the respiratory rate is 10/min or below, or if the patient appears lethargic. In addition, it is important to determine if there are any factors (eg, noise, lights, pain, discomfort) that would interfere with sleep and whether these may be controlled or eliminated.

NURSING DIAGNOSES

Drug-specific nursing diagnoses are highlighted in the Nursing Diagnoses Checklist. Other nursing diagnoses applicable to these drugs are discussed in depth in Chapter 4.

Nursing Diagnoses Checklist

☑ **Risk for Injury** related to sedative or hypnotic effects of drug

☑ **Disturbed Sleep Pattern** related to adverse drug effects

☑ **Risk for Impaired Gas Exchange** related to respiratory depression

---

PLANNING

The expected outcomes for the patient depend on the reason for administration of a sedative or hypnotic but may include an optimal response to drug therapy (eg, sedation or sleep), management of adverse drug reactions, an absence of drug dependence, and an understanding of and compliance with the postdischarge drug regimen (when applicable).

IMPLEMENTATION

Promoting an Optimal Response to Therapy

ENHANCING SLEEP PATTERNS. To promote the effects of the sedative or hypnotic the nurse provides supportive care, such as back rubs, night lights or a darkened room, and a quiet atmosphere. The patient is discouraged from drinking beverages containing caffeine, such as coffee, tea, or cola drinks, which can contribute to wakefulness.

The nurse never leaves hypnotics and sedatives at the patient's bedside to be taken at a later hour; hypnotics and sedatives are controlled substances (see Chap. 1). In addition, the nurse never leaves these drugs unattended in the nurses' station, hallway, or other areas to which patients, visitors, or hospital personnel have direct access. If these drugs are prepared in advance, it is important to place them in a locked cupboard until the time of administration.

When giving these drugs orally, the nurse encourages the patient to drink a full glass of water with the drug. When barbiturates are administered intramuscularly, the nurse gives the drug in the gluteus maximus, vastus lateralis, or other areas where there is little risk of encountering a nerve trunk or major artery. Injection near or into peripheral nerves results in permanent nerve damage. When giving oral paraldehyde, the nurse mixes the drug with cold orange or tomato juice to eliminate some of the pungent taste. When paraldehyde is ordered for rectal administration, the nurse dissolves the dose of the drug (usually 10–20 mL) in one to two parts of oil or isotonic sodium chloride and gives it as a retention enema.

PREVENTING INJURY. After administration of a hypnotic, the nurse raises the side rails and advises the patient to remain in bed and to call for assistance if it is necessary to get out of bed. Patients receiving sedative doses may or may not require this safety measure, depending on the patient's response to the drug. The nurse assesses the patient receiving a sedative dose and determines what safety measures must be taken. The nurse assesses the patient receiving a hypnotic 1 to 2 hours after the drug is given to evaluate the effect of the drug.

Monitoring and Managing Adverse Drug Reactions

It is important that the nurse observes the patient for adverse drug reactions. During periods when the patient is excited or confused, the nurse protects the patient from harm and provides supportive care and a safe environment. The nurse notifies the primary health care provider if the patient fails to sleep, awakens one or more times during the night, or develops an adverse drug reaction. In some instances, supplemental doses of a hypnotic may be ordered if the patient awakens during the night.

Excessive drowsiness and headache the morning after a hypnotic has been given (drug hangover) may occur in some patients. The nurse reports this problem to the primary health care provider because a smaller dose or a different drug may be necessary. The nurse assists the patient with ambulation, if necessary. When getting out of bed the patient is encouraged to rise to a sitting position first, wait a few minutes, then rise to a standing position.

> ❄ **Gerontologic Alert**
>
> *The older adult is at greater risk for oversedation, dizziness, confusion, or* **ataxia** *(unsteady gait) when taking a sedative or hypnotic. The nurse checks elderly and debilitated patients for marked excitement, CNS depression, and confusion. If excitement or confusion occurs, the nurse observes the patient at frequent intervals (as often as every 5–10 minutes may be necessary) for the duration of this occurrence and institutes safety measures to prevent injury. If oversedation, extreme dizziness, or ataxia occurs, the nurse notifies the primary health care provider.*

MONITORING AND MANAGING RESPIRATORY DEPRESSION. These drugs depress the CNS and can cause respiratory depression. The nurse carefully assesses respiratory function (rate, depth, and quality) before administering a sedative, $1/2$ to 1 hour after administering the drug, and frequently thereafter. Toxic reaction of the barbiturates can cause severe respiratory depression, hypoventilation, and circulatory collapse.

> ✳ **Nursing Alert**
>
> *The onset of symptoms of barbiturate toxicity may not occur until several hours after the drug is administered. Symptoms of acute toxicity include CNS and respiratory depression, constriction or paralytic dilation of the pupils, tachycardia, hypotension, lowered body temperature, oliguria, circulatory collapse, and coma. The nurse should report any symptoms of toxicity to the primary health care provider immediately.*

Treatment of barbiturate toxicity is mainly supportive (ie, maintaining a patent airway, oxygen administration, monitoring vital signs and fluid balance). The patient may require treatment for shock, respiratory assistance, administration of activated charcoal, and in severe cases of toxicity, hemodialysis.

MANAGING DRUG DEPENDENCY. Sedatives and hypnotics are best given for no more than 2 weeks and preferably for a shorter time. However, a barbiturate or miscellaneous sedative and hypnotic can cause drug dependency. The nurse must never suddenly discontinue use of these drugs when there is a question of possible dependency. Patients who have been taking a sedative or hypnotic for several weeks should be gradually withdrawn from the drug to prevent withdrawal symptoms. Symptoms of withdrawal include restlessness, excitement, euphoria, and confusion. Withdrawal can result in serious consequences, especially in those with existing diseases or disorders.

Educating the Patient and Family

In educating the patient and family about barbiturates and miscellaneous sedatives and hypnotics, several general points must be considered, as well as teaching about two common abuses of these drugs.

The nurse gives the patient and family an explanation of the prescribed drug and dosage regimen, as well as situations that should be avoided. The nurse develops a teaching plan to include one or more of the following items of information:

GENERAL TEACHING POINTS
- Do not drink any alcoholic beverage 2 hours before, with, or 8 hours after taking the drug.
- If the drug appears to be ineffective, contact the primary health care provider. Do not increase the dose unless advised to do so by the primary health care provider.
- Notify the primary health care provider if any adverse drug reactions occur.
- The primary health care provider usually prescribes these drugs for short-term use only.
- When taking the drug as a sedative, be aware that the drug can impair the mental and physical abilities required for performing potentially dangerous tasks, such as driving a car or operating machinery.
- Observe caution when getting out of bed at night after taking a drug for sleep. Keep the room dimly lit and remove any obstacles that may result in injury when getting out of bed. Never attempt to drive or perform any hazardous task after taking a drug intended to produce sleep.
- Do not use these drugs if you are pregnant, considering becoming pregnant, or breastfeeding.

● Do not use over-the-counter (OTC) cold, cough, or allergy drugs while taking this drug unless their use has been approved by the primary health care provider. Some of these products contain antihistamines or other drugs that also may cause mild to extreme drowsiness. Others may contain an adrenergic drug, which is a mild stimulant, and therefore will defeat the purpose of the drug.

ZALEPLON

● Zaleplon may be taken at bedtime or later in the night if the you have at least 4 hours of bedtime left. You will still wake up naturally without excessive drowsiness in the morning.

● Zaleplon should not be given with a high fat meal or snack because fat interferes with absorption of the drug.

TEACHING ABOUT ABUSE. Sedatives and hypnotics are subject to abuse when taken on an outpatient basis. The most common abuses are increasing the dose of the drug and drinking an alcohol beverage shortly before, with, or shortly after taking the sedative or hypnotic. The nurse emphasizes the importance of not increasing the dosage of the drug and the dangers of consuming alcohol while taking a sedative or hypnotic.

Increasing the Dosage. Sedatives and hypnotics can become less effective after they are taken for a period of time. Thus, there may be a tendency to increase the dose without consulting the primary health care provider. To ensure compliance with the treatment regimen, the nurse emphasizes the importance of not increasing or decreasing the dose unless a change in dosage is recommended by the primary health care provider. In addition, the nurse stresses the importance of not repeating the dose during the night if sleep is interrupted or sleep only lasts a few hours unless the primary health care provider has approved taking the drug more than once per night.

Use With Alcohol. Alcohol is a CNS depressant, as are the sedatives and hypnotics. When alcohol and a sedative or hypnotic are taken together, there is an additive effect and an increase in CNS depression, which has, on occasion, resulted in death. The nurse must emphasize the importance of not drinking alcohol while taking this drug and stress that the use of alcohol and any one of these drugs can result in serious effects.

EVALUATION

● The therapeutic effect is achieved and the sleep pattern improved.

● Adverse drug reactions are identified, reported to the primary health care provider, and managed successfully through appropriate nursing interventions.

● The patient is free of drug dependence.

● The patient and family demonstrate an understanding of the drug regimen.

● The patient verbalizes the importance of complying with the prescribed therapeutic regimen.

● The patient verbalizes an understanding of what to avoid while taking the drug.

● *Critical Thinking Exercises*

1. *Ms. Parker's husband was killed in an automobile accident, and she has had trouble coping with her loss. She complains of being unable to sleep for more than an hour before she wakes. The primary health care provider prescribes a hypnotic, one capsule per night for use during the next 3 weeks. In 2 weeks, she calls the primary health care provider's office and asks for a refill of her prescription. Determine what questions you would you ask Ms. Parker. Explain why you would ask them.*

2. *Mr. Davidson, who is 67 years old, is to be discharged after major bowel surgery. The primary health care provider gives him a prescription for 24 tablets of zolpidem (Ambien). When reading Mr. Davidson's chart you note that he works part time on weekends as a bartender. Discuss what you would emphasize when explaining the prescription to Mr. Davidson.*

3. *Mr. Allen, who is hospitalized in the coronary care unit with a myocardial infarction, is restless and tells you that although he has been able to sleep other nights while in the hospital, he is unable to sleep tonight. Although he has an order for flurazepam (Dalmane) 30 mg HS, analyze what you would investigate before making a decision regarding administration of the hypnotic.*

4. *Discuss and give a rationale for situations or conditions in which sedatives would be contraindicated.*

5. *Explain why sedatives or hypnotics must be given cautiously in older adults.*

● *Review Questions*

1. Ms. Brown has arthritis in her lower back, and the pain keeps her awake at night. She asks if she can have a "sleeping pill." In considering her request the nurse must take into account that _____.

   A. barbiturates, if given in the presence of pain, may cause excitement or delirium

   B. a hypnotic may be given instead of an analgesic to relieve her pain

   C. hypnotics often increase the pain threshold

   D. a hypnotic plus an analgesic is best given in this situation

2. Which of these drugs can be given at bedtime or later during the night if the patient is unable to sleep and has at least 4 hours left to sleep?

   A. temazepam
   B. estazolam
   C. zaleplon
   D. zolpidem

3. When giving a hypnotic to Ms. Green, age 82 years, the nurse is aware that _____.

   A. smaller doses of the drug are usually given to older patients
   B. elderly patients usually require larger doses of a hypnotic
   C. older adults excrete the drug faster than younger adults
   D. dosages of the hypnotic may be increased each night until the desired effect is achieved

4. Which of the following points should be included in a teaching plan for a patient taking a sedative or hypnotic?

   A. An alcoholic beverage may be served 1 to 2 hours before a sedative is taken without any ill effects.
   B. Dosage of the sedative may be increased if sleep is not restful.
   C. These drugs may safely be used for 6 months to 1 year when given for insomnia.
   D. Do not use any over-the-counter cold, cough, or allergy medications while taking a sedative or hypnotic.

5. Which of the following sedatives/hypnotics is a Pregnancy Category X drug?

   A. zolpidem
   B. amobarbital
   C. temazepam
   D. chloral hydrate

● Medication Dosage Problems

1. Triazolam (Halcion) 0.125 mg is prescribed. The drug is available in 0.25-mg tablets. The nurse administers _____.

2. Chloral hydrate (Noctec) 500 mg is prescribed for insomnia. The drug is available in 250-mg tablets. The nurse administers _____.

chapter 27

Central Nervous System Stimulants

Key Terms

analeptics
anorexiants

attention deficit disorder
narcolepsy

Chapter Objectives

On completion of this chapter, the student will:

- List the three types of central nervous system stimulants.
- Discuss the uses, general drug actions, general adverse reactions, contraindications, precautions, and interactions of the central nervous system stimulants.
- Discuss important preadministration and ongoing assessment activities the nurse should perform on the patient taking a central nervous system stimulant.
- List some nursing diagnoses particular to a patient taking a central nervous system stimulant.
- Discuss ways to promote an optimal response to drug therapy, how to manage common adverse drug reactions, and important points to keep in mind when educating patients about the use of central nervous system stimulants.

The central nervous system (CNS) includes the brain and the spinal cord. The CNS processes information to and from the peripheral nervous system and is the center of coordination and control for the entire body. Many drugs stimulate the CNS, but only a few are used therapeutically. This chapter discusses the drugs that stimulate the CNS and the nursing implications related to their administration.

The CNS stimulants include the **analeptics,** drugs that stimulate the respiratory center of the CNS; the amphetamines, drugs with a high abuse potential because of their ability to produce euphoria and wakefulness; and the **anorexiants,** drugs used to suppress the appetite.

ACTIONS

Analeptics

Doxapram (Dopram) and caffeine (combination of caffeine and sodium benzoate) are two analeptics used in medicine. Doxapram increases the depth of respirations by stimulating special receptors located in the carotid arteries and upper aorta. These special receptors (called chemoreceptors) are sensitive to the amount of oxygen in arterial blood. Stimulation of these receptors results in an increase in the depth of the respirations. In larger doses, doxapram increases the respiratory rate by stimulating the medulla.

Caffeine is a mild to potent CNS stimulant, with the degree of its stimulating effect dependent on the dose administered. Caffeine stimulates the CNS at all levels, including the cerebral cortex, the medulla, and the spinal cord. Caffeine has mild analeptic (respiratory stimulating) activity. Other actions include cardiac stimulation (which may produce tachycardia), dilatation of coronary and peripheral blood vessels, constriction of cerebral blood vessels, and skeletal muscle stimulation. Caffeine also has mild diuretic activity.

Modafinil is an analeptic used to treat **narcolepsy** (disorder causing an uncontrollable desire to sleep during normal waking hours even though the individual has a normal nighttime sleeping pattern). The exact mechanism of action is not known, but the drug is thought to bind to dopamine reuptake carrier sites, increasing alpha activity and decreasing delta, theta, and beta activity, thereby reducing the number of sleepiness episodes. It is not associated with cardiac and other systemic stimulatory effects of the other CNS stimulants.

Amphetamines

The amphetamines, such as amphetamine, dextroamphetamine (Dexedrine), and methamphetamine (Desoxyn), are sympathomimetic (ie, adrenergic) drugs that stimulate the CNS (see Chap. 22). Their drug action results in an elevation of blood pressure, wakefulness, and an increase or decrease in pulse rate. The ability of these drugs to act as anorexiants and suppress the appetite is thought to be due to their action on the appetite center in the hypothalamus.

Anorexiants

The anorexiants, such as phentermine and phendimetrazine, are nonamphetamine drugs pharmacologically similar to the amphetamines. Like the amphetamines, their ability to suppress the appetite is thought to be due to their action on the appetite center in the hypothalamus.

USES

The CNS stimulants have limited use in medicine. Examples of CNS stimulants are given in the Summary Drug Table: Central Nervous System Stimulants.

Analeptics

Doxapram is used to treat drug-induced respiratory depression and to temporarily treat respiratory depression in patients with chronic pulmonary disease. This drug also may be used during the postanesthesia period when respiratory depression is caused by anesthesia. It also is used to stimulate deep breathing in patients after anesthesia.

Caffeine and sodium benzoate are administered intramuscularly or intravenously as part of the treatment of respiratory depression caused by CNS depressants, such as narcotic analgesics and alcohol. Because caffeine also has other effects, such as constriction of cerebral arteries and stimulation of skeletal muscles, the use of caffeine for this purpose has largely been replaced by narcotic antagonists for respiratory depression caused by narcotic overdose or other drugs with greater analeptic activity (eg, doxapram). Orally, caffeine, either as a beverage (coffee, tea) or in nonprescription tablet form, may be used by some individuals to relieve fatigue. Caffeine also may be included in some nonprescription analgesics. Modafinil is use to treat narcolepsy to decrease the number of sleepiness episodes during the day.

Amphetamines

Amphetamines may be used in the short-term treatment of exogenous obesity (obesity caused by a persistent calorie intake that is greater than needed by the body). However, their use in treating exogenous obesity has declined because the long-term use of the amphetamines for obesity carries the potential for addiction and abuse.

These drugs may also be helpful in the management of narcolepsy, a disorder manifested by an uncontrollable desire to sleep during normal waking hours even though the individual has a normal nighttime sleeping pattern. The individual with narcolepsy may fall asleep from a few minutes to a few hours many times in one day. This disorder begins in adolescence or in the young adult and persists throughout life.

Amphetamines are used to manage **attention deficit hyperactivity disorder** (ADHD) in children. Children with this disorder exhibit a short attention span, hyperactivity, impulsiveness, and emotional lability. The condition is more prevalent in boys than in girls and poses a problem with school and learning, although these children are usually of normal or above average intelligence. How amphetamines, which are CNS stimulants, calm the hyperactive child is unknown. These drugs reduce motor restlessness, increase mental alertness, provide mood elevation, produce a mild sense of euphoria, and reduce the sense of fatigue. In addition to taking a CNS stimulant, the child with ADHD may also need psychotherapeutic counseling.

Anorexiants

Phendimetrazine and phentermine are chemically related to the amphetamines and are used for short-term treatment of exogenous obesity. These drugs are available only by prescription and have addiction and abuse potential. Some nonprescription diet aids contain phenylpropanolamine, an adrenergic drug that has actions similar to the adrenergic drug ephedrine. These diet aids are not true anorexiants, and those containing phenylpropanolamine have limited appetite-suppressing ability when compared to the anorexiants. Phenylpropanolamine also has little abuse potential and has no addiction potential.

ADVERSE REACTIONS

The adverse reactions associated with the administration of doxapram include excessive CNS stimulation, symptoms of which may include headache, dizziness, apprehension, disorientation, and hyperactivity. Other adverse reactions include nausea, vomiting, cough,

SUMMARY DRUG TABLE CENTRAL NERVOUS SYSTEM STIMULANTS

GENERIC NAME	TRADE NAMES*	USES	ADVERSE REACTIONS	DOSAGE RANGES
Analeptics				
caffeine *kaf-een'*	Caffedrine, Stay Awake, *generic*	Fatigue, drowsiness, as adjunct in analgesic formulation, respiratory depression	Palpitations, nausea, vomiting, insomnia, tachycardia, restlessness	100–200 mg PO q3–4h; caffeine and sodium benzoate: 500 mg–1g IM, IV
doxapram HCL *docks'-a-pram*	Dopram	Drug-induced postanesthesia, drug-induced respiratory depression, acute respiratory insufficiency superimposed on COPD	Dizziness, headache, apprehension, disorientation, nausea, cough, dyspnea, urinary retention	0.5–1 mg/kg IV
modafinil *moe-daf´-in-ill*	Provigil	Narcolepsy	Insomnia, nervousness, headache, tachycardia, anorexia, dizziness, excitement	200–400 mg/d PO
Amphetamines				
amphetamine sulfate *am-fet´-a-meen*	*generic*	Narcolepsy, attention deficit hyperactivity disorder (ADHD), exogenous obesity	Insomnia, nervousness, headache, tachycardia, anorexia, dizziness, excitement	Narcolepsy: 5–60 mg/d PO in divided doses; ADD: 5 mg BID, increase by 10 mg/wk until desired effect; Obesity: 5–30 mg/d PO in divided doses
dexmethylphenidate *dex-meth-thyl-fen-i-date*	Focalin	ADHD	Nervousness, insomnia, loss of appetite, abdominal pain, weight loss, tachycardia, skin rash	2.5 mg PO BID; maximum dosage, 20 mg/d
dextroamphetamine sulfate *dex-troe-am-fet´-a-meen*	Dexedrine, *generic*	Narcolepsy, ADHD, exogenous obesity	Insomnia, nervousness, headache, tachycardia, anorexia, dizziness, excitement	Narcolepsy: 5–60 mg/d PO in divided doses; ADD: up to 40 mg/d PO; obesity: 5–30 mg/d PO in divided doses
methamphetamine *meth-am-fet´-a-meen*	Desoxyn	ADHD	Insomnia, nervousness, headache, tachycardia, anorexia, dizziness, excitement	Up to 25 mg/d PO
methylphenidate HCL *meh-thyl-fen´-ih-date*	Concerta, Metadate ER, Ritalin, *generic*	ADHD, narcolepsy	Nervousness, insomnia, anorexia, dizziness, drowsiness, headache	5–60 mg/day PO
Pemoline *pem´-oh-leen*	Cylert	ADHD	Insomnia, nervousness, headache, tachycardia, anorexia, dizziness, excitement	37.5–112.5 mg/d PO
Anorexiants				
benzphetamine HCL *benz-fe-ta-meen*	Didrex	Obesity	Insomnia, nervousness, headache, dry mouth, palpitations, tachycardia, anorexia, dizziness, excitement	25–50 mg PO 1–3 times/d

SUMMARY DRUG TABLE CENTRAL NERVOUS SYSTEM STIMULANTS (Continued)

GENERIC NAME	TRADE NAMES*	USES	ADVERSE REACTIONS	DOSAGE RANGES
diethylpropion HCl *die-eth´-uhl-pro´-pee-ahn*	Tenuate, *generic*	Obesity	Insomnia, nervousness, headache, palpitations, tachycardia, anorexia, dizziness, excitement	Immediate release: 25 mg PO 3 times/d; Sustained release: 75 mg once daily
phentermine HCl *fen-ter´-meen*	Ionamin, Pro-Fast, *generic*	Obesity	Insomnia, nervousness, headache, tachycardia, anorexia, dizziness, excitement	8 mg PO TID or 15–37.5 mg PO as a single daily dose
sibutramine HCl *si-byoo-tra-meen*	Meridia	Obesity	Insomnia, palpitations, headache, dry mouth, nervousness, tachycardia, anorexia, dizziness, excitement	5–15 mg PO once daily

*The term *generic* indicates the drug is available in generic form.

dyspnea, urinary retention, and variations in the heart rate. Administration of caffeine and sodium benzoate may result in tachycardia, palpitations, nausea, and vomiting.

One of the chief adverse reactions associated with the amphetamines and anorexiants is overstimulation of the CNS, which may result in a variety of adverse reactions, including insomnia, tachycardia, nervousness, headache, anorexia, dizziness, and excitement. In some instances, the intensity of these reactions is dose dependent, but some individuals may experience an intense degree of these symptoms even with low doses. Other individuals experience few symptoms of CNS stimulation.

Nursing Alert

The amphetamines and anorexiants have abuse and addiction potential. Long-term use of amphetamines for obesity may result in tolerance to the drug and a tendency to increase the dose. Extreme psychological dependency may also occur.

The amphetamines and anorexiants are recommended only for short-term use in selected patients for the treatment of exogenous obesity. When used for treatment of children with ADD, long-term use must be followed by gradual withdrawal of the drug.

CONTRAINDICATIONS

The CNS stimulants are contraindicated in patients with known hypersensitivity or severe hypertension, in newborns, and in patients with epilepsy or convulsive

states, pneumothorax, acute bronchial asthma, head injury, or stroke. In addition, the amphetamines are contraindicated in patients with hyperthyroidism and glaucoma. The anorexiants are classified as Pregnancy Category X and should not be used during pregnancy.

PRECAUTIONS

The CNS stimulants are given cautiously in all patients, particularly because the use of these drugs can lead to physical dependence. Some individuals are especially sensitive to the effects of the CNS stimulants. The analeptics and amphetamines are Pregnancy Category B drugs and are not recommended during pregnancy, except when clearly needed. These drugs are used with extreme caution in patients with cardiovascular disease and in women during the early stages of pregnancy.

INTERACTIONS

The amphetamines and the anorexiants should not be given during or within 14 days after administration of monoamine oxidase inhibitors (see Chap. 31) because the patient may experience hypertensive crisis and intracranial hemorrhage. When guanethidine is administered with the amphetamines or the anorexiants, the antihypertensive effect of guanethidine may decrease. Coadministration of the amphetamines or the anorexiants with the tricyclic antidepressants may decrease the effects of the amphetamines or the anorexiants.

NURSING PROCESS

● **The Patient Receiving a Central Nervous System Stimulant**

ASSESSMENT

Assessment of the patient receiving a CNS stimulant depends on the drug, the patient, and the reason for administration.

Preadministration Assessment

The preadministration assessment depends on the type of CNS used and the reason for administration.

ANALEPTICS. When a CNS stimulant is prescribed for respiratory depression, initial patient assessments will include the blood pressure, pulse, and respiratory rate. It is important to note the depth of the respirations and any pattern to the respiratory rate, such as shallow respirations or alternating deep and shallow respirations. The nurse reviews recent laboratory tests (if any), such as arterial blood gas studies. Before administering the drug, the nurse ensures that the patient has a patent airway. Oxygen is usually administered before, during, and after drug administration.

AMPHETAMINES. When an amphetamine is prescribed for any reason, the nurse weighs the patient and takes the blood pressure, pulse, and respiratory rate before starting drug therapy.

The nurse should initially observe the child with ADD for the various patterns of abnormal behavior. The nurse records a summary of the behavior pattern in the patient's chart to provide a comparison with future changes that may occur during therapy.

ANOREXIANTS. When an anorexiant or amphetamine is used as part of the treatment of obesity, the drug is usually prescribed for outpatient use. The nurse obtains and records the blood pressure, pulse, respiratory rate, and weight before therapy is started.

Ongoing Assessment

The ongoing assessment depends on the type of CNS stimulant used and the reason for administration.

ANALEPTICS. After administration of an analeptic, the nurse carefully monitors the patient's respiratory rate and pattern until the respirations return to normal. The nurse monitors the level of consciousness, the blood pressure, and pulse rate at 5- to 15-minute intervals or as ordered by the primary health care provider. The nurse may draw blood for arterial blood gas analysis at intervals to determine the effectiveness of the analeptic, as well as the need for additional drug therapy. It is important to observe the patient for adverse drug reactions and to report their occurrence immediately to the primary health care provider.

ATTENTION DEFICIT DISORDER. If the child is hospitalized, the nurse enters a daily summary of the child's behavior in the patient's record. This provides a record of the results of therapy.

NARCOLEPSY. The nurse observes the patient with narcolepsy during daytime hours. If periods of sleep are noted, the nurse records the time of day they occur and their length.

WEIGHT LOSS. When an amphetamine or anorexiant is prescribed for obesity, the nurse obtains the patient's weight and vital signs at the time of each outpatient visit.

NURSING DIAGNOSES

Drug-specific nursing diagnoses are highlighted in the Nursing Diagnoses Checklist. Other nursing diagnoses applicable to these drugs are discussed in depth in Chapter 4.

PLANNING

The expected outcomes for the patient depend on the reason for administration of a CNS stimulant but may include an optimal response to therapy, management of adverse drug reactions, and an understanding of the drug regimen.

IMPLEMENTATION

Promoting an Optimal Response to Therapy

Respiratory depression can be a serious event requiring administration of a respiratory stimulant. When an analeptic is administered, the nurse notes and records the rate, depth, and character of the respirations before the drug is given to provide a database for evaluation of the effectiveness of drug therapy. Oxygen is usually ordered for before and after administration of a respiratory stimulant. After administration, the nurse monitors respirations closely and records the effects of therapy.

When a CNS stimulant such as dextroamphetamine is administered to treat a child with ADD, the drug regimen will be periodically interrupted to determine if the child still exhibits the symptoms of ADD.

Nursing Diagnoses Checklist

☑ **Risk for Sleep Pattern Disturbance** related to hyperactivity, nervousness, insomnia, other (specify)

☑ **Risk for Injury** related to adverse drug effects (CNS stimulation, drug dependency, other [specify])

Monitoring and Managing Adverse Drug Reactions

The adverse drug reactions that may occur with the use of an amphetamine, such as insomnia and a significant increase in blood pressure and pulse rate, may be serious enough to require discontinuation of the drug. In some instances, the adverse drug effects are mild and may even disappear during therapy. The nurse informs the primary care provider of all adverse reactions.

When use of the CNS stimulants causes insomnia, the nurse administers the drug early in the day (when possible) to diminish sleep disturbances. The patient is encouraged not to nap during the day. Other stimulants, such as coffee, tea, or cola drinks, are avoided. In some patients, nervousness, restlessness, and palpitations may occur. The vital signs are checked every 6 to 8 hours or more often if tachycardia, hypertension, or palpitations occur. Many times these adverse reactions will diminish with continued use as tolerance develops. If tolerance develops, the dosage is not increased.

❄ Gerontologic Alert

Older adults are especially sensitive to the effects of the CNS stimulants and may exhibit excessive anxiety, nervousness, insomnia, and mental confusion. Cardiovascular disorders, common in the older adult, may be worsened by the CNS stimulants. Careful monitoring is important because the presence of these reactions may result in the need to discontinue use of the drug.

Nausea and vomiting may occur with the administration of an analeptic; therefore, the nurse should keep a suction machine nearby should vomiting occur. Urinary retention may be seen with the administration of doxapram; therefore, the nurse measures intake and output and notifies the primary health care provider if the patient is unable to void or the bladder appears distended on palpation.

Long-term treatment with the CNS stimulants can retard growth in children. Children on long-term treatment with the CNS drugs require frequent height and weight measurements to monitor growth. Intermittent therapy is usually advised to prevent tolerance to the drug and to minimize the effect on growth and the development of tolerance.

Educating the Patient and Family

The nurse explains the therapeutic regimen and adverse drug reactions to the patient and family. The type of information included in the teaching plan will depend on the drug and the reason for its use. It is important to emphasize the importance of following the recommended dosage schedule. The nurse may include the following additional teaching points:

- Attention deficit disorder: Give the drug in the morning 30 to 45 minutes before breakfast and before lunch. Do not give the drug in the afternoon. Pemoline is given once daily in the morning. Therapeutic response of pemoline may take 3 to 4 weeks. Insomnia and anorexia usually disappear during continued therapy. Write a daily summary of the child's behavior, including periods of hyperactivity, general pattern of behavior, socialization with others, and attention span. Bring this record to each primary health care provider or clinic visit because this record may help the primary health care provider determine future drug dosages or additional treatment modalities. The primary health care provider may prescribe that the drug be given only on school days when high levels of attention and performance are necessary.
- Narcolepsy: Keep a record of the number of times per day that periods of sleepiness occur, and bring this record to each visit to the primary health care provider or clinic.
- Amphetamines and anorexiants: These drugs are taken early in the day to avoid insomnia. Do not increase the dose or take the drug more frequently, except on the advice of a primary health care provider. These drugs may impair the ability to drive or perform hazardous tasks and may mask extreme fatigue. If dizziness, light-headedness, anxiety, nervousness, or tremors occur, contact the primary care provider. Avoid or decrease the use of coffee, tea, and carbonated beverages containing caffeine (see Patient and Family Teaching Checklist: Using Anorexiants for Weight Loss).
- Caffeine (oral, nonprescription): Avoid the use of oral caffeine-containing products to stay awake if there is a history of heart disease, high blood pressure, or stomach ulcers. These products are intended for occasional use and should not be used if heart palpitations, dizziness, or light-headedness occurs.

EVALUATION

- The parent or child reports that the child's behavior and school performance are improved.
- The patient reports fewer episodes of inappropriate sleep patterns.
- Adverse reactions are identified and managed through appropriate nursing interventions.
- The patient complies with the prescribed drug regimen.
- The patient and family demonstrate an understanding of the drug regimen.
- The patient verbalizes the importance of complying with the prescribed therapeutic regimen.

Patient and Family Teaching Checklist

Using Anorexiants for Weight Loss

The nurse:

✓ Reviews reasons for the drug and prescribed drug regimen, including drug name, dosage, and frequency of administration.

✓ Stresses the importance of taking the drug exactly as prescribed, including not to increase the dose or take more frequently unless instructed to do so by the prescriber.

✓ Reinforces use of drug for short-term therapy only.

✓ Warns about possible addiction, drug tolerance, and psychological dependency.

✓ Reviews possible adverse reactions, especially CNS overstimulation, with instructions to notify the health care provider immediately should any occur.

✓ Instructs to take drug early in day to minimize insomnia.

✓ Cautions about safety measures because of possible impairment in ability to drive or perform hazardous tasks.

✓ Advises to avoid other stimulants, including those containing caffeine such as coffee, tea, and cola drinks; provides a written list of foods to avoid.

✓ Urges to read labels of foods and nonprescription drugs for possible stimulant content.

✓ Reinforces prescribed dietary and exercise program for weight reduction, both verbally and in writing.

✓ Reassures that results of therapy will be monitored by continued follow-up visits with health care provider.

✓ Arranges for follow-up visits as necessary.

● Critical Thinking Exercises

1. *Ms. Stone is given a special diet and prescribed an anorexiant to help her lose 20 lb before she has reconstructive knee surgery. Determine what instructions you would include in a teaching plan for this patient.*

2. *Mr. Trent has narcolepsy and is prescribed amphetamine 10 mg/d. Develop questions you would ask Mr. Trent when he returns to the clinic for evaluation after 1 month of therapy.*

3. *Ms. Allison is prescribed an analeptic for respiratory depression. Discuss what preadministration and ongoing assessments you would make when caring for Ms. Allison.*

4. *Discuss precautions that should be taken when administering the CNS stimulants.*

● Review Questions

1. Initial assessment of the child with attention deficit disorder includes _____.
   A. assessing to which stimuli the child responds the most
   B. determining the child's intelligence
   C. obtaining a summary of the child's behavior pattern
   D. obtaining vital signs

2. When assessing the patient receiving doxapram for chronic pulmonary disease, the nurse observes the patient for adverse drug reactions, which may include _____.
   A. headache, dizziness, variations in heart rate
   B. diarrhea, drowsiness, hypotension
   C. decreased respiratory rate, weight gain, bradycardia
   D. fever, dysuria, constipation

3. When teaching a patient with narcolepsy who is receiving an amphetamine, the nurse instructs the patient to _____.
   A. record the times of the day the medication is taken
   B. take the medication at bedtime as well as in the morning
   C. take the drug with meals
   D. keep a record of how often periods of sleepiness occur

4. When administering an amphetamine, the nurse first checks to see if the patient is taking or has taken an monoamine oxidase (MAO) inhibitor because _____.
   A. a lower dosage of the amphetamine may be needed
   B. a higher dosage of the amphetamine may be needed
   C. if the amphetamine is administered within 14 days of the MAO inhibitor, cardiac arrest may occur
   D. if the amphetamine is administered within 14 days of the MAO inhibitor, an intracranial hemorrhage may occur

● Medication Dosage Problems

1. Phentermine hydrochloride 8 mg three times a day PO is prescribed as an adjunct for weight loss. The total amount of drug the patient will receive daily is _____. Is this an appropriate dose for this drug? _____

2. Modafinil 400 mg is prescribed. The drug is available in 200-mg tablets. The nurse administers _____.

Anticonvulsants

Chapter Objectives

On completion of this chapter, the student will:

- List the five types of drugs used as anticonvulsants.
- Discuss the general drug actions, uses, adverse reactions, contraindications, precautions, and interactions of anticonvulsants.
- Discuss important preadministration and ongoing assessment activities the nurse should perform on the patient receiving an anticonvulsant.
- List some nursing diagnoses particular to a patient taking an anticonvulsant.
- Discuss ways to promote an optimal response to therapy, how to manage common adverse reactions when administering the anticonvulsants, and important points to keep in mind when educating a patient about the use of anticonvulsants.

The terms **convulsion** and seizure are often used interchangeably and basically have the same meaning. A **seizure** may be defined as a periodic attack of disturbed cerebral function. A seizure may also be described as an abnormal disturbance in the electrical activity in one or more areas of the brain. Seizures may be classified as partial (focal) or generalized. Each different type of seizure disorder is characterized by a specific pattern of events, as well as a different pattern of motor or sensory manifestation.

Partial or focal seizures arise from a localized area in the brain and cause specific symptoms. A partial seizure can spread to the entire brain and cause a generalized seizure. Partial seizures include simple seizures in which consciousness is not impaired, **jacksonian seizure**s (a focal seizure that begins with an uncontrolled stiffening or jerking in one part of the body such as finger, mouth, hand, or foot that may progress to a generalized seizure), and psychomotor seizures.

Psychomotor seizures occur most often in children 3 years of age through adolescence. The individual may experience an aura with perceptual alterations, such as hallucinations or a strong sense of fear. Repeated coordinated but inappropriate movements, such as clutching, kicking, picking at clothes, walking in circles, and licking are characteristic. The most common motor symptom is drawing or jerking of the mouth and face.

Generalized seizures include absence, myoclonic, and tonic-clonic. Manifestations of a generalized **tonic-clonic seizure** include alternate contraction (tonic phase) and relaxation (clonic phase) of muscles, a loss of consciousness, and abnormal behavior. **Myoclonic seizure**s involve sudden, forceful contractions involving the musculature of the trunk, neck, and extremities. **Absence seizures,** previously referred to as petit mal seizures, are seizures characterized by a brief loss of consciousness during which physical activity ceases. The seizures typically last a few seconds, occur many times a day, and may go unnoticed by others.

Seizure disorders are generally categorized as idiopathic or acquired. Idiopathic seizures have no known cause; acquired seizure disorders have a known cause, including high fever, electrolyte imbalances, uremia, hypoglycemia, hypoxia, brain tumors, and some drug withdrawal reactions. Once the cause is removed (if it can be removed), the seizures theoretically cease.

an additive CNS depressant effect may occur. Increased effects of the benzodiazepines are seen when the drugs are administered with cimetidine, disulfiram, and oral contraceptives. When the benzodiazepines are administered with theophylline, there is a decreased effect of the benzodiazepines. See Chapter 30 for additional information on the benzodiazepines.

Hydantoins

The hydantoins are contraindicated in patients with known hypersensitivity to the drugs. Phenytoin is contraindicated in patients with sinus bradycardia, sinoatrial block, second and third degree AV block, and Adams-Stokes syndrome; it also is contraindicated during pregnancy (ethotoin and phenytoin are Pregnancy Category D) and lactation. Ethotoin is contraindicated in patients with hepatic abnormalities.

When the hydantoins are used with other CNS depressants (eg, alcohol, narcotic analgesics, and antidepressants), an additive CNS depressant effect may occur. The hydantoins are used cautiously in patients with liver or kidney disease and neurologic disorders. Phenytoin is used cautiously in patients with hypotension, severe myocardial insufficiency, and hepatic impairment.

Phenytoin interacts with many different drugs. For example, isoniazid, chloramphenicol, sulfonamides, benzodiazepines, succinimides, and cimetidine all increase phenytoin blood levels. The barbiturates, rifampin, theophylline, and warfarin decrease phenytoin blood levels. When administering the hydantoins with meperidine, the analgesic effect of meperidine is decreased.

Oxazolidinediones

The oxazolidinediones are contraindicated in patients with known hypersensitivity to the drugs. Trimethadione is classified as a Pregnancy Category D drug and is contraindicated during pregnancy and lactation. Trimethadione is used with caution in patients with eye disorders (eg, retinal or optic nerve disease), liver or kidney disease, and neurologic disorders. When trimethadione is used with other nervous system (CNS) depressants (eg, alcohol, narcotic analgesics, and antidepressants), an additive CNS depressant effect may occur.

Succinimides

The succinimides are contraindicated in patients with known hypersensitivity to the drugs. The succinimides are contraindicated in patients with bone marrow depression or hepatic or renal impairment and during lactation. Ethosuximide is classified as a

Pregnancy Category C drug and is used with caution during pregnancy. As with all anticonvulsants, when the succinimides are used with other CNS depressants (eg, alcohol, narcotic analgesics, and antidepressants), an additive CNS depressant effect may occur.

When the hydantoins are administered with the succinimides there may be an increase in the hydantoin blood levels. Concurrent administration of valproic acid and the succinimides may result in either a decrease or an increase in succinimide blood levels. When primidone in administered with the succinimides, lower primidone levels may occur.

Miscellaneous Anticonvulsants

The miscellaneous anticonvulsants are contraindicated in patients with known hypersensitivity to any of the drugs. Carbamazepine is contraindicated in patients with bone marrow depression or hepatic or renal impairment and during pregnancy (Category D). Valproic acid is not administered to patients with renal impairment or during pregnancy (Category D). Oxcarbazepine (Trileptal), a miscellaneous anticonvulsant, may exacerbate dementia.

The miscellaneous anticonvulsants are used cautiously in patients with glaucoma or increased intraocular pressure; a history of cardiac, renal or liver dysfunction; and psychiatric disorders. When the miscellaneous anticonvulsants are used with other CNS depressants (eg, alcohol, narcotic analgesics, and antidepressants), an additive CNS depressant effect may occur.

When carbamazepine is administered with primidone, decreased primidone levels and higher carbamazepine serum levels may result. Cimetidine administered with carbamazepine may result in an increase in plasma levels of carbamazepine that can lead to toxicity. Blood levels of lamotrigine increase when the agent is administered with valproic acid, requiring a lower dosage of lamotrigine.

NURSING PROCESS

● **The Patient Receiving an Anticonvulsant**

ASSESSMENT

Preadministration Assessment

Seizures that occur in the outpatient setting are almost always seen first by family members or friends, rather than by a member of the medical profession. The occurrence of abnormal behavior patterns or convulsive movements usually prompts the patient to visit the primary health care provider's office or a neurologic clinic. A thorough patient history is necessary to identify the type of seizure disorder. Information the nurse should obtain from those who have observed the seizure is listed in Display 28-1.

Additional patient information should include a family history of seizures (if any) and recent drug therapy (all drugs currently being used). Depending on the type of seizure disorder, other information may be needed, such as a history of a head injury or a thorough medical history.

The nurse obtains the vital signs at the time of the initial assessment to provide baseline data. The primary health care provider may order many laboratory and diagnostic tests, such as an electroencephalogram, computed tomographic scan, complete blood count, and hepatic and renal function tests to confirm the diagnosis and identify a possible cause of the seizure disorder, as well as to provide a baseline during therapy with anticonvulsants.

Ongoing Assessment

Anticonvulsants control, but do not cure, epilepsy. An accurate ongoing assessment is important to obtain the desired effect of the anticonvulsant. The dosage of the anticonvulsant may require frequent adjustments during the initial treatment period. Dosage adjustments are based on the patient's response to therapy (eg, the control of the seizures), as well as the occurrence of adverse reactions. Depending on the patient's response to therapy, a second anticonvulsant may be added to the therapeutic regimen, or one anticonvulsant may be changed to another. Regular serum plasma levels of the anticonvulsant are taken to monitor for toxicity.

The patient's seizures, as well as response to drug therapy, must be observed when a hospitalized patient is receiving an anticonvulsant. The nurse must carefully document each seizure with regard to the time of occurrence, the length of the seizure, and the psychic or motor activity occurring before, during, and after the seizure. Most seizures occur without warning, and the nurse may not see the patient until after the seizure begins or after the seizure is over. However, any observations made during and after the seizure are important and may aid in the diagnosis of the type of seizure, as well as assist the primary health care provider in evaluating the effectiveness of drug therapy.

NURSING DIAGNOSES

Drug-specific nursing diagnoses are highlighted in the Nursing Diagnoses Checklist. Other nursing diagnoses applicable to these drugs are discussed in depth in Chapter 4.

PLANNING

The expected outcomes for the patient depend on the type and severity of the seizure but may include an optimal response to therapy (control of seizure), management of common adverse drug reactions (includes minimizing injury and maintaining normal oral mucous membranes), reduction in anxiety, and an understanding of and compliance with the prescribed therapeutic regimen.

 Nursing Alert

Status epilepticus may result from abrupt discontinuation of the drug, even when the anticonvulsant is being administered in small daily doses.

IMPLEMENTATION

Promoting an Optimal Response to Therapy

When administering an anticonvulsant, the nurse must not omit or miss a dose (except by order of the primary health care provider). An abrupt interruption in therapy by omitting a dose may result in a recurrence of the seizures. In some instances, abrupt withdrawal of an anticonvulsant can result in status epilepticus.

The nurse aids continuity of anticonvulsant administration by making a notation on the care plan, as well as by informing all health care team members of the importance of the drug. If the primary health care provider discontinues the anticonvulsant therapy, the dosage is gradually withdrawn or another drug is gradually substituted.

To prevent gastric upset, the nurse gives oral anticonvulsants with food or soon after eating. Oral suspensions are shaken well before measuring. If the patient appears drowsy, the nurse must use caution when giving an oral preparation because aspiration of the tablet, capsule, or liquid may occur. The nurse tests the swallowing ability of the patient by offering small sips of water before giving the drug. If the patient has difficulty swallowing, the nurse withholds the drug and notifies the primary health care provider as soon as possible. A different route of administration may be necessary. Injury may occur when the patient has a seizure. The nurse takes precautions to prevent falls and other injuries until seizures are controlled by the drug.

BARBITURATES. The barbiturate phenobarbital (Luminal) is commonly used to treat convulsive disorders. When administering the barbiturates by the intravenous (IV) route, it is important not to exceed a rate of 60 mg/min and to administer the drug within 30 minutes of preparation. The nurse monitors the patient carefully during administration of a barbiturate. The blood pressure and respirations are taken frequently. Resuscitation equipment and artificial ventilation equipment are kept nearby.

BENZODIAZEPINES. The dosage of the benzodiazepines is highly individualized, and the nurse must increase the dosage cautiously to avoid adverse reactions, particularly in elderly and debilitated patients. IV diazepam may bring seizures under control quickly. However, patients may have a return of seizure activity because of the short duration of the effects of the drug. The nurse must be prepared to administer another dose of the drug. The nurse must not mix diazepam with other drugs. When used to control seizures, the drug is administered by IV push. The nurse injects IV diazepam slowly, allowing at least 1 minute for each 5 mg of drug.

HYDANTOINS. Phenytoin is the most commonly prescribed anticonvulsant because of its effectiveness and relatively low toxicity. However, a genetically linked inability to metabolize phenytoin has been identified. For this reason, it is important to monitor serum concentrations of the drug on a regular basis to detect signs of toxicity. Phenytoin is administered orally and parenterally. If the drug is administered parenterally, the IV route is preferred over the intramuscular route because erratic absorption of phenytoin causes pain and muscle damage at the injection site.

OXAZOLIDINEDIONES. The oxazolidinediones are used only when other, less-toxic drugs have not been effective in controlling the seizure disorder because they have been associated with fetal abnormalities and serious adverse reactions.

SUCCINIMIDES. The succinimides are easily absorbed in the gastrointestinal tract and are effective in controlling absence or petit mal seizures. These drugs are given with food to prevent gastrointestinal upset.

MISCELLANEOUS ANTICONVULSANTS. Valproic acid (Depakene) is unrelated chemically to the other anticonvulsants. This drug is absorbed rapidly when taken orally. Tablets should not be chewed but swallowed whole to avoid irritation to the mouth and throat. The capsules may be opened and the drug sprinkled on a small amount of food, such as pudding or applesauce. This mixture must be swallowed whole immediately and not chewed. Zonisamide is administered orally once a day or in divided doses. The dose may be increased by 100 mg/day every 1 to 2 weeks until control of the seizures is obtained or the patient reaches the maximum dosage of 600 mg/d.

The nurse may give lamotrigine without regard to meals. However, it is important to give carbamazepine with meals to decrease gastric upset. The nurse can crush the tablets if the patient has difficulty swallowing. However, it is important not to crush or chew extended-released carbamazepine.

Monitoring and Managing Adverse Reactions

Drowsiness is a common adverse reaction of the anticonvulsant drugs, especially early in therapy. Therefore, the nurse should assist the patient with all ambulatory activities. The nurse helps the patient to arise from the bed slowly and sit for a few minutes before standing. Drowsiness decreases with continued use.

BARBITURATES. The barbiturates can produce a hypersensitivity rash. Should a skin rash occur, the nurse must notify the primary health care provider immediately because the primary health care provider may discontinue the drug. The nurse carefully examines all affected areas and provides an accurate description. If pruritus is present, the nurse keeps the patient's nails short, applies an antiseptic cream (if prescribed), and tells the patient to avoid the use of soap until the rash subsides.

> ❄ **Gerontologic Alert**
>
> *The barbiturates may produce marked excitement, depression, and confusion in the elderly. In some individuals the barbiturates produce excitement, rather than depression. The nurse should monitor the older adult carefully during therapy with the barbiturates and report any unusual effects to the primary health care provider.*

BENZODIAZEPINES. Carbamazepine may cause aplastic anemia and agranulocytosis. During treatment blood studies are performed frequently. If evidence of bone marrow depression is obtained (eg, the patient's platelet count and white blood cell count decrease significantly), the primary health care provider is notified because the drug may be discontinued. The nurse reports any unusual bruising or unusual bleeding, fever, sore throat, rash, or mouth ulcers.

 Gerontologic Alert

Older or debilitated adults may require a reduced dosage of diazepam to reduce ataxia and oversedation. The nurse observes these patients carefully. Apnea and cardiac arrest have occurred when diazepam is administered to older adults, very ill patients, and individuals with limited pulmonary reserve.

HYDANTOINS. The nurse must also be alert for the signs of blood dyscrasias, such as sore throat, fever, general malaise, bleeding of the mucous membranes, epistaxis (bleeding from the nose), and easy bruising. These are serious reactions that the nurse must report to the primary health care provider immediately. Routine laboratory tests, such as complete blood counts and differential counts, should be performed periodically. When a blood dyscrasia is present, the skin and mucous membranes are protected from bleeding and easy bruising by using a soft-bristled toothbrush, and the extremities are protected from trauma or injury.

 Nursing Alert

Phenytoin can cause hematologic changes (eg, aplastic anemia, leukopenia, and thrombocytopenia). The nurse should immediately report any of the following: signs of thrombocytopenia (eg, bleeding gums, easy bruising, increased menstrual bleeding, tarry stools) or leukopenia (eg, sore throat, chills, swollen glands, excessive fatigue, or shortness of breath).

Hypersensitivity reactions and Stevens-Johnson syndrome (a serious, sometimes fatal inflammatory disease) have been reported with the use of phenytoin.

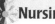 **Nursing Alert**

The nurse informs the primary health care provider immediately if a skin rash occurs. The use of phenytoin is usually discontinued if a skin rash occurs. If the rash is exfoliative (red rash with scaling of the skin), purpuric (small hemorrhages or bruising on the skin), or bullous (skin vesicle filled with fluid, ie, blister) use of the drug is not resumed. If the rash is milder (eg, measles-like), therapy may be resumed after the rash has completely disappeared.

The hydantoins may affect the blood glucose levels. In some patients these drugs have an inhibitory effect on the release of insulin in the body, causing hyperglycemia. The nurse closely monitors blood glucose levels, particularly in patients with diabetes. The nurse reports any abnormalities to the primary health care provider.

Long-term administration of the hydantoins can cause gingivitis and gingival hyperplasia (overgrowth of gum tissue). It is important to periodically inspect the teeth and gums of patients in a hospital or long-term clinical setting who are receiving one of these drugs. The nurse reports any changes in the gums or teeth to the primary health care provider. It is important that oral care be given after each meal and that the mouth and gums be inspected routinely.

The nurse monitors vital signs every 4 hours or as ordered. Any adverse drug reactions or signs of toxicity are reported to the primary health care provider immediately.

 Nursing Alert

When administering phenytoin, the nurse closely monitors the patient for the following signs of drug toxicity: slurred speech, ataxia, lethargy, dizziness, nausea, and vomiting. Phenytoin plasma levels between 10 and 20 mcg/mL give optimal anticonvulsant effect. However, many patients achieve seizure control at lower serum concentration levels. Levels greater than 20 mcg/mL are associated with toxicity. Patients with plasma levels greater than 20 mcg/mL may exhibit nystagmus, and at concentrations greater than 30 mcg/mL, ataxia and mental changes are usually seen.

OXAZOLIDINEDIONES. Drowsiness is the most common adverse reaction and, as with the other anticonvulsants, tends to subside with continued use. Visual disturbances may also occur. The patient with a visual disturbance is assisted with ambulation and oriented carefully to the environment. The nurse ensures that the environment is safe. The patient may be especially sensitive to bright lights and may want the room light to be kept dim. Because photosensitivity can occur, the nurse must keep the patient out of the sun. The nurse instructs the patient to use sunscreens and protective clothing until the individual effects of the drug are known.

SUCCINIMIDES. The succinimides are particularly toxic. The nurse must be alert for signs of blood dyscrasias, such as the presence of fever, sore throat, and general malaise. The nurse reports any of these symptoms immediately because fatal blood dyscrasias have occurred. Routine blood tests may be performed, such as complete blood counts and differential counts.

MISCELLANEOUS ANTICONVULSANTS. A severe and potentially fatal rash can occur in patients taking lamotrigine. The nurse must immediately report any rash in

Nursing Alert

The nurse must report symptoms of succinimide overdosage immediately. Symptoms of overdosage include confusion, sleepiness, unsteadiness, flaccid muscles, slow shallow respirations, nausea, vomiting, hypotension, absent reflexes, and CNS depression leading to coma. It is important to report symptoms to the primary health care provider immediately. Therapeutic serum blood levels of ethosuximide (Zarontin) range from 40 to 100 mcg/mL.

a patient taking lamotrigine to the primary health care provider before the next dose is due. Discontinuation of the drug may be required.

Educating the Patient and Family

When the patient receives a diagnosis of epilepsy, the nurse must assist the patient and the family to adjust to the diagnosis. The nurse should instruct family members in the care of the patient before, during, and after a seizure. The nurse explains the importance of restricting some activities until the seizures are controlled by drugs. Restriction of activities often depend on the age, sex, and occupation of the patient. For example, the nurse should advise a mother with a seizure disorder who has a newborn infant to have help when caring for her child. The nurse also would warn a carpenter about climbing ladders or using power tools. For some patients, the restriction of activities may create problems with such things as employment, management of the home environment, or child care. If a problem is recognized, a referral may be needed to a social worker, discharge planning coordinator, or public health nurse.

The nurse reviews adverse drug reactions associated with the prescribed anticonvulsant with the patient and family members. The patient and family members are instructed to contact the primary health care provider if any adverse reactions occur before the next dose of the drug is due. The patient must not stop taking the drug until the problem is discussed with the primary health care provider.

Some patients, once their seizures are under control (eg, stop occurring or occur less frequently), may have a tendency to stop the drug abruptly or begin to omit a dose occasionally. The drug must never be abruptly discontinued or doses omitted. If the patient experiences drowsiness during initial therapy, a family member should be responsible for administration of the drug.

The nurse should include the following points in a patient and family teaching plan.

- Do not omit, increase, or decrease the prescribed dose.
- Anticonvulsant blood levels must be monitored at regular intervals, even if the seizures are well controlled.

- This drug should never be abruptly discontinued, except when recommended by the primary health care provider.
- If the primary health care provider finds it necessary to stop the drug, another drug usually is prescribed. Start taking this drug immediately (at the time the next dose of the previously used drug was due).
- These drugs may cause drowsiness or dizziness. Observe caution when performing hazardous tasks. Do not drive unless the adverse reactions of drowsiness, dizziness, or blurred vision are not significant. Driving privileges will be given by the primary health care provider based on seizure control.
- Avoid the use of alcohol unless use has been approved by the primary health care provider.
- Carry identification, such as a Medic-Alert tag, indicating drug use and the type of seizure disorder.
- Do not use any nonprescription drug unless use of a specific drug has been approved by the primary health care provider.
- Keep a record of all seizures (date, time, length), as well as any minor problems (eg, drowsiness, dizziness, lethargy), and bring this information to each clinic or office visit.
- Contact the local branches of agencies, such as the Epilepsy Foundation of America, for information and assistance with problems such as legal matters, insurance, driver's license, low-cost prescription services, and job training or retraining.

HYDANTOINS

- Inform the dentist and other primary health care providers of use of this drug.
- Brush and floss the teeth after each meal and make periodic dental appointments for oral examination and care.
- Take the medication with food to reduce gastrointestinal upset.
- Phenytoin suspension must be thoroughly shaken immediately before use.
- Do not use when capsules are discolored.
- Notify the primary health care provider if any of the following occurs: skin rash, bleeding, swollen or tender gums, yellowish discoloration of the skin or eyes, unexplained fever, sore throat, unusual bleeding or bruising, persistent headache, malaise, or pregnancy.

SUCCINIMIDES

- If gastrointestinal upsets occurs, take the drug with food or milk.
- Phensuximide may discolor the urine pink, red, or redbrown. This is not abnormal and will cause no harm.
- Notify the primary health care provider if any of the following occurs: skin rash, joint pain, unexplained fever, sore throat, usual bleeding or bruising, drowsiness, dizziness, blurred vision, or pregnancy.

OXAZOLIDINEDIONES

- This drug may cause photosensitivity. Take protective measures (eg, use sunscreens, wear protective clothing) when exposed to ultraviolet light or sunlight until tolerance is determined.
- Notify the primary care provider if the following reactions occur: visual disturbances, excessive drowsiness or dizziness, sore throat, fever, skin rash, pregnancy, malaise, easy bruising, epistaxis, or bleeding tendencies.
- Avoid pregnancy while taking trimethadione; the drug has caused serious birth defects.

EVALUATION

- The therapeutic effect is achieved, and convulsions are controlled.
- No evidence of injury is seen.
- Adverse reactions are identified, reported to the primary health care provider, and managed successfully through appropriate nursing interventions.
- Oral mucous membranes appear normal.
- The patient verbalizes the importance of complying with the prescribed treatment regimen.
- The patient verbalizes an understanding of treatment modalities and the importance of continued follow-up care.
- The patient and family demonstrate an understanding of the drug regimen.

● *Critical Thinking Exercises*

1. *Ms. Taylor tells you that since she has been taking phenytoin she has had no seizures. In fact, she states that she has omitted one or two doses over the last month because she is "doing so well." Explain your response to Ms. Taylor's statement.*
2. *Mr. Parks, age 32 years, has recently received a diagnosis of epilepsy. He has been taking the anticonvulsant carbamazepine, but his seizures are not yet under control. Mr. Parks asks you how long it will take to "cure" his epilepsy. Determine how you would respond to Mr. Parks.*
3. *Develop a teaching plan educating the family members on what to do when the patient has a seizure.*

● *Review Questions*

1. A patient is prescribed phenytoin for a recurrent convulsive disorder. The nurse informs the patient that the most common adverse reactions are _____.
   A. related to the gastrointestinal system
   B. associated with the reproductive system
   C. associated with kidney function
   D. related to the CNS

2. Which of the following adverse reactions, if observed in a patient prescribed phenytoin, would indicate that the patient may be developing phenytoin toxicity?
   A. severe occipital headache
   B. ataxia
   C. hyperactivity
   D. somnolence

3. When administering phenobarbital to an elderly patient the nurse should monitor the patient for unusual effects of the drug such as _____.
   A. marked excitement
   B. excessive sweating
   C. insomnia
   D. agitation

4. When caring for a patient taking a succinimide for absent seizures, the nurse monitors the patient for blood dyscrasias. Which of the following symptoms would indicate that the patient may be developing a blood dyscrasia?
   A. constipation, blood in the stool
   B. diarrhea, lethargy
   C. sore throat, general malaise
   D. hyperthermia, excitement

5. Which statement would be included when educating the patient taking trimethadione for absence seizures?
   A. Take this drug with milk to enhance absorption.
   B. Wear a sunscreen and protective clothing when exposed to sunlight.
   C. To minimize adverse reactions, take this drug once daily at bedtime.
   D. Visit a dentist frequently because this drug increases the risk of gum disease.

● *Medication Dosage Problems*

1. The nurse is preparing to administer an anticonvulsant for status epilepticus. The primary care provider prescribes Luminal 200 mg IV. The drug is available in a dosage of 60 mg/mL. The nurse administers _____.

2. Zonisamide 200 mg is prescribed. The drug is available in 100-mg tablets. The nurse administers _____.

3. The primary care provider prescribes ethosuximide syrup 500 mg for a patient with absence seizures. The drug is available in a strength of 250 mg/5 mL. The nurse administers _____.

Antiparkinsonism Drugs

Key Terms

blood–brain barrier
choreiform
  movements
dystonic movements

on-off phenomenon
Parkinson's disease
parkinsonism

Chapter Objectives

On completion of this chapter, the student will:

- Define the terms *Parkinson's disease* and *parkinsonism.*
- Discuss the uses, general drug action, adverse drug reactions, contraindications, precautions, and interactions of the antiparkinsonism drugs.
- Discuss important preadministration and ongoing assessment activities the nurse should perform on the patient taking antiparkinsonism drugs.
- List some nursing diagnoses particular to a patient taking antiparkinsonism drugs.
- Discuss ways to promote an optimal response to therapy, how to manage adverse reactions, and important points to keep in mind when educating patients about the use of the antiparkinsonism drugs.

Parkinson's disease, also called paralysis agitans, is a degenerative disorder of the central nervous system (CNS). The disease is thought to be caused by a deficiency of dopamine and an excess of acetylcholine within the CNS. Parkinson's disease affects the part of the brain that controls muscle movement, causing such symptoms as trembling, rigidity, difficulty walking, and problems in balance. It is characterized by fine tremors and rigidity of some muscle groups and weakness of others. Parkinson's disease is progressive, that is the symptoms become worse over time. As the disease progresses, speech becomes slurred, the face has a masklike and emotionless expression, and the patient may have difficulty chewing and swallowing. The patient may have a shuffling and unsteady gait, and the upper part of the body is bent forward. Fine tremors begin in the fingers with a pill-rolling movement, increase with stress, and decrease with purposeful movement. Depression or dementia may occur, causing memory impairment and alterations in thinking.

Parkinson's disease has no cure, but the antiparkinsonism drugs are used to relieve the symptoms and assist in maintaining the patient's mobility and functioning capability as long as possible. For years, levodopa was the drug that provided the mainstay of treatment. Now, there are new drugs that are used either alone or in combination with levodopa. Entacapone (Comtan), pramipexole

(Mirapex), and ropinirole (Requip) are newer drugs used in the treatment of Parkinson's disease. Drug-induced parkinsonism is treated with the anticholinergics benztropine (Cogentin) and trihexyphenidyl (Artane).

Parkinsonism is a term that refers to the symptoms of Parkinson's disease, as well as the Parkinson-like symptoms that may be seen with the use of certain drugs, head injuries, and encephalitis. Drugs used to treat the symptoms associated with parkinsonism are called antiparkinsonism drugs. As with some other types of drugs, it may be necessary to change from one antiparkinsonism drug to another or to increase or decrease the dosage until maximum response is obtained. The Summary Drug Table: Antiparkinsonism Drugs provides a listing of the drugs used to treat Parkinson's disease. Antiparkinsonism drugs discussed in the chapter are classified as dopaminergic agents, anticholinergic drugs, COMT inhibitors, and dopamine receptor agonists (non-ergot).

DOPAMINERGIC DRUGS

Dopaminergic drugs are drugs that affect the dopamine content of the brain. These drugs include levodopa (Larodopa), carbidopa (Ladosyn), amantadine (Symmetrel), and pergolide mesylate (Permax). (See Summary Drug Table: Antiparkinsonism Drugs).

ACTIONS

The symptoms of parkinsonism are caused by a depletion of dopamine in the CNS. Dopamine, when given orally, does not cross the blood–brain barrier and therefore is ineffective. The body's **blood–brain barrier** is a meshwork of tightly packed cells in the walls of the brain's capillaries that screen out certain substances. This unique meshwork of cells in the CNS prohibits large and potentially harmful molecules from crossing into the brain. This ability to screen out certain substances has important implications for drug therapy because some drugs are able to pass through the blood–brain barrier more easily than others.

Levodopa is a chemical formulation found in plants and animals that is converted into dopamine by nerve cells in the brain. Levodopa does cross the blood–brain barrier, and a small amount is then converted to dopamine. This allows the drug to have a pharmacologic effect in patients with Parkinson's disease (Fig. 29-1). Combining levodopa with another drug (carbidopa) causes more levodopa to reach the brain. When more levodopa is available, the dosage of levodopa may be reduced. Carbidopa has no effect when given alone. Sinemet is a combination of carbidopa and levodopa and is available in several combinations (eg, Sinemet 10/100 has 10 mg of carbidopa and 100 mg of levodopa; Sinemet CR is a time-released version of the combined drugs).

The mechanism of action of amantadine (Symmetrel) and selegiline (Eldepryl) in the treatment of parkinsonism is not fully understood.

USES

The dopaminergic drugs are used to treat the signs and symptoms of parkinsonism. As with some other types of drugs, it may be necessary to change from one antiparkinsonism drug to another or to increase or decrease the dosage until maximum response is obtained.

Levodopa has been considered the gold standard drug therapy for Parkinson's disease since it was first used in the 1960s. Carbidopa is always given with levodopa, combined either as one drug or as two separate drugs. When it is necessary to titrate the dose of carbidopa, both carbidopa and levodopa may be given at the same time, but as separate drugs. Sometimes the response with these two drugs can be enhanced by the addition of another drug. For example, selegiline or pergolide may be added to the drug regimen of those being treated with carbidopa and levodopa but who

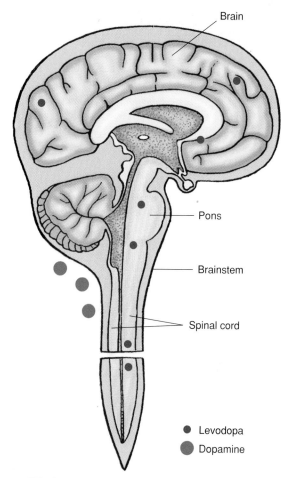

FIGURE 29–1. The blood–brain barrier selectively inhibits certain substances from entering the interstitial spaces of the brain and spinal fluid. It is thought that certain cells within the brain form tight junctions that prevent or slow the passage of certain substances. Levodopa passes the blood–brain barrier, whereas dopamine is unable to pass.

have had a decreased response to therapy with these two drugs.

Amantadine is less effective than levodopa in the treatment of Parkinson's disease but more effective than the anticholinergics. Amantadine may be given alone or in combination with an antiparkinsonism drug with anticholinergic activity. Amantadine is also used as an antiviral drug (see Chap. 14).

ADVERSE REACTIONS

During early treatment with levodopa and carbidopa, adverse reactions are usually not a problem. But as the disease progresses, the response to the drug may become less, and the period of time that each dose is effective begins to decrease, leading to more frequent doses, and more adverse reactions.

The most serious and frequent adverse reactions seen with levodopa include **choreiform movements**

SUMMARY DRUG TABLE ANTIPARKINSONISM DRUGS

GENERIC NAME	TRADE NAME*	USES	ADVERSE REACTIONS	DOSAGE RANGES
Dopaminergic Agents				
amantadine *a-man´-ta-deen*	Symmetrel, *generic*	Parkinson's disease/ drug-induced extrapyramidal reactions, prevention and treatment of influenza A virus	Light-headedness, dizziness, insomnia, confusion, nausea, constipation, dry mouth, orthostatic hypotension, depression	100–400 mg/d PO in divided doses
bromocriptine *broe-moe-krip´-tine*	Parlodel, Parlodel Snap Tabs	Parkinson's disease	Drowsiness, sedation, dizziness, faintness, epigastric distress, anorexia	1.25–100 mg/d PO
carbidopa *kar´-bi-doe-pa*	Lodosyn	Used with levodopa in the treatment of Parkinson's disease	None when given alone; when administered with levodopa, adverse reactions of levodopa	Up to 200 mg/d PO
carbidopa/ levodopa *kar´-bi-doe-pa/* *lee´-voe-doe-pa*	Sinemet CR, Sinemet 10/100, Sinemet 25/100, Sinemet 25/250, *generic*	Parkinson's disease	Same as levodopa	Dosages individualized to obtain therapeutic effect; average dose is 1 tablet PO TID
levodopa *lee´-voe-doe-pa*	Dopar, Larodopa, *generic*	Parkinson's disease	Choreiform or dystonic movements, anorexia, nausea, vomiting, abdominal pain, dysphagia, dry mouth, mental changes, headache, dizziness, increased hand tremor	0.5–8 g/d
pergolide *per´-goe-lide*	Permax	As adjunct to levodopa/carbidopa in Parkinson's disease	Nausea, dyskinesia, dizziness, hallucinations, somnolence, insomnia, peripheral edema, constipation	0.05–3 mg/d PO TID
selegiline *sell-eh´-geh-leen*	Carbex, Eldepryl, *generic*	As adjunct to levodopa/carbidopa in Parkinson's disease	Nausea, hallucinations, confusion, depression, loss of balance, dizziness, nausea	10 mg/d PO in divided doses
Anticholinergic Agents				
benztropine mesylate *benz´-tro-peen*	Cogentin, *generic*	Adjunct therapy in Parkinson's disease	Dry mouth, blurred vision, dizziness, nausea, nervousness, skin rash, urinary retention, dysuria, tachycardia, muscle weakness, disorientation, confusion	0.5–6 mg/d PO, IM, IV
biperiden *by-per´-i-den*	Akineton	Adjunct therapy in Parkinson's disease	Same as benztropine mesylate	2 mg PO 3–4 times/d; maximum dose, 16 mg/24h; 2 mg IM or IV
diphenhydramine *dye-fen-hye´-dra-* *meen*	Benadryl, *generic*	Drug-induced extrapyramidal reactions in Parkinson's disease, allergies	Same as benztropine mesylate	25–50 mg PO q4–6h; 10–400 mg IM, IV
procyclidine *pro-sye´-kli-deen*	Kemadrin	Parkinson's disease	Same as benztropine mesylate	2.5–5 mg PO TID
trihexyphenidyl *trye-hex-ee-fen´-i-dill*	Artane, Trihexy-2, *generic*	Adjunct in the treatment of Parkinson's disease	Same as benztropine mesylate	1–15 mg/d PO in divided doses

SUMMARY DRUG TABLE ANTIPARKINSONISM DRUGS (*Continued*)

GENERIC NAME	TRADE NAME*	USES	ADVERSE REACTIONS	DOSAGE RANGES
COMT Inhibitors				
entacapone *en-tah-kap´-own*	Comtan	As adjunct to levodopa/carbidopa in Parkinson's disease	Orthostatic hypotension, dyskinesia, sleep disorders, dystonia, excessive dreaming, somnolence, confusion, dizziness, nausea, anorexia, diarrhea, muscle cramps	200–1600 mg/d PO
tolcapone *toll-kap´-own*	Tasmar	As adjunct to levodopa/carbidopa in Parkinson's disease	Orthostatic hypotension, dyskinesia, sleep disorders, dystonia, excessive dreaming, somnolence, confusion, dizziness, nausea, anorexia, diarrhea, muscle cramps	100–200 mg PO TID
Dopamine Receptor Agonists, Non-Ergot				
pramipexole *pram-ah-pex´-ole*	Mirapex	Parkinson's disease	Dizziness, somnolence, insomnia, hallucinations, confusion, nausea, dyspepsia, syncope	0.125–1.5 mg PO TID
ropinirole HCL *roe-pin´-o-role*	Requip	Parkinson's disease	Dizziness, somnolence, insomnia, hallucinations, confusion, nausea, dyspepsia, syncope	0.25–1 mg PO TID; maximum dose, 24 mg/d

* The term *generic* indicates the drug is available in generic form.

(involuntary muscular twitching of the limbs or facial muscles) and **dystonic movements** (muscular spasms most often affecting the tongue, jaw, eyes, and neck). Less common but serious reactions include mental changes, such as depression, psychotic episodes, paranoia, and suicidal tendencies. Common and less serious adverse reactions include anorexia, nausea, vomiting, abdominal pain, dry mouth, difficulty in swallowing, increased hand tremor, headache, and dizziness. Carbidopa is used with levodopa and has no effect when given alone.

The most common serious adverse reactions to amantadine are orthostatic hypotension, depression, congestive heart failure, psychosis, urinary retention, convulsions, leukopenia, and neutropenia. Less serious reactions include hallucinations, confusion, anxiety, anorexia, nausea, and constipation. Adverse reactions with selegiline include nausea, hallucinations, confusion, depression, loss of balance, and dizziness.

CONTRAINDICATIONS, PRECAUTIONS, AND INTERACTIONS

The dopaminergic drugs are contraindicated in patients with known hypersensitivity to the drugs. Levodopa is contraindicated in patients with narrow-angle glaucoma, those receiving a monoamine oxidase inhibitor (see Chap. 31), and during lactation. Levodopa is used cautiously in patients with cardiovascular disease, bronchial asthma, emphysema, peptic ulcer disease, renal or hepatic disease, and psychosis. Levodopa and combination antiparkinsonism drugs (eg, carbidopa/levodopa) are classified as Pregnancy Category C and are used with caution during pregnancy and lactation.

Levodopa interacts with many different drugs. When levodopa is used with phenytoin, reserpine, and papaverine, there is a decrease in response to levodopa. The risk of a hypertensive crisis increases when levodopa is used with the monoamine oxidase inhibitors (see Chap. 31). Foods high in pyridoxine (vitamin B_6) or vitamin B_6 preparations reverse the effect of levodopa. However, when carbidopa is used with levodopa, pyridoxine has no effect on the action of levodopa. In fact, when levodopa and carbidopa are given together, pyridoxine may be prescribed to decrease the adverse effects associated with levodopa.

Selegiline is used cautiously in patients with psychosis, dementia, or excessive tremor. When selegiline is administered with levodopa, the effectiveness of levodopa increases. This effect allows for a decrease in the dosage of levodopa. If selegiline is given in doses greater than 10 mg/d there is an increased risk of hypertension, particularly if tyramine-containing foods (eg, beer, wine, aged cheese, yeast products, chicken livers, and pickled herring) are ingested. A potentially serious reaction (confusion, agitation, hypertension, and seizures) can occur when fluoxetine is administered with selegiline. Fluoxetine therapy is discontinued for a least 1 week before treatment with selegiline is initiated.

Amantadine is used cautiously in patients with seizure disorders, hepatic disease, psychosis, cardiac disease, and renal disease. The antihistamines, phenothiazines, disopyramide, and alcohol increase the risk of adverse reactions when administered with amantadine.

ANTICHOLINERGIC DRUGS

ACTIONS

Drugs with anticholinergic activity inhibit acetylcholine (a neurohormone produced in excess in Parkinson's disease) in the CNS. Drugs with anticholinergic activity are generally less effective than levodopa.

USES

Drugs with anticholinergic activity are used as adjunctive therapy in all forms of parkinsonism and in the control of drug-induced extrapyramidal disorders. Examples of drugs with anticholinergic activity include benztropine mesylate (Cogentin), biperiden (Akineton), diphenhydramine, procyclidine (Kemadrin), and trihexyphenidyl (Artane). See Summary Drug Table: Antiparkinsonism Drugs for specific uses of these drugs.

ADVERSE REACTIONS

Frequently seen adverse reactions to drugs with anticholinergic activity include dry mouth, blurred vision, dizziness, mild nausea, and nervousness. These may become less pronounced as therapy progresses. Other adverse reactions may include skin rash, urticaria (hives), urinary retention, dysuria, tachycardia, muscle weakness, disorientation, and confusion. If any of these reactions are severe, the drug may be discontinued for several days and restarted at a lower dosage, or a different antiparkinsonism drug may be prescribed.

CONTRAINDICATIONS, PRECAUTIONS, AND INTERACTIONS

These drugs are contraindicated in those with a hypersensitivity to the anticholinergic drugs, those with glaucoma (angle-closure), pyloric or duodenal obstruction, peptic ulcers, prostatic hypertrophy, achalasia (failure of

the muscles of the lower esophagus to relax causing difficulty swallowing), myasthenia gravis, and megacolon.

These drugs are used with caution in patients with tachycardia, cardiac arrhythmias, hypertension, hypotension, those with a tendency toward urinary retention, those with decreased liver or kidney function, and those with obstructive disease of the urinary system or gastrointestinal tract. The anticholinergic drugs are given with caution to the older adult.

> ### ❄ Gerontologic Alert
>
> Individuals older than 60 years frequently develop increased sensitivity to anticholinergic drugs and require careful monitoring. Confusion and disorientation may occur. Lower doses may be required.

When the anticholinergic drugs are administered with amantadine, there is an increased anticholinergic effect. When digoxin is administered with an anticholinergic drug, digoxin blood levels may be increased, leading to an increased risk for digitalis toxicity. Haloperidol and anticholinergic co-administration may result in worsening of schizophrenic symptoms, decreased haloperidol blood levels, and development of tardive dyskinesia (see Chap. 32). When the anticholinergic drugs are administered with the phenothiazines, there is a decrease in the therapeutic effects of the phenothiazines and an increase in anticholinergic adverse reactions.

COMT INHIBITORS

A newer classification of antiparkinson drugs is the catechol-O-methyltransferase (COMT) inhibitors. Examples of the COMT inhibitors are entacapone (Comtan) and tolcapone (Tasmar).

ACTIONS

These drugs are thought to prolong the effect of levodopa by blocking an enzyme, catechol-O-methyltransferase (COMT), which eliminates dopamine. When given with levodopa, the COMT inhibitors increase the plasma concentrations and duration of action of levodopa.

USES

The COMT inhibitors are used as adjuncts to levodopa/carbidopa in Parkinson's disease. Tolcapone is a potent COMT inhibitor that easily crosses the blood–brain barrier. However, the drug is associated with liver damage and liver failure. Because of the danger to the liver, tolcapone is reserved for people who are not responding to other therapies. Entacapone is a milder COMT inhibitor and is used to help manage fluctuations in the response to levodopa in individuals with Parkinson's disease.

ADVERSE REACTIONS

The adverse reactions most often associated with the administration of the COMT inhibitors include disorientation, confusion, light-headedness, dizziness, dyskinesias, hyperkinesias, nausea, vomiting, hallucinations, and fever. Other adverse reactions are orthostatic hypotension, sleep disorders, excessive dreaming, somnolence, and muscle cramps. A serious and possibly fatal adverse reaction that can occur with the administration of tolcapone is liver failure.

CONTRAINDICATIONS, PRECAUTIONS, AND INTERACTIONS

These drugs are contraindicated in patients with a hypersensitivity to the drugs and during pregnancy (Category C) and lactation. Tolcapone is contraindicated in patients with liver dysfunction. The COMT inhibitors are used with caution in patients with hypertension, hypotension, and decreased hepatic or renal function.

The COMT inhibitors should not be administered with the monoamine oxidase (MAO) inhibitors (see Chap. 31) because there is an increased risk of toxicity. If the COMT inhibitors are administered with norepinephrine, dopamine, dobutamine, methyldopa, or epinephrine, there is a risk of increased heart rate, arrhythmias, and excessive blood pressure changes.

DOPAMINE RECEPTOR AGONISTS (NON-ERGOT)

ACTIONS

The exact mechanism of action of these drugs is not understood. It is thought that these drugs act directly on postsynaptic dopamine receptors of nerve cells in the brain, mimicking the effects of dopamine in the brain.

USES

The dopamine receptor agonists, such as pramipexole (Mirapex) and ropinirole (Requip), are used for the treatment of the signs and symptoms of Parkinson's disease.

ADVERSE REACTIONS

The most common adverse reactions seen with pramipexole and ropinirole include nausea, dizziness, postural hypotension, hallucinations, somnolence, vomiting, confusion, visual disturbances, abnormal involuntary movements, and headache.

CONTRAINDICATIONS, PRECAUTIONS, AND INTERACTIONS

The dopamine receptor agonists are contraindicated in patients with known hypersensitivity to the drugs, severe ischemic heart disease, or peripheral vascular disease. The dopamine receptor agonists are used with caution in patients with dyskinesia, orthostatic hypotension, and hepatic or renal impairment. The dopamine receptor agonists are used cautiously in patients with a history of hallucinations or psychosis, cardiovascular disease, and renal impairment. Both ropinirole and pramipexole are Pregnancy Category C drugs, and safety during pregnancy has not been established.

There is an increased risk of CNS depression when the dopamine receptor agonists are administered with other CNS depressants. When administered with levodopa, the dopamine receptor agonists increase the effects of levodopa (a lower dosage of levodopa may be required). In addition, when the dopamine receptor agonists are administered with levodopa, there is an increased risk of hallucinations. When administered with ciprofloxacin, there is an increased effect of the dopamine receptor agonist.

The phenothiazines may decrease the effectiveness of the dopamine receptor agonists. When pramipexole is administered concurrently with cimetidine, ranitidine, verapamil, and quinidine, there is an increased effect of pramipexole. When ropinirole is administered with the estrogens, particularly estradiol, there may be an increased effect of ropinirole.

NURSING PROCESS

● **The Patient Receiving an Antiparkinsonism Drug**

ASSESSMENT

Preadministration Assessment
Because of memory impairment and alterations in thinking in some patients with parkinsonism, a history obtained from the patient may be unreliable. When necessary, the nurse obtains the health history from a family member. Important data to include is information regarding the symptoms of the disorder, the length of

time the symptoms have been present, the ability of the patient to carry on activities of daily living, and the patient's current mental condition (eg, impairment in memory, signs of depression, or withdrawal).

Before starting the drug therapy, the nurse performs a physical assessment of the patient to provide a baseline for future evaluations of drug therapy. It also is important to include an evaluation of the patient's neurologic status. Display 29-1 describes the assessments the nurse would make when evaluating the neurological status.

Ongoing Assessment

The nurse evaluates the patient's response to drug therapy by neurologic observations (see Display 29-1) and compares these observations with the data obtained during the initial physical assessment. For example, the patient is assessed for clinical improvement of the symptoms of the disease, such as improvement of tremor of head and/or hands at rest, muscular rigidity, mask-like facial expression, and ambulation stability. Although drug response may occur slowly in some patients, these observations aid the primary health care provider in adjusting the dosage of the drug upward or downward to obtain the desired therapeutic results.

NURSING DIAGNOSES

Drug-specific nursing diagnoses are highlighted in the Nursing Diagnoses Checklist. Other nursing diagnoses applicable to these drugs are discussed in depth in Chapter 4.

PLANNING

The expected outcomes for the patient may include an optimal response to drug therapy, management of common adverse drug reactions, absence of injury, and an understanding of and compliance with the prescribed therapeutic regimen.

Nursing Diagnoses Checklist

☑ **Imbalanced Nutrition: Less than Body Requirements** related to adverse drug effects (nausea, vomiting)

☑ **Risk for Injury** related to parkinsonism, adverse drug reactions (dizziness, light-headedness, orthostatic hypotension, loss of balance)

☑ **Impaired Physical Mobility** related to alterations in balance, unsteady gait, dizziness

☑ **Imbalanced Nutrition: Less than Body Requirements** related to adverse drug effects (nausea, vomiting)

☑ **Constipation** related to adverse drug reactions

IMPLEMENTATION

Promoting an Optimal Response to Therapy

Effective management of the patient with parkinsonism requires that the nurse carefully monitor the drug therapy, provide psychological support, and place a strong emphasis on patient and family teaching.

The drugs used to treat parkinsonism also may be used to treat the symptoms of parkinsonism that occur with the administration of some of the psychotherapeutic drugs (see Chap. 32). When used for this purpose, the antiparkinsonism drugs may exacerbate mental symptoms and precipitate a psychosis. The nurse must observe the patient's behavior at frequent intervals. If sudden behavioral changes are noted, the nurse withholds the next dose of the drug and immediately notifies the primary health care provider.

Monitoring and Managing Adverse Drug Reactions

The nurse observes the patient daily for the development of adverse reactions. All adverse reactions are reported to the primary health care provider because a dosage adjustment or change to a different antiparkinsonism drug may be necessary with the occurrence of the more serious adverse reactions.

✳ Nursing Alert

The nurse observes patients receiving levodopa or carbidopa and levodopa for the occurrence of choreiform and dystonic movements, such as facial grimacing, protruding tongue, exaggerated chewing motions and head movements, and jerking movements of the arms and legs. If these occur, the nurse should withhold the next dose of the drug and notify the primary health care provider because it may be necessary to reduce the dosage of levodopa or discontinue use of the drug.

Some adverse reactions, although not serious, may be uncomfortable. An example of a less serious but uncomfortable adverse reaction is dryness of the mouth. The nurse can help relieve dry mouth by offering frequent

---

DISPLAY 29-1 ● Neurologic Evaluation

The neurologic evaluation includes observation for the following:
- Tremors of the hands or head while the patient is at rest
- A masklike facial expression
- Changes (from the normal) in walking
- Type of speech pattern (halting, monotone)
- Postural deformities
- Muscular rigidity
- Drooling, difficulty in chewing or swallowing
- Changes in thought processes
- Ability of the patient to carry out any or all of the activities of daily living (eg, bathing, ambulating, dressing)

sips of water, ice chips, or hard candy (if allowed). If dry mouth is so severe that there is difficulty in swallowing or speaking, or if loss of appetite and weight loss occurs, the dosage of the antiparkinsonism drug may be reduced.

> ### ❋ Nursing Alert
>
> *A serious and potentially fatal adverse reaction to tolcapone is hepatic injury. Regular blood testing to monitor liver function is usually prescribed. The physician may order testing of serum transaminase levels at frequent intervals (eg, every 2 weeks for the first year and every 8 weeks thereafter). Treatment is discontinued if the ALT (SGPT) exceeds the upper normal limit or signs or symptoms of liver failure develop. The patient is observed for persistent nausea, fatigue, lethargy, anorexia, jaundice, dark urine, pruritus, and right upper quadrant tenderness.*

Some patients with parkinsonism communicate poorly and do not tell the primary health care provider or nurse that problems are occurring. The nurse observes the patient with parkinsonism for outward changes that may indicate one or more adverse reactions. For example, a sudden change in the facial expression or changes in posture may indicate abdominal pain or discomfort, which may be caused by urinary retention, paralytic ileus, or constipation. Sudden changes in behavior may indicate hallucinations, depression, or other psychotic episodes.

> ### ❄ Gerontologic Alert
>
> *Hallucinations occur more often in the older adult than in the younger adult receiving the antiparkinsonism drugs, especially when taking the dopamine receptor agonists. The nurse should assess the older adult for signs of visual, auditory, or tactile hallucinations. The incidence of hallucinations appears to increase with age.*

Visual difficulties (eg, adverse reactions of blurred vision and diplopia) may be evidenced by the patient's sudden refusal to read or watch television or by the patient bumping into objects when ambulating. The nurse carefully evaluates any sudden changes in the patient's behavior or activity and reports them to the primary health care provider. The patient with visual difficulties may need assistance with ambulation. The room should be kept well lighted, the use of scatter or throw rugs should be avoided, and any small pieces of furniture or objects that might increase the risk of falling should be removed. The nurse carefully assesses the environment and makes the necessary adjustments to ensure the patient's safety.

Some patients taking the antiparkinsonism drugs experience gastrointestinal disturbances such as nausea, vomiting, or constipation. This can affect the patient's nutritional status. It is a good idea for the nurse to create a calm environment, serve small frequent meals, and serve foods the patient prefers to help improve nutrition. The nurse also may monitor the patient's weight daily. Gastrointestinal disturbances are sometimes helped by taking the drug with meals. Severe nausea or vomiting may necessitate discontinuing the drug and changing to a different antiparkinsonism drug. With continued use of the drug, nausea usually decreases or is resolved. If constipation is a problem, the nurse stresses the need for a diet high in fiber and increasing fluids in the diet. A stool softener may be needed to help prevent constipation.

Minimizing the risk for injury is an important aspect in the care of the patient with parkinsonism. These patients may have difficulty ambulating. Adverse reactions, such as dizziness, muscle weakness, and ataxia (lack of muscular coordination) may further increase difficulty with ambulatory activities. These individuals are especially prone to falls and other accidents because of their disease process and possible adverse drug reactions. The nurse assists the patient in getting out of the bed or a chair, walking, and other self-care activities. In addition, assistive devices such as a cane or walker may be helpful with ambulation. The nurse may suggest that the patient wear shoes with rubber soles to minimize the possibility of slipping. Patients are prone to orthostatic hypotension as a result of the drug regimen. These patients are instructed to arise slowly from a sitting or lying position, especially after sitting or lying for a prolonged time.

The **on-off phenomenon** may occur in patients taking levodopa. In this condition, the patient may suddenly alternate between improved clinical status and loss of therapeutic effect. This effect is associated with long-term levodopa treatment. Low doses of the drug, reserving the drug for severe cases, or the use of a "drug holiday" may be prescribed. Should symptoms occur, the primary health care provider may order a drug holiday that includes complete withdrawal of levodopa for 5 to 14 days, followed by gradually restarting use of the drug at a lower dose.

> ### ❋ Nursing Alert
>
> *Do not abruptly discontinue use of the antiparkinsonism drugs. Neuroleptic malignant-like syndrome may occur when the antiparkinsonism drugs are discontinued or the dosage of levodopa is reduced abruptly. The nurse carefully observes the patient and reports the following symptoms: muscular rigidity, elevated body temperature, and mental changes.*

Educating the Patient and Family

The nurse evaluates the patient's ability to understand the therapeutic drug regimen, ability to care for himself or herself in the home environment, and ability to comply with the prescribed drug therapy. If any type of assistance is needed, the nurse provides a referral to the discharge planning coordinator or social worker.

If the patient requires supervision or help with daily activities and the drug regimen, the nurse encourages the family to create a home environment that is least likely to result in accidents or falls. Changes such as removing throw rugs, installing a handrail next to the toilet, and moving obstacles that can result in tripping or falling can be made at little or no expense to the family.

The nurse should include the following information in the patient and family teaching plan:

- Take this drug as prescribed. Do not increase, decrease, or omit a dose or stop taking the drug unless advised to do so by the primary health care provider. If gastrointestinal upset occurs, take the drug with food.
- If dizziness, drowsiness, or blurred vision occurs, avoid driving or performing other tasks that require alertness.
- Avoid the use of alcohol unless use has been approved by the primary health care provider.
- Relieve dry mouth by sucking on hard candy (unless the patient has diabetes) or frequent sips of water. Consult a dentist if dryness of the mouth interferes with wearing, inserting, or removing dentures or causes other dental problems.
- Inform patients that orthostatic hypotension may develop with or without symptoms of dizziness, nausea, fainting, and sweating. Caution the patient against rising rapidly after sitting or lying down.
- Notify the primary health care provider if any of these problems occur: severe dry mouth, inability to chew or swallow food, inability to urinate, feelings of depression, severe dizziness or drowsiness, rapid or irregular heartbeat, abdominal pain, mood changes, and unusual movements of the head, eyes, tongue, neck, arms, legs, feet, mouth, or tongue.
- Keep all appointments with the primary health care provider or clinic personnel because close monitoring of therapy is necessary.
- When taking levodopa, avoid vitamin B₆ (pyridoxine) because this vitamin may interfere with the action of levodopa (see Home Care Checklist: Avoiding Certain Foods While Taking Levodopa).
- Patients with diabetes: Levodopa may interfere with urine tests for glucose or ketones. Report any abnormal result to the primary care provider before adjusting the dosage of the antidiabetic medication.
- Tolcapone: Keep all appointments with the primary care provider. Liver function tests are performed periodically and are an important part of therapy. Report any signs of liver failure, such as persistent nausea, fatigue, lethargy, anorexia, jaundice, dark urine, pruritus, and right upper quadrant tenderness.

EVALUATION

- The therapeutic effect is achieved and the symptoms of parkinsonism are controlled.
- Adverse reactions are identified, reported to the primary health care provider, and managed successfully through appropriate nursing interventions.
- No evidence of injury is seen.
- The patient verbalizes an understanding of the treatment modalities, adverse reactions, and importance of continued follow-up care.
- The patient and family demonstrate an understanding of the drug regimen.

● Critical Thinking Exercises

1. *Ms. Dennis, age 89 years, has Parkinson's disease and is taking amantadine daily. In discussing her care with the family, determine what information you would include in the teaching plan and what information would be most important for the family to understand. Explain your answer.*

2. *Ms. Whitman is taking two drugs for Parkinson's disease: levodopa and carbidopa. Ms. Whitman questions you as to why she received two drugs while her friend with Parkinson's disease is taking only one drug. Discuss how you would explain this to Ms. Whitman.*

3. *Discuss the special considerations the nurse should be aware of when administering tolcapone.*

4. *Explain what adverse reaction would be more likely to occur in the older adult prescribed a non-ergot dopamine receptor agonist drug. Describe how you would assess for this adverse reaction.*

● Review Questions

1. The most serious adverse reactions seen with levodopa include _____.
   - **A.** choreiform and dystonic movements
   - **B.** depression
   - **C.** suicidal tendencies
   - **D.** paranoia

2. Elderly patients prescribed one of the dopamine receptor agonists are monitored closely for which of the following adverse reactions?
   - **A.** occipital headache
   - **B.** hallucinations
   - **C.** paralytic ileus
   - **D.** cardiac arrhythmias

Home Care Checklist

AVOIDING CERTAIN FOODS WHILE TAKING LEVODOPA

If your patient with parkinsonism is taking levodopa, he must be careful to avoid vitamin B_6 (pyridoxine) because it may interfere with the therapeutic effects of the drug. Most multivitamin supplements contain vitamin B_6. Therefore, be sure to instruct your patient to check with his health care provider before taking any vitamin supplements.

Vitamin B_6 is also found in a wide variety of food sources. It may be impossible to ask the patient to avoid these food sources entirely, but your patient may need to limit or decrease such intake to enhance or maintain the drug's effectiveness. Use the list below to teach your patient about possible food sources of vitamin B_6.

✓	Organ meats	✓	Pork
✓	Chicken	✓	Egg yolk
✓	Fish	✓	Whole grain cereals
✓	Peanuts	✓	Corn
✓	Walnuts	✓	Potatoes
✓	Oats	✓	Bananas
✓	Yeast	✓	Raisins
✓	Wheat germ	✓	Molasses

3. When taking an anticholinergic drug for parkinsonism, the patient would mostly experience which of the following adverse reactions?

   A. constipation, urinary frequency
   B. muscle spasm, convulsions
   C. diarrhea, hypertension
   D. dry mouth, dizziness

4. The patient taking tolcapone for Parkinson's disease is monitored closely for _____.

   A. kidney dysfunction
   B. liver dysfunction
   C. agranulocytosis
   D. the development of an autoimmune disease

● Medication Dosage Problems

1. Levodopa 0.75 g PO is prescribed. The drug is available in 100-mg tablets, 250-mg tablets, and 500-mg tablets. The nurse administers _____.

2. Ropinirole 6 mg PO is prescribed. The drug is available in 2-mg tablets. The nurse administers _____.

pressure and pulse rate, increased rate and depth of respiration, and increased muscle tension. An anxious patient will have cool and pale skin. Physical assessments include the blood pressure on both arms and in a sitting position, pulse, respiratory rate, and weight.

In addition, if possible, the nurse obtains a history of any past drug or alcohol abuse. Individuals with a history of previous abuse are more likely to abuse other drugs, such as the antianxiety drugs. Some patients, such as those with mild anxiety or depression, do not necessarily require inpatient care. These patients are usually seen at periodic intervals in the primary health care provider's office or in a psychiatric outpatient setting. The preadministration assessments of the outpatient are the same as those for the hospitalized patient.

Ongoing Assessment

An ongoing assessment is important for the patient taking an antianxiety drug. The nurse checks the patient's blood pressure before drug administration. If systolic pressure drops 20 mm Hg, the nurse withholds the drug and notifies the primary health care provider. The nurse periodically monitors the patient's mental status and anxiety level during therapy. The nurse assesses for improvement or worsening of behavioral and physical symptoms identified in the preadministration assessment.

The patient is monitored for adverse reactions. The sedation and drowsiness that sometimes occur with the use of an antianxiety drug may decrease as therapy continues. Prolonged therapy (> 3–4 months) may lead to dependence.

When the patient is an outpatient, the nurse observes the patient for a response to therapy at the time of each clinic visit. In some instances, the nurse may question the patient or a family member about the response to therapy. The type of questions asked depends on the patient and the diagnosis and may include questions such as: "How are you feeling," "Do you seem to be less nervous," or "Would you like to tell me how everything is going?" Many times the nurse may need to rephrase questions or direct the conversation toward other subjects until these patients feel comfortable and are able to discuss their therapy.

The nurse can ask the patient or a family member about adverse drug reactions or any other problems occurring during therapy. The nurse then brings these reactions or problems to the attention of the primary health care provider. The nurse documents a general summary of the patient's outward behavior and any complaints or problems in the patient's record. The nurse then compares notations to previous notations and observations.

Nursing Diagnoses Checklist

☑ **Anxiety** related to (individual manifestations)

☑ **Risk for Injury** related to an adverse drug reaction (eg, drowsiness or ataxia)

NURSING DIAGNOSES

Drug-specific nursing diagnoses are highlighted in the Nursing Diagnoses Checklist. Other nursing diagnoses applicable to these drugs are discussed in depth in Chapter 4.

PLANNING

The expected outcomes of the patient may include an optimal response to drug therapy, management of common adverse drug reactions, and a knowledge of and compliance with the prescribed therapeutic regimen.

IMPLEMENTATION

Promoting an Optimal Response to Therapy

The antianxiety drugs are not recommended for long-term use. When the antianxiety drugs are used for short periods (1–2 weeks), tolerance, dependence, or withdrawal symptoms usually do not develop. The nurse reports any signs of tolerance or dependence, such as the patient requesting larger doses of drug or increased anxiety and agitation (see Display 30-1).

When the patient is hospitalized, the nurse develops a nursing care plan to meet the patient's individual needs. Vital signs are monitored at frequent intervals, usually 3 to 4 times daily. In some instances, such as when hypotensive episodes occur, the vital signs are taken more often. The nurse reports any significant change in the vital signs to the primary health care provider.

Parenteral administration is indicated primarily in acute states. When these drugs are given intramuscularly, the nurse gives them in a large muscle mass, such as the gluteus muscle. The nurse observes the patient closely for at least 3 hours after parenteral administration. The patient is kept lying down (when possible) for 30 minutes to 3 hours after the drug is given.

> ### ❄ Gerontologic Alert
>
> *Parenteral (IV or IM) administration to older adults, the debilitated, and those with limited pulmonary reserve requires that the nurse exert extreme care because the patient may experience apnea and cardiac arrest. Resuscitative equipment should be readily available during parenteral (particularly IV) administration.*

The nurse may administer oral antianxiety drugs with food or meals to decrease the possibility of gastrointestinal upset. However, the nurse should use great care when administering these drugs orally because some patients have difficulty swallowing (due to a dry mouth or other causes). The patient may chew sugarless gum, suck on hard candy, or take frequent sips of water to reduce discomfort from dry mouth.

> ### ❄ Gerontologic Alert
>
> *Benzodiazepines are excreted more slowly in older adults, causing a prolonged drug effect. The drugs may accumulate in the blood, resulting in an increase in adverse reactions or toxicity. For this reason, the initial dose should be small, and the nurse should increase dosages gradually until a therapeutic response is obtained.*

However, lorazepam and oxazepam are relatively safe for older adults when given in normal dosages. Buspirone (BuSpar) also is a safe choice for older adults with anxiety because it does not cause excessive sedation, and the risk of falling is not as great. Before buspirone therapy is begun, benzodiazepines and sedatives and hypnotics are gradually withdrawn. Buspirone, unlike most of the benzodiazepines, must be taken regularly and is not effective on an as-needed basis.

Monitoring and Managing Adverse Drug Reactions

During initial therapy the nurse observes the patient closely for adverse drug reactions. Some adverse reactions, such as dry mouth, episodes of postural hypotension, and drowsiness, may need to be tolerated because drug therapy must continue. Nursing interventions to relieve some of these reactions may include offering frequent sips of water, assisting the patient out of the bed or chair, and supervising all ambulatory activities. The nurse should provide total assistance with activities of daily living to the patient experiencing extreme sedation, including help with eating, dressing, and ambulating.

> ### ✳ Nursing Alert
>
> *Benzodiazepine withdrawal may occur when use of the antianxiety drugs is abruptly discontinued after 3 to 4 months of therapy. Occasionally, withdrawal symptoms may occur after as little as 4 to 6 weeks of therapy. Symptoms of benzodiazepine withdrawal include increased anxiety, concentration difficulties, tremor, and sensory disturbances, such as paresthesias, photophobia, hypersomnia, and metallic taste. To help prevent withdrawal symptoms, the nurse must make sure the dosage of the benzodiazepine is gradually decreased over a period of time, usually 4 to 6 weeks.*

Although rare, benzodiazepine toxicity may occur from an overdose of the drug. Benzodiazepine toxicity causes sedation, respiratory depression, and coma. Flumazenil (Romazicon) is an antidote (antagonist) for benzodiazepine toxicity and acts to reverse the sedation, respiratory depression, and coma within 6 to 10 minutes after intravenous administration. The dosage is individualized based on the patient's response, with most patients responding to doses of 0.6 to 1 mg. However, the drug's action is short, and additional doses may be needed. Adverse reactions of flumazenil include agitation, confusion, seizures, and in some cases, symptoms of benzodiazepine withdrawal. Adverse reactions of flumazenil related to the symptoms of benzodiazepine withdrawal are relieved by the administration of the benzodiazepine.

Educating the Patient and Family

The nurse evaluates the patient's ability to assume responsibility for taking drugs at home. The nurse explains any adverse reactions that may occur with a specific antianxiety drug and encourages the patient or family members to contact the primary health care provider immediately if a serious drug reaction occurs.

The nurse should include the following points in a teaching plan for the patient or family member:

- Take the drug exactly as directed. Do not increase, decrease, or omit a dose or discontinue use of this drug unless directed to do so by the primary health care provider.
- Do not discontinue use of the drug abruptly because withdrawal symptoms may occur.
- Do not drive or perform other hazardous tasks if drowsiness occurs.
- Do not take any nonprescription drug unless use of a specific drug has been approved by the primary health care provider.
- Inform physicians, dentists, and other health care providers of therapy with this drug.
- Do not drink alcoholic beverages unless approval is obtained from the primary health care provider.
- If dizziness occurs when changing position, rise slowly when getting out of bed or a chair. If dizziness is severe, always have help when changing positions.
- If dryness of the mouth occurs, relieve it by taking frequent sips of water, sucking on hard candy, or chewing gum (preferably sugarless).
- If constipation occurs, relieve it by eating foods high in fiber, increasing fluid intake, and exercising if condition permits.
- Keep all appointments with the primary health care provider because close monitoring of therapy is essential.
- Report any unusual changes or physical effects to the primary health care provider.

EVALUATION

- The therapeutic effect is achieved, and the patient reports a decrease in feelings of anxiety.
- Adverse reactions are identified, reported to the primary health care provider, and managed successfully through appropriate nursing interventions.
- The patient verbalizes the importance of complying with the prescribed therapeutic regimen.
- The patient and family demonstrate an understanding of the drug regimen.

● *Critical Thinking Exercises*

1. *Ms. Stovall, age 66 years, is hospitalized for congestive heart failure. She is improving, but has been complaining of feelings of anxiety. Her respirations are 32 min, heart rate 88 bpm, and blood pressure 118/60 mm Hg. The primary health care provider prescribes alprazolam 0.25 mg PO TID. What precautions would the nurse expect to be taken because of Ms. Stovall's age? Discuss what assessment findings would indicate increased anxiety.*

2. *The primary health care provider prescribes lorazepam for short-term management of anxiety. What information would be included in a teaching plan for this patient?*

3. *A patient is prescribed buspirone 5 mg PO TID to be taken on an outpatient basis. What assessments would be important for the nurse to make when the patient comes to the clinic for a visit?*

● *Review Questions*

1. Alprazolam is contraindicated in patients with _____.
   A. a psychotic disorder
   B. congestive heart failure

   C. diabetes
   D. hypertension

2. The three types of psychotherapeutic drugs include _____.
   A. antianxiety drugs, tranquilizers, and anxiolytics
   B. antidepressants, psychotropic drugs, and anticonvulsants
   C. antipsychotic drugs, benzodiazepines, and tranquilizers
   D. antianxiety drugs, antidepressants, and antipsychotic drugs

3. Which antianxiety drug must be taken regularly and is not effective on a PRN basis?
   A. lorazepam
   B. buspirone
   C. oxazepam
   D. hydroxyzine

4. The benzodiazepines are pregnancy category _____ drugs that should not be taken while lactating because the infant may _____.
   A. B; seizure
   B. C; develop the floppy infant syndrome
   C. D; become lethargic and lose weight
   D. X; become hypoglycemic

● *Medication Dosage Problems*

1. Hydroxyzine 100 mg IM is prescribed. Available is a vial with 100 mg hydroxyzine per mL. The nurse administers _____.

2. The patient is prescribed 30 mg oxazepam TID orally. The drug is available in 15-mg tablets. The nurse administers _____.

Antidepressant Drugs

Key Terms

antidepressant drugs
depression
dysphoric

orthostatic
hypotension
priapism

Chapter Objectives

On completion of this chapter, the student will:

- Define depression and identify symptoms of a major depressive episode.
- Name the different types of antidepressant drugs.
- Discuss the uses, general drug actions, general adverse reactions, contraindications, precautions, and interactions of the antidepressant drugs.
- Discuss important preadministration and ongoing assessment activities that the nurse should perform on the patient taking antidepressant drugs.
- List some nursing diagnoses particular to a patient taking antidepressant drugs.
- Discuss ways to promote an optimal response to therapy, how to manage common adverse reactions, and important points to keep in mind when educating patients about the use of antidepressant drugs.

Depression is one of the most common psychiatric disorders. It is characterized by feelings of intense sadness, helplessness, worthlessness, and impaired functioning. Those experiencing a major depressive episode exhibit physical and psychological symptoms, such as appetite disturbances, sleep disturbances, and loss of interest in job, family, and other activities usually enjoyed. A major depressive episode is a depressed or **dysphoric** (extreme or exaggerated sadness, anxiety, or unhappiness) mood that interferes with daily functioning and includes five or more of the symptoms listed in Display 31-1.

To be classified as a major depression, these symptoms should occur daily or nearly every day for a period of 2 weeks or more. The symptoms of major depression should not be the result of normal bereavement, such as the loss of a loved one, or disease, such as hypothyroidism.

Depression is treated with the use of **antidepressant drugs**. Psychotherapy is used in conjunction with the antidepressant drugs in treating major depressive episodes. The four types of antidepressants are:

- Tricyclic antidepressants (TCAs)
- Monoamine oxidase inhibitors (MAOIs)

- Selective serotonin reuptake inhibitors (SSRIs)
- A group of miscellaneous, unrelated drugs

ACTIONS

For several years it was thought that the antidepressants blocked the reuptake of the endogenous neurohormones norepinephrine and serotonin, which resulted in stimulation of the central nervous system (CNS). Although the exact mechanism of action is unknown, this theory is now being questioned. New research indicates that the effects of the antidepressants are related to the slower adaptive changes in norepinephrine and serotonin receptor systems. Treatment with the antidepressants is thought to produce complex changes in the sensitivities of both presynaptic and postsynaptic receptor sites. The antidepressants increase the sensitivity of postsynaptic alpha (α)-adrenergic and serotonin receptors and decrease the sensitivity of the presynaptic receptor sites. This enhances the recovery from the depressive episode by normalizing neurotransmission activity.

Patient and Family Teaching Checklist

Promoting Patient Responsibility for Antidepressant Drug Therapy

The nurse:

✓ Explains the reason for drug therapy, including the type of antidepressant prescribed, drug name, dosage, and frequency of administration.

✓ Enlists the aid of family members to ensure compliance with therapy, including checking patient's oral cavity to be sure drug has been swallowed.

✓ Urges the patient to take the drug exactly as prescribed and not to increase or decrease dosage, omit doses, or discontinue use of the drug unless directed to do so by health care provider.

✓ Advises that full therapeutic effect may not occur for several weeks.

✓ Instructs in signs and symptoms of behavioral changes indicative of therapeutic effectiveness or increasing depression and suicidal tendencies.

✓ Reviews measures to reduce the risk for suicide.

✓ Instructs about possible adverse reactions with instructions to notify health care provider should any occur.

✓ Reinforces safety measures such as changing positions slowly and avoiding driving or hazardous tasks.

✓ Advises avoidance of alcohol and use of nonprescription drugs unless use is approved by health care provider.

✓ Encourages patient to inform other health care providers and medical personnel about drug therapy regimen.

✓ Instructs in measures to minimize dry mouth.

✓ Emphasizes importance of avoiding foods containing tyramine (if MAOIs are prescribed) and provides written list of foods to avoid.

✓ Reassures results of therapy will be monitored by periodic laboratory tests and follow-up visits with the health care provider.

✓ Assists with arrangements for follow-up visits.

● Do not drink alcoholic beverages unless approval is obtained from the primary health care provider.

● If dizziness occurs when changing position, rise slowly when getting out of bed or a chair. If dizziness is severe, always have help when changing positions.

● If dryness of the mouth occurs, relieve it by taking frequent sips of water, sucking on hard candy, or chewing gum (preferably sugarless).

● Keep all clinic appointments or appointments with the primary health care provider because close monitoring of therapy is essential.

● Do not take the antidepressants during pregnancy. Notify the primary health care provider if you are pregnant or wish to become pregnant.

● Report to the primary health care provider any unusual changes or physical effects.

● Avoid prolonged exposure to sunlight or sunlamps because an exaggerated reaction to the ultraviolet light may occur (photosensitivity), resulting in sunburn.

● Remember that a high incidence of sexual dysfunction is associated with clomipramine therapy.

● Remember that male patients taking trazodone who experience prolonged, inappropriate, and painful erections should stop taking the drug and notify the primary care provider.

EVALUATION

● The therapeutic effect is achieved.
● No evidence of injury is apparent.
● The patient is able to provide self-care.
● Adverse reactions are identified, reported to the primary health care provider, and managed successfully through appropriate nursing interventions.
● The patient verbalizes an understanding of treatment modalities and importance of continued follow-up care.
● The patient verbalizes the importance of complying with the prescribed therapeutic regimen.
● The patient and family demonstrate understanding of the drug regimen.

● *Critical Thinking Exercises*

1. *Mr. Hopkins has been severely depressed for several months. Two weeks ago the primary care provider prescribed amitriptyline 30 mg orally four times a day. His family is concerned because he is still depressed. They are requesting that the dosage be increased. Discuss what information you would give Mr. Hopkins and his family and what assessments you could make.*

2. *Ms. Jefferson has been taking phenelzine for depression. She reports having a "bad headache" at the back of her head. Determine what assessment would be most important to make. Explain what action, if any, you would take.*

3. *Mr. Jones is prescribed trazodone, and the nurse is preparing discharge instructions. What would be the most important points to cover at the teaching session.*

● *Review Questions*

1. When administering an antidepressant to a patient contemplating suicide, it is most important for the nurse to _____.

   A. have the patient remain upright for at least 30 minutes after taking the antidepressant

   B. assess the patient in 30 minutes for a therapeutic response to the drug

   C. monitor the patient for an occipital headache

   D. inspect the patient's oral cavity to be sure the drug was swallowed

2. Which of the following adverse reactions would the nurse expect to find in a patient taking amitriptyline?

   A. constipation and abdominal cramps

   B. bradycardia and double vision

   C. sedation and dry mouth

   D. polyuria and hypotension

3. The nurse instructs the patient taking a monoamine oxidase inhibitor not to eat foods containing _____.

   A. glutamine

   B. sugar

   C. tyramine

   D. large amounts of iron

4. Which of the following antidepressants would be most likely to cause the patient to have a seizure?

   A. amitriptyline

   B. bupropion

   C. sertraline

   D. venlafaxine

● *Medication Dosage Problems*

1. The primary care provider prescribes trazodone 150 mg PO. Available are 50-mg tablets. The nurse administers _____.

2. The primary care provider prescribes paroxetine 50 mg/d PO. The drug is available as oral suspension with a strength of 10 mg/5 mL. The nurse administers _____.

Antipsychotic Drugs

Chapter Objectives

On completion of this chapter, the student will:

- List the uses, general drug actions, general adverse reactions, contraindications, precautions, and interactions associated with the administration of the antipsychotic drugs.
- Discuss important preadministration and ongoing assessment activities the nurse should perform on the patient taking an antipsychotic drug.
- List some nursing diagnoses particular to a patient taking an antipsychotic drug.
- Discuss ways to promote an optimal response to therapy, how to manage common adverse reactions, and important points to keep in mind when educating patients about the use of the antipsychotic drugs.

Antipsychotic drugs are also called **neuroleptic drugs**. These drugs are given to patients with a psychotic disorder, such as schizophrenia. A **psychotic disorder** is characterized by extreme personality disorganization and the loss of contact with reality. **Hallucinations** (a false perception having no basis in reality) or **delusions** (false beliefs that cannot be changed with reason) are usually present. Other symptoms include disorganized speech, behavior disturbance, social withdrawal, flattened affect (absence of an emotional response to any situation or condition), and anhedonia (finding no pleasure in activities that are normally pleasurable).

Although lithium is not a true antipsychotic drug, it is considered with the antipsychotics because of its use in regulating the severe fluctuations of the manic phase of **bipolar disorder** (a psychiatric disorder characterized by severe mood swings of extreme hyperactivity to depression). During the manic phase, the person experiences altered thought processes, which can lead to bizarre delusions. The drug diminishes the frequency and intensity of hyperactive (manic) episodes.

ACTIONS

The exact mechanism of action of antipsychotic drugs is not well understood. These drugs are thought to act by inhibiting or blocking the release of the neurohormone dopamine in the brain and possibly increasing the firing of nerve cells in certain areas of the brain. These effects may be responsible for the ability of these drugs to suppress the symptoms of certain psychotic disorders. Examples of antipsychotic drugs include chlorpromazine (Thorazine), haloperidol (Haldol), and lithium. Lithium is an antimanic drug; although its exact mechanism is unknown, it appears to alter sodium transport in nerve and muscle cells and inhibits the release of norepinephrine and dopamine. Haloperidol may act to block postsynaptic dopamine receptors in the brain and depress the RAS, including those parts of the brain involved with wakefulness and emesis. The Summary Drug Table: Antipsychotic Drugs gives a more complete listing of the antipsychotic drugs.

SUMMARY DRUG TABLE ANTIPSYCHOTIC DRUGS

GENERIC NAME	TRADE NAME*	USES	ADVERSE REACTIONS	DOSAGE RANGES
chlorpromazine HCL *klor-proe'-ma-zeen*	Thorazine, *generic*	Psychotic disorders, nausea, vomiting, intractable hiccups	Hypotension, postural hypotension, tardive dyskinesia, photophobia, urticaria, nasal congestion, dry mouth, akathisia, dystonia, pseudoparkinsonism, behavioral changes, headache, photosensitivity	Psychiatric disorders: up to 2000 mg/d PO in divided doses, 25 IM; nausea and vomiting: 10–25 mg PO, 25–50 mg IM, 50–100 rectal; hiccups: 25–50 mg PO, IM, IV TID–QID
clozapine *kloe'-za-peen*	Clozaril, *generic*	Severely ill schizophrenic patients with no response to other therapies	Drowsiness, sedation, akathisia, seizures, dizziness, syncope, tachycardia, hypotension, nausea, vomiting	Up to 900 mg/d PO in divided doses
fluphenazine HCL *floo-fen'-a-zeen*	Permitil, Prolixin, *generic*	Psychotic disorders	Drowsiness, extrapyramidal effects, dystonia, akathisia, hypotension	0.5–10 mg/PO in divided doses up to 20 mg/d; 2.5–10 mg/d IM in divided doses
haloperidol *ha-loe-per'-i-dole*	Haldol	Psychotic disorders; Tourette's syndrome, behavior problems in children	Extrapyramidal symptoms, akathisia, dystonia, tardive dyskinesia, drowsiness, headache, dry mouth, orthostatic hypotension	0.5–5 mg PO BID, TID with dosages up to 100 mg/d in divided doses; 2–5 mg IM; children 0.05–0.075 mg/kg/d PO
lithium *lith'-ee-um*	Eskalith, Lithobid, Lithonate, *generic*	Manic episodes of bipolar disorder	Headache, drowsiness, tremors, nausea, polyuria (see Table 32-1)	Based on lithium serum levels; average dose range is 900–1800 mg/d PO in divided doses
loxapine *lox'-a-peen*	Loxitane	Psychotic disorders	Extrapyramidal symptoms, akathisia, dystonia, tardive dyskinesia, drowsiness, headache, dry mouth, orthostatic hypotension	60–250 mg/d PO in divided doses; 12.5–50 mg IM
olanzapine *oh-lan'-za-peen*	Zyprexa	Schizophrenia, short-term treatment of manic episodes of bipolar disorder	Agitation, dizziness, nervousness, akathisia, constipation, fever, weight gain	5–20 mg/d PO
perphenazine *per-fen'-a-zeen*	Trilafon, *generic*	Psychotic disorders	Hypotension, postural hypotension, tardive dyskinesia, photophobia, urticaria, nasal congestion, dry mouth, akathisia, dystonia, pseudoparkinsonism, behavioral changes, headache, photosensitivity	Psychotic disorders: 4–16 mg PO BID to QID, 5–10 mg IM
pimozide *pi'-moe-zide*	Orap	Tourette's syndrome	Parkinson-like symptoms, motor restlessness, dystonia, oculogyric crisis, tardive dyskinesia, dry mouth, diarrhea, headache, rash, drowsiness	Initial dose: 1–2 mg/d PO; maintenance dose: up to 10 mg/d PO

(continued)

Nursing Diagnoses Checklist

- ☑ **Confusion** related to adverse effects of the drug
- ☑ **Risk for Injury** related to an adverse drug reaction (eg, drowsiness, ataxia)
- ☑ **Impaired Physical Mobility** related to adverse drug reactions (eg, drowsiness, ataxia)
- ☑ **Impaired Verbal Communication** related to drug-induced extrapyramidal effects (eg, dystonia)
- ☑ **Risk for Imbalanced Fluid Volume** related to adverse drug effects of lithium

IMPLEMENTATION

Promoting an Optimal Response to Therapy

The nurse develops a nursing care plan to meet the patient's individual needs. It is important to monitor vital signs at least daily. In some instances, such as when hypotensive episodes occur, the nurse should monitor vital signs more frequently. The nurse should report any significant change in the vital signs to the primary health care provider.

Behavioral records should be written at periodic intervals (frequency depends on hospital or unit guidelines). An accurate description of the patient's behavior aids the primary health care provider in planning therapy and thus becomes an important part of nursing management. Patients with poor response to drug therapy may require dosage changes, a change to another psychotherapeutic drug, or the addition of other therapies to the treatment regimen. However, it is important for the nurse to know that full response to antipsychotic drugs takes several weeks.

The nurse may give antipsychotic drugs orally as a single daily dose or in divided doses several times a day. Divided daily doses are recommended when beginning drug therapy, but once-daily dosing may be used with continued therapy. Administration at bedtime helps to minimize the postural hypotension and sedation associated with these drugs. The exact dosage (milligram to milligram) has not been precisely identified. The primary care provider may prescribe small incremental dosage increases until the patient's symptoms are controlled.

 Gerontologic Alert

In elderly or debilitated patients, doses may be instituted at ½ to ⅓ the recommended dose for younger adults and increased more gradually than dose increases in younger adults.

Oral administration requires great care because some patients have difficulty swallowing (because of a dry mouth or other causes). Other patients may refuse to take the drug. The nurse should never force a patient to take an oral drug. If the patient refuses the drug, the nurse contacts the primary health care provider regarding this problem because parenteral administration of the drug may be necessary.

After administration of an oral drug, the nurse inspects the patient's oral cavity to be sure the drug has been swallowed. If the patient resists having his or her oral cavity checked, the nurse reports this refusal to the primary health care provider.

 Gerontologic Alert

Dosages in older adults are usually in the lower range. Because older adults are more susceptible to cardiovascular and neuromuscular reactions to the antipsychotic drugs, the nurse must closely monitor them. It is important to increase the dosages gradually.

Oral liquid concentrates are available for use in patients who can more easily swallow a liquid. These concentrates are light sensitive and dispensed in amber or opaque bottles to help protect the concentrate from light. They are administered mixed in liquids such as fruit juices, tomato juice, milk, or carbonated beverages. Semisolid foods, such as soups or puddings, may also be used. Perphenazine (Trilafon) concentrate should not be mixed with beverages containing caffeine (coffee, cola), tea, or apple juice because of the risk of incompatibility.

When these drugs are given parenterally, the nurse should give the drugs intramuscularly in a large muscle mass, such as the gluteus muscle. The nurse keeps the patient lying down (when possible) for about 30 minutes after the drug is given.

Nursing Alert

In combative patients or those who have serious manifestations of acute psychosis (eg, hallucinations or loss of contact with reality), parenteral administration may be repeated every 1 to 4 hours until the desired effects are obtained or until cardiac arrhythmias or rhythm changes, or hypotension occur.

MANAGING CARE OF THE OUTPATIENT. At the time of each visit of the patient to the primary health care provider's office or clinic, the nurse observes the patient for a response to therapy. In some instances, the nurse may question the patient or a family member about the response to therapy. The questions asked depend on the patient and the diagnosis and may include questions such as

- How are you feeling?
- Do you seem to be less nervous?
- Would you like to tell me how everything is going?

Many times the nurse may need to rephrase questions or direct conversation toward other subjects until these patients feel comfortable and are able to discuss their therapy.

The nurse asks the patient or a family member about adverse drug reactions or any other problems occurring during therapy. The nurse brings these reactions or problems to the attention of the primary health care provider. The nurse should document in the patient's record a general summary of the patient's outward behavior and any complaints or problems. The nurse then compares these notations to previous notations and observations.

LITHIUM. The dosage of lithium is individualized according to serum levels and clinical response to the drug. The desirable serum lithium levels are 0.6 to 1.2 mEq/L. Blood samples are drawn immediately before the next dose of lithium (8–12 hours after the last dose) when lithium levels are relatively stable. During the acute phase the nurse monitors serum lithium levels twice weekly or until the patient's manic phase is under control. During maintenance therapy, the serum lithium levels are monitored every 2 to 4 months.

Monitoring and Managing Adverse Drug Reactions

During initial therapy or whenever the dosage is increased or decreased, the nurse observes the patient closely for adverse drug reactions, including tardive dyskinesia (see Fig. 32-1) and any behavioral changes. It is important to report to the primary health care provider any change in behavior or the appearance of adverse reactions. A further increase or decrease in dosage may be necessary, or use of the drug may need to be discontinued.

> **Nursing Alert**
>
> *When administering the antipsychotic drugs, the nurse observes the patient for extrapyramidal effects, which include muscular spasms of the face and neck, the inability to sleep or sit still, tremors, rigidity, or involuntary rhythmic movements. The nurse notifies the primary health care provider of the occurrence of these symptoms because they may indicate a need for dosage adjustment.*

The patient may need to tolerate some adverse reactions, such as dry mouth, episodes of orthostatic hypotension, and drowsiness because drug therapy must continue. Nursing interventions to relieve some of these reactions may include offering frequent sips of water, assisting the patient out of the bed or chair, and supervising all ambulatory activities. The nurse provides total assistance with activities of daily living to the patient experiencing extreme sedation, including help with eating, dressing, and ambulating. However, the nurse must protect extremely hyperactive patients from injury to themselves or others.

> **Nursing Alert**
>
> *The antipsychotic drugs may cause extreme drowsiness and sedation, especially during the first or second weeks of therapy. This reaction may impair mental of physical abilities. Drowsiness usually diminishes after 2–3 weeks of therapy. However, if the patient continues to be troubled by drowsiness and sedation, the physician may prescribe a lower dosage.*

Tardive dyskinesia can occur in patients taking the antipsychotics. The nurse must remain alert for any signs and symptoms of this condition.

> **Nursing Alert**
>
> *Because there is no known treatment for tardive dyskinesia and because it is irreversible in some patients, the nurse must immediately report symptoms. These include rhythmic, involuntary movements of the tongue, face, mouth, jaw, or the extremities.*

CLOZAPINE. This drug is available only through the Clozaril Patient Management System (a program that combines WBC testing, patient monitoring, and pharmacy and drug distribution services). Only 1 week of this drug is dispensed at a time. Patients taking clozapine are at increased risk for bone marrow suppression. A weekly WBC count is done throughout therapy and for 4 weeks after therapy is discontinued. In addition, the nurse monitors the patient for adverse reactions that indicate bone marrow suppression: lethargy, weakness, fever, sore throat, malaise, mucous membrane ulceration, or "flu-like" complaints.

LITHIUM. Lithium toxicity is closely related to serum lithium levels and can occur even when the drug is administered at therapeutic doses. Adverse reactions are seldom observed at serum lithium levels of less than 1.5 mEq/L, except in the patient who is especially sensitive to lithium. Toxic symptoms may be seen with serum lithium levels of 1.5 mEq/L or greater. Levels should not exceed 2 mEq/L (see Table 32-1). Therefore, the nurse must continually monitor patients taking lithium for signs of toxicity, such as diarrhea, vomiting, nausea, drowsiness, muscular weakness, and lack of coordination. For early symptoms, the primary health care provider may order a dosage reduction or discontinue the drug for 24 to 48 hours and then gradually restart the drug therapy at a lower dosage.

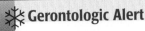

❄ Gerontologic Alert

Older adults are at increased risk for toxicity because of a decreased rate of excretion. Lower dosages may be necessary to decrease the risk of toxicity.

For patients receiving lithium, the nurse increases the oral fluid intake to about 3000 mL/d. It is important to keep fluids readily available and to offer extra fluids throughout waking hours. If there is any question regarding the oral fluid intake, the nurse monitors intake and output.

Educating the Patient and Family

Noncompliance is a problem with some patients once they are discharged to the home setting. It is important for the nurse to accurately evaluate the patient's ability to assume responsibility for taking drugs at home. The administration of antipsychotic drugs becomes a family responsibility if the outpatient appears to be unable to manage his or her own drug therapy.

The nurse explains any adverse reactions that may occur with a specific antipsychotic drug and encourages the patient or family members to contact the primary health care provider immediately if a serious drug reaction occurs.

The nurse includes the following points in a teaching plan for the patient or family member:

- Keep all primary care provider and clinic appointments because close monitoring of therapy is essential.
- Report any unusual changes or physical effects to the primary health care provider.
- Take the drug exactly as directed. Do not increase, decrease, or omit a dose or discontinue use of this drug unless directed to do so by the primary health care provider.
- Do not drive or perform other hazardous tasks if drowsiness occurs.
- Do not take any nonprescription drug unless use of a specific drug has been approved by the primary health care provider.
- Inform physicians, dentists, and other medical personnel of therapy with this drug.
- Do not drink alcoholic beverages unless approval is obtained from the primary health care provider.
- If dizziness occurs when changing position, rise slowly when getting out of bed or a chair. If dizziness is severe, always have help when changing positions.
- If dryness of the mouth occurs, relieve it by taking frequent sips of water, sucking on hard candy, or chewing gum (preferably sugarless).
- Notify your primary care provider if you become pregnant or intend to become pregnant during therapy.

- Immediately report the occurrence of the following adverse reactions: restlessness, inability to sit still, muscle spasms, masklike expression, rigidity, tremors, drooling, or involuntary rhythmic movements of the mouth, face, or extremities. Inform all patients about the risks of extrapyramidal symptoms and tardive dyskinesia. Avoid exposure to the sun. If exposure is unavoidable, wear sunblock, keep arms and legs covered, and wear a sun hat.
- Note that only a 1-week supply of clozapine is dispensed at a time. The drug is obtained through a special program designed to ensure the required blood monitoring. Weekly WBC laboratory tests are required. Immediately report any signs of weakness, fever, sore throat, malaise, or "flu-like" symptoms to the primary care provider.
- Note that olanzapine is available as a tablet to swallow or as an orally disintegrating tablet. When using the orally disintegrating tablet, peel back the foil on the blister. Using dry hands, remove the tablet and place the entire tablet in the mouth. The tablet will disintegrate with or without liquid.
- Remember to take lithium with food or immediately after meals to avoid stomach upset. Drink at least 10 large glasses of fluid each day and add extra salt to food. Prolonged exposure to the sun may lead to dehydration. If any of the following occurs, do not take the next dose and immediately notify the primary health care provider: diarrhea, vomiting, fever, tremors, drowsiness, lack of muscle coordination, or muscle weakness.

EVALUATION

- The therapeutic effect is achieved.
- Adverse reactions are identified, reported to the primary health care provider, and managed successfully through appropriate nursing interventions.
- No evidence of injury is seen.
- The patient verbalizes an understanding of treatment modalities and the importance of continued follow-up care.
- The patient verbalizes the importance of complying with the prescribed therapeutic regimen.
- The patient and family demonstrate understanding of the drug regimen.

● *Critical Thinking Exercises*

1. *Ms. Brown comes to the mental health clinic for a follow-up visit. She is taking lithium to control a bipolar disorder. Ms. Brown tells you that she is concerned because her "hands are always shaking" and "sometimes I walk like I have been drinking alcohol." Explain how you would explore this problem with Ms. Brown.*

2. *As a nurse on the psychiatric unit, you are assigned to discuss extrapyramidal effects at a team conference. Discuss how you would present and explain this topic. Describe the points you would stress.*

3. *Your patient is prescribed clozapine for schizophrenia that has not responded to other drugs. You must discuss this new therapy with the family. Discuss what points to include in this family teaching session.*

● Review Questions

1. A patient taking chlorpromazine (Thorazine) for schizophrenia is also prescribed the antiparkinson drug benztropine. What is the best explanation for adding an antiparkinson drug to the drug regimen?

A. Antiparkinson drugs prevent symptoms of tardive diskinesia, such as involuntary movements of the face and tongue.

B. Antiparkinson drugs promote the effects of chlorpromazine.

C. Antiparkinson drugs are given to reduce the possibility of symptoms such as fine tremors, muscle rigidity, and slow movement.

D. Antiparkinson drugs help to decrease hallucinations and delusions in patients with schizophrenia.

2. Which of the following reactions would the nurse expect to see in a patient experiencing tardive dyskinesia?

A. Muscle rigidity, dry mouth, insomnia

B. Rhythmic, involuntary movements of the tongue, face, mouth, or jaw

C. Muscle weakness, paralysis of the eyelids, diarrhea

D. Dyspnea, somnolence, muscle spasms

3. Which of the following symptoms would indicate to the nurse that a patient taking lithium is experiencing toxicity?

A. Constipation, abdominal cramps, rash

B. Stupor, oliguria, hypertension

C. Nausea, vomiting, diarrhea

D. Dry mouth, blurred vision, difficulty swallowing

4. In giving discharge instructions to a patient taking lithium the nurse stresses that the patient should _____.

A. eat a diet high in carbohydrates and low in proteins

B. increase oral fluid intake to approximately 3000 mL/day

C. have blood drawn before each dose of lithium is administered

D. avoid eating foods high in amines

● Medication Dosage Problems

1. A patient is prescribed haloperidol 3 mg IM. The drug is available in solution of 2 mg/mL. The nurse would administer _____.

2. Thorazine 50 mg PO is prescribed. Use the drug label below to determine the correct dosage. The nurse administers _____.

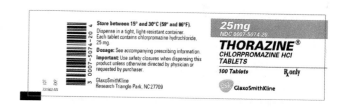

3. Lithium 600 mg is prescribed. Use the drug label below to determine the correct dosage. The nurse administers _____.

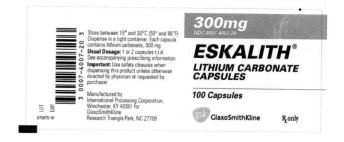

Cholinesterase Inhibitors

Chapter Objectives

On completion of this chapter, the student will:

- Discuss the clinical manifestations of Alzheimer's disease.
- List the uses, general drug actions, general adverse reactions, contraindications, precautions, and interactions associated with the administration of the cholinesterase inhibitors.
- Discuss important preadministration and ongoing assessment activities the nurse should perform on the patient taking a cholinesterase inhibitor.
- List some nursing diagnoses particular to a patient taking a cholinesterase inhibitor.
- Discuss ways to promote an optimal response to therapy, how to manage common adverse reactions, and important points to keep in mind when educating patients about the use of the cholinesterase inhibitors.

Alzheimer's disease (AD) is a progressive deterioration of mental, physical, and cognitive abilities from which there is no recovery. About 2 million Americans have the disease. Almost 50% of individuals in nursing homes and almost half of all people older than 85 years experience the devastating effects of AD. Currently it is the fourth leading cause of death in adults. Specific pathologic changes occur in the cortex of the brain thought to be associated with deficiencies of one or more of the neurohormones, such as acetylcholine or norepinephrine.

Drugs that are used to treat AD do not cure the disease but are aimed at slowing the progression. These drugs are the cholinesterase inhibitors. Examples of the cholinesterase inhibitors include donepezil (Aricept), galantamine hydrobromide (Reminyl), rivastigmine tartrate (Exelon), and tacrine hydrochloride (Cognex). These drugs are used to treat mild to moderate **dementia** (decrease in cognitive functioning) of AD. Other drugs are used for symptomatic relief. For example, wandering, irritability, and aggression in people with AD are treated with the antipsychotics, such as risperidone and olanzapine (see Chap. 32). Other drugs, such as the antidepressants or antianxiety drugs, may be helpful in AD for symptoms of depression and anxiety.

Several herbal remedies are thought to be helpful in AD. **Ginkgo biloba** is a common herb that appears to increase blood flow to the brain and has antioxidant properties. The herb is available over the counter, but there are no standards in the United States to regulate its quality of effectiveness. No one should take this or any other herb for AD without first consulting with the primary care provider. When ginkgo biloba is used with other drugs, such as with warfarin or high doses of vitamin E, there is a risk for increased bleeding.

ACTIONS

Acetylcholine, a natural chemical in the brain, is required for memory and thinking. Individuals with AD slowly lose this chemical, and as the levels of the chemical decrease, the patient experiences problems with memory and thinking. The cholinesterase inhibitors act to increase the level of acetylcholine in the CNS by inhibiting its breakdown and slowing neuronal destruction. However, the disease is progressive, and although these drugs alter the progress of the disease, they do not cure the disease. The life span of a

SUMMARY DRUG TABLE CHOLINESTERASE INHIBITORS

GENERIC NAME	TRADE NAME*	USES	ADVERSE REACTIONS	DOSAGE RANGES
donepezil HCL *doe-nep'-ah-zill*	Aricept	Mild to moderate dementia of the Alzheimer type	Nausea, vomiting, diarrhea, muscle cramps, fatigue, anorexia, syncope	5–10 mg/d PO
galantamine hydrobromide *ga-lan'-ta-meen*	Reminyl	Mild to moderate dementia of the Alzheimer type	Nausea, vomiting, diarrhea, anorexia, weight loss, abdominal pain, headache, dizziness, lethargy, confusion	4 mg BID PO up to 24 mg/d
rivastigmine tartrate *riv-ah-stig'-meen*	Exelon, Exelon Oral Solution	Mild to moderate dementia of the Alzheimer type	Nausea, vomiting, diarrhea, dyspepsia, anorexia, abdominal pain, insomnia, fatigue, skin rash, dizziness, constipation, somnolence, tremor	1.5–12 mg/d BID PO
tacrine HCL *tay'-krin*	Cognex	Mild to moderate dementia of the Alzheimer type	Diarrhea, loss of appetite, clumsiness, nausea, vomiting, fainting, tachycardia, fever, hyper- or hypotension, skin rash, severe abdominal pain, hepatotoxicity	40–160 mg/d in 4 divided doses PO

*The term *generic* indicates the drug is available in generic form.

USES

Cholinesterase inhibitors are used to treat the dementia associated with AD. The effectiveness of these drugs varies from individual to individual. The drugs may noticeably diminish the symptoms of AD, the symptoms could improve only slightly, or the symptoms could continue to progress (only at a slower rate).

Donepezil has the advantage of once-daily administration and appears to be better tolerated than tacrine. Tacrine is particularly harmful to the liver. The new drugs rivastigmine and galantamine, like the other two, are effective in treating mild-to-moderate dementia of AD.

ADVERSE REACTIONS

In most situations, adverse reactions of the cholinesterase inhibitors are mild and are most often experienced early in the treatment. When adverse reactions occur, they tend to disappear gradually as the body gets used to the treatment and generally will not last for more than several days. Adverse reactions of the cholinesterase inhibitors

include anorexia, nausea, vomiting, diarrhea, weight loss, abdominal pain, dizziness, and headache.

Tacrine is particularly damaging to the liver and can result in hepatotoxicity. Because tacrine is more likely to cause adverse reactions and drug interactions, it must be administered more frequently (4 times a day) and is rarely used in current therapy. Donepezil has fewer and milder side effects than tacrine. It is considered the agent of first choice. However, some patients may achieve a better response with one drug than another. Additional adverse reactions are listed in the Summary Drug Table: Cholinesterase Inhibitors.

CONTRAINDICATIONS

The cholinesterase inhibitors are contraindicated in patients with a hypersensitivity to the drugs and during pregnancy (Pregnancy Category B) and lactation.

PRECAUTIONS

These drugs are used cautiously in patients with renal or hepatic disease, bladder obstruction, seizure disorders, sick sinus syndrome, gastrointestinal bleeding, and asthma. Individuals with a history of ulcer disease may have a recurrence of the bleeding.

INTERACTIONS

When the cholinesterase inhibitors are administered with the anticholinergic drugs, there is a potential decrease in activity of the anticholinergic drug. There is an increased risk of toxicity of theophylline when the cholinesterase inhibitors are administered with tacrine. There is a synergistic effect when tacrine is administered with succinylcholine, cholinesterase inhibitors, or cholinergic agonists (eg, bethanechol).

 Herbal Alert: Ginseng

Ginseng has been called the "king of herbs" because of its wide use and the benefits attributed to the herb. In early times in China, ginseng was valued as high as gold. Hundreds of ginseng products (eg, gum, teas, chewing gum, juices) are sold throughout the US. Ginseng is the fourth best selling herb in the US. The primary use of ginseng is to improve energy and mental performance. The benefits of ginseng include improving endurance during exercise, reducing fatigue, boosting stamina and reaction times, and increasing feelings of well-being.

Adverse reactions are rare, but sleeplessness, nervousness, and diarrhea have been reported in individuals taking large amounts of the herb. The herb should not be taken in combination with stimulants including those containing caffeine. Dosage is 200 to 500 mg/day of the standardized extract or 1 to 4 g of powdered root a day. Ginseng is contraindicated in individuals with high blood pressure and during pregnancy.

 Herbal Alert: Ginkgo

Ginkgo is one of the oldest herbs in the world and has many beneficial effects. Ginkgo is taken to improve memory and brain function and to enhance circulation to the brain, heart, limbs, and eyes. Most of the research done on ginkgo has been done on standardized extract ginkgo. The recommended dose is 40 mg standardized extract ginkgo three times a day. The effects of ginkgo may not be seen until after 4 to 24 weeks of treatment. The most common adverse reactions include mild gastrointestinal discomfort, headache, and rash. Excessively large doses have been reported to cause diarrhea, nausea, vomiting, and restlessness. Ginkgo is contraindicated in patients taking monoamine oxidase inhibitors (MAOIs) because of the risk of a toxic reaction. Individuals taking anticoagulants should take ginkgo only on the advice of a primary care provider.

NURSING PROCESS

● **The Patient Receiving a Cholinesterase Inhibitor for Mild-to-Moderate Dementia of Alzheimer's Disease**

ASSESSMENT

Preadministration Assessment

A patient receiving a cholinesterase inhibitor may be treated in the hospital, nursing home, or in an outpatient setting. The patient's cognitive ability and functional ability are assessed before and during therapy. The baseline or initial assessment depends on the stage of AD. The nurse assesses the patient for confusion, agitation, and impulsive behavior. Speech, ability to perform activities of daily living, and self-care ability also are assessed. These assessments will be used by the nurse in the ongoing assessment in monitoring the patient's improvement (if any) after taking the cholinesterase inhibitors. These drugs may slow the progression of the disease but are not a cure for AD.

Before starting therapy for the hospitalized patient, the nurse obtains a complete psychiatric and medical history. With AD, patients often are unable to give a reliable history of their illness. A family member or primary caregiver will be able to verify or give information needed for an accurate assessment. During the time the history is taken, the nurse observes the patient for any behavior patterns that appear to be deviations from normal. Examples of deviations include poor eye contact, failure to answer questions completely, inappropriate answers to questions, a monotone speech pattern, and inappropriate laughter, sadness, or crying. These patients are in varying stages of decline. Display 33-1 identifies the stages of AD and the associated clinical manifestations. The nurse documents the patient's cognitive ability using Display 33-1 as a guide.

Late dementia or the final phase of AD may last from a few months to several years while the patient becomes increasingly immobile and dysfunctional.

Physical assessments include obtaining blood pressure measurements on both arms with the patients in a sitting position, pulse, respiratory rate, and weight. The functional ability of the patient is also important.

DISPLAY 33-1 ● Clinical Manifestations of Alzheimer's Disease

EARLY PHASE—MILD COGNITIVE DECLINE
- Increased forgetfulness
- Decreased performance in social settings
- Evidence of memory deficit when interviewed
- Mild to moderate anxiety

EARLY DEMENTIA PHASE—MODERATELY SEVERE COGNITIVE DECLINE
- Needs assistance for activities of daily living
- Unable to recall important aspects of current life
- Difficulty making choices (ie, what clothes to wear, what to eat)
- Able to recall major facts (ie, their name and family member's names)
- Need assistance for survival

LATE DEMENTIA PHASE—SEVERE COGNITIVE DECLINE
- Incontinent of urine
- No verbal ability
- No basic psychomotor skills
- Needs assistance when bathing, toileting, and feeding

The initial assessments of the outpatient are basically the same as those for the hospitalized patient. The nurse obtains a complete medical history and a history of the symptoms of AD from the patient (if possible), a family member, or the patient's hospital records. During the initial interview, the nurse observes the patient for what appear to be deviations from a normal behavior pattern. The nurse also should assess the patient's vital signs and body weight.

Ongoing Assessment

Ongoing assessment of patients taking the cholinesterase inhibitors includes both mental and physical assessments. Cognitive and functional abilities are assessed using Display 33-1 as a guide. Initial assessments will be compared with the ongoing assessments to monitor the patient's improvement (if any) after taking the cholinesterase inhibitors.

NURSING DIAGNOSES

Drug-specific nursing diagnoses are highlighted in the Nursing Diagnoses Checklist. Other nursing diagnoses applicable to these drugs are discussed in depth in Chapter 4.

PLANNING

The expected outcomes for the patient may include an optimal response to drug therapy, management of common adverse drug reactions, an absence of injury, and compliance with the prescribed therapeutic regimen.

IMPLEMENTATION

Promoting an Optimal Response to Therapy

The nurse develops a nursing care plan to meet the patient's individual needs. It is important to monitor vital signs at least daily. The nurse should report any significant change in the patient's vital signs to the primary health care provider.

Behavioral records should be written at periodic intervals (frequency depends on hospital or unit guidelines). An accurate description of the patient's behavior and cognitive ability aids the primary health care provider in planning therapy and thus becomes an important part of nursing management. Patients with poor response to drug therapy may require dosage changes, discontinuation of the drug therapy, or the addition of other therapies to the treatment regimen. However, it is important for the nurse to know that response to these drugs may take several weeks. The symptoms that the patient is experiencing may get better or remain the same, or the patient may experience only a small response to therapy. It is important to remember that a treatment that slows the progression of symptoms in AD is a successful treatment.

Donepezil is administered orally once daily at bedtime. It can be taken with or without food. Galantamine is administered orally twice daily, preferably with morning and evening meals.

Rivastigmine is administered as a tablet or oral solution twice daily. When rivastigmine is administered as an oral solution, the nurse removes the oral dosing syringe provided in the protective container. The syringe provided is used to withdraw the prescribed amount. The dosage may be swallowed directly from the syringe or first mixed with a small glass of water, cold fruit juice, or soda.

Tacrine is administered orally 3 or 4 times a day, preferably on an empty stomach 1 hour before or 2 hours after meals. For best results the drug should be administered around the clock.

Monitoring and Managing Adverse Reactions

When taking the cholinesterase inhibitors, patients may experience nausea and vomiting. Although this can occur with all of the cholinesterase inhibitors, patients taking rivastigmine appear to have more problems with nausea and severe vomiting. Nausea and vomiting should be reported to the primary health care provider because the primary care provider may discontinue use of the drug and then restart the drug therapy at the lowest dose possible. Restarting therapy at the lower dose helps to reduce the nausea and vomiting.

Weight loss and eating problems related to the inability to swallow are two major problems in the late stage of AD. These problems coupled with the anorexia and nausea associated with administration of the cholinesterase inhibitors present a challenge for the nurse or the caregiver. Mealtime should be simple and calm. The patient should be offered a well-balanced diet with foods that are easy to chew and digest. Frequent, small meals may be tolerated better than three regular meals. Offering foods of different consistency and flavor is important in case the patient can handle one form better than another. Fluid intake of 6 to 8 glasses of water daily is encouraged to prevent dehydration. In later stages, the patient may be fed through a feeding syringe, or the caregiver can encourage chewing action by pressing gently on the bottom of the patient's chin and on the lips.

Nursing Diagnoses Checklist

✓ **Imbalanced Nutrition: Less than Body Requirements** related to adverse reactions (eg, anorexia, nausea)

✓ **Risk for Injury** related to an adverse drug reaction (eg, dizziness, syncope, clumsiness) or disease process

✓ **Impaired Physical Mobility** related to adverse drug reactions (eg, dizziness, syncope) or disease process

Physical decline and the adverse reactions of dizziness and syncope place the patient at risk for injury. The patient may require assistance by the nurse when ambulating. Assistive devices such as walkers or canes may reduce falls. To minimize the risk of injury, the patient's environment should be controlled and safe. Encouraging the use of bedrails, keeping the bed in low position, using night lights, and frequenting monitoring by the nurse or caregiver will reduce the risk of injury. The patient should wear an identification tag, such as a medical alert bracelet.

When administering tacrine, the nurse must monitor the patient for liver damage. This is best accomplished by monitoring **alanine aminotransferase** (ALT) levels. ALT is an enzyme found predominately in the liver. Disease or injury to the liver causes a release of this enzyme into the bloodstream, resulting in elevated ALT levels. In patients taking tacrine, ALT levels should be obtained weekly from at least week 4 to week 16 after the initiation of therapy. After week 16, transaminase levels are monitored every 3 months.

> ### ✴ Nursing Alert
>
> *The nurse immediately reports any elevated alanine aminotransferase (ALT) level to the primary health care provider. The primary health care provider may want to continue monitoring the ALT level or discontinue use of the drug because of the danger of hepatotoxicity. However, abrupt discontinuation may cause a decline in cognitive functioning.*

Within 6 weeks of the discontinuation of cholinesterase inhibitor therapy, individuals lose any benefit they have received from the drugs.

Educating the Patient and Family

The patient with AD may understand and comprehend the extent and severity of this disease early on in the disease process, but as cognitive abilities decrease, the nurse will focus on educating the family and major caregiver of the patient. Depending on the degree of cognitive decline, the nurse will discuss the drug regimen with the patient, family member, and/or caregiver. It is important for the nurse to accurately evaluate the patient's ability to assume responsibility for taking drugs at home. The administration of drugs to the patient with AD becomes a family responsibility if the outpatient appears to be unable to manage his or her own drug therapy.

The nurse explains any adverse reactions that may occur with a specific antipsychotic drug and encourages the caregiver or family members to contact the primary health care provider immediately if a serious drug reaction occurs.

The nurse includes the following points in a teaching plan for the patient or family member:

- Keep all appointments with the primary care provider or clinic because close monitoring of therapy is essential. Dose changes may be needed to achieve the best results.
- Report any unusual changes or physical effects to the primary health care provider.
- Take the drug exactly as directed. Do not increase, decrease, or omit a dose or discontinue use of this drug unless directed to do so by the primary health care provider.
- Do not drive or perform other hazardous tasks if drowsiness occurs. As soon as the diagnosis of AD is made, patients should not be permitted to drive.
- Do not take any nonprescription drug unless use of a specific drug has been approved by the primary health care provider.
- Inform physicians, dentists, and other medical personnel of therapy with this drug.
- Keep track of when the drug is taken. In the early stages of forgetfulness, a mark on the calendar each time the medicine is taken or use of a pill counter that holds the medicine for each day of the week may be used to help the patient remember to take the medication or if the medication has been taken for the day.
- Notify the primary care provider if the following adverse reactions are experienced for more than a few days: nausea, diarrhea, difficulty sleeping, vomiting, or loss of appetite.
- Immediately report the occurrence of the following adverse reactions: severe vomiting, dehydration, changes in neurologic functioning, or yellowing of the skin or eyes.
- Notify the primary health care provider if you have a history of ulcers, feel faint, experience severe stomach pains, vomit blood or material that resembles coffee grounds, or have bloody or black stools.
- Remember that these drugs do not cure AD but slow the mental and physical degeneration associated with the disease.
- Remember that during tacrine therapy the ALT level must be monitored at intervals prescribed by the primary health care provider.

EVALUATION

- The therapeutic effect is achieved.
- Adverse reactions are identified, reported to the primary health care provider, and managed successfully through appropriate nursing interventions.
- No evidence of injury is seen.
- The patient (if possible), family member, or caregiver demonstrates understanding of the drug regimen.

● *Critical Thinking Exercises*

1. *A patient is prescribed tacrine (Cognex) for mild dementia related to AD. The nurse has a meeting with the patient and family. What patient assessments would you need to make before discussing the drug regimen with the patient? What would you include in a teaching plan for the patient and family?*

2. *A patient with AD is taking donepezil (Aricept). She attends an adult day care center during the day. She is not eating well and recently has lost 5 pounds. If you are the nurse at the center, what actions would you take and why would you take these particular actions?*

● *Review Questions*

1. Adverse reactions that the nurse would assess for in a patient taking rivastigmine (Exelon) include _____.

   A. occipital headache
   B. vomiting
   C. hyperactivity
   D. hypoactivity

2. When administering tacrine (Cognex) to a patient with AD the nurse would expect which of the laboratory examinations most likely to be prescribed _____.

   A. a complete blood count
   B. cholesterol levels
   C. transaminase levels
   D. electrolytes

3. Which of the following nursing diagnoses would the nurse most likely place on the care plan of a patient with AD that is related to adverse reactions of the cholinesterase inhibitors?

   A. Imbalanced nutrition
   B. Confusion
   C. Risk for suicide
   D. Bowel incontinence

4. The nurse correctly administers donepezil (Aricept) _____.

   A. three times daily around the clock.
   B. twice daily 1 hour before meals or 2 hours after meals.
   C. once daily in the morning.
   D. once daily at bedtime.

● *Medication Dosage Problems*

1. Rivastigmine (Exelon) oral solution 6 mg PO is prescribed. The drug is available as an oral solution of 2 mg/mL. The nurse administers _____.

2. Galantamine (Reminyl) 4 mg PO is prescribed for a patient with AD. On hand are 8-mg tablets. The nurse administers _____.

Antiemetic and Antivertigo Drugs

Key Terms

antiemetic
antivertigo
chemoreceptor trigger
   zone (CTZ)

nausea
vertigo
vestibular neuritis
vomiting

Chapter Objectives

On completion of this chapter, the student will:

- Define the terms nausea, vomiting, antiemetic, and antivertigo.
- Discuss the general drug actions, uses, adverse reactions, contraindications, precautions, and interactions of antiemetic and antivertigo drugs.
- Discuss important preadministration and ongoing assessment activities the nurse should perform on the patient receiving an antiemetic or antivertigo drug.
- List nursing diagnoses particular to a patient receiving an antiemetic or antivertigo drug.
- Use the nursing process when administering an antiemetic or antivertigo drug.

An **antiemetic** drug is used to treat or prevent **nausea** (unpleasant gastric sensation usually preceding vomiting) or **vomiting** (forceful expulsion of gastric contents through the mouth). An **antivertigo** drug is used to treat or prevent **vertigo** (a feeling of a spinning or rotation-type motion) that may occur with motion sickness, Ménière's disease of the ear, middle and inner ear surgery, and other disorders.

Vomiting caused by drugs, radiation, and metabolic disorders usually occurs because of stimulation of the **chemoreceptor trigger zone** (CTZ), a group of nerve fibers located on the surface of the fourth ventricle of the brain. When these fibers are stimulated by chemicals, such as drugs or toxic substances, impulses are sent to the vomiting center located in the medulla. The vomiting center may also be directly stimulated by disorders such as gastrointestinal irritation, motion sickness, and **vestibular neuritis** (inflammation of the vestibular nerve).

ACTIONS

These drugs appear to act primarily by inhibiting the CTZ or by depressing the sensitivity of the vestibular apparatus of the inner ear. Those that act on the CTZ are more effective for vomiting caused by stimulation of the CTZ, whereas those that act on the vestibular apparatus of the inner ear are more effective for vertigo associated with motion sickness and middle and inner ear surgeries.

USES

Antiemetic Drugs

An antiemetic is used to prevent (prophylaxis) or treat nausea and vomiting. An example of prophylactic use is the administration of an antiemetic before surgery to prevent vomiting during the immediate postoperative period when the patient is recovering from anesthesia. Another example is giving an antiemetic before administration of one or a combination of antineoplastic drugs (drugs used in the treatment of cancer; see Chap. 55), which have a high incidence of causing vomiting.

Dronabinol is the only currently available derivative of THC, which is a derivative of the active substance found in marijuana. Dronabinol is a second-line antiemetic and is used after treatment with other antiemetics has failed.

Other causes of nausea and vomiting that may be treated with an antiemetic include radiation therapy for a malignancy, bacterial and viral infections, nausea and vomiting caused by drugs, Ménière's disease and other ear disorders, and neurological diseases and disorders. Some of these drugs also are used to treat the nausea and vomiting seen with motion sickness. Some antiemetics also are antivertigo drugs (see the Summary Drug Table: Antiemetic and Antivertigo Drugs).

Antivertigo Drugs

An antivertigo drug is used to treat vertigo, which is usually accompanied by light-headedness, dizziness, and weakness. The individual often has difficulty walking. Some of the causes of vertigo include high alcohol consumption during a short time, certain drugs, inner ear disease, and postural hypotension. Motion sickness (seasickness, carsickness) has similar symptoms but is caused by repetitive motion (eg, riding in an airplane, boat, or car). Both vertigo and motion sickness may result in nausea and vomiting.

It is important to note that antivertigo drugs are essentially antiemetics because many of these preparations, whether used for motion sickness or vertigo, also have direct or indirect antiemetic properties. They prevent the nausea and vomiting that occur because of stimulation of the vestibular apparatus in the ear. Stimulation of this apparatus results in vertigo, which is often followed by nausea and vomiting.

ADVERSE REACTIONS

The most common adverse reactions seen with these drugs are varying degrees of drowsiness. Additional adverse reactions for each drug are listed in the Summary Drug Table: Antiemetic and Antivertigo Drugs.

CONTRAINDICATIONS

The antiemetic and antivertigo drugs are contraindicated in patients with known hypersensitivity to these drugs, those in a coma, or those with severe central nervous system (CNS) depression. In general, these drugs are not recommended during pregnancy, lactation, or for uncomplicated vomiting in young children. Metoclopramide is contraindicated in patients with a seizure disorder, breast cancer, pheochromocytoma, or gastrointestinal obstruction. Prochlorperazine is contraindicated in patients with bone marrow depression, blood dyscrasia, Parkinson's disease, or severe liver or cardiovascular disease. Thiethylperazine is classified as Pregnancy Category X and is contraindicated during pregnancy.

PRECAUTIONS

Severe nausea and vomiting should not be treated with antiemetic drugs alone. The cause of the vomiting must be investigated. Antiemetic drugs may hamper the diagnosis of disorders such as brain tumors, appendicitis, intestinal obstruction, or drug toxicity (eg, digitalis toxicity). Delayed diagnosis of any of these disorders could have serious consequences for the patient.

Antiemetics and antivertigo drugs are used cautiously in patients with glaucoma or obstructive disease of the gastrointestinal or genitourinary system, those with renal or hepatic dysfunction, and in older men with possible prostatic hypertrophy. Promethazine is used cautiously in patients with hypertension, sleep apnea, or epilepsy. Trimethobenzamide is used cautiously in children with a viral illness because it may increase the risk of Reye's syndrome.

Perphenazine, prochlorperazine, promethazine, scopolamine, chlorpromazine, and trimethobenzamide are Pregnancy Category C drugs. The pregnancy category of diphenidol is unknown. Other antiemetics and antivertigo drugs are classified as Pregnancy Category B (except for thiethylperazine, which is classified as Pregnancy Category X).

INTERACTIONS

The antiemetics and antivertigo drugs may have additive effects when used with alcohol and other CNS depressants such as sedatives, hypnotics, antianxiety drugs, opiates, and antidepressants. There may be additive anticholinergic effects (see Chap. 25) when administered with drugs that have anticholinergic activity such as the antihistamines, antidepressants, phenothiazines, and disopyramide. The antacids decrease absorption of the antiemetics.

When ondansetron is administered with rifampin, blood levels of ondansetron may be reduced, decreasing the antiemetic effect. Dimenhydrinate may mask the signs and symptoms of ototoxicity when administered with ototoxic drugs, such as the aminoglycosides (see Chap. 10), causing irreversible hearing damage. When lithium is administered with prochlorperazine, the risk of extrapyramidal reactions increases (see Chap. 32).

NURSING PROCESS

● **The Patient Receiving an Antiemetic or Antivertigo Drug**

ASSESSMENT

Preadministration Assessment

As part of the preadministration assessment for a patient receiving a drug for nausea and vomiting, the nurse documents the number of times the patient has vomited and the approximate amount of fluid lost. Before starting therapy, the nurse takes vital signs and assesses for signs of fluid and electrolyte imbalances (see Chap. 58).

Ongoing Assessment

If vomiting is severe, the nurse observes the patient for signs and symptoms of electrolyte imbalance. The nurse monitors the blood pressure, pulse, and respiratory rate every 2 to 4 hours or as ordered by the primary health care provider. The nurse carefully measures the intake and output (urine, emesis) until vomiting ceases and the patient is able to take oral fluids in sufficient quantity. The nurse documents in the patient's chart each time the patient has an emesis. The nurse notifies the primary health care provider if there is blood in the emesis or if vomiting suddenly becomes more severe.

The nurse also may need to measure the patient's weight daily to weekly in those with prolonged and repeated episodes of vomiting (eg, those receiving chemotherapy for malignant disease).

The nurse assesses the patient at frequent intervals for the effectiveness of the drug to relieve symptoms (eg, nausea, vomiting, or vertigo). The nurse notifies the primary health care provider if the drug fails to relieve or diminish symptoms.

NURSING DIAGNOSES

Drug-specific nursing diagnoses are highlighted in the Nursing Diagnoses Checklist. Other nursing diagnoses applicable to these drugs are discussed in depth in Chapter 4.

Nursing Diagnoses Checklist

✓ **Risk for Fluid Volume Deficit** related to nausea and vomiting

✓ **Risk for Injury** related to adverse drug effects of drowsiness

✓ **Altered Nutrition: Less than Body Requirements** related to impaired ability to ingest and retain food and fluids

---

PLANNING

The expected outcomes for the patient depend on the reason the antiemetic or antivertigo drug is administered but may include an optimal response to drug therapy, management of symptoms, absence of injury, and an understanding of the drug regimen.

IMPLEMENTATION

Promoting an Optimal Response to Therapy

If the patient is unable to retain the oral form of the drug, the nurse may give it parenterally or as a rectal suppository (if the prescribed drug is available in these forms). If only the oral form has been ordered and the patient is unable to retain the drug, the nurse contacts the primary health care provider regarding an order for a parenteral or suppository form of this or another antiemetic drug.

Buclizine may be taken without water. The patient is instructed to place the tablet in the mouth and allow it to dissolve or to chew or swallow the tablet whole. When given for motion sickness, one 50-mg dose is usually effective. For more extensive travel, a second 50-mg dose may be taken after 4 to 6 hours. When administering scopolamine, one transdermal system is applied behind the ear approximately 4 hours before the antiemetic effect is needed. About 1 g of scopolamine will be administered every 24 hours for 3 days. If the disk detaches from the body, discard it and place a fresh one behind the opposite ear. (See Patient and Family Teaching Checklist: Applying Transdermal Scopolamine.)

PREVENTION OF NAUSEA IN PATIENTS WITH CANCER. Granisetron (Kytril), ondansetron (Zofran), dolasetron (Anzemet), and dronabinol (Marinol) are examples of antiemetics used to prevent nausea and vomiting after cancer (antineoplastic) chemotherapy. The nurse administers these drugs on the day the chemotherapy is given. The nurse may give granisetron and ondansetron intravenously. The nurse mixes the drug according to the manufacturer's directions and administers it about 30 minutes before administration of an antineoplastic drug. The nurse may give ondansetron orally 30 minutes before antineoplastic therapy, as well as for 1 to 2 days after, to prevent or relieve nausea and vomiting. The nurse gives dolasetron orally within 1 hour before chemotherapy. It is important to give dronabinol, which has abuse potential, orally 1 to 3 hours before administration of an antineoplastic drug, then every 2 to 4 hours after chemotherapy. These drugs have been effective in relieving or eliminating nausea and vomiting after antineoplastic therapy.

Managing Patient Symptoms

Dehydration is a serious concern in the patient experiencing nausea and vomiting. It is important to observe

Patient and Family Teaching Checklist

Applying Transdermal Scopolamine

The nurse:

✔ Instructs the patient to apply the transdermal scopolamine system behind the ear.

✔ Explains that after application of the system, the hands are washed *thoroughly* with soap and water and dried. The importance of thorough hand washing to prevent any traces of the drug from coming in contact with the eyes is emphasized.

✔ Teaches that the disk will last about 3 days, at which time the patient may apply another disk, if needed.

✔ Instructs the patient to discard the used disk and thoroughly wash and dry the hands and previous application site.

✔ Instructs the patient to apply the new disk behind the opposite ear and to again thoroughly wash and dry the hands.

✔ Emphasizes that only one disk at a time is used.

✔ Makes sure that the patient has a thorough knowledge of the adverse reactions that may occur with the use of this system: dizziness, dry mouth, and blurred vision.

✔ Stresses the importance of observing caution when driving or performing hazardous tasks.

the patient for signs of dehydration, which include poor skin turgor, dry mucous membranes, decrease in or absence of urinary output, concentrated urine, restlessness, irritability, increased respiratory rate, and confusion. If the patient is able to take and retain small amounts of oral fluids, the nurse offers sips of water at frequent intervals. In addition, it is important to observe the patient for signs of electrolyte imbalance, particularly sodium and potassium deficit (see Chap. 58). If signs of dehydration or electrolyte imbalance are noted, the nurse contacts the primary health care provider because parenteral administration of fluids or fluids with electrolytes may be necessary.

❄ Gerontologic Alert

Observations for fluid and electrolyte disturbances are particularly important in the aged or chronically ill patient in whom severe dehydration may develop in a short time. The nurse must immediately report symptoms of dehydration, such as dry mucous membranes, decreased urinary output, concentrated urine, restlessness, or confusion in the older adult.

Nausea, vomiting, vertigo, and dizziness are disagreeable sensations. The nurse changes the patient's bedding and patient's clothing or gown as needed because the odor of vomitus may only intensify these sensations. The nurse provides the patient with an emesis basin and checks the basin at frequent intervals. If an emesis occurs, the nurse empties the basin and measures and documents the vomitus in the patient's chart. The nurse may give the patient a damp washcloth and a towel to wipe the hands and face as needed. It also is a good idea to give the patient mouthwash or frequent oral rinses to remove the disagreeable taste that accompanies vomiting.

☀ Nursing Alert

Many of these drugs cause variable degrees of drowsiness. The nurse advises the patient to seek help when getting out of bed if drowsiness occurs.

Preventing Injury

Administration of these drugs may result in varying degrees of drowsiness. To prevent accidental falls and other injuries, the nurse assists the patient who is allowed out of bed with ambulatory activities. If extreme drowsiness is noted, the nurse instructs the patient to remain in bed and provides a call light for assistance.

Educating the Patient and Family

When an antiemetic or antivertigo drug is prescribed for outpatient use, the nurse includes the following information in a patient teaching plan:

● Avoid driving or performing other hazardous tasks when taking this drug because drowsiness may occur with use.

● Contact the primary health care provider if nausea, vomiting, or vertigo persists or worsens.

● Use only as directed. Do not increase the dose or frequency of use unless told to do so by the primary health care provider.

● Avoid the use of alcohol and other sedative-type drugs unless use has been approved by the primary health care provider.

● Take the drug about 1 hour before travel for motion sickness. Buclizine may be taken without water. Place the tablet in the mouth and allow it to dissolve or chew or swallow the tablet whole.

● Take granisetron (Kytril), dronabinol (Marinol), or ondansetron (Zofran) before antineoplastic chemotherapy (oral, intravenous) about 30 minutes before the chemotherapy treatment. Take dolasetron mesylate (Anzemet) orally at least 1 hour before chemotherapy. After the treatment, take the prescribed antiemetic at the time recommended by the primary health care provider or printed on the drug container.

- Follow the directions for application of transdermal scopolamine that are supplied with the drug (see Patient and Family Teaching Checklist: Applying Transdermal Scopolamine).

EVALUATION

- The therapeutic effect is achieved; nausea or vertigo is controlled.
- Adverse reactions are identified, reported to the primary health care provider, and managed successfully through appropriate nursing interventions.
- No evidence of a fluid volume deficit or electrolyte imbalance is seen.
- No evidence of injury is apparent.
- The patient verbalizes the importance of complying with the prescribed treatment regimen.
- The patient or family demonstrates an understanding of the drug regimen.

● Critical Thinking Exercises

1. *Ms. Davis was prescribed meclizine (Antivert-50) 50 mg for motion sickness. On return from a long car ride she tells you that the medicine did not help. Explain what questions you would ask to determine if Ms. Davis followed the prescribed drug regimen.*

2. *Mr. Collins is prescribed transdermal scopolamine to relieve motion sickness. Discuss the rationale you would give him to stress the importance of washing his hands after applying or removing the transdermal system.*

3. *Discuss the ongoing assessment needs of a patient receiving an antiemetic before chemotherapy for cancer.*

4. *In assessing Ms. Potter, age 52 years, in the emergency department you find that she has a decreased urinary output, concentrated urine, and poor skin turgor and is confused. She reports nausea and states she has been "vomiting all morning." Explain what is the most important information obtained from your assessment of Ms. Potter. Determine what action you would take first.*

● Review Questions

1. What is the most common adverse reaction the nurse would expect in a patient receiving an antiemetic?
   A. Occipital headache
   B. Drowsiness
   C. Edema
   D. Nausea

2. When explaining how to use transdermal scopolamine the nurse tells the patient to apply the system to _____.
   A. a nonhairy region of the chest
   B. on the upper back
   C. behind the ear
   D. on the forearm

3. When an antivertigo drug is prescribed for a patient experiencing motion sickness, the nurse advises the patient to _____.
   A. avoid driving or performing hazardous tasks
   B. administer the drug at least 6 hours before travel
   C. take the drug with food immediately before traveling
   D. take the drug at the first sign of motion sickness

4. Which of these drugs is a Pregnancy Category X drug and should not be administered to a pregnant woman?
   A. Dimenhydrinate
   B. Scopolamine
   C. Promethazine
   D. Thiethylperazine

● Medication Dosage Problems

1. Ondansetron 4 mg is prescribed. The drug is available as a solution of 2 mg/mL. The nurse administers _____.

2. Diphenhydramine 50 is prescribed. The drug is available in 25-mg tablets. The nurse administers _____.

3. Compazine 2.5 mg PO is prescribed. Use the drug label below to prepare the correct dosage. The nurse would administer _____.

Store between 15° and 30°C (59° and 86°F). Dispense in a tight, light-resistant container. Each tablet contains prochlorperazine, 5 mg, as the maleate. **Usual Dosage:** 10 to 40 mg daily. See accompanying prescribing information. **Important:** Use safety closures when dispensing this product unless otherwise directed by physician or requested by purchaser.

GlaxoSmithKline
Research Triangle Park, NC 27709
731561-AD

NDC 0007-3366-20   **5mg**

COMPAZINE®
PROCHLORPERAZINE
as the maleate TABLETS
100 Tablets

gsk GlaxoSmithKline   ℞ only

Anesthetic Drugs

Anesthesia is a loss of feeling or sensation. Anesthesia may be induced by various drugs that are able to bring about partial or complete loss of sensation. There are two types of anesthesia: local anesthesia and general anesthesia. **Local anesthesia**, as the term implies, is the provision of a pain-free state in a specific area (or region). With a local anesthetic, the patient is fully awake but does not feel pain in the area that has been anesthetized. However, some procedures done under local anesthesia may require the patient to be sedated. Although not fully awake, sedated patients may still hear what is going on around them. **General anesthesia** is the provision of a pain-free state for the entire body. When a general anesthetic is given, the patient loses consciousness and feels no pain. Reflexes, such as the swallowing and gag reflexes, are lost during deep general anesthesia (Fig. 35-1). An **anesthesiologist** is a physician with special training in administering anesthesia. A nurse **anesthetist** is a nurse with special training who is qualified to administer anesthetics.

LOCAL ANESTHESIA

The various methods of administering a local anesthetic include topical application, local infiltration, or regional anesthesia.

Topical Anesthesia

Topical anesthesia involves the application of the anesthetic to the surface of the skin, open area, or mucous membrane. The anesthetic may be applied with a cotton swab or sprayed on the area. This type of anesthesia may be used to desensitize the skin or mucous membrane to the injection of a deeper local anesthetic. In some instances, topical anesthetics may be applied by the nurse.

Local Infiltration Anesthesia

Local infiltration anesthesia is the injection of a local anesthetic drug into tissues. This type of anesthesia may be used for dental procedures, the suturing of small wounds, or making an incision into a small area, such as that required for removing a superficial piece of tissue for biopsy.

Regional Anesthesia

Regional anesthesia is the injection of a local anesthetic around nerves so that the area supplied by these nerves will not send pain signals to the brain. The anesthetized area is usually larger than the area affected by

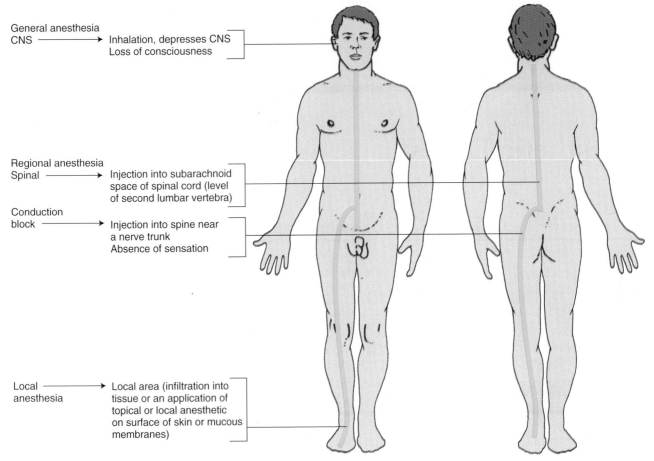

General anesthesia
CNS ——————→ Inhalation, depresses CNS
Loss of consciousness

Regional anesthesia
Spinal ——————→ Injection into subarachnoid
space of spinal cord (level
of second lumbar vertebra)

Conduction
block ——————→ Injection into spine near
a nerve trunk
Absence of sensation

Local ——————→ Local area (infiltration into
anesthesia   tissue or an application of
topical or local anesthetic
on surface of skin or mucous
membranes)

FIGURE 35-1. Sites and mechanisms of action of drugs used for anesthesia.

local infiltration anesthesia. Spinal anesthesia and conduction blocks are two types of regional anesthesia.

Spinal Anesthesia

Spinal anesthesia is a type of regional anesthesia that involves the injection of a local anesthetic drug into the subarachnoid space of the spinal cord, usually at the level of the second lumbar vertebra. There is a loss of feeling (anesthesia) and movement in the lower extremities, lower abdomen, and perineum.

Conduction Blocks

A **conduction block** is a type of regional anesthesia produced by injection of a local anesthetic drug into or near a nerve trunk. Examples of a conduction block include an **epidural block** (injection of a local anesthetic into the space surrounding the dura of the spinal cord); a **transsacral** (caudal) **block** (injection of a local anesthetic into the epidural space at the level of the sacrococcygeal notch); and **brachial plexus block** (injection of a local anesthetic into the brachial plexus). Epidural, especially, and transsacral blocks are often used in obstetrics. A brachial plexus block may be used for surgery of the arm or hand.

Preparing the Patient for Local Anesthesia

Depending on the procedure performed, preparing the patient for local anesthesia may or may not be similar to preparing the patient for general anesthesia. For example, administering a local anesthetic for dental surgery or for suturing a small wound may require that the nurse explain to the patient how the anesthetic will be administered, take a patient's allergy history, and when applicable, prepare the area to be anesthetized, which may involve cleaning the area with an antiseptic or shaving the area. Other local anesthetic procedures may require the patient to be in a fasting state because a sedative may also be administered. The nurse may administer an intravenous sedative such as the antianxiety drug diazepam (Valium) (see Chap. 30) during some local anesthetic procedures, such as cataract surgery or surgery performed under spinal anesthesia.

Administering Local Anesthesia

The physician or dentist administers a local injectable anesthetic. Table 35-1 lists the more commonly used local anesthetics.

TABLE 35-1	EXAMPLES OF LOCAL ANESTHETICS

GENERIC NAME	TRADE NAME*
articaine HCl	Septocaine
bupivacaine HCl	Marcaine HCl, *generic*
chloroprocaine HCl	Nesacaine, Nescaine-MPF
lidocaine HCl	Dilocaine, Xylocaine, *generic*
mepivacaine HCl	Carbocaine, Isocaine HCl
prilocaine HCl	Citanest HCl
procaine HCl, injectable	Novocain, *generic*
ropivacaine	Naropin
tetracaine HCl	Pontocaine HCl

*The term *generic* indicates the drug is available in generic form.

Nursing Responsibilities When Caring for a Patient Receiving Local Anesthesia

When applicable, the nurse may be responsible for applying a dressing to the area. Depending on the reason for using local anesthesia, the nurse also may be responsible for observing the area for bleeding, oozing, or other problems after the administration of the anesthetic.

PREANESTHETIC DRUGS

A **preanesthetic drug** is one given before the administration of anesthesia. The nurse usually gives a preanesthetic drug before the administration of general anesthesia but on occasion may give it before injection of the local anesthetic to sedate the patient. The preanesthetic may consist of one drug or a combination of drugs.

Purpose of Preanesthetic Drugs

The general purpose of the preanesthetic drug is to prepare the patient for anesthesia. The more specific purposes of these drugs include the following:

- Narcotic or antianxiety drug—to decrease anxiety and apprehension immediately before surgery. The patient who is calm and relaxed can be anesthetized more quickly, usually requires a smaller dose of an induction drug, may require less anesthesia during surgery, and may have a smoother anesthesia recovery period (awakening from anesthesia).
- Cholinergic blocking drug—to decrease secretions of the upper respiratory tract. Some anesthetic gases and volatile liquids are irritating to the lining of the respiratory tract and thereby increase mucous secretions. The cough and swallowing reflexes are lost during general anesthesia, and excessive secretions can pool in the lungs, resulting in pneumonia or atelectasis during the postoperative period. The

administration of a cholinergic blocking drug, such as glycopyrrolate (Robinul) dries up secretions of the upper respiratory tract and lessens the possibility of excessive mucous production.
- Antiemetic—to lessen the incidence of nausea and vomiting during the immediate postoperative recovery period.

❄ Gerontologic Alert

Preanesthetic drugs may be omitted in those 60 years or older because many of the medical disorders for which these drugs are contraindicated are seen in older individuals. For example, atropine and glycopyrrolate, drugs that can be used to decrease secretions of the upper respiratory tract, are contraindicated in certain medical disorders, such as prostatic hypertrophy, glaucoma, and myocardial ischemia. Other preanesthetic drugs that depress the central nervous system (CNS), such as narcotics, barbiturates, and antianxiety drugs with or without antiemetic properties, may be contraindicated in the older individual.

Selection of Preanesthetic Drugs

The preanesthetic drug is usually selected by the anesthesiologist and may consist of one or more drugs (Table 35-2). A narcotic (see Chap. 19), antianxiety drug (see Chap. 30), or barbiturate (see Chap. 26) may be given to

TABLE 35-2	EXAMPLES OF PREANESTHETIC DRUGS

GENERIC NAME	TRADE NAME*
Narcotics	
droperidol	Inapsine
fentanyl	Sublimaze, *generic*
meperidine hydrochloride	Demerol, *generic*
morphine sulfate	Duramorph, *generic*
Barbiturates	
pentobarbital	Nembutal Sodium, *generic*
secobarbital	*generic*
Cholinergic-Blocking Drugs	
atropine sulfate	*generic*
glycopyrrolate	Robinul, *generic*
scopolamine	*generic*
Antianxiety Drugs With Antiemetic Properties	
hydroxyzine	Atarax, Vistaril, *generic*
Antianxiety Drugs	
chlordiazepoxide	Librium, *generic*
diazepam	Valium, *generic*
midazolam	Versed

*The term *generic* indicates the drug is available in generic form.

relax or sedate the patient. Barbiturates are used only occasionally; narcotics are usually preferred for sedation. A cholinergic blocking drug (see Chap. 25) is given to dry secretions in the upper respiratory tract. Scopolamine and glycopyrrolate also have mild sedative properties, and atropine may or may not produce some sedation. Antianxiety drugs have sedative action; when combined with a narcotic, they allow for a lowering of the narcotic dosage because they also have the ability to potentiate the sedative action of the narcotic. Diazepam (Valium), an antianxiety drug, is one of the more commonly used drugs for preoperative sedation.

Nursing Responsibilities When Caring for a Patient Receiving a Preanesthetic Drug

The nurse evaluates the patient's physical status and gives an explanation of the anesthesia. In some hospitals, the anesthesiologist examines the patient the day or evening before surgery, although this may not be possible in emergency situations. Some hospitals use members of the operating room or postanesthesia recovery room staff to visit the patient the night before or the morning of surgery to explain certain facts, such as the time of surgery, the effects of the preanesthetic drug, preparations for surgery, and the postanesthesia recovery room. Proper explanation of anesthesia, the surgery itself, and the events that may occur in preparation for surgery, as well as care after surgery, require a team approach. The nurse's responsibilities include the following:

- The nurse describes or explains the preparations for surgery ordered by the physician. Examples of preoperative preparations include fasting from midnight (or the time specified by the physician), enemas, shaving of the operative site, use of a hypnotic for sleep the night before, and the preoperative injection about 30 minutes before going to surgery.
- The nurse describes or explains immediate postoperative care, such as the postanesthesia recovery room or a special postoperative surgical unit and the activities of the physicians and nurses during this period. The nurse tells the patient that his or her vital signs will be monitored frequently and that other equipment, such as intravenous fluids and monitors, may be used.
- The nurse describes, explains, and demonstrates postoperative patient activities, such as deep breathing, coughing, and leg exercises.
- The nurse tailors the preoperative explanations to fit the type of surgery scheduled. Not all of these teaching points may be included in every explanation.

GENERAL ANESTHESIA

The administration of general anesthesia requires the use of one or more drugs. The choice of anesthetic drug depends on many factors, including:

- The general physical condition of the patient
- The area, organ, or system being operated on
- The anticipated length of the surgical procedure

The anesthesiologist selects the anesthetic drugs that will produce safe anesthesia, **analgesia** (absence of pain), and in some surgeries, effective skeletal muscle relaxation. General anesthesia is most commonly achieved when the anesthetic vapors are inhaled or administered intravenously (IV). Volatile liquid anesthetics produce anesthesia when their vapors are inhaled. **Volatile liquid**s are liquids that evaporate on exposure to air. Examples of volatile liquids include halothane, desflurane, and enflurane. Gas anesthetics are combined with oxygen and administered by inhalation. Examples of gas anesthetics are nitrous oxide and cyclopropane.

Drugs Used for General Anesthesia

Methohexital and Thiopental

Methohexital (Brevital) and thiopental (Pentothal), which are ultrashort-acting barbiturates, are used for:

- Induction of anesthesia
- Short surgical procedures with minimal painful stimuli
- In conjunction with or as a supplement to other anesthetics
- Control of convulsive states (thiopental)

These drugs have a rapid onset and a short duration of action. They depress the central nervous system (CNS) to produce hypnosis and anesthesia but do not produce analgesia. Recovery after a small dose is rapid.

Etomidate

Etomidate (Amidate), a nonbarbiturate, is used for induction of anesthesia. Etomidate also may be used to supplement other anesthetics, such as nitrous oxide, for short surgical procedures. It is a hypnotic without analgesic activity.

Propofol

Propofol (Diprivan) is used for induction and maintenance of anesthesia. It also may be used for sedation during diagnostic procedures and procedures that use a local anesthetic. This drug also is used for continuous sedation of intubated or respiratory-controlled patients in intensive care units.

Midazolam

Midazolam (Versed), a short-acting benzodiazepine CNS depressant, is used as a preanesthetic drug to relieve anxiety; for induction of anesthesia; for conscious sedation before minor procedures, such as endoscopic procedures; and to supplement nitrous oxide and oxygen for short surgical procedures. When the drug is used for induction anesthesia, the patient gradually loses consciousness during a period of 1 to 2 minutes.

Sevoflurane

Sevoflurane (Ultane) is an inhalational analgesic. It is used for induction and maintenance of general anesthesia in adult and pediatric patients for inpatient and outpatient surgical procedures.

Ketamine

Ketamine (Ketalar) is a rapid-acting general anesthetic. It produces an anesthetic state characterized by profound analgesia, cardiovascular and respiratory stimulation, normal or enhanced skeletal muscle tone, and occasionally mild respiratory depression. Ketamine is used for diagnostic and surgical procedures that do not require relaxation of skeletal muscles, for induction of anesthesia before the administration of other anesthetic drugs, and as a supplement to other anesthetic drugs.

Cyclopropane

An anesthetic gas, cyclopropane has a rapid onset of action and may be used for induction and maintenance of anesthesia. Skeletal muscle relaxation is produced with full anesthetic doses. Cyclopropane is supplied in orange cylinders. Disadvantages of cyclopropane are difficulty in detecting the planes of anesthesia, occasional laryngospasm, cardiac arrhythmias, and postanesthesia nausea, vomiting, and headache. Cyclopropane and oxygen mixtures are explosive, which limits the use of this gas anesthetic.

Ethylene

Ethylene is an anesthetic gas with a rapid onset of action and a rapid recovery from its anesthetic effects. It provides adequate analgesia but has poor muscle-relaxant properties. The advantages of ethylene include minimal bronchospasm, laryngospasm, and postanesthesia vomiting. A disadvantage of ethylene is hypoxia. This gas is supplied in red cylinders. Mixtures of ethylene and oxygen are flammable and explosive.

Nitrous Oxide

Nitrous oxide is the most commonly used anesthetic gas. It is a weak anesthetic and is usually used in combination with other anesthetic drugs. It does not cause skeletal muscle relaxation. The chief danger in the use of nitrous oxide is hypoxemia. Nitrous oxide is nonexplosive and is supplied in blue cylinders.

Enflurane

Enflurane (Ethrane) is a volatile liquid anesthetic that is delivered by inhalation. Induction and recovery from anesthesia are rapid. Muscle relaxation for abdominal surgery is adequate, but greater relaxation may be necessary and may require the use of a skeletal muscle relaxant. Enflurane may produce mild stimulation of respiratory and bronchial secretions when used alone. Hypotension may occur when anesthesia deepens.

Halothane

Halothane (Fluothane) is a volatile liquid given by inhalation for induction and maintenance of anesthesia. Induction and recovery from anesthesia are rapid, and the depth of anesthesia can be rapidly altered. Halothane does not irritate the respiratory tract, and an increase in tracheobronchial secretions usually does not occur. Halothane produces moderate muscle relaxation, but skeletal muscle relaxants may be used in certain types of surgeries. This anesthetic may be given with a mixture of nitrous oxide and oxygen.

Isoflurane

Isoflurane (Forane) is a volatile liquid given by inhalation. It is used for induction and maintenance of anesthesia.

Methoxyflurane

Methoxyflurane (Penthrane), a volatile liquid, provides analgesia and anesthesia. It is usually used in combination with nitrous oxide but may also be used alone. It does not produce good muscle relaxation, and a skeletal muscle relaxant may be required.

Desflurane

Desflurane (Suprane), a volatile liquid, is used for induction and maintenance of anesthesia. A special vaporizer is used to deliver this anesthetic because delivery by mask results in irritation of the respiratory tract.

Fentanyl and Droperidol

The narcotic analgesic fentanyl (Sublimaze) and the neuroleptic (major tranquilizer) droperidol (Inapsine) may be used together as a single drug called Innovar. The combination of these two drugs results in **neuroleptanalgesia**, which is characterized by general quietness, reduced motor activity, and profound analgesia. Complete loss of consciousness may not occur unless other anesthetic drugs are used. A combination of fentanyl and droperidol may be used for the tranquilizing effect and analgesia for surgical and diagnostic procedures. It may also be used as a preanesthetic for the induction of anesthesia and in the maintenance of general anesthesia.

Droperidol may be used alone as a tranquilizer, as an antiemetic to reduce nausea and vomiting during the immediate postanesthesia period, as an induction drug, and as an adjunct to general anesthesia. Fentanyl may be used alone as a supplement to general or regional anesthesia. It may also be administered alone or with other drugs as a preoperative drug and as an analgesic during the immediate postoperative (recovery room) period.

Remifentanil Hydrochloride

Remifentanil (Ultiva) is used for induction and maintenance of general anesthesia and for continued analgesia during the immediate postoperative period. This drug is used cautiously in patients with a history of hypersensitivity to fentanyl.

Skeletal Muscle Relaxants

The various skeletal muscle relaxants that may be used during general anesthesia are listed in Table 35-3. These drugs are administered to produce relaxation of the skeletal muscles during certain types of surgeries, such as those involving the chest or abdomen. They may also be used to facilitate the insertion of an endotracheal tube. Their onset of action is usually rapid (45 seconds to a few minutes), and the duration of action is 30 minutes or more.

TABLE 35-3	Examples of Muscle Relaxants Used During General Anesthesia
GENERIC NAME	**TRADE NAME***
atracurium besylate	Tracrium
cisatracurium besylate	Nimbex
doxacurium chloride	Nuromax
metocurine iodide	Metubine Iodine, *generic*
mivacurium chloride	Mivacron
pancuronium bromide	Pavulon, *generic*
pipecuronium bromide	Arduan
rapacuronium bromide	Raplon
rocuronium bromide	Zemuron
succinylcholine chloride	Anectine, *generic*
tubocurarine chloride	*generic*
vecuronium bromide	Norcuron, *generic*

*The term *generic* indicates that the drug is available in generic form.

Stages of General Anesthesia

General surgical anesthesia is divided into the following stages:

- Stage I—analgesia
- Stage II—delirium
- Stage III—surgical analgesia
- Stage IV—respiratory paralysis

Display 35-1 describes the stages of general anesthesia more completely.

With newer drugs and techniques, the stages of anesthesia may not be as prominent as those described in Display 35-1. In addition, movement through the first two stages is usually very rapid.

Anesthesia begins with a loss of consciousness. This is part of the induction stage (stage I). The patient is now relaxed and can no longer see or hear what is going on. After consciousness is lost, additional anesthetic drugs are administered. Some of these drugs are also used as part of the induction phase, as well as for deepening anesthesia. Depending on the type of surgery, an endotracheal tube also may be inserted into the trachea to provide an adequate airway and to assist in the administration of oxygen and other anesthetic drugs. The endotracheal tube is removed during the postanesthesia period once the gag and swallowing reflexes have returned. If an intravenous line was not inserted before the patient's

---

DISPLAY 35-1 ● Stages of General Anesthesia

STAGE I

Induction is a part of stage I anesthesia. It begins with the administration of an anesthetic drug and lasts until consciousness is lost. With some induction drugs, such as the short-acting barbiturates, this stage may last only 5 to 10 seconds.

STAGE II

Stage II is the stage of delirium and excitement. This stage is also brief. During this stage, the patient may move about and mumble incoherently. The muscles are somewhat rigid, and the patient is unconscious and cannot feel pain. During this stage, noises are exaggerated and even quiet sounds may seem extremely loud to the patient. If surgery were attempted at this stage, there would be a physical reaction to painful stimuli, yet the patient would not remember sensing pain. During these first two stages of anesthesia, the nurse and other health care professionals avoid any unnecessary noise or motion.

STAGE III

Stage III is the stage of surgical analgesia and is divided into four parts, planes, or substages. The anesthesiologist differentiates these planes by the character of the respirations, eye movements, certain reflexes, pupil size, and other factors. The levels of the planes range from plane 1 (light) to plane 4 (deep). At plane 2 or 3, the patient is usually ready for the surgical procedure.

STAGE IV

Stage IV is the stage of respiratory paralysis and is a rare and dangerous stage of anesthesia. At this stage, respiratory arrest and cessation of all vital signs may occur.

arrival in surgery, it is inserted by the anesthesiologist before the administration of an induction drug.

Nursing Responsibilities During the Administration of General Anesthesia

Preanesthesia

Before surgery, the nurse has the following responsibilities:

- Performing the required tasks and procedures as prescribed by the physician and hospital policy the day or evening before or the morning of surgery and recording these tasks on the patient's chart. Examples of these tasks include administration of a hypnotic the night before surgery, shaving the operative area, taking vital signs, seeing that the operative consent is signed, checking to see if all jewelry or metal objects are removed, administering enemas, inserting a catheter, inserting a nasogastric tube, and teaching.
- Checking the chart for any recent, abnormal laboratory tests. If a recent, abnormal laboratory test was attached to the patient's chart shortly before surgery, the nurse must make sure that the surgeon and the anesthesiologist are aware of the abnormality. The nurse can attach a note to the front of the chart and contact the surgeon or anesthesiologist by telephone.
- Placing a list of known or suspected drug allergies or idiosyncrasies on the front of the chart.
- Administering the preanesthetic (preoperative) drug.
- Instructing the patient to remain in bed and placing the side rails up once the preanesthetic drug has been given.

☀ Nursing Alert

Preanesthetic drugs must be administered on time to produce their intended effects. Failure to give the preanesthetic drug on time may result in events such as increased respiratory secretions caused by the irritating effect of anesthetic gases and the need for an increased dose of the induction drug because the preanesthetic drug has not had time to sedate the patient.

Postanesthesia: Recovery Room

After surgery, the nurse has the following responsibilities, which vary according to where the nurse first sees the postoperative patient:

- Admitting the patient to the unit according to hospital procedure or policy.
- Checking the airway for patency, assessing the respiratory status, and giving oxygen as needed.

- Positioning the patient to prevent aspiration of vomitus and secretions.
- Checking blood pressure, pulse, intravenous lines, catheters, drainage tubes, surgical dressings, and casts.
- Reviewing the patient's surgical and anesthesia records.
- Monitoring the blood pressure, pulse, and respiratory rate every 5 to 15 minutes until the patient is discharged from the area.
- Checking the patient every 5 to 15 minutes for emergence from anesthesia. Suctioning is provided as needed.
- Exercising caution in administering narcotics. The nurse must check the patient's respiratory rate, blood pressure, and pulse before these drugs are given and 20 to 30 minutes after administration (see Chap. 20). The physician is contacted if the respiratory rate is below 10 before the drug is given or if the respirations fall below 10 after the drug is given.
- Discharging the patient from the area to his or her room or other specified area. The nurse must record all drugs administered and nursing tasks performed before the patient leaves the postanesthesia recovery room.

● *Critical Thinking Exercises*

1. *Mr. Cantu's family asks you why a drug is being given before he goes to surgery for a bowel resection. When checking the chart, you note that Mr. Cantu has an order for meperidine HCl (Demerol) 50 mg IM and glycopyrrolate (Robinul) 0.35 mg IM 30 minutes before surgery. Describe how you would explain to the family the purpose of the preanesthetic drugs that are to be given to Mr. Cantu.*

2. *A nurse you are working with complains she was reprimanded and asked to fill out an incident report for not giving a preanesthetic drug on time. She states that she feels she is being unfairly accused of an error because the drug was given 10 minutes before the patient was taken to surgery. Justify why this is a potentially serious error.*

3. *Discuss the most important responsibilities of the nurse in the recovery room after a patient has undergone general anesthesia.*

● *Review Questions*

1. When planning preoperative care, the nurse expects that a preanesthetic medication usually is given _____ before the patient is transported to surgery.

   A. 20 minutes
   B. 30 minutes
   C. 40 minutes
   D. 60 minutes

2. Which of the following drugs is the most commonly used gas for general anesthesia?
   A. Ehylene
   B. Eflurane
   C. Nitrous oxide
   D. Sevoflurane

3. Neuroleptanalgesia is used to promote general quietness, reduced motor activity, and profound analgesia. Which of the following two drugs are used in combination to accomplish neuroleptanalgesia?
   A. Fentanyl and droperidol
   B. Morphine and glycopyrrolate
   C. Atropine and meperidine
   D. Fentanyl and midazolam

4. One use of skeletal muscle relaxants as part of general anesthesia is to _____.
   A. prevent movement during surgery
   B. facilitate insertion of the endotracheal tube
   C. allow for deeper anesthesia
   D. produce additional anesthesia

● *Medication Dosage Problems*

1. As a preoperative medication for a patient going to surgery, the anesthesiologist prescribes meperidine HCl (Demerol) 50 mg IM. Meperidine is available in solution of 50 mg/mL. The nurse prepares to administer _____.

2. Glycopyrrolate (Robinul) is prescribed for a patient as part of the preoperative preparation for surgery. The drug dose recommendation is 0.002 mg/lb. The patient weighs 150 pounds. The nurse expects the primary care provider to prescribe _____.

chapter **36**

Antihistamines and Decongestants

Key Terms

anticholinergic effects
antihistamine

decongestant
histamine

Chapter Objectives

On completion of this chapter, the student will:

- Describe the uses, general drug action, general adverse reactions, contraindications, precautions, and interactions of the antihistamines and decongestants.
- Discuss important preadministration and ongoing assessment activities the nurse should perform on the patient taking an antihistamine or a decongestant.
- List some nursing diagnoses particular to a patient taking an antihistamine or a decongestant.
- Discuss ways to promote an optimal response to therapy, how to manage common adverse reactions, and important points to keep in mind when educating a patient about the use of an antihistamine or a decongestant.

The respiratory system consists of the upper and lower airways, the lungs, and the thoracic cavity. The function of the respiratory system is to provide a mechanism for the exchange of oxygen and carbon dioxide in the lungs. Any change in the respiratory status has the potential to affect every other body system because all cells need an adequate supply of oxygen for optimal functioning. This chapter focuses on drugs used to treat some of the more common disorders affecting the respiratory system, particularly allergies and the congestion associated with certain respiratory disorders.

ANTIHISTAMINES

Histamine is a substance present in various tissues of the body, such as the heart, lungs, gastric mucosa, and skin (Fig. 36-1). The highest concentration of histamine is found in the basophil (a type of white blood cell) and mast cells that are found near capillaries. Histamine is produced in response to injury. It acts on areas such as the vascular system and smooth muscle, producing dilatation of arterioles and an increased permeability of capillaries and venules. Dilatation of the arterioles results in localized redness. An increase in the permeability of

small blood vessels produces an escape of fluid from these blood vessels into the surrounding tissues, which produces localized swelling. Thus, the release of histamine produces an inflammatory response. Histamine is also released in allergic reactions or hypersensitivity reactions, such as anaphylactic shock.

Antihistamines are drugs used to counteract the effects of histamine on body organs and structures. Examples of antihistamines include diphenhydramine (Benadryl), loratadine (Claritin), fexofenadine (Allegra), and cetirizine (Zyrtec). A new antihistamine, desloratadine (Clarinex), is the active metabolite of loratadine and is intended to eventually replace loratadine (Claritin). Topical corticosteroid nasal sprays such as fluticasone propionate (Flonase) or triamcinolone acetonide (Nasacort AQ) are also used for nasal allergy symptoms. See Chapter 56 for more information on the topical corticosteroids.

ACTIONS

Antihistamines block most, but not all, of the effects of histamine. They do this by competing for histamine at histamine receptor sites, thereby preventing histamine

325

retention, pyloroduodenal obstruction, or hyperthyroidism.

INTERACTIONS

There is an increase in anticholinergic effects when antihistamines are administered with the monamine oxidase inhibitors (MAOIs) and additive sedative effects if administered with central nervous system depressants (eg, narcotic analgesics or alcohol). When cimetidine and loratadine are administered together there is a risk for increased loratadine levels.

NURSING PROCESS

● **The Patient Receiving an Antihistamine**

ASSESSMENT

Preadministration Assessment
The preadministration assessment of the patient receiving these drugs depends on the reason for use. Examples of assessments the nurse may perform include an assessment of the involved areas (eyes, nose, and upper and lower respiratory tract) if the patient is receiving an antihistamine for the relief of symptoms of an allergy. If promethazine (Phenergan) is used with a narcotic to enhance the effects and reduce the dosage of the narcotic, the nurse should take the patient's blood pressure, pulse, and respiratory rate before giving the drug.

Ongoing Assessment
The nurse usually gives these drugs in the outpatient setting. If the patient is in the hospital or clinic, the nurse observes the patient for the expected effects of the antihistamine and for adverse reactions. The nurse reports adverse reactions to the primary health care provider. In some instances, drowsiness or sedation may occur. When the drug is given to relieve preoperative anxiety, these adverse reactions are expected and are allowed to occur.

If the antihistamine is given for a serious situation, such as a blood transfusion reaction or a severe drug allergy, the nurse assesses the patient at frequent intervals until the symptoms appear relieved and for about 24 hours after the incident.

NURSING DIAGNOSES

Drug-specific nursing diagnoses are highlighted in the Nursing Diagnoses Checklist. Other nursing diagnoses applicable to these drugs are discussed in depth in Chapter 4.

Nursing Diagnoses Checklist

☑ **Impaired Oral Mucous Membranes** related to adverse drug effects (dry mouth, nose, and throat)

☑ **Risk for Injury** related to adverse drug reactions (drowsiness, dizziness, disturbed coordination)

PLANNING

The expected outcomes of the patient vary according to the reason the drug was administered and may include an optimal response to drug therapy, management of common adverse drug reactions, and an understanding of and compliance with the prescribed therapeutic regimen.

IMPLEMENTATION

Promoting an Optimal Response to Therapy
Most antihistamines are given orally with food to prevent gastrointestinal upset. The nurse gives loratadine to the patient whose stomach is empty, at least 2 hours after meals or 1 hour before meals. Loratadine disintegrating tablets can be administered with or without water and are placed on the tongue where the tablet disintegrates rapidly. When administering the antihistamines parenterally, the nurse should give the drug deep intramuscularly, rather than subcutaneously, because many of the antihistamines are irritating to subcutaneous tissue.

 Nursing Alert

The nurse must not administer antihistamines to patients with lower respiratory tract diseases. If the nurse administers these drugs to patients with disorders such as asthma, the drying effect on the respiratory tract may cause thickening of the respiratory secretions and make expectoration more difficult.

Monitoring and Managing Adverse Reactions
Dryness of the mouth, nose, and throat may occur. The nurse offers the patient frequent sips of water to relieve these symptoms.

❄ **Gerontologic Alert**

Older adults are more likely to experience anticholinergic effects (eg, dryness of the mouth, nose, and throat), dizziness, sedation, hypotension, and confusion from the antihistamines. A dosage reduction may be necessary if these symptoms persist.

If the patient experiences dizziness or drowsiness, it is important to provide assistance with ambulation. If drowsiness is severe or if other problems such as dizziness or a disturbance in muscle coordination occur, the patient may require assistance with ambulation and other activities. The nurse places the call light within easy reach and instructs the patient to call before attempting to get out of bed or ambulate. The nurse informs the patient that this adverse reaction may lessen with continued use of the drug.

Educating the Patient and Family

The nurse reviews the dosage regimen and possible adverse drug reactions with the patient. The following points are included in the patient teaching plan:

- Do not drive or perform other hazardous tasks if drowsiness occurs. This effect may diminish with continued use.
- Avoid the use of alcohol, as well as other drugs that cause sleepiness or drowsiness, while taking these drugs.
- These drugs may cause dryness of the mouth and throat. Frequent sips of water, hard candy, or chewing gum (preferably sugarless) may relieve this problem.
- If gastric upset occurs, take this drug with food or meals. Loratadine should be taken on an empty stomach, if possible. If the gastric upset is not relieved, discuss this with the primary health care provider.
- Avoid ultraviolet light or sunlight because of the possibility of photosensitivity. Wear sunglasses, protective clothing, and a sunscreen when exposed to sunlight.
- Do not crush or chew sustained-release preparations.

EVALUATION

- The therapeutic effect is achieved.
- Adverse reactions are identified, reported to the primary health care provider, and managed successfully through nursing interventions.
- No evidence of injury is seen.
- Mucous membranes are kept moist.
- The patient demonstrates an understanding of the drug regimen and adverse effects of the drug.

DECONGESTANTS

A **decongestant** is a drug that reduces swelling of the nasal passages, which, in turn, opens clogged nasal passages and enhances drainage of the sinuses. These drugs are used for the temporary relief of nasal congestion caused by the common cold, hay fever, sinusitis, and other respiratory allergies.

ACTIONS

The nasal decongestants are sympathomimetic drugs, which produce localized vasoconstriction of the small blood vessels of the nasal membranes. Vasoconstriction reduces swelling in the nasal passages (decongestive activity). Nasal decongestants may be applied topically, and a few are available for oral use. Examples of nasal decongestants include phenylephrine (Neo-Synephrine) and oxymetazoline (Afrin), which are available as nasal sprays or drops, and pseudoephedrine (Sudafed), which is taken orally. Additional nasal decongestants are listed in the Summary Drug Table: Systemic and Topical Nasal Decongestants.

USES

Decongestants are used to treat the congestion associated with rhinitis, hay fever, allergic rhinitis, sinusitis, and the common cold. In addition, they are used in adjunctive therapy of middle ear infections to decrease congestion around the eustachian tube. Nasal inhalers may relieve ear block and pressure pain during air travel. Many can be administered orally as well as topically, but topical application is more effective than the oral route.

ADVERSE REACTIONS

When used topically in prescribed doses, there are usually minimal systemic effects in most individuals. On occasion, nasal burning, stinging, and dryness may be seen. When the topical form is used frequently or if the liquid is swallowed, the same adverse reactions seen with the oral decongestants may occur.

Use of oral decongestants may result in tachycardia and other cardiac arrhythmias, nervousness, restlessness, insomnia, blurred vision, nausea, and vomiting.

CONTRAINDICATIONS

The decongestants are contraindicated in patients with known hypersensitivity, hypertension, and severe coronary artery disease. These drugs are also contraindicated in patients taking monoamine oxidase inhibitors (MAOIs). Naphazoline is contraindicated in patients with glaucoma.

PRECAUTIONS

The decongestants are used cautiously in patients with hyperthyroidism, diabetes mellitus, prostatic hypertrophy, ischemic heart disease, and glaucoma. Safe use of the

2. *Discuss important teaching points that should be included in developing a teaching plan for a patient taking a nasal decongestant. Determine what teaching points would be the most important. Provide a rationale for your answer.*

● Review Questions

1. Which of the following is a common adverse reaction seen when administering an antihistamine?

   A. Sedation
   B. Blurred vision
   C. Headache
   D. Hypertension

2. Antihistamines are not routinely given to patient with lower respiratory disorders because _____.

   A. the depressant effects may cause a hypotensive crisis
   B. stimulation of the central nervous system may occur, resulting in paradoxical excitement
   C. the effects of these drugs on the respiratory tract may cause secretions to thicken
   D. antihistamines may irritate the bronchi, causing bronchospasm

3. When antihistamines are administered to patients receiving central nervous system depressants, the nurse monitors the patient for _____.

   A. an increase in anticholinergic effects
   B. excessive sedation
   C. seizure activity
   D. loss of hearing

4. A patient receives a prescription for phenylephrine (Neo-Synephrine). The nurse explains that overuse of this drug may _____.

   A. result in hypotensive episodes
   B. decrease sinus drainage
   C. cause rebound nasal congestion
   D. dilate capillaries in the nasal mucosa

● Medication Dosage Problems

1. Loratadine (Claritin) 10 mg is prescribed. The drug is available in a syrup containing 1 mg/mL. The nurse prepares to administer _____.

2. A patient is to receive 50 mg of diphenhydramine hydrochloride orally. The drug is available in 25-mg tablets. The nurse administers _____.

Bronchodilators and Antiasthma Drugs

Within the past few years a number of new drugs have been introduced to treat respiratory disorders, such as bronchial asthma and disorders that produce chronic airway obstruction. This chapter discusses the bronchodilators, drugs that have been around for a long time but are still effective in specific instances, and the newer antiasthma drugs that have proven to be highly effective in the prophylaxis (prevention) of breathing difficulty.

Asthma is a reversible obstructive disease of the lower airway. With asthma there is increasing airway obstruction caused by bronchospasm and bronchoconstriction, inflammation and edema of the lining of the bronchioles, and the production of thick mucus that can plug the airway (see Fig. 37-1). There are three types of asthma:

1. Extrinsic (also referred to as allergic asthma and caused in response to an allergen such as pollen, dust, and animal dander)
2. Intrinsic asthma (also called nonallergic asthma and caused by chronic or recurrent respiratory infections, emotional upset, and exercise)
3. Mixed asthma (caused by both intrinsic and extrinsic factors)

Extrinsic or allergic asthma causes the IgE inflammatory response. With exposure, the IgE antibodies are produced and attach to mast cells in the lung. Reexposure to the antigen causes them to bind to the IgE antibody, releasing histamine and other mast cell products. The release of these products causes bronchospasm, mucous membrane swelling, and excessive mucous production. Gas exchange is impaired, causing carbon dioxide to be trapped in the alveoli so that oxygen is unable to enter. Figure 37-2 identifies the asthmatic pathway from both intrinsic and extrinsic stimulus.

Other disorders of the lower respiratory tract include emphysema (lung disorder in which the terminal bronchioles or alveoli become enlarged and plugged with mucus) and chronic bronchitis (chronic inflammation and possibly infection of the bronchi). Chronic obstructive pulmonary disease (COPD) is the name given collectively to emphysema and chronic bronchitis because the obstruction to the airflow is present most of the time. Asthma that is persistent and present for most of the time may also be referred to as COPD.

The nurse observes the patient for adverse drug reactions. If adverse reactions occur, the nurse withholds the next dose and contacts the primary health care provider.

Occasionally the patient may experience an acute bronchospasm either as a result of the disease, after exposure to an allergen, or as an adverse reaction to some antiasthma drugs, such as cromolyn inhalation.

An inhaled sympathomimetic, such as albuterol, may be prescribed initially. Salmeterol, a long-acting β-agonist, is contraindicated because of its slowed onset of action. During an acute bronchospasm, the nurse checks the blood pressure, pulse, respiratory rate, and response to the drug every 15 to 35 minutes until the patient's condition stabilizes and respiratory distress is relieved.

✳ Nursing Alert

Acute bronchospasm causes severe respiratory distress and wheezing from the forceful expiration of air and is considered a medical emergency. It is characterized by severe respiratory distress, dyspnea, forceful expiration, and wheezing. The nurse must report these symptoms to the primary health care provider immediately.

NURSING DIAGNOSES

Drug-specific nursing diagnoses are highlighted in the Nursing Diagnoses Checklist. Other nursing diagnoses applicable to these drugs are discussed in depth in Chapter 4.

PLANNING

The expected outcomes for the patient depend on the specific reason for administering the drug but may include an optimal response to therapy, management of common adverse drug reactions, and an understanding of and compliance with the prescribed treatment regimen.

Nursing Diagnoses Checklist

☑ **Ineffective Airway Clearance** related to narrowed airway passages, thick or excessive mucus

☑ **Ineffective Breathing Pattern** related to narrowed airway passage, thick or excessive mucus

☑ **Risk for Impaired Oral Mucous Membrane** related to adverse reactions of the bronchodilating and antiasthma inhalants

☑ **Anxiety** related to adverse reactions of the bronchodilators (sympathomimetic drugs)

IMPLEMENTATION

Promoting an Optimal Response to Therapy

Nursing care of the patient receiving a bronchodilating drug or an antiasthma drug requires careful monitoring of the patient and proper administration of the various drugs. These drugs may be given orally, parenterally, or topically by inhalation or nebulization (see Chap. 2). In general, the nurse gives the drugs around the clock to maintain therapeutic blood levels. If the drug is to be administered once a day, the nurse should give it in the morning. Dosages are individualized for each patient, which allows the smallest effective dose to be given. The nurse can give oral preparations with food or milk if gastric upset occurs.

If the nurse is responsible for administering the medication by nebulization, it is important to place the patient in a location where he can sit comfortably for 10 to 15 minutes. The compressor is plugged in and the medication mixed as directed, or the prepared unit dose vial is emptied into the nebulizer. Different types of medication are not mixed without checking with the physician or the pharmacist. The mask or mouthpiece is assembled and the tubing connected to the compressor. The patient is placed in a comfortable, upright position with the mask over the nose and mouth. The mask must fit properly so that the mist does not flow up into the eyes. If using a mouthpiece instead of a mask, have the patient place the mouthpiece into the mouth. The compressor is turned on and the patient instructed to take slow, deep breaths. If possible, the patient should hold his breath for 10 seconds before slowly exhaling. The treatment is continued until the medication chamber is empty. After treatment, the mask is washed with hot, soapy water, rinsed well, and allowed to air dry.

PATIENTS TAKING SYMPATHOMIMETICS. Some of the sympathomimetics are extremely potent drugs. The nurse exercises great care in reading the primary health care provider's order when preparing these drugs for administration. Doses of drugs such as epinephrine are measured in tenths of a milliliter. A tuberculin syringe is used for measuring and administering these drugs by the parenteral route.

The nurse may administer epinephrine subcutaneously for an acute bronchospasm. Therapeutic effects occur within 5 minutes after administration and last as long as 4 hours.

Salmeterol is a long-acting inhaled bronchodilator and is not used to treat acute asthma symptoms. It does not replace the fast-acting inhalers for sudden symptoms. Salmeterol should not be used more frequently than twice daily (morning and evening).

Formoterol fumarate (Foradil Aerolizer) is administered only by oral inhalation using the Aerolizer Inhaler.

The usual dosage is one 12-μg capsule of formoterol every 12 hours. When using the Aerolizer Inhaler, the patient must not exhale into the device. When beginning treatment with this drug, the patient is instructed to discontinue the regular use of the short-acting β₂-agonist and use that agent only for relief of acute asthma symptoms.

PATIENTS TAKING XANTHINE DERIVATIVES. For acute respiratory symptoms, rapid theophyllinization using one of the xanthine derivatives may be required. **Theophyllinization** is accomplished by giving the patient a higher initial dose, called a loading dose, to bring blood levels to a therapeutic range more quickly than waiting several days for the drug to exert a therapeutic effect. The nurse may give loading doses orally or intravenously (IV) during a period of 12 to 24 hours. It is important to closely monitor the patient for signs of theophylline toxicity. See "Monitoring and Managing Adverse Reactions."

For patients receiving a xanthine derivative such as theophylline, the dosage is individualized and based on improvement of the patient's condition and serum theophylline drug levels.

The nurse can give some of these drugs (for example, aminophylline or theophylline) IV, either direct IV or as an IV infusion. When giving theophylline or aminophylline IV, the nurse monitors the patient for hypotension, cardiac arrhythmias, and tachycardia. If a bronchodilator is given IV, the nurse administers it through an infusion pump. The nurse checks the IV infusion site at frequent intervals because these patients may be extremely restless, and extravasation can occur.

If theophylline or another xanthine derivative is given as a rectal suppository, the nurse checks the patient every 15 to 30 minutes to be sure the suppository has been retained. If the patient is unable to retain the suppository, the nurse contacts the primary health care provider because another route of administration may be necessary.

When immediate-release products are used, the nurse administers the drug every 6 hours. In some adults, intervals of 8 hours between dosing may be satisfactory.

PATIENTS TAKING LEUKOTRIENE RECEPTOR ANTAGONISTS AND LEUKOTRIENE FORMATION INHIBITORS. The nurse should never administer these during an acute asthma attack. These agents are used for the management of chronic asthma and are not bronchodilators. If used during an acute attack, these drugs may worsen the attack.

These drugs are administered orally. Montelukast is administered once daily in the evening; zafirlukast is administered twice daily 1 hour before meals or 2 hours after meals. Zileuton is administered four times daily.

PATIENTS TAKING CORTICOSTEROID INHALANTS. If the patient is receiving a sympathomimetic bronchodilator by inhalation and a corticosteroid such as triamcinolone by inhalation, the nurse administers the bronchodilator first, waits several minutes, then administers the corticosteroid inhalant. When administering two inhalations of the same drug, it is advisable to wait at least 1 minute between puffs.

PATIENTS TAKING MAST CELL STABILIZERS. The mast cell stabilizers, such as cromolyn (Intal), may be added to the patient's existing treatment regimen (eg, bronchodilators). When added to the existing regimen, the other medications (ie, corticosteroids) are decreased gradually when the patient experiences a therapeutic response to cromolyn (2–4 weeks) and asthma is under good control. The corticosteroids or other antiasthma drugs may be reinstituted based on the patient's symptoms. If use of the mast cell stabilizers must be discontinued for any reason, the dosage is gradually tapered.

When administered orally, cromolyn is given 1/2 hour before meals and at bedtime. The oral form of the drug comes in an ampule. The ampule is opened and the contents poured into a glass of water. The nurse stirs the mixture thoroughly. The patient must drink all of the mixture. The drug may not be mixed with any other substance (eg, fruit juice, milk, or foods).

The drugs may be administered by a metered-dose inhaler (see Patient and Family Teaching Checklist: Teaching the Patient to Use a Metered-Dose Inhaler). If an aerosol inhaler is used for administration, the nurse teaches the patient how to use this method of delivering the drug to the lungs.

When a therapeutic response occurs, the dosage may be reduced to a maintenance dose.

Monitoring and Managing Adverse Reactions

SYMPATHOMIMETIC DRUGS. Patients who have difficulty breathing and are receiving a sympathomimetic drug may experience extreme anxiety, nervousness, and restlessness, which may be caused by their breathing difficulty or the action of the sympathomimetic drug. In these patients, it may be difficult for the primary health care provider to determine if the patient is having an adverse drug reaction or if the problem is related to the respiratory disorder. The nurse can reassure the patient that the drug being administered will most likely relieve the respiratory distress in a short time. Patients who are extremely apprehensive are observed more frequently until their respirations are near normal. The nurse closely monitors the patient's blood pressure and pulse during therapy and reports any significant changes. The nurse speaks and acts in a calm manner, being careful not to increase the anxiety or nervousness caused by the sympathomimetic drug. Explaining the effects of the

Home Care Checklist

USING A PEAK FLOW METER

Patients receiving bronchodilators or antiasthma drugs often need to monitor their lung function at home with a peak flow meter. Doing so provides the patient and the physician with valuable information about the status of the patient's condition and the effectiveness of therapy. Often, trends in the readings can detect changes in the patient's airway and airflow even before any signs and symptoms are experienced. This allows possible intervention before a major problem arises.

Because a variety of meters are commercially available, the nurse explains about the type of meter that will be used, how often the peak flow should be checked, and the ranges for the readings along with instructions on what to do for each range. The nurse uses the following steps to instruct the patient on the use of the peak flow meter:

✓ Check to make sure that the indicator is at the lowest level of the scale.

✓ Stand upright to allow the best inhalation possible. (Be sure to remove gum or food from your mouth.)

✓ Inhale as deeply as you can and then place your lips around the mouthpiece, making sure that you have a tight seal.

✓ Exhale as forcibly and as quickly as possible in one large "huff."

✓ Watch the indicator rise on the scale, noting where it stops. The number below the indicator's position is your peak flow reading.

✓ Repeat the procedure two more times.

✓ Compare the three readings. Record the highest reading along with the date and time. Do not calculate an average.

✓ Keep a written record of your readings and bring it with you on follow-up visits.

✓ Measure the peak flow rate close to the same time each day. (Your physician may provide you with a suggested time. Some patients measure the peak flow rate twice daily between 7 and 9 AM and between 6 and 8 PM. Others measure the peak flow rate before or after taking their medication.)

✓ Follow the medication instructions written on your record sheet next to the zone color of your reading (see Display 37-2) provided by your physician.

✓ Clean your meter with mild soap and hot water after use.

---

thorough explanation of its use (see Patient and Family Teaching Checklist: Teaching the Patient to Use a Metered-Dose Inhaler).

 Nursing Alert

The nurse should not assume that the patient understands how to use an aerosol inhaler correctly. Many patients, even with repeated instruction, do not use the proper technique to administer the drug by inhalation. Along with verbal instructions, the nurse should have the patient demonstrate the use of the inhaler to evaluate if he or she is using the proper technique. It is important to repeat instructions at each follow-up visit.

Because each brand is slightly different, the nurse carefully reviews any instruction sheets with the patient and provides information about how the unit is assembled, used, and cleaned.

In addition, the patient may use a peak flow meter at home to monitor the effectiveness of the drug regimen or breathing status. The nurse teaches the patient how to use the peak flow meter and when to notify the primary health care provider (see Home Care Checklist: Using a Peak Flow Meter). A commonly used method to interpret peak flow rates is to relate the three zones to the traffic light colors: green, yellow, and red. See Display 37-2 for information about the three-zone system. The physician may give the patient an action plan to determine what action to take for each of the three zones (see Fig. 37-3).

The nurse also includes the following general points in the patient teaching plan:

● Take the drug exactly as prescribed by the primary health care provider.
● If symptoms become worse, do not increase the dose or frequency of use unless directed to do so by the primary health care provider.

DISPLAY 37-2 ● Monitoring Peak Flow Readings

Many primary care health providers recommend a three-zone system. This system is based on your personal best peak flow rate—the highest peak flow measurement you can achieve on a day when your asthma is under good control—and it divides peak flow readings into three zones. The green zone ranges from 80% to 100%* of your personal best. The yellow zone, from 50% to 80%*. And the red zone is anything below 50%*.

*These percentages are given as an example. Your doctor will tailor your zones to your individual needs and peak flow patterns.

THINK OF THESE ZONES AS TRAFFIC SIGNALS

 ● Green means "go." Continue your regular activities and follow your maintenance asthma medication plan.

 ● Yellow means "caution." Additional medication may be needed (either for an acute episode, or if your condition remains stable, as part of your maintenance plan).

 ● Red means "stop." This is a danger zone. Notify the primary care health provider immediately. Use the medication prescribed when peak flow readings indicate that asthma is not in good control.

The goal is to stay in the green zone as long as possible and to take action whenever you enter the yellow zone, so you **never** enter the red zone. The primary care health provider will adjust the color-coded zone indicators on your personal best peak flow meter to remind you of your red, yellow, and green zones, as well as fill out your action plan with your medication instructions.

- If gastrointestinal upset occurs, take this drug with food or milk (oral form).
- Drink 6 to 8 glasses of water each day to decrease the thickness of secretions.
- Do not use nonprescription drugs (some may contain sympathomimetic drugs) unless use has been approved by the primary health care provider.
- Avoid smoking (when applicable). Smoking may make it difficult to adjust the dosage and may worsen breathing problems.
- Do not puncture metered dose inhalers or store them near heat or open flame; the contents of such inhalers are under pressure. Never throw the container into a fire or incinerator. If an unusual smell or taste is noted with use of the inhaler, discontinue use and contact the primary care provider.

SYMPATHOMIMETICS

- Do not exceed the recommended dosage.
- These drugs may cause nervousness, insomnia, and restlessness (especially the sympathomimetics). Contact the primary health care provider if the symptoms become severe.
- Contact the primary care provider if palpitations, tachycardia, chest pain, muscle tremors, dizziness, headache, flushing, or difficulty with urination or breathing occur.

- Salmeterol is not meant to relieve acute asthmatic symptoms. Notify the physician immediately if salmeterol becomes less effective for symptom relief, if more inhalations than usual are needed, or if more than the maximum number of inhalations of short-acting bronchodilators are needed.
- Formoterol fumarate (Foradil Aerolizer) is administered only by oral inhalation using the Aerolizer Inhaler. When using the Aerolizer Inhaler, do not exhale into the device. Always store formoterol capsules in the blister and remove immediately before use. Always discard the capsule and Aerolizer Inhaler by the expiration date included in the manufacturer's instructions. When treatment with formoterol begins, discontinue the regular use of the short-acting β$_2$-agonist and use it only for relief of acute asthma symptoms. Do not substitute formoterol for inhaled oral corticosteroids and do not reduce the use of the corticosteroids.

XANTHINE DERIVATIVES

- Remember that frequent monitoring of theophylline serum levels is important.
- Avoid foods that contain xanthine, such as colas, coffee, chocolate, and charcoal-prepared foods.
- If gastrointestinal upset occurs, take the drug with food. Do not chew or crush coated or sustained-release tablets.
- Do not change from one brand to another without consulting your physician.

CORTICOSTEROID INHALANTS

- Corticosteroid Inhalant—Rinse mouth with water without swallowing after each dose to reduce the risk of oral candidiasis. Carry a warning card indicating the need for supplemental systemic steroids in the event of stress or severe asthmatic attack that is unresponsive to bronchodilators. Do not stop therapy abruptly. These drugs are not bronchodilators and do not contain medication to provide rapid relief of breathing difficulties during an asthma attack. If taking bronchodilators by inhalation, use the bronchodilator several minutes before the corticosteroid to enhance application of the steroid into the bronchial tract. See Patient and Family Teaching Checklist: Teaching the Patient to Use a Metered-Dose Inhaler.
- Corticosteroid Inhaled Powder—Hold the inhaler upright and twist off the cover. Twist the grip to the right as far as it will go, listen for the click, and then twist it back. Exhale and place the mouthpiece between lips; slightly tilt head back and inhale deeply and forcefully. Remove inhaler from the mouth and hold breath for about 10 seconds. Rinse the mouth with water after each use to help reduce dry mouth and hoarseness.

ASTHMA ACTION PLAN FOR _____ Doctor's Name _____ Date _____

Doctor's Phone Number _____ Hospital/Emergency Room Phone Number _____

GREEN ZONE: Doing well

- No cough, wheeze, chest tightness, or shortness of breath during the day or night
- Can do usual activities

And, if peak flow meter is used,
Peak flow: more than _____
(80% or more of my best peak flow)

My best peak flow is: _____

Take These Long-Term-Control Medicines Each Day (Include an anti-inflammatory)

Medicine	How much to take	When to take it

☐ | ☐ 2 or ☐ 4 puffs | 5 to 60 minutes before exercise
Before exercise

YELLOW ZONE: Asthma is getting worse

- Cough, wheeze, chest tightness, or shortness of breath, or
- Waking at night due to asthma, or
- Can do some, but not all, usual activities

–Or–

Peak flow: _____ to _____
(50%–80% of my best peak flow)

FIRST → **Add: Quick-Relief Medicine—and keep taking your GREEN ZONE medicine**

_____ (short-acting beta₂-agonist)
☐ 2 or ☐ 4 puffs, every 20 minutes for up to 1 hour
☐ Nebulizer, once

SECOND → If your symptoms (and peak flow, if used) return to *GREEN ZONE* after 1 hour of above treatment:
☐ Take the quick-relief medicine every 4 hours for 1 to 2 days.
☐ Double the dose of your inhaled steroid for _____ (7-10) days.

–Or–

If your symptoms (and peak flow, if used) do not return to *GREEN ZONE* after 1 hour of above treatment:

☐ Take: _____ (short-acting beta₂-agonist) ☐ 2 or ☐ 4 puffs or ☐ Nebulizer

☐ Add: _____ (oral steroid) _____ mg. per day For _____ (3-10) days.

☐ Call the doctor ☐ before/ ☐ within _____ hours after taking the oral steroid.

RED ZONE: Medical Alert!

- Very short of breath, or
- Quick-relief medicines have not helped, or
- Cannot do usual activities, or
- Symptoms are same or get worse after 24 hours in Yellow Zone

–Or–

Peak flow: less than _____
(50% of my best peak flow)

Take this medicine:

☐ _____ (short-acting beta₂-agonist) ☐ 4 or ☐ 6 puffs or ☐ Nebulizer

☐ _____ (oral steroid) _____ mg.

Then call your doctor *NOW*. Go to the hospital or call for an ambulance if:
☐ You are still in the red zone after 15 minutes AND
☐ You have not reached your doctor.

↑ ☐ Take ☐ 4 or ☐ 6 puffs of your quick-relief medicine *AND*
☐ Go to the hospital or call for an ambulance (_____) **NOW!**

DANGER SIGNS

- Trouble walking and talking due to shortness of breath
- Lips or fingernails are blue

FIGURE 37–3. Example of an action plan for asthma.

LEUKOTRIENE RECEPTOR AGONISTS AND LEUKOTRIENE FORMATION INHIBITORS

- Zafirlukast—Take this drug regularly as prescribed, even during symptom-free times. Do not use to treat acute episodes of asthma.
- Montelukast—Take once daily in the evening, even when free of symptoms. Contact physician if the asthma is not well controlled. This drug is not for the treatment of an acute attack. Avoid taking aspirin and the NSAIDs while taking montelukast.
- Zileuton—This drug is not a bronchodilator, so do not use it for an acute episode of asthma. Contact the physician if bronchodilators are needed more often than usual or if more than the maximum number of inhalations for a 24-hour period is needed. This drug can interact with other drugs; consult a physician before starting or stopping any prescription or non-prescription drug. Have liver enzyme tests monitored on a regular basis. Immediately report any symptoms of liver dysfunction, such as upper right quadrant pain, nausea, fatigue, lethargy, pruritus, and jaundice.

MAST CELL STABILIZERS

- Inform the primary health care provider if asthma symptoms do not improve within 4 weeks of initiating treatment. The primary health care provider may discontinue the drug therapy.
- Cromolyn—When taken to prevent exercise-induced asthma, this drug should be taken approximately 15 minutes before activity but no earlier than 1 hour before the expected activity.
- Cromolyn—When taken orally, this drug should be taken at least 30 minutes before meals and at bedtime. The drug is prepared by opening the ampule and squeezing the liquid contents into a glass of water. The nurse stirs the solution, and the patient is instructed to drink the entire amount. Do not mix the drug with any other food or beverage.

EVALUATION

- The therapeutic effect is achieved, and breathing is easier and more effective.
- Adverse reactions are identified, reported to the primary health care provider, and managed successfully.
- The patient demonstrates an understanding of the drug regimen and use of the nebulizer or aerosol inhalator.

● *Critical Thinking Exercises*

1. *Mr. Potter, age 57 years, is admitted to the pulmonary unit in acute respiratory distress. The primary health care provider orders IV aminophylline. In developing a care plan for Mr. Potter, you select the nursing diagnosis Ineffective Airway Clearance. Suggest nursing interventions that would be most important in managing this problem.*

2. *Ms. Smith, age 68 years, returned to the clinic for a follow-up visit after receiving a diagnosis of COPD. She is taking theophylline daily and using a metered-dose inhaler 4 times a day. Determine what assessments would be most important for you to make at this time.*
3. *Discuss what to include in a teaching plan for a patient taking montelukast for asthma.*

● *Review Questions*

1. Which of the following laboratory exams would the nurse expect to be ordered for a patient taking aminophylline?
   - **A.** Thyroid levels
   - **B.** Alanine aminotransferase
   - **C.** Electrolytes
   - **D.** Serum aminophylline levels

2. When the sympathomimetics are administered to older adults there is an increased risk of _____.
   - **A.** gastrointestinal effects
   - **B.** nephrotoxic effects
   - **C.** neurotoxic effects
   - **D.** cardiovascular effects

3. When zileuton is prescribed, the nurse expects which laboratory test to be checked periodically?
   - **A.** Urine for culture and sensitivity (C&S)
   - **B.** Complete blood count (CBC)
   - **C.** Prothrombin test (PT)
   - **D.** Alanine aminotransferase (ALT)

4. When administering aminophylline, a xanthine derivative bronchodilating drug, the nurse monitors the patient for adverse reactions, which include _____.
   - **A.** restlessness, nervousness
   - **B.** hypoglycemia, hypothyroidism
   - **C.** bradycardia, bronchospasm
   - **D.** somnolence, lethargy

5. The nurse correctly administers montelukast (Singulair) _____.
   - **A.** once daily in the evening
   - **B.** twice daily in the morning and evening
   - **C.** three times a day with meals
   - **D.** once daily in the morning

● *Medication Dosage Problems*

1. A patient is to have 0.25 mg of terbutaline SC. The drug is available for injection in a solution of 1 mg/mL. The nurse administers _____.
2. The patient is prescribed zafirlukast 20 mg PO BID. The drug is available in 10-mg tablets. The nurse administers _____. How many milligrams of zafirlukast will the patient receive each day?

chapter 38

Antitussives, Mucolytics, and Expectorants

Key Terms

antitussive
coughing
expectorant

mucolytic
nonproductive cough
productive cough

Chapter Objectives

On completion of this chapter, the student will:

- Define the terms antitussive, mucolytic, and expectorant.
- Describe the uses, general drug actions, adverse reactions, contraindications, precautions and interactions of antitussive, mucolytic, and expectorant drugs.
- Discuss important preadministration and ongoing assessment activities the nurse should perform on patients receiving an antitussive, mucolytic, or expectorant drug.
- List some nursing diagnoses particular to a patient taking an antitussive, mucolytic, or expectorant drug.
- Discuss ways to promote an optimal response to therapy, how to manage common adverse reactions, and important points to keep in mind when educating the patient about the use of an antitussive, mucolytic, or expectorant drug.

Upper respiratory infections are among the most common afflictions of humans. The drugs used to treat the discomfort associated with an upper respiratory infection include antitussives, mucolytics, and expectorants. Many of these drugs are available as nonprescription (over-the-counter) drugs, whereas others are available only by prescription.

ANTITUSSIVES

Coughing is the forceful expulsion of air from the lungs. A cough may be productive or nonproductive. With a **productive cough,** secretions from the lower respiratory tract are expelled. A **nonproductive cough** is a dry, hacking one that produces no secretions. An **antitussive** is a drug used to relieve coughing. Many antitussive drugs are combined with another drug, such as an antihistamine or expectorant, and sold as nonprescription cough medicine. Other antitussives, either

alone or in combination with other drugs, are available by prescription only.

ACTIONS

Some antitussives depress the cough center located in the medulla and are called centrally acting drugs. Codeine and dextromethorphan are examples of centrally acting antitussives. Other antitussives are peripherally acting drugs, which act by anesthetizing stretch receptors in the respiratory passages, thereby decreasing coughing. An example of a peripherally acting antitussive is benzonatate (Tessalon).

USES

Antitussives are used to relieve a nonproductive cough. When the cough is productive of sputum, it should be treated by the primary health care provider who, based on a physical examination, may or may not prescribe or recommend an antitussive.

SUMMARY DRUG TABLE ANTITUSSIVE, MUCOLYTIC, AND EXPECTORANT DRUGS

GENERIC NAME	TRADE NAME*	USES	ADVERSE REACTIONS	DOSAGE RANGES
Antitussives				
Narcotic				
codeine sulfate *koe'-deen*	generic	Suppression of nonproductive cough, relief of mild to moderate pain	Sedation, nausea, vomiting, dizziness, constipation, CNS depression	10–20 mg PO q4–6h; maximum dosage 120 mg/d
Nonnarcotic				
benzonatate *ben-zoe'-naa-tate*	Tessalon Perles, generic	Symptomatic relief of cough	Sedation, headache, mild dizziness, constipation, nausea, GI upset, skin eruptions, nasal congestion	Adults and children older than 10 years: 100 mg TID (up to 600 mg/d)
dextromethorphan HBr *dex-troe-meth-or'-fan*	Drixoral Cough Liquid Caps, Robitussin Pediatric, Sucrets, Suppress, Trocal	Symptomatic relief of cough	Sedation, headache, mild dizziness, constipation, nausea, GI upset, skin eruptions, nasal congestion	Adults and children older than 12 years: 10–30 mg q4–8h, sustained release (SR) 60 mg q12h PO; children 6–12 years: 5–10 mg q4h or 15 mg q6–8h, SR 30 mg q12h PO; children 2–6 years: 2.5–7.5 mg q4–8h, SR 15 mg q12h PO
dextromethorphan HBr and benzocaine	Spec-T, Tetra-Formula, Cough X, Vicks Formula 44 Cough	Symptomatic relief of cough	Same as dextromethorphan HBr	Varies, depending on formulation; take as directed on package
diphenhydramine HCl *dye-fen-hye'-dra-meen*	Benadryl, generic	Symptomatic relief of cough, allergies, sleep aid, motion sickness, Parkinson's disease	Sedation, headache, mild dizziness, constipation, nausea, GI upset, skin eruptions, postural hypotension	Adults: 25 mg q4h PO not to exceed 150 mg/d; children (6–12 years): 25 mg PO q4h (not to exceed 75 mg/d); children 2–6 years old, 6.25 mg q4h (not to exceed 25 mg/d)
Mucolytic				
acetylcysteine *a-se-teel-sis'-tay-een*	Mucomyst, generic	Reduction of viscosity of mucus in acute and chronic bronchopulmonary disease, tracheostomy care, atelectasis due to mucus obstruction	Stomatitis, nausea, vomiting, fever, drowsiness, bronchospasm, irritation of the trachea and bronchi	10 mL of 20% solution or 2–20 mL of 10% solution q2–6h
Expectorants				
guaifenesin (glyceryl guaiacolate) *gwye-fen'-e-sin*	Fenesin, Humibid LA, Liquibid Muco-Fen-LA, Tussin, generic	Relief of dry, nonproductive cough, and in the presence of mucus in the respiratory tract	Nausea, vomiting, dizziness, headache, rash	Adults and children 12 years and older: 100–400 mg PO q4h; children 6–12 years: 100–200 mg q4h PO; children 2–6 years: 50–100 mg q4h
potassium iodide *poe-tass'-ee-um-eye-o-dide*	Pima, SSKI, generic	Symptomatic relief of chronic pulmonary diseases for which tenacious mucus complicates the problem	Iodine sensitivity or iodinism (sore mouth, metallic taste, increased salivation, nausea, vomiting, epigastric pain, parotid swelling, and pain)	300–1000 mg PO after meals BID or TID, up to 1.5 g PO TID
terpin hydrate *ter'-pin-high'-drate*	generic	Symptomatic relief of dry, nonproductive cough	Drowsiness, nausea, vomiting or abdominal pain	85–170 mg TID or QID PO

*The term *generic* indicates the drug is available in generic form.

ADVERSE REACTIONS

Use of codeine may result in respiratory depression, euphoria, light-headedness, sedation, nausea, vomiting, and hypersensitivity reactions. The more common adverse reactions associated with the antitussives are listed in the Summary Drug Table: Antitussive, Mucolytic, and Expectorant Drugs. When used as directed, nonprescription cough medicines containing two or more ingredients have few adverse reactions. However, those that contain an antihistamine may cause drowsiness.

CONTRAINDICATIONS

Antitussives are contraindicated in patients with known hypersensitivity to the drugs. The narcotic antitussives (those with codeine) are contraindicated in premature infants or during labor when delivery of a premature infant is anticipated. Codeine is a Pregnancy Category C drug except in the pregnant woman at term or when taken for extended periods, when it is considered a Pregnancy Category D drug.

PRECAUTIONS

All antitussives are given with caution to patients with a persistent or chronic cough or when the cough is accompanied by excessive secretion. Individuals with a high fever, rash, persistent headache, nausea, or vomiting should take antitussives only when advised to do so by the primary health care provider. Antitussives containing codeine are used with caution in patients having an acute asthmatic attack, those with COPD, and those with pre-existing respiratory disorders. Administration of codeine may obscure the diagnosis in patients with acute abdominal conditions.

Antitussives containing codeine are classified as Pregnancy Category C (during pregnancy) and Pregnancy Category D (during labor) drugs. Safe use of non-narcotic antitussives during pregnancy has not been established. They are used with caution and only when clearly needed during pregnancy and lactation.

The narcotic antitussives are used cautiously in patients with head injury and increased intracranial pressure, acute abdominal disorders, convulsive disorders, hepatic or renal impairment, prostatic hypertrophy, and asthma or other respiratory conditions.

INTERACTIONS

Other central nervous system (CNS) depressants and alcohol may cause additive depressant effects when administered with antitussives containing codeine.

When dextromethorphan is administered with the monoamine oxidase inhibitors (see Chap. 31), patients may experience hypotension, fever, nausea, jerking motions to the leg, and coma.

NURSING PROCESS

● **The Patient Receiving an Antitussive Drug**

ASSESSMENT

Preadministration Assessment
A hospitalized patient may occasionally have an antitussive preparation prescribed, especially when a nonproductive cough causes discomfort or threatens to cause more serious problems, such as raising pressure in the eye (increased intraocular pressure) after eye surgery or increasing intracranial pressure in those with CNS disorders. During the preadministration assessment, the nurse documents the type of cough (productive, nonproductive) and describes the color and amount of any sputum present. The nurse takes and records vital signs because some patients with a productive cough may have an infection.

Ongoing Assessment
During the ongoing assessment, the nurse observes for a therapeutic effect (eg, coughing decreases). The nurse auscultates lung sounds and takes vital signs periodically. When a patient has a cough, the nurse describes and records in the chart the type of cough (productive or nonproductive of sputum) and the frequency of coughing. The nurse also notes and records whether the cough interrupts sleep or causes pain in the chest or other parts of the body.

NURSING DIAGNOSES

Drug-specific nursing diagnoses are highlighted in the Nursing Diagnoses Checklist. Other nursing diagnoses applicable to these drugs are discussed in depth in Chapter 4.

PLANNING

The expected outcomes for the patient may include an optimal response to therapy and an understanding of and compliance with the prescribed treatment regimen.

Nursing Diagnoses Checklist

☑ **Ineffective Airway Clearance** related to congestion or coughing

☑ **Disturbed Sleep Pattern** related to coughing at night

☑ **Risk for Ineffective Therapeutic Regimen Management** related to lack of knowledge of drug regimen, adverse drug effects

IMPLEMENTATION

Promoting an Optimal Response to Therapy

The nurse gives antitussives orally. When the nurse gives the drug as a tablet, the patient should swallow the drug whole and not chew it. Chewing of benzonatate tablets may result in a local anesthetic effect (oropharyngeal anesthesia) with possible choking.

One problem associated with the use of an antitussive is related to its drug action. Although not an adverse reaction, depression of the cough reflex can cause a pooling of secretions in the lungs. A pooling of the secretions that are normally removed by coughing may result in more serious problems, such as pneumonia and atelectasis. For this reason, using an antitussive for a productive cough is often contraindicated.

Another problem can arise from the use of nonprescription cough medicine for self-treatment of a chronic cough. Indiscriminate use of antitussives by the general public may prevent early diagnosis and treatment of serious disorders, such as lung cancer and emphysema.

> ### ✷ Nursing Alert
>
> *The nurse should advise the patient taking a nonprescription cough medicine that if a cough lasts more than 10 days or is accompanied by fever, chest pain, severe headache, or skin rash, the patient should consult the primary health care provider.*

PROMOTING SLEEP. The nurse notes whether coughing keeps the patient awake at night or if the patient has difficulty falling asleep after being awakened by coughing. If sleep is frequently interrupted by coughing, the problem is discussed with the primary health care provider.

Educating the Patient and Family

The nurse discourages the indiscriminate use of nonprescription cough medicines, especially when coughing produces sputum. The nurse advises the patient to read the label carefully, follow the dosage recommendations, and consult the primary health care provider if the cough persists for more than 10 days or if fever or chest pain occurs. If an antitussive is prescribed for use at home, the nurse includes the following information in a teaching plan:

- Do not exceed the recommended dose.
- If chills, fever, chest pain, or sputum production occurs, contact the primary health care provider as soon as possible.
- Drink plenty of fluids. A fluid intake of 1500 to 2000 mL is recommended.
- If taking oral capsules, do not chew or break open the capsules; swallow them whole.
- If the cough is not relieved or becomes worse, contact the primary health care provider.

- Avoid irritants such as cigarette smoke, dust, or fumes to decrease irritation to the throat. Take frequent sips of water, suck on sugarless hard candy, or chew gum to diminish coughing.
- Remember than codeine may impair mental or physical abilities required for the performance of potentially hazardous tasks. Observe caution when driving or performing tasks requiring alertness, coordination, or physical dexterity. Do not use with alcohol or other CNS depressants (eg, antidepressants, hypnotics, sedatives, tranquilizers). Codeine may cause orthostatic hypotension when rising too quickly from a sitting or lying position. Do not take for persistent or chronic cough, such as occurs with smoking, asthma, or emphysema or when the cough is accompanied by excessive secretions, except when under the supervision of a physician.

EVALUATION

- The therapeutic effect is achieved and coughing is relieved.
- The patient sleeps through the night.
- The patient and family demonstrate an understanding of the drug regimen.

MUCOLYTICS AND EXPECTORANTS

A **mucolytic** is a drug that loosens respiratory secretions. An **expectorant** is a drug that aids in raising thick, tenacious mucus from the respiratory passages.

ACTIONS

A drug with mucolytic activity appears to reduce the viscosity (thickness) of respiratory secretions by direct action on the mucus. An example of a mucolytic drug is acetylcysteine (Mucomyst).

Expectorants increase the production of respiratory secretions, which in turn appears to decrease the viscosity of the mucus. This helps to raise secretions from the respiratory passages. An example of an expectorant is guaifenesin.

USES

The mucolytic acetylcysteine may be used as part of the treatment of bronchopulmonary diseases such as emphysema. It is primarily given by nebulization but also may be directly instilled into a tracheostomy to liquefy (thin) secretions. The mucolytic drugs are effective as adjunctive therapy in chronic bronchopulmonary diseases, such as chronic emphysema, emphysema with bronchitis, chronic asthma, tuberculosis, and bronchiectasis, and acute bronchopulmonary diseases, such as pneumonia and tracheobronchitis. It is also used in pulmonary conditions of cystic fibrosis and in tracheostomy care. Acetylcysteine has an additional use in preventing liver damage caused by acetaminophen overdosage.

Expectorants are used to help raise respiratory secretions. An expectorant may also be included along with one or more additional drugs, such as an antihistamine, decongestant, or antitussive, in some prescription and nonprescription cough medicines.

ADVERSE REACTIONS

The more common adverse reactions associated with mucolytic and expectorant drugs are listed in the Summary Drug Table: Antitussive, Mucolytic, and Expectorant Drugs.

CONTRAINDICATIONS

The expectorants and mucolytics are contraindicated in patients with known hypersensitivity. The expectorant potassium iodide is contraindicated during pregnancy (Pregnancy Category D).

PRECAUTIONS

The expectorants are used cautiously in patients with persistent cough that may be caused by a serious condition needing medical evaluation. Acetylcysteine is used cautiously in those with severe respiratory insufficiency or asthma and in older adults or debilitated patients. The expectorants are used cautiously during pregnancy and lactation. Acetylcysteine is a Pregnancy Category B drug; guaifenesin is a Pregnancy Category C drug.

INTERACTIONS

No significant interactions have been reported when the expectorants are used as directed. The exception is iodine products. Lithium and other antithyroid drugs may potentiate the hypothyroid effects of these drugs if used concurrently with iodine products. When potassium-containing medications and potassium-sparing diuretics are administered with iodine products, the patient may experience hypokalemia, cardiac arrhythmias, or cardiac arrest. Thyroid function tests may also be altered by iodine.

NURSING PROCESS

● **The Patient Receiving a Mucolytic or an Expectorant**

ASSESSMENT

Preadministration Assessment

Before administering the drug, the nurse assesses the respiratory status of the patient. The nurse documents lung sounds, amount of dyspnea (if any), and consistency of sputum (if present). A description of the sputum is important as a baseline for future comparison.

Ongoing Assessment

After administering the drug, the nurse notes any increase in sputum or change in consistency. The nurse documents, on the patient's chart, a description of the sputum raised. Patients with thick, tenacious mucus may have difficulty breathing. It is important to notify the primary health care provider if the patient has difficulty breathing because of an inability to raise sputum and clear the respiratory passages.

Immediately before and after treatment with the mucolytic acetylcysteine, the nurse auscultates the lungs and records the findings of both assessments on the patient's chart. Between treatments, the nurse evaluates the patient's respiratory status and records these findings on the patient's chart. These evaluations aid the primary health care provider in determining the effectiveness of therapy. If any problem occurs during or after treatment, or if the patient is uncooperative, the nurse discusses the problem with the primary health care provider.

When expectorants are given to those with chronic pulmonary disease, the nurse evaluates the effectiveness of drug therapy (ie, the patient's ability to raise sputum) and records this finding in the patient's chart.

NURSING DIAGNOSES

Drug-specific nursing diagnoses are highlighted in the Nursing Diagnoses Checklist. Other nursing diagnoses applicable to these drugs are discussed in depth in Chapter 4.

PLANNING

The expected outcomes for the patient may include an optimal response to drug therapy and an understanding of and compliance with the drug regimen.

Nursing Diagnoses Checklist

✓ **Ineffective Breathing Pattern** related to thick, tenacious sputum

✓ **Risk for Ineffective Therapeutic Regimen Management** related to lack of knowledge of drug regimen, adverse drug effects, treatment modalities

Patient and Family Teaching Checklist

Using Respiratory Equipment at Home

The nurse:

✓ Contacts the respiratory care provider to arrange for equipment delivery to the patient's home.

✓ Describes equipment such as compressor, filter, tubing, aerosol cup, and mask or mouthpiece to be used for therapy, including rationale for use and need for electrical power source.

✓ Reviews the drug therapy regimen, including the prescribed drug and solution strength, dosage, amount and type of diluent, if required, and frequency of administration.

✓ Demonstrates step-by-step procedure for equipment setup and drug preparation and administration.

✓ Evaluates return demonstration of procedure.

✓ Recommends sitting or high Fowler's position to maximize lung expansion and drug dispersion.

✓ Instructs to observe for misting as evidence of proper equipment function.

✓ Encourages slow, even breathing during treatment and coughing and expectorating as necessary.

✓ Stresses the importance of continuing treatment until the entire drug has evaporated and misting has ceased.

✓ Reviews the signs and symptoms of possible adverse reactions and impaired respiratory function, including changes in cough, color and amount of sputum, shortness of breath, or difficulty breathing and stresses the need to notify health care provider at once should any occur.

✓ Instructs to rinse equipment after each use with warm or cool water and allow to air dry.

✓ Recommends storing equipment parts in clean plastic bag or container.

✓ Reviews manufacturer's instructions for daily cleaning of equipment parts and routine maintenance of compressor.

✓ Provides written list for trouble-shooting problems such as changing filter, tightening connections, or replacing aerosol cup.

✓ Explains use of any additional drug therapy.

✓ Stresses need for fluid intake to liquefy secretions.

✓ Emphasizes importance of periodic laboratory tests and follow-up visits with health care provider to evaluate effectiveness of therapy.

IMPLEMENTATION

Promoting an Optimal Response to Therapy

When the mucolytic acetylcysteine is administered by nebulization, the nurse explains the treatment to the patient and demonstrates how the nebulizer will be used. The nurse remains with the patient during the first few treatments, especially when the patient is elderly or exhibits anxiety. The nurse supplies the patient with tissues and places a paper bag for disposal of the tissues within the patient's reach. If acetylcysteine is ordered to be inserted into a tracheostomy, the nurse must make sure suction equipment is at the bedside to be immediately available for aspiration of secretions.

When acetylcysteine is administered for acetaminophen overdosage, the drug is given as soon as the overdosage is discovered. Treatment should begin as soon as possible after overdose and within 24 hours of ingestion.

Educating the Patient and Family

Acetylcysteine usually is administered in the hospital but may be prescribed for the patient being discharged and renting or buying respiratory therapy equipment for use at home (see Patient and Family Teaching Checklist: Using Respiratory Equipment at Home). The nurse gives the patient or a family member full instruction in the use and maintenance of the equipment, as well as the technique of administration of acetylcysteine.

When an expectorant is prescribed, the nurse instructs the patient to take the drug as directed and to contact the primary health care provider if any unusual symptoms or other problems occur during use of the drug or if the drug appears to be ineffective.

EVALUATION

● The therapeutic effect is achieved, and secretions are thinned and easily expectorated.

● The patient and family demonstrate an understanding of the drug regimen and use of equipment to administer the drug (mucolytic).

● *Critical Thinking Exercises*

1. *Your neighbor, Mr. Peterson, tells you that he has had a chronic cough for the past several months and asks you what the best "cough medicine" to buy is. Describe the advice you would give to Mr. Peterson.*

2. *Ms. Moore, a patient in a nursing home, has had a cough for the past 3 weeks. Ms. Moore's physician is aware of her problem and has ordered an expectorant but told her that he wants her to cough and raise sputum. Ms. Moore's family asks you if something can be given to their mother to stop her from coughing. Explain how you would discuss this problem and explain the prescribed therapy with Ms. Moore's family.*

3. *Discuss any precautions the nurse would consider when the expectorants are administered. Give a rationale for your answer.*

● Review Questions

1. Antitussives are given with caution to patients with _____.

   A. an unproductive cough
   B. a chronic cough
   C. hypertension
   D. hypotension

2. Which of these drugs is classified as an expectorant?

   A. Guaifenesin
   B. Codeine
   C. Dextromethorphan
   D. Diphenhydramine

3. Which of the following statements is appropriate for the nurse to include in discharge instructions for a patient taking an antitussive?

   A. Increase the dosage if the drug does not relieve the cough.
   B. Limit fluids to less than 1000 mL each day.
   C. Expect the cough to worsen during the first few days of treatment.
   D. Frequent sips of water and sugarless hard candy may diminish coughing.

4. Which of these drugs would be prescribed for a patient with an acetaminophen overdosage?

   A. Acetylcysteine
   B. Guaifenesin
   C. Benzonatate
   D. Dextromethorphan

● Medication Dosage Problems

1. A patient is prescribed 200 mg of guaifenesin syrup. The drug is available in a syrup of 200 mg/5 mL. The nurse administers _____.

2. Codeine 10 mg is prescribed for a patient with a severe unproductive cough. The drug is available as an oral solution of 10 mg/5 mL. The nurse administers _____.

c h a p t e r **39**

Cardiotonics and Miscellaneous Inotropic Drugs

Key Terms

atrial fibrillation
cardiac glycosides
cardiac output
digitalis glycosides
digitalis toxicity
digitalization
heart failure
hypokalemia

left ventricular
  dysfunction
neurohormonal
  activity
positive inotropic
  action
right ventricular failure

Chapter Objectives

On completion of this chapter, the student will:

- Discuss heart failure in relationship to left ventricular failure, right ventricular failure, neurohormonal activity, and treatment options.
- Discuss the uses, general drug action, general adverse reactions, contraindications, precautions, and interactions of the cardiotonic and inotropic drugs.
- Discuss the use of other drugs with positive inotropic action.
- Discuss important preadministration and ongoing assessment activities the nurse should perform on the patient taking a cardiotonic or inotropic drug.
- List some nursing diagnoses particular to a patient taking a cardiotonic or inotropic drug.
- Identify the symptoms of digitalis toxicity.
- Discuss ways to promote an optimal response to therapy, how to manage common adverse reactions, and important points to keep in mind when administering a cardiotonic drug.

The cardiotonics are drugs used to increase the efficiency and improve the contraction of the heart muscle, which leads to improved blood flow to all tissues of the body. The drugs have long been used to treat congestive heart failure (CHF), a condition in which the heart cannot pump enough blood to meet the tissue needs of the body. While the term "congestive heart failure" continues to be used by some, a more accurate term is simply "heart failure."

About 4.5 million Americans have heart failure (HF). It is the most frequent cause of hospitalization for individuals older than 65 years. Some patients, with treatment, may lead nearly normal lives, whereas more than 50% of individuals with severe HF die each year. HF is a complex clinical syndrome that can result from any number of cardiac or metabolic disorders such as ischemic heart disease, hypertension, or hyperthyroidism. Any condition that impairs the ability of the ventricle to pump blood can lead to HF. In HF, the heart

fails in its ability to pump enough blood to meet the needs of the body or can do so only with an elevated filling pressure. Recently it was discovered that HF causes a number of neurohormonal changes as the body tries to compensate for the increased workload of the heart. Display 39-1 discusses this neurohormonal response.

The sympathetic nervous system increases the secretions of the catecholamines (neurohormones epinephrine and norepinephrine), which results in increased heart rate and vasoconstriction. The activation of the renin-angiotensin-aldosterone (RAA) system occurs because of decreased perfusion to the kidneys. As the RAA system is activated, increased levels of angiotensin II and aldosterone occur, which increases the blood pressure, adding to the workload of the heart. These increases in neurohormonal activity cause a remodeling (restructuring) of the cardiac muscle cells, leading to hypertrophy of the heart, increased need for oxygen, and cardiac necrosis, which worsens the HF. The tissue of the heart is changed

357

in a manner to increase the cellular mass of cardiac tissue, change the shape of the ventricle(s), and reduce the heart's ability to contract effectively.

Heart failure is best described as denoting the area of initial ventricle dysfunction: left-sided (left ventricular) dysfunction and right-sided (right ventricular) dysfunction. Left ventricular dysfunction leads to pulmonary symptoms such as dyspnea and moist cough. Right ventricular dysfunction leads to neck vein distention, peripheral edema, weight gain, and hepatic engorgement. Because both sides of the heart work together, ultimately both sides are affected in HF. Typically the left side of the heart is affected first, followed by right ventricular involvement.

The most common symptoms associated with HF include:

Left Ventricular Dysfunction
- Shortness of breath with exercise or difficulty breathing when lying flat
- Dry, hacking cough or wheezing
- Orthopnea (difficulty breathing while lying flat)
- Restlessness and anxiety

Right Ventricular Dysfunction
- Swollen ankles, legs, or abdomen, leading to pitting edema
- Anorexia
- Nausea
- Nocturia (the need to urinate frequently at night)
- Weakness
- Weight gain as the result of fluid retention

  Other symptoms include:

- Palpitations, fatigue, or pain when performing normal activities
- Tachycardia or irregular heart rate
- Dizziness or confusion

Left ventricular dysfunction, also called left ventricular systolic dysfunction, is the most common form of heart failure and results in decreased cardiac output and decreased ejection fraction (the amount of blood that the ventricle ejects per beat in relationship to the amount of blood available to eject). Typically, the ejection fraction should be greater than 60%. With left ventricular systolic dysfunction, the ejection fraction in less than 40%, and the heart is enlarged and dilated.

Until recently, the cardiotonics and a diuretic were the treatment of choice for HF. However, other drugs such as the angiotensin-converting enzyme (ACE) inhibitors, and beta blockers have become the treatment of choice during the last several years. See Figure 39-1 for an example of a method of determining treatment for left ventricular systolic dysfunction. See Chapters 23, 42, and 46 for more information on the beta blockers, ACE inhibitors, and diuretics, respectively.

CARDIOTONICS

Digoxin (Lanoxin) is the most commonly used cardiotonic drug. Other terms used to identify the cardiotonics are **cardiac glycosides** or **digitalis glycosides**. The digitalis or cardiac glycosides are obtained from the leaves of the purple foxglove plant or the *Digitalis purpurea* and the *Digitalis lanata*.

Miscellaneous drugs with positive inotropic action such as inamrinone and milrinone (Primacor) are nonglycosides used in the short-term management of HF. Although in the past the cardiotonics were the mainstay in the treatment of HF, currently they are used as the fourth line of treatment for patients who continue to experience symptoms after using the ACE inhibitors, diuretics, and beta blockers. See the Summary Drug Table: Cardiotonics and Miscellaneous Inotropic Drugs for information concerning these drugs.

ACTIONS

Digitalis acts in two ways:

1. Increases cardiac output through positive inotropic activity
2. Decreases the conduction velocity through the atrioventricular (AV) and sinoatrial (SA) nodes in the heart

Increased Cardiac Output

Cardiotonic drugs increase the force of the contraction of the muscle (myocardium) of the heart. This is called a **positive inotropic action**. When the force of contraction of the myocardium is increased, the amount of blood leaving the left ventricle at the time of each contraction is increased. When the amount of blood leaving the left ventricle is increased, **cardiac output** (the amount of blood leaving the left ventricle with each contraction) is increased.

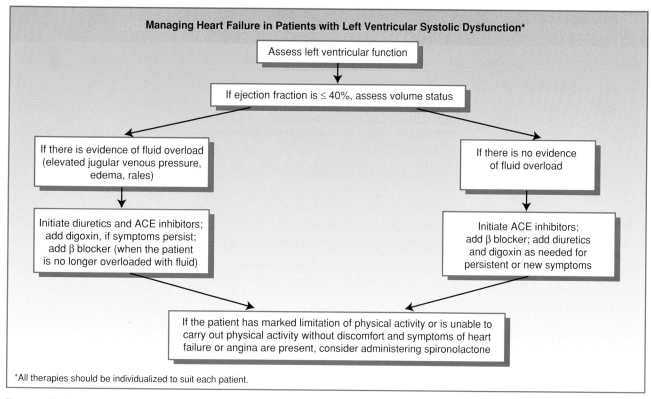

FIGURE 39-1. Management of left ventricular systolic dysfunction. (Adapted from Ammon, S. [2001]. Managing patients with heart failure, *AJN 101* [12] 35.)

The most profound effect of a cardiotonic drug occurs in patients with HF. In HF, the heart, weakened by disease or age, cannot pump a sufficient amount of blood to meet the demands of the body. The weakened heart results in a decrease in the amount of oxygenated blood leaving the left ventricle during each myocardial contraction (a decrease in cardiac output). A marked decrease in cardiac output deprives the kidneys, brain, and other vital organs of an adequate blood supply. The weakened heart is unable to pump enough circulated blood back into the heart. The blood accumulates or congests in the body's tissues. With congestion, legs and ankles swell. Fluid collects in the lungs, and the individual finds it increasingly hard to breathe, especially when lying down. When the kidneys are deprived of an adequate blood supply, they are unable to effectively remove water, electrolytes, and waste products from the bloodstream. Excess fluid (edema) may occur in the lungs or tissues, increasing the congestion. The body then attempts to make up for this deficit by increasing the heart rate, which in turn circulates more blood through the kidneys, brain, and other vital organs. In many instances, an increase in the heart rate ultimately fails to deliver an adequate amount of blood to the kidneys and other vital organs. An increased heart rate also places added strain on the heart's muscle, which may further weaken the heart. Untreated, congestion worsens and may prevent the heart form pumping enough blood to keep the individual alive.

When a cardiotonic drug is administered, the positive inotropic action increases the force of the contraction, resulting in an increased cardiac output. When cardiac output is increased, the blood supply to the kidneys and other vital organs is increased. Water, electrolytes, and waste products are removed in adequate amounts, and the symptoms of inadequate heart action or HF are relieved. In most instances, the heart rate also decreases. This occurs because vital organs are now receiving an adequate blood supply because of the increased force of myocardial contraction.

Depression of the Sinoatrial and Atrioventricular Nodes

The cardiotonics affect the transmission of electrical impulses along the pathway of the conduction system of the heart. The conduction system of the heart is a group of specialized nerve fibers consisting of the SA node, the AV node, the bundle of His, and the branches of Purkinje (Fig. 39-2). Each heartbeat (or contraction of the ventricles) is the result of an electrical impulse that normally starts in the SA node, is then received by the AV node, and travels down the bundle of His and through the Purkinje fibers (see Fig. 39-2). The heartbeat can be felt as a pulse at the wrist and other areas of the body where an artery is close to the surface or lies near a bone. When the electrical impulse reaches the

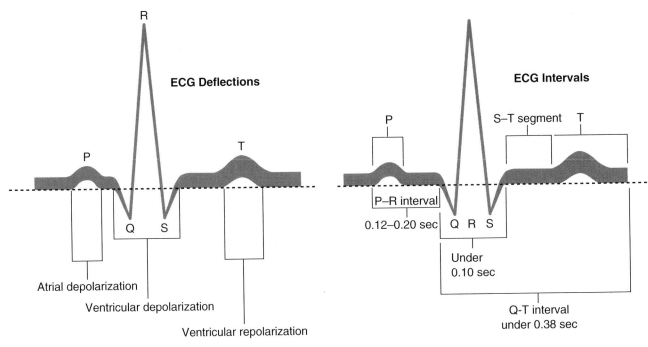

FIGURE 40-3. Normal QRS complex.

the primary health care provider's order or on nursing judgment and are based on the patient's general condition. The nurse closely observes the patient for a response to drug therapy, signs of CHF, the development of a new cardiac arrhythmia, or worsening of the arrhythmia being treated.

The nurse should immediately report to the primary health care provider any significant changes in the blood pressure, the pulse rate or rhythm, respiratory difficulty, change in respiratory rate or rhythm, or change in the patient's general condition.

> ### ☀ Nursing Alert
>
> *When giving an oral antiarrhythmic drug, the nurse withholds the drug and notifies the primary health care provider immediately when the pulse rate is above 120 bpm or below 60 bpm. In some instances, the primary health care provider may establish additional or different guidelines for withholding the drug.*

Continual cardiac monitoring assists the nurse in assessing the patient for adverse drug reactions. If the patient is acutely ill or is receiving one of these drugs parenterally, the nurse measures and records the fluid intake and output. The primary health care provider may order subsequent laboratory tests to monitor the patient's progress for comparison with tests performed in the preadministration assessment, such as an ECG, renal and hepatic function tests, complete blood count, serum enzymes, and serum electrolytes. The nurse reports to the primary care provider any abnormalities or significant

interval changes of the ECG, such as prolongation of the PR or QT interval or widening of the QRS complex. (See Fig. 40-3 for a diagram of a normal QRS complex.) In addition, when subsequent laboratory tests are ordered, the nurse reviews the results and reports any abnormalities to the primary health care provider.

NURSING DIAGNOSES

Drug-specific nursing diagnoses are highlighted in the Nursing Diagnoses Checklist. Other nursing diagnoses applicable to these drugs are discussed in depth in Chapter 4.

PLANNING

The expected outcomes for the patient may include obtaining an optimal therapeutic response to drug therapy, management of adverse drug reactions, and an understanding of and compliance with the postdischarge drug regimen.

> ### Nursing Diagnoses Checklist
>
> ☑ **Ineffective Tissue Perfusion: Peripheral** related to adverse drug reactions (hypotension)
>
> ☑ **Decreased Cardiac Output** related to adverse drug reactions (drug-induced arrhythmias)
>
> ☑ **Activity Intolerance** related to weakness and fatigue
>
> ☑ **Risk for Injury** related to adverse drug reactions (dizziness, light-headedness)

IMPLEMENTATION

Promoting an Optimal Response to Therapy

ADMINISTERING QUINIDINE. When quinidine is administered orally the drug is not crushed or chewed. Gastrointestinal upset can be reduced if the drug is given with food. The nurse must monitor serum quinidine levels during administration of the drug. Normal therapeutic levels range between 2 and 6 μg/mL. Toxic effects of quinidine usually occur at levels greater than 8 μg/mL.

ADMINISTERING PROCAINAMIDE. If procainamide is given IV, the nurse maintains continuous and close cardiac monitoring. When the drug is given IV, the nurse discontinues the drug immediately if changes in the ECG pattern occur. IV administration is by IV piggyback. Hypotension may be seen with IV administration; therefore, the blood pressure must be monitored every 15 minutes while the drug is being infused. The nurse keeps the patient supine during IV administration to minimize hypotension. If hypotension should occur, the drug therapy is discontinued, and the primary IV line is run at a rate to keep the vein open until the primary health care provider sees the patient. Although not the route of choice, the drug may be administered by IM injection. When the drug is given IM, the gluteus muscle is used and the injection sites are rotated.

When the drug is given orally, the nurse instructs the patient not to chew the capsule or tablet but to swallow it whole. For faster absorption, the drug is given with a full glass of water when the patient's stomach is empty, either 1 hour before or 2 hours after meals. If gastrointestinal upset occurs, the nurse can administer the drug with or immediately after meals. Sustained-released tablets should not be crushed or divided.

ADMINISTERING DISOPYRAMIDE. Disopyramide is administered to the patient with a full glass of water either 1 hour before or 2 hours after meals. If patients are receiving procainamide or quinidine, the manufacturer suggests that disopyramide therapy not be started for 6 to 12 hours after the last dose of quinidine and 3 to 6 hours after the last dose of procainamide. When the patient is to switch from taking the regular capsules to taking extended-release capsules, 6 hours should lapse after the last capsule before therapy is begun with the extended-release capsules.

ADMINISTERING LIDOCAINE. Lidocaine is most often administered IV either continuously diluted in D_5W or direct IV as a loading dose. When administered as a loading dose, the drug is given during a period of 1 minute with the dose repeated once after 5 minutes. The arrhythmia is usually controlled within 24 hours of continuous administration. The infusion is discontinued when the heart rhythm is stable or at the earliest sign of lidocaine toxicity. Blood lidocaine levels greater than 7 μg/mL are potentially toxic.

ADMINISTERING TOCAINIDE AND MEXILETINE. Tocainide and mexiletine are administered at 8-hour intervals and with food (or an antacid) to prevent gastrointestinal upset. In addition, administering tocainide with food may offer some protection against toxicity because the absorption rate is slowed in the presence of food.

ADMINISTERING FLECAINIDE AND PROPAFENONE. The nurse closely observes the patient for a response to drug therapy, signs of CHF, the development of a new cardiac arrhythmia, or worsening of the arrhythmia being treated. When flecainide is being administered, other antiarrhythmic drugs should be discontinued for at least two to four half-lives (time required for the blood level of a drug to decrease by 50%) of the drug being discontinued before flecainide therapy is begun. In general, when a drug therapy is discontinued, four to five half-lives are needed to eliminate the drug from the body. It is advisable to hospitalize the patient during withdrawal of the antiarrhythmic drug before initiating flecainide therapy because life-threatening arrhythmias may occur.

Propafenone is administered orally every 8 hours. Any previously given antiarrhythmic drug should be discontinued before propafenone therapy is started. Dosage changes are done 3 to 4 days apart because of the length of time the drug remains active in the body.

ADMINISTERING PROPRANOLOL. Cardiac monitoring is recommended when the drug is given IV because severe bradycardia and hypotension may be seen. The nurse obtains written instructions from the primary health care provider for propranolol administration. For example, the primary health care provider may want the drug to be withheld for a systolic blood pressure less than 90 mm Hg or a pulse rate less than 50 bpm.

ADMINISTERING BRETYLIUM. Bretylium is used in the emergency treatment of life-threatening ventricular arrhythmias. Because of its adverse reactions, bretylium is used when the arrhythmia is unresponsive to the other antiarrhythmic drugs. Baseline data will come from routine assessments made before the emergency. The nurse administers this drug IM or IV and uses continuous cardiac monitoring. The patient is placed in a supine position with suction equipment readily available in the event vomiting should occur.

✳ **Nursing Alert**

A transient increase in arrhythmias and hypertension may occur within 1 hour after initial therapy with bretylium is begun. The nurse should take the blood pressure and respiratory rate every 5 to 15 minutes and obtain the pulse rate from the cardiac monitor. These activities are continued until the arrhythmia is corrected.

To discontinue use of the drug, the dosage should be gradually reduced during a period of 3 to 5 days. After administering the drug, the nurse observes the patient closely. An oral antiarrhythmic drug may be prescribed to provide continued stability to the cardiac muscle.

ADMINISTERING VERAPAMIL. This drug is used to manage supraventricular arrhythmias and rapid ventricular rates in atrial flutter or fibrillation. Continuous cardiac monitoring is necessary during IV administration. The nurse notifies the primary health care provider if bradycardia or hypotension occurs. Patients receiving a cardiac glycoside (eg, digoxin) concurrently with verapamil must be monitored for an increased risk of digitalis toxicity. Verapamil is administered orally with food to minimize gastric upset.

Monitoring and Managing Adverse Reactions

Nursing judgment is necessary in reporting other adverse reactions to the primary health care provider. For example, the patient with a dry mouth is in no danger, even though the condition is uncomfortable. Although the occurrence of this is reported to the primary health care provider, it is not of an emergency nature. In some instances, minor adverse reactions must be tolerated by the patient. However, the patient with severe bradycardia or prolonged nausea and vomiting is in a potentially dangerous situation. The nurse contacts the primary health care provider immediately because additional treatment may be necessary.

Proarrhythmic effects (worsening of the existing arrhythmia or causation of a new arrhythmia) may occur, such as severe ventricular tachycardia or ventricular fibrillation. It is often difficult to distinguish proarrhythmic effects from the patient's preexisting arrhythmia.

> **❄ Nursing Alert**
>
> *Antiarrhythmic drugs are capable of causing new arrhythmias, as well as an exacerbation of existing arrhythmias. The nurse must report any new arrhythmia or exacerbation of an existing arrhythmia to the primary health care provider immediately.*

Some of the antiarrhythmic drugs may cause dizziness and light-headedness, especially during early therapy. The nurse provides assistance to patients not on complete bed rest with ambulatory activities until these symptoms are no longer present.

> **❄ Gerontologic Alert**
>
> *When older adults take the antiarrhythmic drugs, they are at greater risk for adverse reactions such as the development of additional arrhythmias or aggravation of existing arrhythmias, hypotension, and congestive heart failure (CHF). A dosage reduction may be indicated. Careful monitoring by the nurse is necessary for early identification and management of adverse reactions. The nurse monitors the intake and output and reports any signs of CHF, such as increase in weight, decrease in urinary output, or shortness of breath.*

Some antiarrhythmic drugs such as quinidine, procainamide, mexiletine, tocainide, or verapamil may cause agranulocytosis. The nurse reports any signs of agranulocytosis such as fever, chills, sore throat, or unusual bleeding or bruising. A complete blood count is usually ordered every 2 to 3 weeks during the first 3 months of therapy. If a decrease in the blood levels of leukocytes, platelets, or hematocrit occurs, use of the drug is discontinued. Blood levels usually return to normal within 1 month after use of the antiarrhythmic drug is discontinued.

ADMINISTERING QUINIDINE. The nurse monitors the patient for the most common adverse reactions seen with quinidine, which include nausea, vomiting, abdominal pain, diarrhea, or anorexia. **Cinchonism** is the term used to describe quinidine toxicity, and it occurs with high blood levels of quinidine (> 8 μg/mL). The nurse must report any quinidine levels greater than 8 μg/mL and the occurrence of any of the following signs or symptoms of cinchonism: ringing in the ears (tinnitus), hearing loss, headache, nausea, dizziness, vertigo, and light-headedness. These symptoms may also appear after a single dose. The patient is kept in a supine position throughout IV administration to minimize hypotension. If a widening of the QRS complex of 50% or more occurs, the nurse immediately notifies the primary care provider, who may order that the drug therapy be discontinued.

ADMINISTERING PROCAINAMIDE. Adverse reactions with procainamide therapy include nausea, loss of appetite, and vomiting. Small meals eaten frequently may be better tolerated than three full meals. Administering the drug with meals may decrease gastrointestinal effects.

ADMINISTERING DISOPYRAMIDE. Because of the cholinergic blocking effects of disopyramide (see Chap. 25), urinary retention may occur. The nurse monitors the urinary output closely, especially during the initial period of therapy. If the patient's intake is sufficient but the output is low, the lower abdomen is palpated for bladder distention. If urinary retention occurs, catheterization may be necessary.

Dryness of the mouth and throat caused by the cholinergic blocking action of this drug also may occur. The nurse provides an adequate amount of fluid and instructs the patient to take frequent sips of water to relieve this problem. In addition, postural hypotension may occur during the first few weeks of disopyramide therapy. The patient is advised to make position changes slowly. In some instances, the patient may require assistance in getting out of the bed or chair.

ADMINISTERING LIDOCAINE. Lidocaine is an emergency drug used in the treatment of life-threatening ventricular arrhythmias. Constant cardiac monitoring is essential when this drug is administered by the IV or intramuscular (IM) route. The administration of lidocaine is titrated to the patient's response and within institutional protocols. The nurse must observe the patient closely for signs of respiratory depression, bradycardia, change in mental status, respiratory arrest, convulsions, and hypotension. An oropharyngeal airway and suction equipment are kept at the bedside in case convulsions should occur.

If pronounced bradycardia occurs, the primary health care provider may order emergency measures, such as the administration of IV atropine (see Chap. 25) or isoproterenol (see Chap. 22). Any sudden change in mental state should be reported to the primary health care provider immediately because a decrease in the dosage may be necessary.

The nurse monitors the blood pressure and respiratory rate every 2 to 5 minutes when the drug is given IV and every 5 to 10 minutes when the drug is given IM. The pulse rate and rhythm are monitored continually by means of the cardiac monitor. The primary health care provider is contacted immediately if there are any changes in the vital signs or the ECG pattern or if respiratory problems or convulsions occur.

ADMINISTERING TOCAINIDE AND MEXILETINE. The dosage of these drugs must be individualized; therefore, the nurse monitors vital signs at frequent intervals during initial therapy. The nurse reports any changes in the pulse rate or rhythm to the primary health care provider. Onset of tremors is an indicator the maximum dosage of both tocainide and mexiletine has been reached. Adverse effects related to the central nervous system or gastrointestinal tract may occur during initial therapy and must be reported to the primary health care provider.

ADMINISTERING FLECAINIDE AND PROPAFENONE. When administering flecainide, the nurse must carefully monitor the patient for cardiac arrhythmias. Therapeutic serum levels fall between 0.2 and 1 µg/mL. Life support equipment, including pacemaker, should be kept on stand-by during administration.

During the initiation of therapy, patients taking propafenone must be monitored carefully. To minimize adverse reactions, dosage is increased slowly at a minimum of 3- to 4-day intervals. Periodic ECG monitoring is necessary to evaluate the effects on cardiac conduction.

ADMINISTERING PROPRANOLOL. The nurse monitors the ECG frequently for cardiac arrhythmias. Patients receiving IV propranolol must have continuous cardiac monitoring. The nurse must monitor the blood pressure and pulse frequently during the dosage adjustment period and periodically throughout therapy.

ADMINISTERING BRETYLIUM. The nurse monitors cardiac rhythm and blood pressure continuously during administration. Hypotension and postural hypotension occur in about 50% of the patients receiving bretylium. If systolic pressure is less than 75 mm Hg, the nurse should notify the primary health care provider. The patient is kept supine until tolerance of postural hypotension develops. The nurse instructs the patient to change position slowly. Most individuals adjust to blood pressure changes within a few days.

ADMINISTERING VERAPAMIL. The nurse monitors the patient's blood pressure and cardiac rhythm carefully while the drug is being titrated (dosage increased or decreased based on an established criteria by the primary care provider). Dosage may be increased more rapidly in a hospitalized setting. The nurse must assess the cardiac rhythm (ECG) regularly during stabilization of the dosage and periodically during long-term therapy.

Educating the Patient and Family

The nurse explains the adverse drug effects that may occur to the patient and family. To ensure compliance with the prescribed drug regimen, the nurse emphasizes the importance of taking these drugs exactly as prescribed. It may be necessary to teach the patient or a family member how to take the pulse rate. The nurse advises the patient to report any changes in the pulse rate or rhythm to the primary health care provider (see Patient and Family Teaching Checklist: Self-Monitoring Pulse Rate With Antiarrhythmic Therapy).

The nurse emphasizes the following points when teaching the patient and the family:

● Take the drug at the prescribed intervals. Do not omit a dose or increase or decrease the dose unless advised to do so by the primary health care provider. Do not stop taking the drug unless advised to do so by the primary health care provider.
● Do not take any nonprescription drug unless the use of a specific drug is approved by the primary health care provider.

SUMMARY DRUG TABLE   ANTIHYPERTENSIVE DRUGS (*Continued*)

GENERIC NAME	TRADE NAME*	USES	ADVERSE REACTIONS	DOSAGE RANGES
Drugs Used for Hypertensive Crisis				
diazoxide, parenteral *di-az-ok´-side*	Hyperstat IV, *generic*	Hypertensive crisis	Dizziness, weakness, nausea, vomiting, sodium and water retention, hypotension, myocardial ischemia	1–3 mg/kg IV bolus; maximum dosage: 150 mg
nitroprusside sodium *nye-troe-pruss´-ide*	Nitropress, *generic*	Hypertensive crisis	Apprehension, headache, restlessness, nausea, vomiting, palpitations, diaphoresis	3 mcg/kg per minute, not to exceed infusion rate of 10 mcg/min (if blood pressure is not reduced within 10 min, discontinue administration)

*The term *generic* indicates the drug is available in generic form.

because use may cause fetal and neonatal injury or death. These drugs are Pregnancy Category C during the first trimester of pregnancy and Pregnancy Category D during the second and third trimesters.

PRECAUTIONS

Antihypertensive drugs are used cautiously in patients with renal or hepatic impairment or electrolyte imbalances, during lactation and pregnancy, and in older patients. ACE inhibitors are used cautiously in patients with sodium depletion, hypovolemia, or coronary or cerebrovascular insufficiency and those receiving diuretic therapy or dialysis. The angiotensin II receptor agonists are used cautiously in patients with renal or hepatic dysfunction, hypovolemia, or volume or salt depletion, and patients receiving high doses of diuretics.

INTERACTIONS

The hypotensive effects of most antihypertensive drugs are increased when administered with diuretics and other antihypertensives. Many drugs can interact with the antihypertensive drugs and decrease their effectiveness (eg, antidepressants, monoamine oxidase inhibitors, antihistamines, and sympathomimetic bronchodilators). When the ACE inhibitors are administered with the NSAIDs, their antihypertensive effect may be decreased. Absorption of the ACE inhibitors may be decreased when administered with the antacids. Administration of potassium-sparing diuretics or potassium supplements concurrently with the ACE inhibitors may cause hyperkalemia. When the angiotensin II receptor agonists are administered with

NSAIDs or phenobarbital, their antihypertensive effects may be decreased.

❀ Herbal Therapy Alert

Various herbs and supplements, such as hawthorn extracts, garlic, onion, ginkgo biloba, vitamin E, and aspirin, may be used by herbalists for hypertension. Although these substances may lower blood pressure in some individuals, their use is not recommended because the effect is slight and usually too gentle to affect moderate to severe hypertension. However, several studies have demonstrated that hypertensive patients may benefit from daily doses of calcium (800 mg) or magnesium (300 mg). Patients should consult the primary health care provider before taking any herbal remedy.

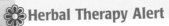

NURSING PROCESS

● The Patient Receiving an Antihypertensive Drug

ASSESSMENT

Preadministration Assessment

Before therapy with an antihypertensive drug is started, the nurse obtains the blood pressure (see Fig. 42-3) and pulse rate on both arms with the patient in standing, sitting, and lying positions. The nurse correctly identifies all readings (eg, the readings on each arm and the three positions used to obtain the readings) and records these on the patient's chart. The nurse also obtains the patient's weight, especially if a diuretic is part of therapy or if the primary care provider prescribes a weight-loss regimen.

Ongoing Assessment

Monitoring and recording the blood pressure is an important part of the ongoing assessment, especially

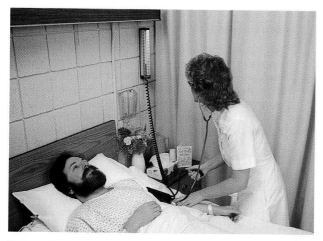

FIGURE 42-3. The nurse takes the patient's blood pressure prior to administering an antihypertensive drug.

early in therapy. The primary care provider may need to adjust the dose of the drug upward or downward, try a different drug, or add another drug to the therapeutic regimen if the patient does not have an adequate response to drug therapy.

Each time the blood pressure is obtained, the nurse uses the same arm and the patient is placed in the same position (eg, standing, sitting, or lying down). In some instances, the primary care provider may order the blood pressure taken in one or more positions, such as standing and lying down. The nurse monitors the blood pressure and pulse every 1 to 4 hours if the patient has severe hypertension, does not have the expected response to drug therapy, or is critically ill.

> ### ☀ Nursing Alert
>
> *The blood pressure and pulse rate must be obtained immediately before each administration of an antihypertensive drug and compared with previous readings. If the blood pressure is significantly decreased from baseline values, the nurse should not give the drug but should notify the primary health care provider. In addition, the primary health care provider must be notified if there is a significant increase in the blood pressure.*

The nurse obtains daily weights during the initial period of drug therapy. Patients taking an antihypertensive drug will occasionally retain sodium and water, resulting in edema and weight gain. The nurse assesses the patient's weight and examines the extremities for edema. The nurse reports weight gain of 2 lb or more per day and any evidence of edema in the hands, fingers, feet, legs, or sacral area. The patient is also weighed at regular intervals if a weight-reduction diet is used to lower the blood pressure or if the patient is receiving a thiazide or related diuretic as part of antihypertensive therapy.

> ### Nursing Diagnoses Checklist
>
> ☑ **Risk for Deficient Fluid Volume** related to administration of a diuretic as an antihypertensive drug (when appropriate)
>
> ☑ **Risk for Injury** related to dizziness or light-headedness secondary to postural or orthostatic hypotensive episodes
>
> ☑ **Decreased Cardiac Output** related to adverse drug reactions, other factors (specify)

NURSING DIAGNOSES

Drug-specific nursing diagnoses are highlighted in the Nursing Diagnoses Checklist. Other nursing diagnoses applicable to these drugs are discussed in depth in Chapter 4.

PLANNING

The expected outcomes for the patient may include an optimal response to therapy (blood pressure maintained in an acceptable range), management of common adverse drug reactions, and an understanding of and compliance with the prescribed therapeutic regimen.

IMPLEMENTATION

Promoting an Optimal Response to Therapy
ADMINISTERING ANTIADRENERGIC DRUGS. Clonidine is available as an oral tablet (Catapres) and transdermal patch (Catapres-TTS). The nurse applies the transdermal patch to a hairless area of intact skin on the upper arm or torso; the patch is kept in place for 7 days. The adhesive overlay is applied directly over the system to ensure the patch remains in place for the required time. A different body area is selected for each application. If the patch loosens before the 7 days, the edges can be reinforced with nonallergenic tape. The date the patch was placed and the date the patch is to be removed can be written on the surface of the patch with a fiber-tipped pen. (See Chapter 23 for additional information concerning the antiadrenergic drugs.)

ADMINISTERING VASODILATING DRUGS. The nurse must carefully monitor the patient receiving minoxidil because the drug increases the heart rate. The primary care provider is notified if any of the following occur:

* Heart rate of 20 bpm or more above the normal rate
* Rapid weight gain of 5 lb or more
* Unusual swelling of the extremities, face, or abdomen
* Dyspnea, angina, severe indigestion, or fainting

ADMINISTERING CALCIUM CHANNEL BLOCKERS. The nurse may give these drugs without regard to meals. If gastrointestinal upset occurs, the drug may be administered with meals. Bepridil and verapamil are best given with meals or milk because of the tendency of these two drugs to cause gastric upset. The sustained-release capsules should not be crushed, opened, or chewed. Verapamil capsules (not sustained released) may be opened and the contents sprinkled in liquid or on soft foods. Diltiazem may be crushed and mixed with food or fluids for patients who have difficulty swallowing. Sublingual nifedipine may be administered by puncturing the capsule with a sterile needle. The contents can then be squeezed into the buccal pouch.

ADMINISTERING ACE INHIBITORS. The nurse administers captopril and moexipril 1 hour before or 2 hours after meals to enhance absorption. Some patients taking an ACE inhibitor experience a dry cough that does not subside until the drug therapy is discontinued. This reaction may need to be tolerated. If the cough becomes too bothersome, the primary care provider may discontinue use of the drug.

The ACE inhibitors may cause a significant drop in blood pressure after the first dose. This effect can be minimized by discontinuing the diuretic therapy (if the patient is taking a diuretic) or by increasing salt intake for at least 1 week before treatment with the ACE inhibitors is begun or beginning treatment with small doses. After the first dose of an ACE inhibitor, the nurse monitors the blood pressure every 15 to 30 minutes for at least 2 hours and afterward until the blood pressure is stable for 1 hour.

ADMINISTERING ANGIOTENSIN II RECEPTOR ANTAGONISTS. Women of childbearing age must use a reliable contraceptive while taking the angiotensin II receptor antagonists. The primary care provider is notified if pregnancy is suspected. The most serious consequences of these drugs occur during the second and third trimesters of pregnancy.

ADMINISTERING DRUGS FOR HYPERTENSIVE EMERGENCIES. Nitroprusside and diazoxide are drugs used to treat patients with a hypertensive emergency (a systolic pressure of 120 mm Hg or more). When these drugs are used, the nurse frequently monitors the blood pressure, heart rate, and electrocardiogram throughout the course of therapy. Continuous monitoring is preferred. The primary care provider will order the parameters for the blood pressure maintenance.

Nitroprusside infusion bottles are wrapped in aluminum foil or other opaque material to protect the drug from light. The administration tubing does not require a covering. If the solution is protected from light, it remains stable for up to 24 hours. The newly prepared solution normally has a very light brownish tint. The nurse should discard the solution if the mixture becomes blue, green, or dark red.

❋ Nursing Alert

When diazoxide or nitroprusside is used for a hypertensive emergency, the nurse places the patient in a supine position immediately before, as well as after, administration of the drug. The rate of infusion (nitroprusside) or rate of direct IV administration (diazoxide) and the patient's blood pressure are monitored closely during and after administration of the drug because severe hypotension can occur. The blood pressure and pulse rate may need to be monitored every 15 minutes until the blood pressure is reduced to safe levels. The systolic pressure should not drop below 60 mm Hg.

❄ Gerontologic Alert

Older adults are particularly sensitive to the hypotensive effects of nitroprusside. To minimize the hypotensive effects, the drug is initially given in lower dosages. Older adults require more frequent monitoring during the administration of nitroprusside.

Monitoring and Managing Adverse Drug Reactions

The nurse observes the patient for adverse drug reactions because their occurrence may require a change in the dose or the drug. The nurse should notify the primary care provider if any adverse reactions occur. In some instances, the patient may have to tolerate mild adverse reactions, such as dry mouth or mild anorexia.

❋ Nursing Alert

Should it be necessary to discontinue antihypertensive therapy, the nurse should never discontinue use of the drug abruptly. The dosage is gradually reduced over 2 to 4 days to avoid rebound hypertension (a rapid rise in blood pressure).

MANAGING FLUID VOLUME DEFICIT. The patient receiving a diuretic is observed for dehydration and electrolyte imbalances. A fluid volume deficit is most likely to occur if the patient fails to drink a sufficient amount of fluid. This is especially true in the elderly or confused patient. To prevent a fluid volume deficit, the nurse encourages patients to drink adequate oral fluids (up to 3000 mL/d, unless contraindicated).

Electrolyte imbalances that may be seen during therapy with a diuretic include **hyponatremia** (low blood sodium) and **hypokalemia** (low blood potassium), although other imbalances may also be seen. See Chapter 58 and Display 58–2 for the signs and symptoms of electrolyte imbalances. The primary care provider is notified if any signs or symptoms of an electrolyte imbalance occur.

MINIMIZING THE RISK FOR INJURY. Dizziness or weakness along with postural hypotension can occur with the administration of antihypertensive drugs. If postural

Home Care Checklist

PREVENTING ORTHOSTATIC HYPOTENSION

Many patients receiving antihypertensive therapy commonly receive more than one drug, placing them at risk for orthostatic hypotension. If it occurs, your patient may fall and be injured. So teach the following measures to follow while in the acute care facility and at home:

✓ Change your position slowly.

✓ Sit at the edge of the bed or chair for a few minutes before standing up.

✓ Stand for a few minutes before starting to walk.

✓ Ask for assistance when necessary.

✓ If you feel dizzy or light-headed, sit or lie down immediately.

✓ Make sure to drink adequate amounts of fluid throughout the day.

hypotension should occur, the nurse advises the patient to rise slowly from a sitting or lying position. The nurse explains that when rising from a lying position, sitting on the edge of the bed for 1 or 2 minutes often minimizes these symptoms. The nurse informs the patient that rising slowly from a chair and then standing for 1 to 2 minutes also minimizes the symptoms of postural hypotension. When symptoms of postural hypotension, dizziness, or weakness occur, the nurse assists the patient in getting out of bed or a chair and with ambulatory activities.

Educating the Patient and Family

Nurses can do much to educate others on the importance of having their blood pressure checked at periodic intervals. This includes people of all ages because hypertension is not a disease seen only in older individuals. Once hypertension is detected, patient teaching becomes an important factor in successfully returning the blood pressure to normal or near normal levels.

To ensure lifetime compliance with the prescribed therapeutic regimen, the nurse emphasizes the importance of drug therapy, as well as other treatments recommended by the primary care provider. The nurse describes the adverse reactions that may be seen with a particular antihypertensive drug and advises the patient to contact the primary care provider if any should occur.

The primary care provider may want the patient or family to monitor blood pressure during therapy. The nurse teaches the technique of taking a blood pressure and pulse rate to the patient or family member, allowing sufficient time for supervised practice. The nurse instructs the patient to keep a record of the blood pressure and to bring this record to each visit to the primary care provider's office or clinic.

The nurse includes the following points in a teaching plan for the patient receiving an antihypertensive drug:

- Never discontinue use of this drug except on the advice of the primary care provider. These drugs control but do not cure hypertension. Skipping doses of the drug or voluntarily discontinuing the drug may cause severe, rebound hypertension.
- Avoid the use of any nonprescription drugs (some may contain drugs that are capable of increasing the blood pressure) unless approved by the primary care provider.
- Avoid alcohol unless its use has been approved by the primary care provider.
- This drug may produce dizziness or light-headedness when rising suddenly from a sitting or lying position. To avoid these effects, rise slowly from a sitting or lying position (see Home Care Checklist: Preventing Orthostatic Hypotension).
- If the drug causes drowsiness, avoid hazardous tasks such as driving or performing tasks that require alertness. Drowsiness may disappear with time.
- If unexplained weakness or fatigue occurs, contact the primary care provider.
- Contact the primary care provider if adverse drug effects occur.
- Follow the diet restrictions recommended by the primary care provider. Do not use salt substitutes unless a particular brand of salt substitute is approved by the primary care provider.
- Notify the primary care provider if the diastolic pressure suddenly increases to 130 mm Hg or higher; you may have malignant hypertension.

EVALUATION

- The therapeutic effect is achieved and blood pressure controlled.
- Adverse reactions are identified, reported to the primary care provider, and managed successfully through nursing interventions.
- Fluid volume deficit is corrected (when appropriate).
- No evidence of injury is seen.
- The patient complies with the prescribed drug regimen.
- The patient and family demonstrate an understanding of the drug regimen.
- The patient verbalizes the importance of complying with the prescribed therapeutic regimen.

● *Critical Thinking Exercises*

1. *Discuss important preadministration assessments that should be performed on a patient prescribed captopril for hypertension.*
2. *While working in the medical clinic of a hospital associated health care satellite, the primary care provider asks you to explain to a patient what can be done to avoid dizziness and light-headedness when rising from a sitting or lying down position. When talking to the patient, you discover that he understands little English. Discuss how you might communicate to this patient what he can do to decrease the symptoms of postural and orthostatic hypotension.*
3. *Mr. Bates, who has been treated for hypertension, is admitted for treatment of a kidney stone. On admission, he had severe pain and his blood pressure was 160/96 mm Hg. For the past 2 days, his blood pressure has been between 140/92 and 148/92 mm Hg. When taking his blood pressure before giving him an oral antihypertensive drug, you find that it now is 118/82 mm Hg. Analyze the situation and discuss what actions you would take.*
4. *Develop a teaching plan for a patient prescribed verapamil for hypertension. Discuss what information you would need from the patient before developing this plan. Identify important points to include in the plan.*
5. *Ms. Jones is admitted to the emergency department in hypertensive crisis. Nitroprusside therapy is begun, and you are asked to monitor this patient. Discuss important points that the nurse should keep in mind when administering this drug. Identify methods you would use to monitor the patient and prevent complications.*

● *Review Questions*

1. The nurse instructs the patient using the transdermal system (Catapres TTS) _____.

   A. to place the patch on the torso and keep it in place for 24 hours
   B. to change placement of the patch every day after bathing
   C. to place the patch on the upper arm or torso and keep it in place for 7 days
   D. avoid getting the patch wet because it might detach from the skin

2. To avoid symptoms associated with orthostatic hypotension, the nurse advises the patient to _____.

   A. sleep in a slide-lying position
   B. avoid sitting for prolong periods
   C. change position slowly
   D. get up from a sitting position quickly

3. After the first dose of an ACE inhibitor, the nurse monitors _____.

   A. the patient for a hypotensive crisis
   B. the vital signs every 4 hours or more often if the patient reports being dizzy
   C. the blood pressure every hour until it is stable
   D. the blood pressure every 15 to 30 minutes for at least 2 hours

4. When discontinuing use of an antihypertensive drug, the nurse _____.

   A. monitors the blood pressure every hour for 8 hours after the drug therapy is discontinued
   B. expects the primary care provider to order that the drug dosage be gradually decreased during a period of 2 to 4 days to avoid rebound hypertension
   C. checks the blood pressure and pulse every 30 minutes after discontinuing the drug therapy
   D. expects to taper the dosage of the drug during a period of 2 weeks to avoid a return of hypertension

5. When administering an antihypertensive drug for a hypertensive emergency, the nurse _____.

   A. weighs the patient before administering the drug
   B. places the patient in a supine position
   C. darkens the room to decrease stimuli
   D. places the patient in a high Fowler's position

● *Medication Dosage Problems*

1. Nadolol (Corgard) 80 mg PO is prescribed. The drug is available in 20-mg tablets. The nurse administers _____.

2. Diltiazem 180 mg is prescribed. The drug is available in 60-mg, 90-mg, and 120-mg tablets. Which tablet would you select? _____ How many tablets would you administer? _____

Antihyperlipidemic Drugs

Key Terms

atherosclerosis
bile acid sequestrants
catalyst
cholesterol
high-density
  lipoproteins (HDL)
HMG-CoA reductase
  inhibitors

hyperlipidemia
lipids
lipoprotein
low-density
  lipoproteins (LDL)
rhabdomyolysis
triglycerides

Chapter Objectives

On completion of this chapter, the student will:

- Discuss cholesterol, HDL, LDL, and triglyceride levels and how they contribute to the development of heart disease.
- Discuss therapeutic life changes and how they affect cholesterol levels.
- Discuss the general actions, uses, adverse reactions, contraindications, precautions, and interactions of antihyperlipidemic drugs.
- Discuss important preadministration and ongoing assessment activities the nurse should perform on the patient taking an antihyperlipidemic drug.
- List some nursing diagnoses particular to a patient taking an antihyperlipidemic drug.
- Discuss ways to promote an optimal response to therapy, how to manage common adverse reactions, and important points to keep in mind when educating patients about the use of an antihyperlipidemic drug.

Hyperlipidemia is an increase (*hyper*) in the **lipids** (*lipi*), which are a group of fats or fatlike substances in the blood (*demia*). **Cholesterol** and the **triglycerides** are the two lipids in the blood. Elevation of one or both of these lipids is seen in hyperlipidemia. Serum cholesterol levels above 240 mg/dL and triglyceride levels above 150 mg/dL are associated with atherosclerosis. **Atherosclerosis** is a disorder in which lipid deposits accumulate on the lining of the blood vessels, eventually producing degenerative changes and obstruction of blood flow. Atherosclerosis is considered to be a major contributor in the development of heart disease.

Triglycerides and cholesterides are insoluble in water and must be bound to a lipid-containing protein (**lipoprotein**) for transportation throughout the body. Although several lipoproteins are found in the blood, this chapter will focus on the low-density lipoproteins (LDL), the high-density lipoproteins (HDL), and cholesterol. **Low-density lipoproteins** (LDL) transport cholesterol to the peripheral cells. When the cells have all of the cholesterol they need, the excess cholesterol is discarded into the blood. This can result in an excess of cholesterol, which can penetrate the walls of the arteries, resulting in atherosclerotic

plaque formation. Elevation of the LDL increases the risk for heart disease. **High-density lipoproteins** (HDL) take cholesterol from the peripheral cells and bring it to the liver, where it is metabolized and excreted. The higher the HDL, the lower the risk for development of atherosclerosis. Therefore, it is desirable to see an increase in the HDL (the "good" lipoprotein) because of the protective nature of its properties against the development of atherosclerosis and a decrease in the LDL. A laboratory examination of blood lipids, called a lipoprotein profile, provides valuable information on the important cholesterol levels, such as:

- Total cholesterol
- LDL (the harmful lipoprotein)
- HDL (the protective lipoprotein)
- Triglycerides

Table 43-1 provides an analysis of cholesterol levels. HDL cholesterol protects against heart disease, so the higher the numbers the better. An HDL level less than 40 mg/dL is low and considered a major risk factor for heart disease. Triglyceride levels that are borderline (150–190 mg/dL) or high (above 190 mg/dL) may need treatment in some individuals.

TABLE 43-1	Cholesterol Level Analysis
TOTAL CHOLESTEROL LEVEL*	**CATEGORY**
Less than 200 mg/dL	Desirable
200–239 mg/dL	Borderline
240 mg/dL and above	High
LDL CHOLESTEROL LEVEL*	**LDL CHOLESTEROL CATEGORY**
Less than 100 mg/dL	Optimal
100–129 mg/dL	Near optimal/above optimal
130–159 mg/dL	Borderline
160–189 mg/dL	High
190 mg/dL and above	Very high

*Cholesterol levels are measured in milligrams (mg) of cholesterol per deciliter (dL) of blood.

An increase in serum lipids is believed to contribute to or cause atherosclerosis, a disease characterized by deposits of fatty plaques on the inner walls of arteries. These deposits result in a narrowing of the lumen (inside diameter) of the artery and a decrease in blood supply to the area served by the artery. When these fatty deposits occur in the coronary arteries, the patient experiences coronary artery disease. Lowering blood cholesterol levels can arrest or reverse atherosclerosis in the vessels and can significantly decrease the incidence of heart disease.

Hyperlipidemia, particularly elevated serum cholesterol and LDL levels, is a risk factor in the development of atherosclerotic heart disease. Other risk factors, besides cholesterol levels, play a role in the development of hyperlipidemia. Additional risk factors include:

- Family history of early heart disease (father before the age of 55 years and mother before the age of 55 years)
- Cigarette smoking
- High blood pressure
- Age (men older than 45 years and women older than 55 years)
- Low HDL levels
- Obesity
- Diabetes

In general, the higher the LDL level and the more risk factors involved, the greater the risk for heart disease. The main goal of treatment in patients with hyperlipidemia is to lower the LDL to a level that will reduce the risk of heart disease.

The primary care provider may initially seek to control the cholesterol level by encouraging therapeutic life changes (TLC). This includes a cholesterol-lowering diet (TLC diet), physical activity, quitting smoking (if applicable), and weight management. The TLC diet is a low-saturated fat and low cholesterol-eating plan that includes less than 200 mg of dietary cholesterol per day. In addition, 30 minutes of physical activity each day is recommended in the TLC. Walking a brisk pace for 30 minutes a day 5 to 7 days a week can help raise the HDL and lower LDL. Added benefits of a healthy diet and exercise program include a reduction of body weight. If TLC does not result in bringing blood lipids to therapeutic levels, the primary health care provider may add one of the antihyperlipidemic drugs to the treatment plan. The TLC is continued along with the drug regimen.

In addition to control of the dietary intake of fat, particularly saturated fatty acids, antihyperlipidemic drug therapy is used to lower serum levels of cholesterol and triglycerides. The primary health care provider may use one drug or, in some instances, more than one antihyperlipidemic drug for those with poor response to therapy with a single drug. Three types of antihyperlipidemic drugs are currently in use, as well as one miscellaneous antihyperlipidemic drug (see Summary Drug Table: Antihyperlipidemic Drugs for a complete listing of the drugs). The various types of drugs used to treat hyperlipidemia are:

- Bile acid sequestrants
- HMG-CoA reductase inhibitors
- Fibric acid derivatives
- Niacin

The target LDL level for treatment is less that 130 mg/dL. If the response to drug treatment is adequate, lipid levels are monitored every 4 months. If the response is inadequate, another drug or a combination of two drugs is used. Antihyperlipidemic drugs decrease cholesterol and triglyceride levels in several ways. Although the end result is a lower lipid blood level, each has a slightly different action.

ACTIONS

Bile Acid Sequestrants

Cholestyramine (Questran) and colestipol (Colestid) are examples of bile acid sequestrants. Bile, which is manufactured and secreted by the liver and stored in the gallbladder, emulsifies fat and lipids as these products pass through the intestine. Once emulsified, fats and lipids are readily absorbed in the intestine. These drugs bind to bile acids to form an insoluble substance that cannot be absorbed by the intestine, so it is secreted in the feces. With increased loss of bile acids, the liver uses cholesterol to manufacture more bile. This is followed by a decrease in cholesterol levels.

SUMMARY DRUG TABLE ANTIHYPERLIPIDEMIC DRUGS

GENERIC NAME	TRADE NAME*	USES	ADVERSE REACTIONS	DOSAGE RANGES
Bile Acid Sequestrants				
cholestyramine *koe-less'-tir-a-meen*	LoCHOLEST, Prevalite, Questran, Questran Light, *generic*	Hyperlipidemia, relief of pruritus associated with partial biliary obstruction	Constipation (may lead to fecal impaction), exacerbation of hemorrhoids, abdominal pain, distention and cramping, nausea, increased bleeding related to vitamin K malabsorption, vitamin A and D deficiencies	4 g PO 1–6 times/d; individualize dosage based on response
colestipol HCl *koe-les'-ti-pole*	Colestid	Hyperlipidemia	Constipation (may lead to fecal impaction), exacerbation of hemorrhoids, abdominal pain, distention and cramping, nausea, increased bleeding related to vitamin K malabsorption, vitamin A and D deficiencies	Granules: 5–30 g/d PO in divided doses; tablets: 2–16 g/d
colesevelam HCl *ko-leh-sev'-eh-lam*	Welchol	Adjunctive therapy used alone or with an HMG-CoA inhibitor to decrease elevated LDL cholesterol	Constipation (may lead to fecal impaction), exacerbation of hemorrhoids, abdominal pain, distention and cramping, nausea, increased bleeding related to vitamin K malabsorption, vitamin A and D deficiencies	3–6 tablets/d PO
HMG-CoA Reductase Inhibitors				
atorvastatin *ah-tor'-va-stah-tin*	Lipitor	Hyperlipidemia, reduction of elevated total and LDL cholesterol levels; increase HDL-C in patients with hypercholesterolemia	(Usually mild) headache, flatulence, abdominal pain, cramps, constipation, nausea	10–80 mg/d PO
fluvastatin *flue-va-sta'-tin*	Lescol, Lescol XL	Hyperlipidemia and mixed dyslipidemia, reduction of elevated total and LDL cholesterol levels, to slow progression of coronary artery disease (CAD), along with diet and exercise	(Usually mild) headache, flatulence, abdominal pain, cramps, constipation, nausea	20–80 mg/d PO
lovastatin *loe-va-sta'-tin*	Mevacor	Hyperlipidemia, reduction of elevated total and LDL cholesterol levels, to slow progression of CAD along with diet and excercise	(Usually mild) headache, flatulence, abdominal pain, cramps, constipation, nausea	10–80 mg/d PO in single or divided doses
pravastatin *prah-va-sta'-tin*	Pravachol	Hyperlipidemia, reduction of elevated total and LDL cholesterol levels, prevention of first MI, to slow progression of CAD, reduce risk of stroke, TIA, and MI	(Usually mild) headache, flatulence, abdominal pain, cramps, constipation, nausea	10–40 mg/d PO

(continued)

SUMMARY DRUG TABLE ANTIHYPERLIPIDEMIC DRUGS (Continued)

GENERIC NAME	TRADE NAME*	USES	ADVERSE REACTIONS	DOSAGE RANGES
simvastatin *sim-va-stah'-tin*	Zocor	Hyperlipidemia, reduction of elevated total and LDL cholesterol levels	(Usually mild) headache, flatulence, abdominal pain, cramps, constipation, nausea	5–80 mg/d PO
Fibric Acid Derivatives				
clofibrate *klo-fye'-brate*	Atromid-S, *generic*	Hyperlipidemia	Nausea, vomiting, GI upset, impotence, myalgia (muscle cramping and aching), increased or decreased angina, cardiac arrhythmias, fatigue, rash	2 g/d PO in divided doses
fenofibrate *fen-oh-figh'-brate*	Tricor	Hyperlipidemia, hypertriglyceridemia	Nausea, constipation, diarrhea, abnormal liver function tests, respiratory problems, rhinitis, abdominal pain, back pain, headache, asthenia, flu syndrome	54–160 mg/d PO
gemfibrozil *jem-fi'-broe-zil*	Lopid, *generic*	Hyperlipidemia, hypertriglyceridemia, reduction of coronary heart disease risk	Dyspepsia, abdominal pain, diarrhea, nausea, vomiting, rash, vertigo, headache	1200 mg/d PO in 2 divided doses 30 min before morning and evening meal
Miscellaneous Preparations				
niacin *nye'-a-sin* (nicotinic acid)	Niaspan	Adjunctive treatment for hyperlipidemia	Generalized flushing sensation of warmth, severe itching and tingling, nausea, vomiting, abdominal pain	1–2 g PO BID, TID; extended release: 500–2000 mg/d PO

*The term *generic* indicates the drug is available in generic form.

HMG-CoA Reductase Inhibitors

Another group of antihyperlipidemic drugs are called **HMG-CoA reductase inhibitors.** HMG-CoA (3-hydroxy-3-methyglutaryl coenzyme A) reductase is an enzyme that is a **catalyst** (a substance that accelerates a chemical reaction without itself undergoing a change) in the manufacture of cholesterol. These drugs appear to have one of two activities, namely, inhibiting the manufacture of cholesterol or promoting the breakdown of cholesterol. This drug activity lowers the blood levels of cholesterol and serum triglycerides and increases blood levels of HDLs. Examples of these drugs are fluvastatin (Lescol), lovastatin (Mevacor), and simvastatin (Zocor).

Fibric Acid Derivatives

Fibric acid derivatives, the third group of antihyperlipidemic drugs, work in a variety of ways. Clofibrate (Atromid-S), acts to stimulate the liver to increase breakdown of very–low-density lipoproteins (VLDL) to low-density lipoproteins (LDL), decreasing liver synthesis of VLDL and inhibiting cholesterol formation. Fenofibrate (Tricor) acts by reducing VLDL and stimulating the catabolism of triglyceride-rich lipoproteins, resulting in a decrease in plasma triglyceride and cholesterol. Gemfibrozil (Lopid) increases the excretion of cholesterol in the feces and reduces the production of triglycerides by the liver, thus lowering serum lipid levels.

Miscellaneous Antihyperlipidemic Drug: Niacin

The mechanism by which niacin (nicotinic acid) lowers blood lipids is not fully understood.

USES

Bile Acid Sequestrants

The bile acid sequestrants are used as adjunctive therapy for the reduction of elevated serum cholesterol in patients with hypercholesterolemia who do not have an adequate response to a diet and exercise program. Cholestyramine may also be used to relieve pruritus associated with partial biliary obstruction.

HMG-CoA Reductase Inhibitors

These drugs, along with a diet restricted in saturated fat and cholesterol, are used to treat hyperlipidemia when diet and other nonpharmacologic treatments alone have not resulted in lowered cholesterol levels.

Fibric Acid Derivatives

While the fibric acid derivatives have antihyperlipidemic effects, their use varies depending on the drug. For example, Clofibrate (Atromid-S) and gemfibrozil (Lopid) are used to treat individuals with very high serum triglyceride levels who present a risk of abdominal pain and pancreatitis and who do not experience a response to diet modifications. Clofibrate is not used for the treatment of other types of hyperlipidemia and is not thought to be effective for prevention of coronary heart disease. Fenofibrate (Tricor) is used as adjunctive treatment for the reduction of LDL, total cholesterol, and triglycerides in patients with hyperlipidemia.

Miscellaneous Antihyperlipidemic Drug: Niacin

Niacin is used as adjunctive therapy for the treatment of very high serum triglyceride levels in patients who present a risk of pancreatitis (inflammation of the pancreas) and who do not experience an adequate response to dietary control.

ADVERSE REACTIONS

Bile Acid Sequestrants

A common problem associated with the administration of the bile acid sequestrants is constipation. Constipation may be severe and may occasionally result in fecal impaction. Hemorrhoids may be aggravated. Additional adverse reactions include vitamin A and D deficiencies, bleeding tendencies (including gastrointestinal bleeding) caused by a depletion of vitamin K, nausea, abdominal pain, and distention.

HMG-CoA Reductase Inhibitors

HMG-CoA reductase inhibitors are usually well tolerated. Adverse reactions, when they do occur, are often mild and transient and do not require discontinuing therapy. The more common adverse reactions include nausea, vomiting, constipation, abdominal pain or cramps, and

headache. A rare, but more serious, adverse reaction is rhabdomyolysis.

Fibric Acid Derivatives

The adverse reactions associated with fibric acid derivatives include nausea, vomiting, gastrointestinal upset, and diarrhea. Clofibrate, fenofibrate, and gemfibrozil may increase cholesterol excretion into the bile, leading to cholelithiasis (stones in the gallbladder) or cholecystitis (inflammation of the gallbladder). If cholelithiasis is found, use of the drug is discontinued. Fenofibrate may also result in abnormal liver function tests, respiratory problems, back pain, and headache. Gemfibrozil may cause dyspepsia, skin rash, vertigo, and headache. See the Summary Drug Table: Antihyperlipidemic Drugs for additional adverse reactions.

Miscellaneous Antihyperlipidemic Drug: Niacin

Nicotinic acid may cause nausea, vomiting, abdominal pain, diarrhea, severe generalized flushing of the skin, a sensation of warmth, and severe itching or tingling.

CONTRAINDICATIONS, PRECAUTIONS, AND INTERACTIONS

Bile Acid Sequestrants

The bile acid sequestrants are contraindicated in patients with known hypersensitivity to the drugs. Bile acid sequestrants are also contraindicated in those with complete biliary obstruction. These drugs are used cautiously in patients with a history of liver or kidney disease. Bile acid sequestrants are used cautiously during pregnancy (Pregnancy Category C) and lactation (decreased absorption of vitamins may affect the infant).

The bile acids sequestrants, particularly cholestyramine, can decrease the absorption of numerous drugs. For this reason, the bile acid sequestrants should be administered alone and other drugs given at least 1 hour before or 4 hours after administration of the bile acid sequestrants. There is an increased risk of bleeding when the bile acid sequestrants are administered with oral anticoagulants. The dosage of the anticoagulant is usually decreased. The bile acid sequestrants may bind with digoxin, thiazide diuretics, penicillin, propranolol, tetracyclines, folic acid, and the thyroid hormones, resulting in decreased effects of these drugs.

HMG-CoA Reductase Inhibitors

The HMG-CoA reductase inhibitors are contraindicated in individuals with hypersensitivity to the drugs, serious liver disorders, and during pregnancy (Pregnancy

Category X) and lactation. The HMG-CoA reductase inhibitors are used cautiously in patients with a history of alcoholism, acute infection, hypotension, trauma, endocrine disorders, visual disturbances, and myopathy.

The HMG-CoA reductase inhibitors have an additive effect when used with the bile acid sequestrants, which may provide an added benefit in treating hypercholesterolemia that does not respond to a single-drug regimen. There is an increased risk of myopathy (disorders of the striated muscle) when the HMG-CoA reductase inhibitors are administered with erythromycin, niacin, or cyclosporine. When the HMG-CoA reductase inhibitors are administered with oral anticoagulants, there is an increased anticoagulant effect.

Fibric Acid Derivatives

The fibric acid derivatives are contraindicated in patients with hypersensitivity to the drugs and those with significant hepatic or renal dysfunction or primary biliary cirrhosis because these drugs may increase the already elevated cholesterol. The drugs are used cautiously during pregnancy (Pregnancy Category C) and lactation and in patients with peptic ulcer disease or diabetes. Although it rarely occurs, when the fibric acid derivatives, particularly gemfibrozil, are administered with the HMG-CoA reductase inhibitors, there is an increased risk for rhabdomyolysis (see Nursing Alert). When clofibrate, fenofibrate, or gemfibrozil is administered with the anticoagulants, there is an increased risk for bleeding.

Miscellaneous Antihyperlipidemic Drug: Niacin

Niacin is contraindicated in patients with known hypersensitivity to niacin, active peptic ulcer, hepatic dysfunction, and arterial bleeding. The drug is used cautiously in patients with renal dysfunction, high alcohol consumption, unstable angina, gout, and pregnancy (Category C).

✻ Herbal Alert: Garlic

Garlic has been used for many years throughout the world. The benefits of garlic on cardiovascular health are the best known and most extensively researched benefits of the herb. Its benefits include lowering serum cholesterol and triglyceride levels, improving the ratio of HDL to LDL cholesterol, lowering blood pressure, and helping to prevent the development of atherosclerosis. The recommended dosages of garlic are 600 to 900 mg/day of the garlic powder tablets, 10 mg of garlic oil "perles," or one moderate-sized fresh clove of garlic a day. Adverse reactions include mild stomach upset or irritation that can usually be alleviated by taking the supplements with food. Although no serious reactions have occurred in pregnant women taking garlic, its use is not recommended. Garlic is excreted in breast milk and may cause colic in some infants.

NURSING PROCESS

● The Patient Receiving an Antihyperlipidemic Drug

ASSESSMENT

Preadministration Assessment

In many individuals, hyperlipidemia has no symptoms and the disorder is not discovered until laboratory tests reveal elevated cholesterol and triglyceride levels, elevated LDL levels, and decreased HDL levels. Often, these drugs are initially prescribed on an outpatient basis, but initial administration may occur in the hospitalized patient. Serum cholesterol levels (ie, a lipid profile) and liver functions tests are obtained before the drugs are administered.

The nurse takes a dietary history, focusing on the types of foods normally included in the diet. Vital signs and weight are recorded. The skin and eyelids are inspected for evidence of xanthomas (flat or elevated yellowish deposits) that may be seen in the more severe forms of hyperlipidemia.

Ongoing Assessment

The patient will usually take these drugs on an outpatient basis and come to the clinic or the primary health care provider's office for periodic monitoring. Frequent monitoring of blood cholesterol and triglyceride levels is done as a part of the ongoing assessment.

✸ Nursing Alert

Sometimes a paradoxical elevation of blood lipid levels occurs. Should this happen, the primary health care provider is notified because the primary health care provider may prescribe a different antihyperlipidemic drug.

During the ongoing assessment, the nurse checks vital signs and assesses bowel functioning because an adverse reaction to these drugs is constipation. Constipation may become serious if not treated.

When administering the HMG-CoA reductase inhibitors and the fibric acid derivatives, the nurse monitors the patient's liver function by obtaining serum transaminase levels before the drug regimen is started, at 6 and 12 weeks, then periodically thereafter because of the possibility of liver dysfunction with the drugs. If aspartate aminotransferase (AST) levels increase to three times normal, the primary care provider in notified immediately because the HMG-CoA reductase inhibitor therapy may be discontinued.

Because the maximum effects of these drugs are usually seen within 4 weeks, periodic lipid profiles are performed to determine the therapeutic effect of the drug regimen. The primary health care provider may increase the dosage, add another antihyperlipidemic drug, or discontinue the drug therapy, depending on the patient's response to therapy.

NURSING DIAGNOSES

Drug-specific nursing diagnoses are highlighted in the Nursing Diagnoses Checklist. Other nursing diagnoses applicable to these drugs are discussed in depth in Chapter 4.

PLANNING

The expected outcomes for the patient may include a therapeutic response to therapy (lowered blood lipid levels), management of common adverse drug reactions, and an understanding of the dietary measures necessary to reduce lipid and lipoprotein levels.

IMPLEMENTATION

Promoting an Optimal Response to Therapy

Because hyperlipidemia is often treated on an outpatient basis, the nurse explains the drug regimen and possible adverse reactions. If printed dietary guidelines are given to the patient, the nurse emphasizes the importance of following these recommendations. Drug therapy usually is discontinued if the antihyperlipidemic drug is not effective after 3 months of treatment.

Bile acid sequestrants may interfere with the digestion of fats and prevent the absorption of the fat-soluble vitamins (vitamins A, D, E, and K) and folic acid. When the bile acid sequestrants are used for long-term therapy, vitamins A and D may be given in a water-soluble form or administered parenterally. If bleeding tendencies occur as the result of vitamin K deficiency, parenteral vitamin K is administered for immediate treatment, and oral vitamin K is given for prevention of a deficiency in the future.

Monitoring and Managing Adverse Reactions

BILE ACID SEQUESTRANTS. Patients taking the antihyperlipidemic drugs, particularly the bile acid sequestrants, may experience constipation. The drugs can produce or severely worsen preexisting constipation. The nurse instructs the patient to increase fluid intake, eat foods high in dietary fiber, and exercise daily to help prevent constipation. If the problem persists or becomes

severe, a stool softener or laxative may be required. Some patients require decreased dosage or discontinuation of the drug therapy.

> **Gerontologic Alert**
>
> *Older adults are particularly prone to constipation when taking the bile acid sequestrants. The nurse should monitor older adults closely for hard dry stools, difficulty passing stools, and any complaints of constipation. An accurate record of bowel movements must be kept.*

HMG-CoA REDUCTASE INHIBITORS AND FIBRIC ACID DERIVATIVES. The antihyperlipidemic drugs, particularly the HMG-CoA reductase inhibitors, have been associated with skeletal muscle effects leading to rhabdomyolysis. **Rhabdomyolysis** is a very rare condition in which muscle damage results in the release of muscle cell contents into the bloodstream. Rhabdomyolysis may precipitate renal dysfunction or acute renal failure. The nurse is alert for unexplained muscle pain, muscle tenderness, or weakness, especially if they are accompanied by malaise or fever. These symptoms should be reported to the primary health care provider because the drug may be discontinued.

NIACIN. Patients taking nicotinic acid may experience moderate to severe generalized flushing of the skin, a sensation of warmth, and severe itching or tingling. Although these reactions are most often seen at higher dose levels, some patients may experience them even when small doses of nicotinic acid are administered. The sudden appearance of these reactions may frighten the patient.

> **Nursing Alert**
>
> *The nurse should advise the patient taking nicotinic acid to put the call light on if discomfort is experienced. Contact the primary health care provider before the next dose is due should this adverse reaction occur. If the patient is in severe discomfort, the nurse should contact the primary health care provider immediately. The nurse advises outpatients to contact their primary health care provider if these reactions are severe or cause extreme discomfort.*

Educating the Patient and Family

The nurse stresses the importance of following the diet recommended by the primary health care provider because drug therapy alone will not significantly lower cholesterol and triglyceride levels. The nurse provides a copy of the recommended diet and reviews the contents of the diet with the patient and family. If necessary, the

Patient and Family Teaching Checklist

Using Diet and Drugs to Control High Blood Cholesterol Levels

The nurse:

✔ Reviews the reasons for the drug and prescribed drug therapy, including drug name, form and method of preparation, correct dose, and frequency of administration.

✔ Emphasizes that drug therapy alone will not significantly lower blood cholesterol levels.

✔ Stresses importance of taking drug exactly as prescribed.

✔ Reinforces the importance of adhering to prescribed diet.

✔ Provides a written copy of dietary plan and reviews contents.

✔ Contacts dietitian for assistance with diet teaching.

✔ Answers questions and offers suggestions for ways to reduce dietary fat intake.

✔ Instructs in possible adverse reactions and signs and symptoms to report to primary health care provider.

✔ Reviews measures to minimize gastrointestinal upset.

✔ Explains possible need for vitamin A and D therapy and high-fiber foods if patient is receiving bile acid sequestrant.

✔ Reassures that results of therapy will be monitored by periodic laboratory and diagnostic tests and follow-up with primary health care provider.

nurse refers the patient or family member to a teaching dietitian, a dietary teaching session, or a lecture provided by a hospital or community agency (see Patient and Family Teaching Checklist: Using Diet and Drugs to Control High Blood Cholesterol Levels). The nurse develops a teaching plan to include the following information:

BILE ACID SEQUESTRANTS

- Take the drug before meals unless the primary health care provider directs otherwise.
- Cholestyramine powder: The prescribed dose must be mixed in 4 to 6 fluid ounces of water or noncarbonated beverage and shaken vigorously. The powder can also be mixed with highly fluid soups or pulpy fruits (applesauce, crushed pineapple). The powder should not be ingested in the dry form. Other drugs are taken 1 hour before or 4 to 6 hours after cholestyramine. Cholestyramine is available combined with the artificial sweetener, aspartame (Questran Light), for patients with diabetes or those who are concerned with weight gain.

- Colestipol granules: The prescribed dose must be mixed in liquids, soup, cereals, carbonated beverages, or pulpy fruits. The granules will not dissolve. Therefore, when mixing with a liquid, slowly stir the preparation until ready to drink. Take the entire drug, rinse the glass with a small amount of water, and drink.
- Colesevelam: Mix the granules in liquids, soups, cereals, or pulpy fruits. Do not take dry. Mix the prescribed amount in a glassful of liquid. Carbonated beverages should be stirred slowly in a large glass. The tablets are taken twice daily without regard to meals.
- Constipation, flatulence, nausea, and heartburn may occur and may disappear with continued therapy. The primary health care provider is notified if these effects become bothersome or if unusual bleeding occurs.

HMG-CoA INHIBITORS

- Lovastatin is taken once daily, preferably with the evening meal. Fluvastatin, pravastatin, and simvastatin are taken, without regard to meals, once daily in the evening or at bedtime.
- If fluvastatin or pravastatin is prescribed with a bile acid sequestrant, take fluvastatin 2 hours after the bile acid sequestrant and pravastatin at least 4 hours afterward.
- Contact the primary health care provider as soon as possible if nausea; vomiting; muscle pain, tenderness, or weakness; fever; upper respiratory infection; rash; itching; or extreme fatigue occurs.

FIBRIC ACID DERIVATIVES

- Clofibrate: If gastrointestinal upset occurs, take the drug with food. Notify the primary health care provider if chest pain, shortness of breath, palpitations, nausea, vomiting, fever, chills, or sore throat occurs.
- Gemfibrozil: Dizziness or blurred vision may occur. Observe caution when driving or performing hazardous tasks. Notify the primary health care provider if epigastric pain, diarrhea, nausea, or vomiting occurs.

MISCELLANEOUS PREPARATION

- Nicotinic acid: Take this drug with meals. This drug may cause mild to severe facial flushing, feeling of warmth, severe itching, or headache. These symptoms usually subside with continued therapy, but contact the primary health care provider as soon as possible if symptoms are severe. The primary health care provider may prescribe aspirin (325 mg) to be taken about 30 minutes before nicotinic acid to decrease the flushing reaction. If dizziness occurs, avoid sudden changes in posture.

EVALUATION

- The therapeutic effect is achieved and serum lipid levels are decreased.
- Adverse reactions are identified, reported to the primary health care provider, and managed successfully through successful nursing interventions.
- The patient and family demonstrate an understanding of the treatment regimen.

● *Critical Thinking Exercises*

1. *A patient in the medical clinic is taking cholestyramine (Questran) for hyperlipidemia. The primary health care provider has prescribed TLC for the patient. The patient is on a low-fat diet and walks daily for exercise. His major complaint at this visit is constipation, which is very bothersome to him. Discuss how you would approach this situation with the patient. What information would you give the patient concerning his constipation?*
2. *Discuss the important points to include in a teaching plan for a patient who is prescribed atorvastatin (Lipitor).*
3. *Describe the important aspects of the ongoing assessment when administering fluvastatin to a patient.*

● *Review Questions*

1. Which of the following adverse reactions is most common in a patient taking a bile acid sequestrant?
   A. Anorexia
   B. Vomiting
   C. Constipation
   D. Headache

2. Lovastatin (Mevacor) is best taken _____.
   A. once daily, preferably with the evening meal
   B. three times daily with meals
   C. at least 1 hour before or 2 hours after meals
   D. twice daily without regard to meals

3. When assessing a patient taking cholestyramine (Questran) for vitamin K deficiency, the nurse would _____.
   A. check the patient for bruising
   B. keep a record of the patient's intake and output
   C. monitor the patient for myalgia
   D. keep a dietary record of foods eaten

4. A patient taking niacin reports flushing after each dose of the niacin. Which of the following drugs would the nurse expect to be prescribed to help alleviate the flushing?
   A. Demerol
   B. Aspirin
   C. Vitamin K
   D. Benadryl

5. Which of the following points would the nurse include when teaching a patient about drug and diet therapy for hyperlipidemia?
   A. Fluids are taken in limited amounts when eating a low-fat diet.
   B. The medication should be taken at least 1 hour before meals.
   C. Medication alone will not lower cholesterol.
   D. Meat is not allowed on a low-fat diet.

● *Medication Dosage Problems*

1. A patient is prescribed 10 mg simvastatin (Zocor) PO daily for high cholesterol. The drug is available in 5-mg tablets. The nurse administers _____.

2. The primary care provider prescribes fenofibrate (Tricor) for the treatment of hypertriglyceridemia. The patient is now taking 200 mg/d PO. Is this an appropriate dosage? If not, what action would you take? If the dose is appropriate, how many capsules would you administer if the drug is available in 54-mg capsules?

chapter **44**

Anticoagulant and Thrombolytic Drugs

Key Terms

fibrolytic drugs
hemostasis
Homans' sign
protamine sulfate

prothrombin
thrombolytic drugs
thrombosis
thrombus

Chapter Objectives

On completion of this chapter, the student will:

- Discuss hemostasis and thrombosis.
- Discuss the uses, general drug actions, adverse reactions, contraindications, precautions, and interactions of warfarin, heparin preparations, and the thrombolytic drugs.
- Discuss important preadministration and ongoing assessment activities the nurse should perform on the patient taking an anticoagulant or thrombolytic drug.
- List some nursing diagnoses particular to a patient taking an anticoagulant or thrombolytic drug.
- Discuss ways to promote an optimal response to therapy, how to manage common adverse reactions, and important points to keep in mind when educating patients about the use of an anticoagulant or thrombolytic drug.

Anticoagulants are used to prevent the formation and extension of a **thrombus** (blood clot). Anticoagulants have no direct effect on an existing thrombus and do not reverse any damage from the thrombus. However, once the presence of a thrombus has been established, anticoagulant therapy can prevent additional clots from forming. Although they do not thin the blood, they are sometimes called blood thinners by patients. The anticoagulants are a group of drugs that include warfarin (a coumarin derivative), anisindione (an indandione derivative), and fractionated and unfractionated heparin.

Whereas the anticoagulants prevent thrombus formation, thrombolytic drugs dissolve blood clots that have already formed within the walls of a blood vessel. These drugs reopen blood vessels after they become occluded. Another term used to identify the thrombolytic drugs is **fibrolytic drugs**. Each of these groups of drugs is discussed in this chapter. Before these drugs are discussed, a basic understanding of hemostasis and thrombus formation is needed.

HEMOSTASIS

Hemostasis is the process that stops bleeding in a blood vessel. Normal hemostasis involves a complex process of extrinsic and intrinsic factors. Figure 44-1 shows the coagulation pathway and factors involved. The coagulation cascade is so named because as each factor is activated it acts as a catalyst that enhances the next reaction, with the net result being a large collection of fibrin that forms a plug in the vessel. Fibrin is the insoluble protein that is essential to clot formation.

THROMBOSIS

Thrombosis is the formation of a clot. A thrombus may form in any vessel, artery, or vein when blood flow is impeded. For example, a venous thrombus can

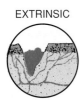

EXTRINSIC

Tissue injury—Facto

INTRINSIC

Platelets Thrombor
Factors VIII, IX, XI,

FIGURE 44-1. The
clot. Formation of
substances. Clotting
before the next step
complete and a fib
formation are in the
the extrinsic pathw
circulating blood.

SUMMARY DRUG TABLE ANTICOAGULANTS (*Continued*)

GENERIC NAME	TRADE NAME*	USES	ADVERSE REACTIONS	DOSAGE RANGES
tinzaparin sodium *ten-zah´-pear-in*	Innohep	Treatment of acute, symptomatic DVT with or without pulmonary emboli when given with warfarin sodium	Hemorrhage, bruising, thrombo-cytopenia, hyperkalemia, hypersensitivity, fever, pain and erythema at injection site	175 anti-Xa IU/kg/d SC once daily; 175 IU/kg/d SC once daily until the patient has been successfully anticoagulated with warfarin
Anticoagulant Antagonists				
phytonadione (vitamin K) *fye-toe-na-dye´-on*	Aqua-mephyton, Mephyton, *generic*	Prevention and treatment of hypopro-thrombinemia associated with excessive doses of oral anticoagulants	Gastric upset, unusual taste, flushing, rash, urticaria, erythema, pain and/or swelling at injection site	PO, IM, 2.5–10 mg, may repeat PO in 12–48 h or in 6–8 h after parenteral dose
protamine sulfate *proe´-ta-meen*	Generic	Acute management of heparin overdosage (neutralizes heparin)	Dyspnea, bradycardia, hypotension, hypertension, bleeding, hypersensitivity reactions	Dose is determined by amount of heparin in body and the time that has elapsed since the heparin was given; the longer the interval, the smaller the dose required. Adult and pediatric: 1mg IV neutralizes 90 USP units of heparin derived from lung tissue or 115 USP units of heparin derived from intestinal mucosa

*The term *generic* indicates the drug is available in generic form.

---

by the liver. This results in the depletion of clotting factors II (**prothrombin**), VII, IX, and X. It is the depletion of prothrombin (see Fig. 44-1), a substance that is essential for the clotting of blood, that accounts for most of the action of warfarin.

USES

Warfarin is used for:

- Prevention (prophylaxis) and treatment of DVT
- Prevention and treatment of atrial fibrillation with embolization
- Prevention and treatment of PE
- As part of the treatment of MI
- Prevention of thrombus formation after valve replacement

In most situations, warfarin is the drug of choice, with anisindione reserved for those who are unable to take warfarin.

ADVERSE REACTIONS

The principal adverse reaction associated with warfarin is bleeding, which may range from very mild to severe. Bleeding may be seen in many areas of the body, such as the bladder, bowel, stomach, uterus, and mucous membranes. Other adverse reactions are rare but may include nausea, vomiting, alopecia (loss of hair), urticaria (severe skin rash), abdominal cramping, diarrhea, rash, hepatitis (inflammation of the liver), jaundice (yellowish discoloration of the skin and mucous membranes), and blood dyscrasias (disorders).

CONTRAINDICATIONS

Warfarin is contraindicated in patients with known hypersensitivity to the drug, hemorrhagic disease, tuberculosis, leukemia, uncontrolled hypertension, gastrointestinal (GI) ulcers, recent surgery of the eye or

---

develop as the
flow), injury
coagulation. Vo
the lower extr
stasis. Deep v
lower extremi
venous throm
because of at
atrial fibrillatio
fibrin, platelet
thrombus, inc
thrombus deta
and is carrie
becomes an e
reaches a vess
If the embol
pulmonary vei
(PE). Similarly
vessel supplyi
myocardial in
are used prop
risk for clot fo

central nervous system, aneurysms, or severe renal or hepatic disease, and during pregnancy and lactation. Use during pregnancy (Pregnancy Category X) can cause fetal death.

PRECAUTIONS

Warfarin is used cautiously in patients with fever, heart failure, diarrhea, malignancy, hypertension, renal or hepatic disease, psychoses, or depression. Women of childbearing age must use a reliable contraceptive to prevent pregnancy.

INTERACTIONS

The effects of warfarin may increase when administered with acetaminophen, NSAIDs, beta blockers, disulfiram, isoniazid, chloral hydrate, loop diuretics, aminoglycosides, cimetidine, tetracyclines, and cephalosporins. Oral contraceptives, ascorbic acid, barbiturates, diuretics, and vitamin K decrease the effects of warfarin. Because the effects of warfarin are influenced by many drugs, the patient must notify the nurse or the primary health care provider when taking a new drug or discontinuing

---

✿ Herbal Alert: Warfarin Interaction

Warfarin, a drug with a narrow therapeutic index, has the potential to interact with many herbal remedies. For example, warfarin should not be combined with any of the following herbs because they may have additive or synergistic activity and increase the risk for bleeding: celery, chamomile, clove, dong quai, feverfew, garlic, ginger, ginkgo biloba, ginseng, green tea, onion, passion flower, red clover, St. John's wort, and tumeric. Any herbal remedy should be used with caution in patients taking warfarin.

Much of the information on drug–herb interactions is speculative. Herb–drug interactions are sporadically reported and difficult to determine. Because herbal supplements are not regulated by the Food and Drug Administration (FDA), products lack standardization, purity, and potency. In addition, multiple ingredients in products and batch-to-batch variation make it difficult to determine if reactions occur as the result of the herb. To assist with the identification of herb–drug interactions, nurses should report any potential interactions to the FDA through its MedWatch program (see Appendix A). Because the absorption, metabolism, distribution, and elimination characteristics of most herbal products are poorly understood, many herb–drug interactions are speculative. It is especially important to take special care when patients are taking any drugs with a narrow therapeutic index (the difference between the minimum therapeutic and minimum toxic drug concentrations is small—such as warfarin) and herbal supplements.

---

use of any drug, both prescription and over-the-counter preparations.

NURSING PROCESS

● The Patient Receiving Warfarin

ASSESSMENT

Preadministration Assessment

Before administering the first dose of warfarin, the nurse questions the patient about all drugs taken during the previous 2 to 3 weeks (if the patient was recently admitted to the hospital). If the patient took any drugs before admission, the nurse notifies the primary health care provider before the first dose is administered. Usually, the prothrombin time (PT) is ordered and the international normalized ratio (INR) determined before therapy is started. The first dose of warfarin is not given until blood for a baseline PT/INR is drawn. The dosage is individualized based on the results of the PT or the INR.

If the patient has a DVT, it usually occurs in a lower extremity. The nurse examines the extremity for color and skin temperature. The nurse also checks for a pedal pulse, noting the rate and strength of the pulse. It is important to record any difference between the affected extremity and the unaffected extremity. The nurse notes areas of redness or tenderness and asks the patient to describe current symptoms. The affected extremity may appear edematous and exhibit a positive **Homans' sign** (pain in the calf when the foot is dorsiflexed). A positive Homans' sign is suggestive of DVT.

Ongoing Assessment

During the course of therapy, the nurse continually assesses the patient for any signs of bleeding and hemorrhage. Areas of assessment include the gums, nose, stools, urine, or nasogastric drainage (see "Promoting an Optimal Response to Therapy").

The nurse examines the skin temperature and color in the patient with a DVT for signs of improvement. The nurse takes and records vital signs every 4 hours or more frequently, if needed.

Patients receiving warfarin for the first time often require daily adjustment of the dose, which is based on the daily PT/INR results. The nurse withholds the drug and notifies the primary health care provider if the PT exceeds 1.2 to 1.5 times the control value or the INR ratio exceeds 3. A daily PT is performed until it stabilizes and when any other drug is added to or removed from the patient's drug regimen. After the PT has stabilized, it is monitored every 4 to 6 weeks.

See Display 44-1 for more information on the laboratory examinations for monitoring warfarin.

DISPLAY 44-1 ● Understanding Prothrombin Time and International Normalized Ratio

Prothrombin time (also called protime) and the International Normalized Ratio are used to monitor the patient's response to warfarin therapy. The daily dose of the oral anticoagulant is based on the patient's daily PT/INR. In the past, recommended therapeutic ranges for PT were 1.5 to 2.5 times the control value. However, today most laboratories use less sensitive substances for testing, and adjustments must be made to reflect this decreased sensitivity. When using the less sensitive substance, the therapeutic range of the PT is 1.2 to 1.5 times the control value. Studies indicate that levels greater than 2 times the control value do not provide additional therapeutic effects in most patients and are associated with a higher incidence of bleeding.

Most laboratories report results for the INR along with the patient's PT and the control value. The INR was devised as a way to standardize PT values and represents a way to "correct" the routine PT results from different laboratories using various sources of thromboplastin and methods of preparation for the test. The INR is determined by a mathematical equation comparing the patient's PT with the standardized PT value. Some institutions may use only PT, others PT/INR, and some may use INR. The INR is maintained between 2 and 3.

Nursing Alert

Optimal therapeutic results are obtained when the patient's PT is 1.2 to 1.5 times the control value. In certain instances, for example as in recurrent systemic embolism, a PT of 1.5 to 2 may be prescribed. Studies indicate that diet can influence the PT/INR values. In patients receiving warfarin, a diet high in vitamin K may decrease the PT/INR and increase the risk of clot formation. A diet low in vitamin K may prolong the PT/INR and increase the risk of hemorrhage. Significant changes in vitamin K intake may necessitate warfarin dosage adjustment. The key to vitamin K management for patients receiving warfarin is maintaining a consistent daily intake of vitamin K. To avoid large fluctuations in vitamin K intake, patients receiving warfarin should be aware of the vitamin K content of food (see Home Care Checklist: Ensuring Appropriate Vitamin K Intake). For example, green leafy vegetables and some vegetable oils (soybean and canola oil) are high in vitamin K. The use of these oils in food preparation may increase the intake of vitamin K enough to cause the PT/INR results to fluctuate. Root vegetables, fruits, cereals, dairy products, and meats are generally low in vitamin K.

Nursing Alert

Patients who have fluctuations in PT/INR levels should be asked about their food intake and any recent dietary changes. A careful assessment of the foods eaten during the last several days is necessary to determine the patient's intake of vitamin K.

NURSING DIAGNOSES

Drug-specific nursing diagnoses are highlighted in the Nursing Diagnoses Checklist. Other nursing diagnoses applicable to these drugs are discussed in depth in Chapter 4.

PLANNING

The expected outcomes for the patient may include an optimal response to therapy, management of common adverse drug reactions, and an understanding of the postdischarge drug regimen.

IMPLEMENTATION

Promoting an Optimal Response to Therapy

Before administering each dose of warfarin, the nurse checks the prothrombin flow sheet or the laboratory report to determine the current PT or INR (PT/INR) results (see Nursing Alerts below). The patient also is checked for any evidence of bleeding.

To hasten the onset of the therapeutic effect, a higher dosage (loading dose) may be prescribed for 2 to 4 days, followed by a maintenance dosage adjusted according to the daily PT/INR. Otherwise, the drug takes 3 to 5 days to reach therapeutic levels. When rapid anticoagulation is required, heparin is preferred as a loading dose, followed by maintenance dose of warfarin based on the PT or INR.

Nursing Diagnoses Checklist

✓ **Risk for Injury** related to adverse drug effects

✓ **Ineffective Tissue Perfusion** related to adverse drug reactions

Although the drug is most often administered orally, warfarin injection may be used as an alternative route for patients who are unable to receive oral drugs. The intravenous dosage is the same as that for the oral drug. Intravenous warfarin is administered as a slow bolus injection during a period of 1 to 2 minutes. Warfarin is not recommended for intramuscular injection. After the drug is reconstituted, it is stable for 4 hours at room temperature. The vial is not recommended for multiple use, and any unused solution should be discarded.

Monitoring and Managing Adverse Drug Reactions

Bleeding can occur any time during therapy with warfarin, even when the PT appears to be within a safe limit (eg, 1.2–1.5 times the control value). All nursing personnel and medical team members should be made aware of any patient receiving warfarin and the observations necessary with administration. The nurse checks the following for signs of bleeding:

- Urinal, bedpan, catheter drainage unit—Inspect the urine for a pink to red color and the stool for signs of GI bleeding (bright red to black stools). Visually check the catheter drainage every 2 to 4 hours and when the unit is emptied. Oral anticoagulants may impart a red-orange color to alkaline urine, making hematuria difficult to detect visually. A urinalysis may be necessary to determine if blood is in the urine.

- Emesis basin, nasogastric suction units—Visually check the nasogastric suction unit every 2 to 4 hours and when the unit is emptied. Check the emesis basin each time it is emptied.
- Skin, mucous membranes—Inspect the patient's skin daily for evidence of easy bruising or bleeding. Be alert for bleeding from minor cuts and scratches, nosebleeds, or excessive bleeding after intramuscular (IM), subcutaneous (SC), or intravenous (IV) injections or after a venipuncture. After oral care, check the toothbrush and gums for signs of bleeding.

☀ Nursing Alert

The nurse should withhold the drug and contact the primary health care provider immediately if any of the following occurs:

- *The PT exceeds 1.5 times the control value.*
- *There is evidence of bleeding.*
- *The INR is greater than 3.*

The nurse must apply prolonged pressure to needle or catheter sites after venipuncture, removal of central or peripheral IV lines, and IM and SC injections. Laboratory personnel or those responsible for drawing blood for laboratory tests are made aware of anticoagulant therapy because prolonged pressure on the venipuncture site is necessary. All laboratory requests require a notation stating the patient is receiving anticoagulant therapy.

MANAGING WARFARIN OVERDOSAGE. Symptoms of overdosage of warfarin include blood in the stool (melena); petechiae (pinpoint-size red hemorrhagic spots on the skin); oozing from superficial injuries, such as cuts from shaving or bleeding from the gums after brushing the teeth; or excessive menstrual bleeding. The nurse must immediately report to the primary health care provider any of these adverse reactions or evidence of bleeding.

If bleeding occurs or if the PT exceeds 1.5 times the control value or the INR exceeds 3, the primary health care provider may either discontinue the anticoagulant therapy for a few days or order vitamin K_1 (phytonadione), an oral anticoagulant antagonist, which must always be readily available when a patient is receiving warfarin. Because warfarin interferes with the synthesis of vitamin K_1-dependent clotting factors, the administration of vitamin K_1 reverses the effects of warfarin by providing the necessary ingredient to enhance clot formation and stop bleeding. However, withholding one or two doses of warfarin may quickly bring the PT to an acceptable level.

The nurse must assess the patient for additional evidence of bleeding until the PT is below 1.5 times the control value or until the bleeding episodes cease. The PT generally returns to a safe level within 6 hours of administration of vitamin K_1. Administration of whole blood or plasma may be necessary if severe bleeding occurs because of the delayed onset of vitamin K_1.

Educating the Patient and Family

The nurse provides a full explanation of the drug regimen to patients taking warfarin, including an explanation of the problems that can occur during therapy. A thorough review of the dose regimen, possible adverse drug reactions, and early signs of bleeding tendencies help the patient cooperate with the prescribed therapy. The nurse should include the following points in a patient and family teaching plan:

- Follow the dosage schedule prescribed by the primary health care provider.
- The PT or INR will be monitored periodically. Keep all primary health care provider and laboratory appointments because dosage changes may be necessary during therapy.
- Do not take or stop taking other drugs except on the advice of the primary health care provider. This includes nonprescription drugs, as well as those prescribed by a primary health care provider or dentist.
- Inform the dentist or other primary health care providers of therapy with this drug before any treatment or procedure is started or drugs are prescribed.
- Take the drug at the same time each day.
- Do not change brands of anticoagulants without consulting a physician or pharmacist.
- Avoid alcohol unless use has been approved by the primary health care provider. Advise the patient to limit foods high in vitamin K, such as leafy green vegetables, beans, broccoli, cabbage, cauliflower, cheese, fish, and yogurt. Vegetables with large amounts of vitamin K can interfere with the anticoagulant's effect (see Home Care Checklist: Ensuring Appropriate Vitamin K Intake).
- If evidence of bleeding should occur, such as unusual bleeding or bruising, bleeding gums, blood in the urine or stool, black stool, or diarrhea, omit the next dose of the drug and contact the primary health care provider immediately. (Anisindione may cause a red-orange discoloration of alkaline urine.)
- Use a soft toothbrush and consult a dentist regarding routine oral hygiene, including the use of dental floss. Use an electric razor when possible to avoid small skin cuts.
- Women of childbearing age must use a reliable contraceptive to prevent pregnancy.

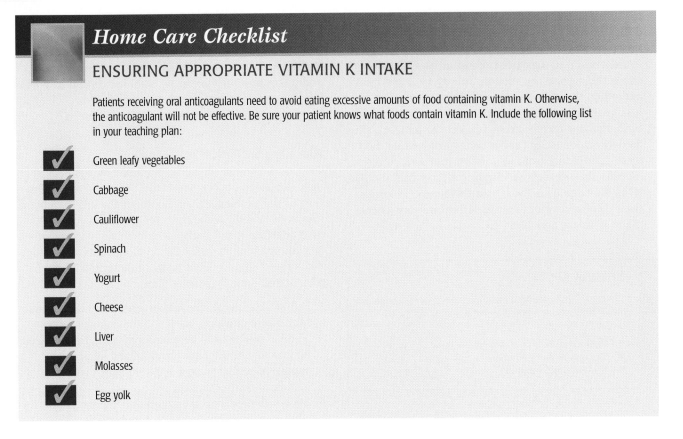

Home Care Checklist

ENSURING APPROPRIATE VITAMIN K INTAKE

Patients receiving oral anticoagulants need to avoid eating excessive amounts of food containing vitamin K. Otherwise, the anticoagulant will not be effective. Be sure your patient knows what foods contain vitamin K. Include the following list in your teaching plan:

- ✓ Green leafy vegetables
- ✓ Cabbage
- ✓ Cauliflower
- ✓ Spinach
- ✓ Yogurt
- ✓ Cheese
- ✓ Liver
- ✓ Molasses
- ✓ Egg yolk

● Wear or carry identification, such as a medical alert tag, Alert, to inform medical personnel and others of therapy with this drug.

EVALUATION

- The therapeutic drug effect is achieved.
- Adverse reactions are identified, reported to the primary health care provider, and managed successfully using appropriate nursing interventions.
- The patient demonstrates an understanding of the drug regimen.
- The patient verbalizes the importance of complying with the prescribed therapeutic regimen.
- The patient lists or describes early signs of bleeding.

FRACTIONATED AND UNFRACTIONATED HEPARIN

Heparin preparations are available as heparin sodium and the low-molecular-weight heparins (fractionated heparins). Heparin is not a single drug, but rather a mixture of high and low-molecular-weight drugs. Fragments of heparin with low molecular weights are available as low-molecular-weight heparin (LMWH). Examples of LMWHs are dalteparin (Fragmin), enoxaparin (Lovenox), and tinzaparin (Innohep). LMWHs

produce very stable responses when administered at the recommended doses. Because of this stability, frequent laboratory monitoring, as with heparin, is not necessary. In addition, bleeding is less likely to occur with LMWHs than with heparin.

ACTIONS

Heparin inhibits the formation of fibrin clots, inhibits the conversion of fibrinogen to fibrin, and inactivates several of the factors necessary for the clotting of blood. Heparin cannot be taken orally because it is inactivated by gastric acid in the stomach; therefore, it must be given by injection. Heparin has no effect on clots that have already formed and aids only in preventing the formation of new blood clots (thrombi). The LMWHs act to inhibit clotting reactions by binding to antithrombin III, which inhibits the synthesis of factor Xa and the formation of thrombin.

USES

Heparin is used for:

- Prevention and treatment of venous thrombosis, PE, peripheral arterial embolism;
- Atrial fibrillation with embolus formation;

- Prevention of postoperative venous thrombosis (DVT) and PE in certain patients undergoing surgical procedures, such as major abdominal surgery;
- Prevention of clotting in arterial and heart surgery, in blood transfusions and dialysis procedures, and in blood samples for laboratory purposes;
- Prevention of a repeat cerebral thrombosis in some patients who have experienced a stroke;
- Treatment of coronary occlusion, acute MI, and peripheral arterial embolism;
- Prevention of clotting in equipment used for extracorporeal (occurring outside the body) circulation;
- Diagnosis and treatment of disseminated intravascular coagulation, a severe hemorrhagic disorder.
- Maintenance of patency of IV catheters (very low doses of 10 to 100 units [U]).

The LMWHs are used to prevent DVT after certain surgical procedures, such as hip or knee replacement surgery or abdominal surgery. The drugs are also used for ischemic complications of unstable angina and MI (for specific uses of each drug see the Summary Drug Table: Anticoagulants).

ADVERSE REACTIONS

Hemorrhage is the chief complication of heparin administration. Hemorrhage can range from minor local bruising to major hemorrhaging from any organ. Thrombocytopenia (low levels of platelets in the blood) may occur, causing bleeding from the small capillaries and resulting in easy bruising, petechiae, and hemorrhage into the tissues.

Other adverse reactions include local irritation when heparin is given via the SC route. Hypersensitivity reactions may also occur with any route of administration and include fever, chills, and urticaria. More serious hypersensitivity reactions include an asthma-like reaction and an anaphylactoid reaction.

The LMWHs cause fewer adverse reactions than heparin. Bleeding related to the LMWHs is possible but has generally been low. See the Summary Drug Table: Anticoagulants for additional adverse reactions associated with the LMWHs.

CONTRAINDICATIONS

Heparin preparations are contraindicated in patients with known hypersensitivity to the drug, active bleeding (except when caused by disseminated intravascular coagulation), hemorrhagic disorders, severe thrombocytopenia, or recent surgery (except for the LMWHs used after certain surgical procedures to prevent thromboembolic complications) and during pregnancy (Pregnancy Category C).

The LMWHs are contraindicated in patients with a hypersensitivity to the drug, heparin, or pork products and inpatients with active bleeding or thrombocytopenia.

PRECAUTIONS

Treatment with heparin preparations is approached cautiously in the elderly, in patients with severe renal or kidney disease, diabetes, diabetic retinopathy, ulcer disease, or uncontrolled hypertension, and in all patients with a potential site for bleeding or hemorrhage. The LMWHs are used with caution in patients who are at increased risk of hemorrhage, such as those with severe uncontrolled hypertension, diabetic retinopathy, bacterial endocarditis, congenital or acquired bleeding disorders, GI disease, or hemorrhagic stroke and shortly after brain, spinal, or ophthalmological surgery.

INTERACTIONS

When heparin is administered with the NSAIDs, aspirin, penicillin, or the cephalosporins, there may be an increase in clotting times, thereby increasing the risk for bleeding. During heparin administration, serum transaminase (aspartate, alanine) levels may be falsely elevated. Careful interpretation is required because these laboratory tests may be used to help diagnose certain disorders, such as liver disease or MI. **Protamine sulfate,** a heparin antagonist, is incompatible with certain antibiotics such as penicillin and the cephalosporins. Use of the LMWHs with the following drugs may increase the risk of bleeding: aspirin, salicylates, NSAIDs, and thrombolytics.

NURSING PROCESS

● **The Patient Receiving Heparin**

ASSESSMENT

Preadministration Assessment
Before administering the first dose of heparin, the nurse obtains the patient's vital signs. The most commonly used test to monitor heparin is activated partial thromboplastin time (APTT). Blood is drawn for laboratory studies before giving the first dose of heparin to obtain baseline data. (See the discussion on preadministration assessment for the oral anticoagulants.)

Ongoing Assessment
The ongoing assessment of a patient receiving heparin requires close observation and careful monitoring. The nurse assesses vital signs every 2 to 4 hours or more frequently during administration.

The dosage of heparin is adjusted according to daily APTT monitoring. A therapeutic dosage is attained when the APTT is 1.5 to 2.5 times the normal. The LMWHs have little or no effect on the APTT values. Special monitoring of clotting times is not necessary when administering the drugs.

Periodic platelet counts, hematocrit, and tests for occult blood in the stool should be performed throughout the entire course of heparin therapy.

It is also important that the nurse monitor for any indication of hypersensitivity reaction. The nurse reports reactions, such as chills, fever, or hives, to the primary health care provider. When heparin is given to prevent the formation of a thrombus, the nurse observes the patient for signs of thrombus formation every 2 to 4 hours. Because the signs and symptoms of thrombus formation vary and depend on the area or organ involved, the nurse should evaluate and report any complaint the patient may have or any change in the patient's condition to the primary health care provider.

NURSING DIAGNOSES

Drug-specific nursing diagnoses are highlighted in the Nursing Diagnoses Checklist. Other nursing diagnoses applicable to these drugs are discussed in depth in Chapter 4.

PLANNING

The expected outcomes for the patient may include an optimal response to drug therapy, management of common adverse drug reactions, and an understanding of the therapeutic regimen.

IMPLEMENTATION

Promoting an Optimal Response to Therapy

Heparin preparations, unlike warfarin, must be given by the parenteral route, preferably SC or IV. The onset of anticoagulation is almost immediate after a single dose. Maximum effects occur within 10 minutes of administration. Clotting time will return to normal within 4 hours unless subsequent doses are given.

Blood coagulation tests are usually ordered before and during heparin therapy, and the dose of heparin is adjusted to the test results. Optimal results of therapy are obtained when the APTT is 1.5 to 2.5 times the control value. The LMWHs do not require close monitoring of blood coagulation tests.

Nursing Diagnoses Checklist

✓ **Ineffective Tissue Perfusion** related to adverse drug effects
✓ **Risk for Injury**

A complete blood count, platelets, and stools for occult blood may be ordered periodically throughout therapy. Thrombocytopenia may occur during heparin administration. A mild, transient thrombocytopenia may occur 2 to 3 days after heparin therapy is begun. This early development of thrombocytopenia tends to resolve itself despite continued therapy. The nurse reports a platelet count of less than 100,000 mm^3 immediately because the primary care provider may choose to discontinue the heparin therapy.

ADMINISTERING HEPARIN PREPARATIONS. The dosage of heparin is measured in units and is available in various dosage strengths as units per milliliter (U/mL), for example, 10,000 U/mL. When selecting the strength used for administration, choose the strength closest to the prescribed dose. For example, if 5000 U is ordered, and the available strengths are 1000, 5000, 7500, 20,000, and 40,000 U/mL, use 1 mL of the 5000 U/mL for administration.

Heparin may be given by intermittent IV administration, continuous IV infusion, and the SC route. Intramuscular administration is avoided because of the possibility of the development of local irritation, pain, or hematoma (a collection of blood in the tissue). A solution of dilute heparin may be used to maintain patency of an IV site used for intermittent administration of any drug given by the IV route.

Intermittent IV administration requires the use of an adapter or heparin lock to provide ready access to a vein without having to maintain a continuous infusion. A solution of dilute heparin consisting of 10 to 100 U/mL may be ordered for injection into the heparin lock before and after the administration of the intermittent dose of heparin or any other drug administered by the intermittent IV route. This is called a heparin lock flush. The lock flush solution aids in preventing small clots from obstructing the needle of the intermittent administration set. To prevent incompatibility of heparin with other drugs, the heparin lock set is flushed with sterile water or sterile normal saline before and after any drug is given through the IV line. The primary health care provider or institutional policy dictates the use and type of lock flush solution.

Each time heparin is given, the nurse inspects the needle site for signs of inflammation, pain, and tenderness along the pathway of the vein. If these should occur, the use of this site is discontinued and a new intermittent set is inserted at a different site. Coagulation tests are usually performed 30 minutes before the scheduled dose and from the extremity opposite the infusion site.

An infusion pump must be used for the safe administration of heparin by continuous IV infusion. The nurse checks the infusion pump every 1 to 2 hours to ensure that it is working properly. The needle site is inspected for signs of inflammation, pain, and tenderness along the pathway of the vein. If these should occur, the infusion is discontinued and restarted in another vein.

⁕ Nursing Alert

Blood coagulation tests for those receiving heparin by continuous IV infusion are taken at periodic intervals (usually every 4 hours) determined by the primary health care provider. If the patient is receiving long-term heparin therapy, blood coagulation tests may be performed at less frequent intervals.

⁕ Nursing Alert

If the patient is receiving heparin by intermittent or continuous IV infusion, other drugs administered by the IV route are not given through the IV tubing or injection port or piggybacked into the continuous IV line unless the primary health care provider orders the drug given in this manner. In addition, the nurse should never mix other drugs with heparin when heparin is given by any route.

When heparin is given by the SC route, administration sites are rotated and the site used is recorded on the patient's chart. The recommended sites of administration are those on the abdomen, but areas within 2 inches of the umbilicus are avoided because of the increased vascularity of that area. Other areas of administration are the buttocks and lateral thighs. The nurse gives the injection at a 90-degree angle. The site is not massaged after giving the injection, but the nurse applies firm pressure to the injection site until all oozing of blood has stopped.

The "bunch" technique may be used when administering heparin SC. When using the bunch method, the nurse grasps the tissue around the selected site to form a tissue roll that is about 0.5 inch in diameter. The nurse inserts the needle into the tissue roll at a 90-degree angle and injects the drug. The nurse then releases the tissue roll. It is not necessary to aspirate before injecting the drug. The application of firm pressure after the injection helps to prevent hematoma formation. Each time heparin is given by this route, the nurse inspects all recent injection sites for signs of inflammation (redness, swelling, tenderness) and hematoma formation. When administering heparin by the SC route, an APTT test is performed 4 to 6 hours after the injection.

ADMINISTERING THE LOW-MOLECULAR-WEIGHT HEPARIN. The LMWHs are administered by the SC route only. Dalteparin is given by the SC route 1 to 2 hours before surgery and once daily for 5 to 10 days after surgery. The first dose of enoxaparin is administered via the SC route within the first 12 to 24 hours after surgery and continued for 7 to 10 days. When enoxaparin is administered in patients having abdominal surgery, the first dose is via the SC route 2 hours before surgery and as long as 12 days after surgery. Tinzaparin is administered via the SC route within 12 to 24 hours after surgery with administration continuing as long as 14 days.

The nurse gives these drugs deep into the SC tissue in the abdomen (avoiding the navel) with the site rotated at the time of each injection. Alternate sites are the buttocks or upper thighs. The nurse places the patient in a supine position. To avoid the loss of the drug, the air bubble is not expelled from the syringe before injection. The drug is administered alternately between left and right anterolateral and left and right posterolateral abdominal wall. The injection site is varied daily. When the drug is administered, the skin is lifted between the thumb and forefinger (as in the bunch technique). The entire length of the needle is inserted into the skin fold at a 45- to 90-degree angle, with the skin fold held throughout the injection. To minimize bruising, the injection site is not rubbed after the drug is administered. Bruising may be decreased by using an ice cube to massage the site before injection of the drug. Prefilled syringes or enoxaparin are available for patients taking the drug at home.

Monitoring and Managing Adverse Drug Reactions

Bleeding at virtually any site can occur during therapy with any heparin preparation, even the LMWHs. The nurse monitors the patient's vital signs every 2 to 4 hours or as ordered by the primary health care provider.

⁕ Nursing Alert

The nurse should immediately report evidence of bleeding in any patient receiving heparin: bleeding gums, epistaxis (nosebleed), easy bruising, black tarry stools, hematuria (blood in the urine), oozing from wounds or IV sites, or decrease in blood pressure.

❄ Gerontologic Alert

There is an increased incidence of bleeding in individuals older than 60 years (particularly older women) when heparin is administered. The nurse should carefully monitor older patients for evidence of bleeding.

MANAGING OVERDOSAGE. If a decided drop in blood pressure or rise in the pulse rate occurs, the nurse notifies the primary health care provider because this may indicate internal bleeding. Because hemorrhage may begin as a slight bleeding or bruising tendency, the nurse frequently observes the patient for these occurrences (see discussion of warfarin). At times, hemorrhage can occur without warning. If bleeding should occur, the primary health care provider may decrease the dose, discontinue the heparin therapy for a time, or order the administration of protamine sulfate.

In most instances, discontinuation of the drug is sufficient to correct overdosage because the duration of action of heparin is short. However, if hemorrhaging is severe, the primary health care provider may order protamine sulfate, the specific heparin antagonist or antidote. Protamine sulfate is also used to treat overdosage of the LMWHs. Protamine sulfate has an immediate onset of action and a duration of 2 hours. It counteracts the effects of heparin and brings blood coagulation tests to within normal limits. The drug is given slowly via the IV route during a period of 10 minutes.

> ### ✳ Nursing Alert
>
> *Protamine sulfate can result in severe hypotension and ana-phylactic reaction. When administering protamine sulfate, the nurse should make sure that resuscitation equipment is read-ily available.*

If administration of this drug is necessary, the nurse monitors the patient's blood pressure and pulse rate every 15 to 30 minutes for 2 hours or more after administration of the heparin antagonist. The nurse immediately reports to the primary health care provider any sudden decrease in blood pressure or increase in the pulse rate. The nurse observes the patient for new evidence of bleeding until blood coagulation tests are within normal limits. To replace blood loss, the primary health care provider may order blood transfusions or fresh frozen plasma.

Educating the Patient and Family

Although heparin is given in the hospital, the LMWHs can be administered at home by a home health nurse, the patient, or a family member. The patient or a family member is taught how to administer the drug by the SC route (see technique under Promoting an Optimal Response to Therapy). Prefilled syringes are available, making administration more convenient. The nurse instructs the patient to apply firm pressure after the injection to prevent hematoma formation. Each time the drug is given, the nurse inspects all recent injection sites for signs of inflammation (redness, swelling, tenderness) and hematoma formation.

The nurse includes the following in a patient and family teaching plan:

- Report any signs of active bleeding immediately.
- Regular coagulation blood tests are critical for safe monitoring of the drug (except the LMWHs).
- Avoid IM injections while receiving anticoagulant therapy.
- Use a soft toothbrush when cleaning the teeth and an electric razor for shaving.
- Do not take any prescription or nonprescription drugs without consulting the primary health care provider. Drugs containing alcohol, aspirin, or ibuprofen may alter the effects of heparin.
- Advise your dentist or primary health care provider of anticoagulant therapy before any procedure or surgery.
- Carry appropriate identification with information concerning drug therapy or wear a medical alert tag at all times.

EVALUATION

- The therapeutic drug effect is achieved.
- Adverse drug reactions are identified, reported to the primary health care provider, and managed successfully through appropriate nursing interventions.
- No evidence of bleeding is seen.
- The patient verbalizes an understanding of treatment modalities.

THROMBOLYTIC DRUGS

Thrombolytics are a group of drugs used to dissolve certain types of blood clots and reopen blood vessels after they have been occluded. Examples of thrombolytics include alteplase* recombinant (Activase), reteplase recombinant (Retavase), streptokinase (Streptase), tenecteplase (TNKase), and urokinase (Abbokinase). Before these drugs are used, their potential benefits must be carefully weighed against the potential dangers of bleeding.

ACTIONS ●

Although the exact action of the thrombolytic drugs is slightly different, these drugs break down fibrin clots by converting plasminogen to plasmin (fibrinolysin). Plasmin is an enzyme that breaks down the fibrin of a blood clot. This reopens blood vessels after their occlusion and prevents tissue necrosis.

USES ●

These drugs are used to treat an acute MI by lysing (dissolving) a blood clot in a coronary artery. These drugs are also effective in lysing clots causing PE and DVT. Urokinase is also used to treat PE and to clear IV

---

*Alteplase is a tissue plasminogen activator (tPA) that is produced by recombinant DNA. Recombinant DNA is obtained by using gene splicing. Specific DNA segments of one organism are placed in the DNA of another organism. The genetic material of the recipient organism then reproduces itself and contains genetic material of its own plus the genetic material from the donor organism.

SUMMARY DRUG TABLE THROMBOLYTICS

GENERIC NAME	TRADE NAME*	USES	ADVERSE REACTIONS	DOSAGE RANGES
alteplase, recombinant *al´-te-plaz*	Activase	Acute myocardial infarction (AMI), acute ischemic stroke, pulmonary embolism (PE)	Bleeding (GU, gingival, retroperitoneal), and epistaxis, ecchymosis	AMI: total dose of 100 mg IV given as 60 mg 1st h, 20 mg 2nd h and 20 mg over 3rd h; for patients < 65 kg, decrease dose to 1.25 mg/kg
reteplase, recombinant *ret´-ah-plaze*	Retavase	AMI	Bleeding (GI, GU, or at injection site), intracranial hemorrhage, anemia	10 plus 10 U double bolus IV over 2 min each with the 2nd bolus given 30 min after the 1st
streptokinase *strep-toe-kye´-nase*	Streptase	AMI, DVT, PE, embolism	Minor bleeding (superficial and surface) and major bleeding (internal and severe)	Lysis of coronary artery thrombosis, 20,000 IU directly into vein; PE, DVT, embolism: 250,000 IU IV over 30 min followed by 100,000 IU for 24–72 h
tenecteplase *teh-nek´-ti-plaze*	TNKase	AMI	Bleeding (GI, GU, or at injection site), intracranial hemorrhage, anemia	Dosage based on weight, not to exceed 50 mg IV
urokinase *yoor-oh´-kye-nase*	Abbokinase	PE, lysis of coronary artery thrombi, IV catheter clearance	Minor bleeding (superficial and surface) and major bleeding (internal and severe)	PE: 4400 IU/kg IV over 10 min, followed by 4400 IU/kg/hr for 12 h; lysis of thrombi: 6000 IU/min IV for 2 h; IV catheter clearance: see packaged instructions

*The term *generic* indicates that drug is available in generic form.

catheter cannulas obstructed by a blood clot. See the Summary Drug Table: Thrombolytics for a more complete listing of the use of these drugs.

ADVERSE REACTIONS

Bleeding is the most common adverse reaction seen with the use of these drugs. Bleeding may be internal and involve areas such as the GI tract, genitourinary tract, and the brain. Bleeding may also be external (superficial) and may be seen at areas of broken skin, such as venipuncture sites and recent surgical wounds. Allergic reactions may also be seen.

CONTRAINDICATIONS

Thrombolytic drugs are contraindicated in patients with known hypersensitivity, active bleeding, history of stroke, aneurysm, and recent intracranial surgery.

PRECAUTIONS

These drugs are used cautiously in patients who have recently undergone major surgery (within 10 days or less), such as coronary artery bypass graft, or experienced stroke, trauma, vaginal or cesarean section delivery, GI bleeding, or trauma within the last 10 days; those who have hypertension, diabetic retinopathy, or any condition in which bleeding is a significant possibility; and patients currently receiving oral anticoagulants. All of the thrombolytic drugs discussed in this chapter are classified in Pregnancy Category C, with the exception of urokinase, which is a Pregnancy Category B drug.

INTERACTIONS

Administration of the thrombolytic drugs with aspirin, dipyridamole, or the anticoagulants may increase the risk of bleeding.

NURSING PROCESS

● The Patient Receiving a Thrombolytic Drug

ASSESSMENT

Preadministration Assessment

During the preadministration assessment the nurse interviews the patient or family and notes any history of conditions that might contraindicate the use of a thrombolytic drug (see Contraindications). The nurse identifies any history of bleeding tendencies, heart disease, or allergic reactions to any drugs. In addition, a history of any drugs currently being taken is obtained. The nurse reports any relevant information to the primary health care provider before the drug is administered. Initial patient assessments include vital signs and a review of the diagnostic tests performed to establish a diagnosis. Most of these patients are admitted or transferred to an intensive care unit because close monitoring for 48 hours or more after therapy is necessary.

Ongoing Assessment

The most important aspect of the ongoing assessment is the possibility of bleeding. The nurse must assess the patient for bleeding every 15 minutes during the first 60 minutes of therapy, every 15 to 30 minutes for the next 8 hours, and at least every 4 hours until therapy is completed. Vital signs are taken at least every 4 hours for the duration of therapy.

The nurse must continually assess the patient for anaphylactic reactions (difficulty breathing, wheezing, fever, swelling around the eyes, hives, or itching) particularly with anistreplase or streptokinase. Resuscitation equipment is immediately available.

NURSING DIAGNOSES

Drug-specific nursing diagnoses are highlighted in the Nursing Diagnoses Checklist. Other nursing diagnoses applicable to these drugs are discussed in depth in Chapter 4.

PLANNING

The expected outcomes for the patient may include an optimal response to therapy (which includes a decrease in pain), management of common adverse reactions, and an understanding of the therapeutic regimen.

Nursing Diagnoses Checklist

- ✓ **Ineffective Tissue Perfusion** related to adverse drug reactions
- ✓ **Risk for Injury** related to adverse drug reactions
- ✓ **Pain** related to obstruction of blood vessel

IMPLEMENTATION

Promoting an Optimal Response to Therapy

For optimal therapeutic effect the thrombolytic drugs are used as soon as possible after the formation of a thrombus, preferably within 4 to 6 hours or as soon as possible after the symptoms are identified. The greatest benefit in mortality is seen when the drugs are administered within 4 hours, but studies indicate that significant benefit has been reported when the agents were used within the first 24 hours. The nurse must follow the primary health care provider's orders precisely regarding dosage and time of administration. These drugs are available in powder form and must be reconstituted according to the directions in the package insert.

Tenecteplase (TNKase) is the first thrombolytic drug that can be administered during a period of 5 seconds in a single dose. The drug is administered intravenously only and offers the fastest administration of a thrombolytic in the treatment of an acute MI. Specific instructions for reconstitution come with the drug. The drug is reconstituted immediately before use because it contains no antibacterial preservatives.

If pain is present, the primary health care provider may order a narcotic analgesic. Once the clot is dissolved and blood flows freely through the obstructed blood vessel, severe pain usually decreases.

When using urokinase to clear an occluded IV catheter, the nurse follows the manufacturer's instructions in the packaged insert. The nurse avoids using excessive pressure when the drug is injected into the catheter. Excessive force could rupture the catheter or expel the clot into the circulation. It is important to remember that if the catheter is occluded by substances other than blood fibrin clots, such as drug precipitates, urokinase is not effective.

✳ Nursing Alert

Streptokinase is not used for restoring IV catheter patency. Serious adverse reactions, including hypotension, hypersensitivity apnea, and bleeding, have occurred when the drug is used for this purpose.

Monitoring and Managing Adverse Drug Reactions

Bleeding is the most common adverse reaction. Throughout administration of the thrombolytic drug, the nurse assesses for signs of bleeding and hemorrhage (see earlier discussion on warfarin). Internal bleeding may involve the GI tract, genitourinary tract, intracranial sites, or respiratory tract. Symptoms of internal bleeding may include abdominal pain, coffee-ground emesis, black tarry stools, hematuria, joint pain, and spitting or coughing up of blood. Superficial bleeding may occur at venous or arterial puncture sites or recent surgical incision sites. As fibrin is lysed during therapy, bleeding from recent injection sites may occur. The nurse must carefully monitor all potential bleeding sites (including catheter insertions sites, arterial and venous puncture sites, cutdown sites, and needle puncture sites). For minor bleeding at a puncture site, the nurse can usually control bleeding by applying pressure for at least 30 minutes at the site, followed by the application of a pressure dressing. The puncture site is checked frequently for evidence of further bleeding. Intramuscular injections and nonessential handling of the patient are avoided during treatment. Venipunctures are done only when absolutely necessary.

> ### ☀ Nursing Alert
>
> *Heparin may be given along with and/or after administration with a thrombolytic drug to prevent another thrombus from forming. However, administration of an anticoagulant increases the risk for bleeding. The patient must be monitored closely for internal and external bleeding.*

If uncontrolled bleeding is noted or the bleeding appears to be internal, the nurse stops the drug and immediately contacts the primary health care provider because whole blood, packed red cells, or fresh, frozen plasma may be required. Vital signs are monitored every hour or more frequently for at least 48 hours after the drug use is discontinued. The nurse contacts the primary health care provider if there is a marked change in one or more of the vital signs. Any signs of an allergic (hypersensitivity) reaction, such as difficulty breathing, wheezing, hives, skin rash, and hypotension, are reported immediately to the primary health care provider.

Educating the Patient and Family

The nurse includes the following in the patient and family teaching plan:

- Explains the purpose of the drug and the method of administration.
- Explains the need for continuous monitoring before and after administration of the thrombolytic drug.
- Instructs the patient to report any evidence of hypersensitivity reaction (rash, difficulty breathing) or evidence of bleeding or bruising.
- Explains the need for bed rest and minimal handling during therapy.

EVALUATION

- The therapeutic effect achieved; lysis of thrombi or emboli occurs and the catheter or cannula is patent.
- Pain is relieved.

- Adverse reactions are identified, reported to the primary health care provider, and managed using appropriate nursing interventions.
- The patient and family demonstrate an understanding of treatment and techniques necessary to monitor therapy.

● Critical Thinking Exercises

1. *Ms. Jackson, age 56 years, is hospitalized with a venous thrombosis. The primary health care provider orders SC heparin. In developing a care plan for Ms. Jackson, discuss the nursing interventions that would be most important to prevent complications while administering heparin. Provide a rationale for each intervention.*

2. *Mr. Harris, age 72 years, is a widower who has lived alone since his wife died 5 years ago. He has been prescribed warfarin to take at home after his dismissal from the hospital. Determine which questions concerning the home environment would be important to ask Mr. Harris to prepare him to care for himself and prevent any complications associated with the warfarin.*

3. *A patient enters the emergency department with an acute MI. Thrombolytic therapy is begun with streptokinase. Discuss ongoing assessments that are important for the nurse to perform.*

4. *Discuss the use of laboratory tests in monitoring heparin administration.*

● Review Questions

1. The patient is receiving the first dose of warfarin. Before administering the drug, the nurse _____.

   A. administers a loading of heparin
   B. has the laboratory draw blood for a serum potassium level
   C. takes the apical pulse
   D. checks to see that blood has been drawn for a baseline prothrombin time

2. The nurse monitors the prothrombin time (PT) during therapy. Optimal PT for warfarin therapy is _____.

   A. more than 15 seconds
   B. less than 25 seconds
   C. 1.8 to 2 times the control value
   D. 1.2 to 1.5 times the control value

3. There is an increased risk for bleeding when the patient receiving heparin is also taking _____.

   A. allopurinol
   B. an NSAID
   C. digoxin
   D. furosemide

4. In which of the following situations would the nurse expect a LMWH to be prescribed?
   A. to prevent a DVT
   B. for a patient with disseminated intravascular coagulation
   C. to prevent hemorrhage
   D. for a patient with atrial fibrillation

5. If bleeding is noted while a patient is receiving a thrombolytic drug, the patient may receive _____.
   A. heparin
   B. whole blood or fresh, frozen plasma

C. a diuretic
D. protamine sulfate

● Medication Dosage Problems

1. The patient is prescribed 5000 U heparin. The drug is available as a solution of 7500 U/mL. The nurse administers _____.

2. Warfarin 5 mg is prescribed. On hand are 2.5-mg tablets. The nurse administers _____.

Agents Used in the Treatment of Anemia

Chapter Objectives

On completion of this chapter, the student will:

- Describe the different types of anemia
- List the drugs used in the treatment of anemia.
- Discuss the actions, uses, general adverse reactions, contraindications, precautions, and interactions of the agents used to treat anemia.
- Discuss important preadministration and ongoing assessment activities the nurse should perform on a patient receiving an agent used to treat anemia.
- Identify nursing diagnoses particular to a patient receiving an agent used to treat anemia.
- Discuss ways to promote an optimal response to therapy and important points to keep in mind when educating patients about the use of an agent used to treat anemia.

Anemia is a decrease in the number of red blood cells (RBCs), a decrease in the amount of hemoglobin in RBCs, or both a decrease in the number of RBCs and hemoglobin. When there is an insufficient amount of hemoglobin to deliver oxygen to the tissues, anemia exists. There are various types and causes of anemia. For example, anemia can be the result of blood loss, excessive destruction of RBCs, inadequate production of RBCs, and deficits in various nutrients, such as in iron deficiency anemia. Once the type and cause have been identified, the primary health care provider selects a method of treatment.

The anemias discussed in this chapter include iron deficiency anemia, anemia in patients with chronic renal disease, pernicious anemia, and anemia resulting from a folic acid deficiency. Table 45-1 defines these anemias. Drugs used in treatment of anemia are summarized in the Summary Drug Table: Drugs Used in the Treatment of Anemia.

DRUGS USED IN THE TREATMENT OF IRON DEFICIENCY ANEMIA

Iron deficiency anemia is by far the most common type of anemia. Iron is a component of hemoglobin, which is in RBCs. It is the iron in the hemoglobin of RBCs that picks up oxygen from the lungs and carries it to all body tissues. Iron is stored in the body and is found mainly in the reticuloendothelial cells of the liver, spleen, and bone marrow. When the body does not have enough iron to supply the body's needs, the resulting condition is **iron deficiency anemia.**

ACTIONS AND USES

Iron salts, such as ferrous sulfate or ferrous gluconate, are used in the treatment of iron deficiency anemia, which occurs when there is a loss of iron that is greater than the available iron stored in the body. Iron preparations act by elevating the serum iron concentration, which replenishes hemoglobin and depleted iron stores.

Iron dextran is a parenteral iron that is also used for the treatment of iron deficiency anemia. It is primarily used when the patient cannot take oral drugs or when the patient experiences gastrointestinal intolerance to oral iron administration. Other iron preparations, both oral and parenteral, used in the treatment of iron deficiency anemia can be found in the Summary Drug Table: Drugs Used in the Treatment of Anemia.

TABLE 45-1	Anemias
TYPE OF ANEMIA	**DESCRIPTION**
Iron deficiency	Anemia characterized by an inadequate amount of iron in the body to produce hemoglobin
Anemia in chronic renal failure (CRF)	Anemia resulting from a reduced production of erythropoietin, a hormone secreted by the kidney that stimulates the production of red blood cells (RBCs)
Pernicious anemia	Anemia resulting from lack of secretions by the gastric mucosa of the intrinsic factor essential to the formation of RBCs and the absorption of vitamin B_{12}
Folic acid deficiency	A slowly progressive type of anemia occurring because of the lack of folic acid, a component necessary in the formation of RBCs

ADVERSE REACTIONS

Iron salts occasionally cause gastrointestinal irritation, nausea, vomiting, constipation, diarrhea, headache, backache, and allergic reactions. The stools usually appear darker (black). Iron dextran is given by the parenteral route. Hypersensitivity reactions, including fatal anaphylactic reactions, have been reported with the use of this form of iron. Additional adverse reactions include soreness, inflammation, and sterile abscesses at the intramuscular (IM) injection site. Intravenous (IV) administration may result in phlebitis at the injection site. When iron is administered via the IM route, a brownish discoloration of the skin may occur. Patients with rheumatoid arthritis may experience an acute exacerbation of joint pain, and swelling may occur when iron dextran is administered.

CONTRAINDICATIONS, PRECAUTIONS, AND INTERACTIONS

Drugs used to treat anemia are contraindicated in patients with known hypersensitivity to the drug or any component of the drug. Iron compounds are contraindicated in patients with any anemia except iron deficiency anemia. Iron compounds are used cautiously in patients with tartrazine or sulfite sensitivity because some iron compounds contain these substances. Oral iron preparations are Pregnancy Category B drugs; iron dextran is a Pregnancy Category C drug. The iron preparations are used cautiously during pregnancy and lactation. Iron dosages of 15 to 30 mg/d are sufficient to meet the needs of pregnancy. Iron dextran is used cautiously in patients with cardiovascular

disease, a history of asthma or allergies, and rheumatoid arthritis (may exacerbate joint pain).

The absorption of oral iron is decreased when the agent is administered with antacids, tetracyclines, penicillamine, and the fluoroquinolones. When iron is administered with levothyroxine, there may be a decrease in the effectiveness of levothyroxine. When administered orally, iron deceases the absorption of levodopa. Ascorbic acid increases the absorption of oral iron. Iron dextran administered concurrently with chloramphenicol increases serum iron levels.

DRUGS USED IN THE TREATMENT OF ANEMIA ASSOCIATED WITH CHRONIC RENAL FAILURE

Anemia may occur in patients with chronic renal failure as the result of the inability of the kidney to produce erythropoietin. Erythropoietin is a glycoprotein hormone synthesized mainly in the kidneys and used to stimulate and regulate the production of erythrocytes or red blood cells (RBCs). Failure to produce the needed erythrocytes results in anemia. Two examples of drugs used to treat anemia associated with chronic renal failure are epoetin alfa (Epogen) and darbepoetin alfa (Aranesp).

ACTIONS AND USES

Epoetin alfa is a drug that is produced using recombinant DNA technology. The drug acts in a manner similar to that of natural erythropoietin. Epoetin alfa is used to treat anemia associated with chronic renal failure, anemia in patients with cancer who are receiving chemotherapy, and in patients with anemia who are undergoing elective nonvascular surgery. Darbepoetin alfa (Aranesp) is an erythropoiesis-stimulating protein produced in Chinese hamster ovary cells by recombinant DNA technology. Darbepoetin stimulates erythropoiesis by the same manner as natural erythropoietin. The drug is used to treat anemia associated with chronic renal failure in patients receiving dialysis as well as for patients who are not receiving dialysis. These drugs elevate or maintain RBC levels and decrease the need for transfusions.

ADVERSE REACTIONS

Epoetin alfa (erythropoietin; EPO) and darbepoetin alfa are usually well tolerated. The most common adverse reactions include hypertension, headache, tachycardia, nausea, vomiting, diarrhea, skin rashes, fever, myalgia, and skin reaction at the injection site. See the Summary Drug Table: Drugs Used in the Treatment of Anemia for more information on these drugs.

SUMMARY DRUG TABLE DRUGS USED IN THE TREATMENT OF ANEMIA

GENERIC NAME	TRADE NAME*	USES	ADVERSE REACTIONS	DOSAGE RANGES
darbepoetin alfa *dar-bah-poe-e´-tin*	Aranesp	Anemia associated with chronic renal failure	Hypertension, hypotension, headache, diarrhea, vomiting, nausea, myalgia, infection, cardiac arrhythmias, cardiac arrest	0.45 mcg/kg IV, SC weekly
epoetin alfa (Erythropoietin; (EPO) *e-po-e´-tin*	Epogen, procrit	Anemia associated with chronic renal failure, anemia related to zidovudine therapy in HIV-infected patients, anemia in cancer patients receiving chemotherapy, anemia in patients who undergo elective nonvascular surgery	Hypertension, headache, tachycardia, nausea, vomiting, skin rashes, fever, skin reaction at injection site	Individualized dosage CRF 50–100 U/kg (3 times weekly IV or SC), maintenance based on HCT, generally 25 U/kg 3 times weekly; zidovudine-treated HIV-infected patients: 100 U/kg 3 times weekly; cancer: 150 U/kg 3 times weekly; surgery: 300 U/kg/d SC x 10 d before surgery, on day of surgery and 4 days after surgery
ferrous fumarate (33% elemental iron) *fair´-us*	Feostat, *generic*	Prevention and treatment of iron deficiency anemia	GI irritation, nausea, vomiting, constipation, diarrhea, allergic reactions	Daily requirements: males, 10 mg/d PO; females, 18 mg/d PO; during pregnancy and lactation, 30–60 mg/d PO; replacement in deficiency states, 90–300 mg/d (6 mg/kg/d) PO for 6–10 months
ferrous gluconate (11.6% elemental iron)	Fergon, *generic*	Prevention and treatment of iron deficiency anemia	GI irritation, nausea, vomiting, constipation, diarrhea, allergic reactions	Daily requirements: males, 10 mg/d PO; females, 18 mg/d PO; during pregnancy and lactation, 30–60 mg/d PO; replacement in deficiency states, 90–300 mg/d (6 mg/kg/d) PO for 6–10 months
ferrous sulfate (20% elemental iron)	Feosol, Fer-In-Sol, *generic*	Prevention and treatment of iron deficiency anemia	GI irritation, nausea, vomiting, constipation, diarrhea, allergic reactions	Daily requirements: males, 10 mg/d PO; females, 18 mg/d PO; during pregnancy and lactation, 30–60 mg/d PO; replacement in deficiency states, 90–300 mg/d (6 mg/kg/d) PO for 6–10 months
folic acid *foe´-lik*	Folvite, *generic*	Megaloblastic anemia due to deficiency of folic acid	Allergic sensitization	Up to 1 mg/d PO, IM, IV, SC
iron dextran	DexFerrum, InFeD, *generic*	Iron deficiency anemia	Anaphylactoid reactions, soreness and inflammation at injection site, chest pain, arthralgia, backache, convulsions, pruritus, abdominal pain, nausea, vomiting, dyspnea	Dosage based on body weight and grams percent (g/dL) of hemoglobin IV, IM

(continued)

SUMMARY DRUG TABLE DRUGS USED IN THE TREATMENT OF ANEMIA (Continued)

GENERIC NAME	TRADE NAME*	USES	ADVERSE REACTIONS	DOSAGE RANGES
iron sucrose	Venofer	Iron deficiency anemia	Hypotension, cramps, leg cramps, nausea, headache, vomiting, diarrhea, dizziness	100 mg elemental iron slow IV or during dialysis session
leucovorin calcium *loo-koe-vor´-in*	Wellcovorin, *generic*	Treatment of megaloblastic anemia leucovorin rescue after high-dose methotrexate therapy in osteosarcoma	Allergic sensitization, urticaria, anaphylaxis	Megaloblastic anemia: 1 mg/d IM rescue after methotrexate therapy: 12–15 g/m^2 PO or parenterally then 10 mg/m^2 q6h for 72 h; check serum creatinine after 24 h; if 50% greater than the pretreatment level, increase leucovorin dose to 100 mg/m^2 until serum methotrexate level is $<5 \times 10^{-8}$ M
sodium ferric gluconate complex	Ferrlecit	Iron deficiency	Flushing, hypotension, syncope, tachycardia, dizziness, pruritus, dyspnea, conjunctivitis, hyperkalemia	125 mg of elemental iron IV over at least 10 min
vitamin B$_{12}$ (cyanocobalamin) *sye-an-oh-koe-bal´-a-min*	*generic*	B$_{12}$ deficiencies as seen in pernicious anemia, GI pathology; also used when requirements for the vitamin are increased; Schilling's test	Mild diarrhea, itching, edema, anaphylaxis	Schilling's test: 100–1000 mcg/d x 2 wk, then 100-1000 mcg IM q mo

*The term *generic* indicates the drug is available in generic form.
GI, gastrointestinal; HIV, human immunodeficiency virus.

CONTRAINDICATIONS, PRECAUTIONS, AND INTERACTIONS

Epoetin alfa is contraindicated in patients with uncontrolled hypertension, those needing an emergency transfusion, or those with a hypersensitivity to human albumin. Darbepoetin alfa (Aranesp) is contraindicated in patients with uncontrolled hypertension or in those allergic to the drug.

Epoetin alfa and darbepoetin alfa are used with caution in patients with hypertension, heart disease, congestive heart failure, or a history of seizures. Both of these drugs are Pregnancy Category C drugs and are used cautiously during pregnancy and lactation.

DRUGS USED IN THE TREATMENT OF FOLIC ACID DEFICIENCY ANEMIA

Folic acid is required for the manufacture of RBCs in the bone marrow. Folic acid is found in leafy green vegetables, fish, meat, poultry, and whole grains. A deficiency of folic acid results in **megaloblastic anemia.** Megaloblastic anemia is characterized by the presence of large, abnormal, immature erythrocytes circulating in the blood.

ACTION AND USES

Folic acid is used in the treatment of megaloblastic anemias that are caused by a deficiency of folic acid. Although not related to anemia, studies indicate there is a decreased risk for neural tube defects if folic acid is taken before conception and during early pregnancy. Neural tube defects occur during early pregnancy, when the embryonic folds forming the spinal cord and brain join together. Defects of this type include anencephaly (congenital absence of brain and spinal cord), spina bifida (defect of the spinal cord), and meningocele (a saclike protrusion of the meninges in the spinal cord or skull). The United States Public Health Service recommends the use of folic acid for all women of childbearing age to decrease the incidence of neural tube defects. Dosages during pregnancy and lactation are as great as 0.8 mg/d.

Leucovorin is a derivative (and active reduced form) of folic acid. The oral and parenteral forms of this drug are used in the treatment of megaloblastic anemia. Leucovorin may also be used to diminish the hematologic effects of (intentional) massive doses of methotrexate, a drug used in the treatment of certain types of cancer (see Chap. 55). Leucovorin "rescues" normal cells from the destruction caused by methotrexate and allows them to survive. This technique of administering leucovorin after a large dose of methotrexate is called **folinic acid rescue** or **leucovorin rescue.** Occasionally, high doses of methotrexate are administered to select patients. Leucovorin is then used either at the time methotrexate is administered or a specific number of hours after the methotrexate has been given to decrease the toxic effects of the methotrexate. Leucovorin may be ordered to be given via the IV, IM, or oral route.

ADVERSE REACTIONS

Few adverse reactions are associated with the administration of folic acid and leucovorin. Rarely, parenteral administration may result in allergic hypersensitivity.

CONTRAINDICATIONS, PRECAUTIONS, AND INTERACTIONS

Folic acid and leucovorin are contraindicated for the treatment of pernicious anemia or for other anemias for which vitamin B_{12} is deficient. Folic acid is a Pregnancy Category A drug and is generally considered safe for use during pregnancy. Pregnant women are more likely to experience folate acid deficiency because folic acid requirements are increased during pregnancy. Pregnant women with a folate deficiency are at increased risk for complications of pregnancy and fetal abnormalities. The recommended daily allowance (RDA) of folate during pregnancy is 0.4 mg/d and during lactation, 0.26 to 0.28 mg/d. Although fetal harm appears remote, the drug should be used cautiously and only within the RDAs. Use of aminosalicylic with folic acid may decrease serum folate levels. Folic acid utilization is decreased when folate is administered with methotrexate. Signs of folic acid deficiency may occur when sulfasalazine is administered concurrently. An increase in seizure activity may occur when folic acid is administered with the hydantoins.

Leucovorin is a Pregnancy Category C drug and is used cautiously during pregnancy.

Leucovorin decreases the effectiveness of the anticonvulsants. There is an increased risk of 5-fluorouracil toxicity when the drug is administered with leucovorin.

DRUGS USED IN THE TREATMENT OF PERNICIOUS ANEMIA

Vitamin B_{12} is essential to growth, cell reproduction, the manufacture of myelin (which surrounds some nerve fibers), and blood cell manufacture. The **intrinsic factor,** which is produced by cells in the stomach, is necessary for the absorption of vitamin B_{12} in the intestine. A deficiency of the intrinsic factor results in abnormal formation of erythrocytes because of the body's failure to absorb vitamin B_{12}, a necessary component for blood cell formation. The resulting anemia is a type of megaloblastic anemia called **pernicious anemia.**

ACTIONS AND USES

Vitamin B_{12} (cyanocobalamin) is used to treat a vitamin B_{12} deficiency. A vitamin B_{12} deficiency may be seen in:

- Strict vegetarians
- Persons who have had a total gastrectomy or subtotal gastric resection (when the cells producing the intrinsic factor are totally or partially removed)
- Persons who have intestinal diseases, such as ulcerative colitis or sprue
- Persons who have gastric carcinoma
- Persons who have a congenital decrease in the number of gastric cells secreting intrinsic factor

Vitamin B_{12} is also used to perform the Schilling test, which is used to diagnose pernicious anemia.

> ☀ **Nursing Alert**
>
> *Pernicious anemia must be diagnosed and treated as soon as possible because vitamin B_{12} deficiency that is allowed to progress for more than 3 months may result in degenerative lesions of the spinal cord.*

A deficiency of this vitamin caused by a low dietary intake of vitamin B_{12} is rare because the vitamin is found in meats, milk, eggs, and cheese. The body is also able to store this vitamin; a deficiency, for any reason, will not occur for 5 to 6 years.

ADVERSE REACTIONS

Mild diarrhea and itching have been reported with the administration of vitamin B_{12}. Other adverse reactions that may be seen include a marked increase in RBC production, acne, peripheral vascular thrombosis, congestive heart failure, and pulmonary edema.

CONTRAINDICATIONS, PRECAUTIONS, AND INTERACTIONS

Vitamin B_{12} is contraindicated in patients allergic to cobalt. Vitamin B_{12} is a Pregnancy Category A drug if administered orally and a Pregnancy Category C drug if given parenterally. Vitamin B_{12} is administered cautiously during pregnancy and in patients with pulmonary disease and anemia. Alcohol, aminosalicylic acid, neomycin, and colchicine may decrease the absorption of oral vitamin B_{12}.

NURSING PROCESS

● The Patient Receiving a Drug Used in the Treatment of Anemia

ASSESSMENT

Preadministration Assessment

The nurse obtains a general health history and asks about the symptoms of the anemia. The primary health care provider may order laboratory tests to determine the type, severity, and possible cause of the anemia. At times, it may be easy to identify the cause of the anemia, but there are also instances where the cause of the anemia is obscure.

The nurse takes the vital signs to provide a baseline during therapy. Other physical assessments may include the patient's general appearance and, in the severely anemic patient, an evaluation of the patient's ability to carry out the activities of daily living. General symptoms of anemia include fatigue, shortness of breath, sore tongue, headache, and pallor.

If iron dextran is to be given, an allergy history is necessary because this drug is given with caution to those with significant allergies or asthma. The patient's weight and hemoglobin level are required for calculating the dosage.

Ongoing Assessment

During the ongoing assessment the nurse takes the vital signs daily; more frequent monitoring may be needed if the patient is moderately to acutely ill or if the patient is taking epoetin alfa (because of the increased risk of hypertension). The nurse monitors the patient for adverse reactions and reports any occurrence of adverse reactions to the primary health care provider before the next dose is due. However, the nurse immediately reports severe adverse reactions.

When the patient is receiving iron salt therapy, the nurse informs the patient that the color of the stool will become darker or black. If diarrhea or constipation occurs, the nurse notifies the primary health care provider.

If iron dextran is administered, the nurse informs the patient that soreness at the injection site may occur. Injection sites are checked daily for signs of inflammation, swelling, or abscess formation.

The nurse assesses the patient for relief of the symptoms of anemia (fatigue, shortness of breath, sore tongue, headache, pallor). Some patients may note a relief of symptoms after a few days of therapy. Periodic laboratory tests are necessary to monitor the results of therapy.

> **Nursing Alert**
>
> *When monitoring the patient taking epoetin, the nurse reports any increase in the hematocrit of 4 points within any 2-week period because an exacerbation of hypertension is associated with an excessive rise of hematocrit. Hematocrit is decreased by decreasing or withholding the epoetin alfa dose.*

NURSING DIAGNOSES

Drug-specific nursing diagnoses are highlighted in the Nursing Diagnoses Checklist. Other nursing diagnoses applicable to these drugs are discussed in depth in Chapter 4.

PLANNING

The expected outcomes for the patient may include an optimal response to therapy, management of constipation, adequate nutritional status, and an understanding of and compliance with the prescribed treatment regimen.

IMPLEMENTATION

Promoting an Optimal Response to Therapy

IRON. Iron salts are preferably given between meals with water but can be given with food or meals if gastrointestinal upset occurs. If the patient is receiving other drugs, the nurse checks with the hospital pharmacist regarding the simultaneous administration of iron salts with other drugs.

Oral iron solutions may cause temporary staining of the teeth. The solution is diluted with 2 to 4 oz of water or juice and drunk through a straw. The stool may appear darker or black; this is a normal occurrence and not a reason for concern.

Iron dextran is given via the IM or IV route. Before iron dextran is administered, a test dose may be done by

> **Nursing Diagnoses Checklist**
>
> ☑ **Altered Nutrition: Less than Body Requirements** related to lack of iron, folic acid, other (specify) in the diet
>
> ☑ **Constipation** related to adverse reaction to iron therapy

Draw up an additional 0.2 mL of air within the syringe.

Attach a needle that is at least 1¹/₂ to 2 inches long.

Don gloves.

Position the client on the abdomen or side depending on which injection site is used.

Using the side of your hand, pull the tissue laterally about 1 inch (2.5 cm) until it is taut.

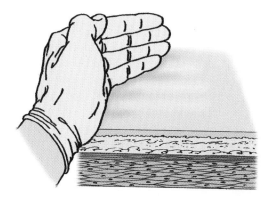

Swab the site with an alcohol pledget.

Insert the needle at a 90-degree angle while continuing to hold the tissue laterally.

Steady the barrel of the syringe with the fingers and use the thumb to manipulate the plunger.

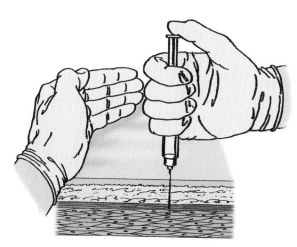

Aspirate for a blood return.

Instill the medication by depressing the plunger with the thumb.

Wait 10 seconds with the needle in place and the skin still held taut.

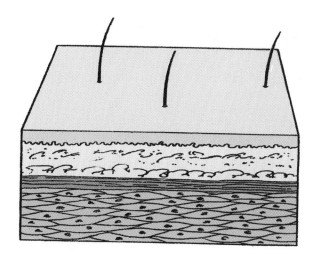

Withdraw the needle and immediately release the taut skin.

Apply direct pressure to the injection site with a gauze square, but do not rub it.

Cover the injection site with a Band-Aid.

Discard the syringe without recapping the needle.

Remove your gloves and wash your hands.

Document the medication administration.

FIGURE 45-1. Administering iron dextran using the Z-track technique.

administering 0.5 mL of iron dextran IV at a gradual rate during a period of 30 seconds or more. A test dose is also performed before administering the first dose of iron dextran IM by injecting 0.5 mL into the upper outer quadrant. The nurse monitors the patient for an allergic response for at least 1 hour after the test dose and before administering the remaining dose.

After the test dose, the prescribed dosage of iron is administered IM. The drug is given into the muscle mass of the upper outer quadrant (never into an arm or other area) using the Z-track method (see Fig. 45-1) to prevent leakage into the subcutaneous (SC) tissue. A large-bore needle is required. If the patient is standing, have the patient place weight on the leg not receiving the injection.

EPOETIN ALFA. When epoetin alfa is administered to a patient with hypertension, the nurse monitors the blood pressure closely. The nurse reports any rise in the systolic or diastolic pressure of 20 mm Hg or more to the primary health care provider. The hematocrit is usually measured before each dose during therapy with epoetin alfa.

The drug is given three times weekly IV or SC, or if the patient is receiving dialysis, the drug is administered into the venous access line. The drug is mixed gently during preparation for administration. Shaking may denature the glycoprotein. The vial is used for only one dose; any remaining or unused portion is discarded.

> ### Nursing Alert
>
> *This drug is not used for treatment of severe anemia or as a substitute for emergency transfusion. However, supplemental iron may be ordered during therapy with epoetin.*

LEUCOVORIN. When leucovorin is administered after a large dose of methotrexate, the timing of the administration is outlined by the primary health care provider. It is essential that the leucovorin be given at the exact time ordered because the purpose of folinic acid rescue is to allow a high dose of a toxic drug to remain in the body for only a limited time.

VITAMIN B$_{12}$. Patients with pernicious anemia are treated with vitamin B$_{12}$ by the parenteral route (IM) weekly stabilized. The parenteral route is used because the vitamin is ineffective orally due to the absence of the intrinsic factor in the stomach, which is necessary for utilization of vitamin B$_{12}$. After stabilization, maintenance (usually monthly) injections are necessary for life.

Monitoring and Managing Adverse Reactions

When the patient is receiving iron dextran, the nurse monitors closely for a hypersensitivity reaction. Epinephrine is kept on standby in the event of severe anaphylactic reaction.

> ### Nursing Alert
>
> *Parenteral iron has resulted in fatal anaphylactic-type reactions. The nurse reports any of the following adverse reactions: dyspnea, urticaria, rashes, itching, and fever.*

MANAGING CONSTIPATION. Constipation may be a problem when a patient is taking oral iron preparations. The nurse instructs the patient to increase fluid intake to 10 to 12 glasses of water per day (if the condition permits), eat a diet high in fiber, and increase activity. An active lifestyle and regular exercise (if condition permits) help to decrease the constipating effects of iron. If constipation persists, the primary health care provider may prescribe a stool softener.

MAINTAINING ADEQUATE NUTRITION. A special diet (eg, foods high in iron or foods high in folic acid) may be prescribed. If the diet is taken poorly, the nurse notes this on the patient's chart and discusses the problem with the primary health care provider.

The nurse recommends a balanced diet with an emphasis on foods that are high in iron (eg, organ meats, lean red meats, cereals, dried beans, and leafy green vegetables), folic acid (eg, green leafy vegetables, liver, and yeast) or vitamin B$_{12}$ (eg, beef, pork, organ meats, eggs, milk, and milk products). The nurse monitors the amount of food eaten at meals. If appetite is poor or eating is inadequate to maintain normal nutrition, a consult with the dietitian may be necessary. Small portions of food may be more appealing than large or moderate portions. The nurse provides a pleasant atmosphere and allows ample time for eating.

Educating the Patient and Family

The nurse explains the medical regimen thoroughly to the patient and family and emphasizes the importance of following the prescribed treatment regimen. The nurse includes the following points in a patient and family teaching plan:

IRON SALT

- Take this drug with water on an empty stomach. If gastrointestinal upset occurs, take the drug with food or meals.
- Do not take antacids, tetracyclines, penicillamine, or fluoroquinolones at the same time or 2 hours before or after taking iron without first checking with the primary health care provider.
- This drug may cause a darkening of the stools, constipation, or diarrhea. If constipation or diarrhea becomes severe, contact the primary health care provider.
- Mix the liquid iron preparation with water or juice and drink through a straw to prevent staining of the teeth.
- Avoid the indiscriminate use of advertised iron products. If a true iron deficiency occurs, the cause must be determined and therapy should be under the care of a health care provider.
- Have periodic blood tests during therapy to determine the therapeutic response.
- Patients with rheumatoid arthritis may experience an acute exacerbation of joint pain, and swelling may occur with iron dextran therapy.

EPOETIN ALFA

- Keep all appointments with the primary health care provider. The drug is administered three times per week (via the SC or IV route or via a dialysis access line). Periodic blood tests are performed to determine the effects of the drug and to determine dosage.

● Strict compliance with antihypertensive drug regimen is important in patients with known hypertension during epoetin therapy.

● Report numbness, tingling of extremities, severe headache, dyspnea, or chest pain. Joint pain may occur but can be controlled with analgesics.

FOLIC ACID

● Avoid the use of multivitamin preparations unless such use has been approved by the primary health care provider.

● Follow the diet recommended by the primary health care provider because diet and drug are necessary to correct a folic acid deficiency.

EPOETIN ALFA

● The drug will be administered three times weekly and can be given only via the IV or SC route or via venous access during dialysis.

● Keep appointments for blood testing, which is necessary to determine the effects of the drug on the blood count and to determine dosage.

● The following adverse reactions may occur: dizziness, headache, fatigue, joint pain, nausea, vomiting, or diarrhea. Report any of these reactions.

LEUCOVORIN

● Megaloblastic anemia—Adhere to the diet prescribed by the primary health care provider. If the purchase of foods high in protein (which can be expensive) becomes a problem, discuss this with the primary health care provider.

● Folinic acid rescue—Take this drug at the exact prescribed intervals. If nausea and vomiting, occur, contact the primary health care provider immediately.

VITAMIN B$_{12}$

● Nutritional deficiency of vitamin B$_{12}$—Eat a balanced diet that includes seafood, eggs, meats, and dairy products.

● Pernicious anemia—Lifetime therapy is necessary. Eat a balanced diet that includes seafood, eggs, meats, and dairy products. Avoid contact with infections, and report any signs of infection to the primary health care provider immediately because an increase in dosage may be necessary.

● Adhere to the treatment regimen and keep all appointments with the clinic or primary health care provider. The drug is given at periodic intervals (usually monthly for life). In some instances, par-

enteral self-administration or parenteral administration by a family member is allowed (instruction in administration is necessary).

EVALUATION

● The therapeutic effect of the drug is achieved.
● The patient has normal bowel movements.
● An adequate nutritional intake is achieved.
● The patient and family demonstrate an understanding of the drug regimen.
● The patient verbalizes the importance of complying with the prescribed treatment regimen.

● *Critical Thinking Exercises*

1. *Ms. Clepper, age 32 years, has received a diagnosis of pernicious anemia. Although the primary health care provider has explained the diagnosis and the treatment, the patient is confused and frightened. She questions you stating, "I just don't understand what is happening in my body to cause me to feel so weak and tired. How is the treatment going to work?" Discuss ways in which you would handle this situation with Ms. Clepper. Determine what to tell her that would decrease her anxiety and increase her understanding.*

2. *Mr. Garcia, age 54 years, has chronic renal failure. He undergoes dialysis three times a week. The physician orders epoetin alfa to be administered. Discuss the preadministration and ongoing assessments for Mr. Garcia. During a discussion with you, Mr. Garcia asks why he is receiving this drug. Discuss how you would answer Mr. Garcia's question.*

● *Review Questions*

1. Which is the most common type of anemia?
   A. Iron deficiency anemia
   B. Folic acid anemia
   C. Pernicious anemia
   D. Megaloblastic anemia

2. Which of the following substances would decrease the absorption of oral iron?
   A. Antacids
   B. Levothryoxine
   C. Ascorbic acid
   D. Vitamin B$_{12}$

3. Folic acid and leucovorin are contraindicated in which of the following conditions?
   A. Hypothyroidism
   B. Hyperthyroidism
   C. Pernicious anemia
   D. Pregnancy

foods high in potassium in the daily diet. See Home Care Checklist: Preventing Potassium Imbalances for a listing of foods high in potassium. Sometimes a potassium-sparing diuretic is prescribed along with a thiazide diuretic to keep potassium levels within normal limits. If excessive electrolyte loss occurs, the primary care provider may reduce the dosage or withdraw the drug temporarily until the electrolyte imbalance is corrected.

CARDIAC ARRHYTHMIAS AND DIZZINESS. Patients receiving a diuretic (particularly a loop or thiazide diuretic) and a digitalis glycoside concurrently require frequent monitoring of the pulse rate and rhythm because of the possibility of cardiac arrhythmias. Any significant changes in the pulse rate and rhythm are immediately reported to the primary health care provider.

Some patients experience dizziness or light-headedness, especially during the first few days of therapy or when a rapid diuresis has occurred. Patients who are dizzy but are allowed out of bed are assisted by the nurse with ambulatory activities until these adverse drug effects disappear.

Educating the Patient and Family

The patient and the family require a full explanation of the prescribed drug therapy, including when to take the drug (diuretics taken once a day are best taken early in the morning), if the drug is to be taken with food, and the importance of following the dosage schedule printed on the container label. The nurse also explains the onset and duration of the drug's diuretic effect. The patient and family must also be made aware of the signs and symptoms of fluid and electrolyte imbalances and adverse reactions that may occur when using a diuretic.

To ensure compliance with the prescribed drug regimen, the nurse stresses the importance of diuretic therapy in treating the patient's disorder. If the patient states that taking a diuretic at a specific time will be a problem, the nurse questions the patient in an attempt to identify the difficulty associated with drug therapy. Once a problem is identified, the nurse can identify solutions or make suggestions. The nurse includes the following points in a patient teaching plan:

- Do not stop taking the drug or omit doses, except on the advice of a primary health care provider.
- If gastrointestinal upset occurs, take the drug with food or milk.
- Take the drug early in the morning (once-a-day dosage) unless directed otherwise to minimize the effects on nighttime sleep. Twice-a-day dosing should be administered early in the morning (eg, 7:00 AM and early afternoon (eg, 2:00 PM) or as directed by the primary care provider. These drugs will initially cause an increase in urination, which should subside after a few weeks.

- Avoid alcohol and nonprescription drugs unless their use has been approved by the primary health care provider. Hypertensive patients should be careful to avoid medications that increase blood pressure, such as over-the-counter drugs for appetite suppression and cold symptoms.
- Notify the primary health care provider if any of the following should occur: muscle cramps or weakness, dizziness, nausea, vomiting, diarrhea, restlessness, excessive thirst, general weakness, rapid pulse, increased heart rate or pulse, or gastrointestinal distress.
- If dizziness or weakness occurs, observe caution while driving or performing hazardous tasks, rise slowly from a sitting or lying position, and avoid standing in one place for an extended time.
- Weigh yourself weekly or as recommended by the primary health care provider. Keep a record of these weekly weights and contact the primary health care provider if weight loss exceeds 3 to 5 lb a week.
- If foods or fluids high in potassium are recommended by the primary health care provider, eat the amount recommended. Do not exceed this amount or eliminate these foods from the diet for more than 1 day, except when told to do so by the primary health care provider (see Home Care Checklist: Preventing Potassium Imbalances).
- After a time, the diuretic effect of the drug may be minimal because most of the body's excess fluid has been removed. Continue therapy to prevent further accumulation of fluid.
- Thiazide and related diuretics, loop diuretics, potassium-sparing diuretics, carbonic anhydrase inhibitors, triamterene: Avoid exposure to sunlight or ultraviolet light (sunlamps, tanning beds) because exposure may cause exaggerated sunburn (photosensitivity reaction). Wear sunscreen and protective clothing until tolerance is determined.
- Loop and thiazide diuretics: patients with diabetes mellitus: Blood glucometer test results for glucose may be elevated (blood) or the urine positive for glucose. Contact the primary health care provider if results of home testing of blood glucose levels increase or if urine tests positive for glucose.
- Potassium-sparing diuretics: Avoid eating foods high in potassium and avoid the use of salt substitutes containing potassium. Read food labels carefully. Do not use a salt substitute unless a particular brand has been approved by the primary health care provider. Avoid the use of potassium supplements. Male patients taking spironolactone may experience gynecomastia. This is usually reversible when therapy is discontinued.
- Thiazide diuretics may cause gout attacks. Contact the primary care provider if significant, sudden joint pain occurs.

● Carbonic anhydrase inhibitors: During treatment for glaucoma, contact the primary health care provider immediately if eye pain is not relieved or if it increases. When a patient with epilepsy is being treated for seizures, a family member of the patient should keep a record of all seizures witnessed and bring this to the primary health care provider at the time of the next visit. Contact the primary health care provider immediately if the seizures increase in number.

EVALUATION

● The therapeutic effect is achieved.
● Adverse reactions are identified, reported to the primary health care provider, and managed successfully thorough appropriate nursing interventions.
● Fluid volume deficit (if present) is corrected.
● No evidence of injury is seen.
● The patient verbalizes the importance of complying with the prescribed treatment regimen.
● The patient and family demonstrate an understanding of the drug regimen.

● *Critical Thinking Exercises*

1. *Mr. Walsh, age 46 years, sees his primary health care provider and is prescribed a thiazide diuretic for hypertension. He tells you that it will be inconvenient for him to take his drug in the morning and he would prefer to take it at night. Other than asking him why taking the drug in the evening is more convenient, discuss what other questions you would ask Mr. Walsh. Analyze the situation to determine what explanation regarding present and future actions of this diuretic you would tell this patient.*

2. *Mr. Rodriguez, age 68 years, is taking amiloride for hypertension. He and his wife stopped by the clinic for a routine blood pressure check. Mrs. Rodriguez states that her husband has been confused and very irritable for the last 2 days. He complains of nausea and has had several "loose" stools. Discuss what actions you would take, giving a rationale for each action.*

3. *Ms. Palmer, age 88 years, is a resident in a nursing home. Her primary health care provider prescribes a thiazide diuretic for CHF. The nurse in charge advises you to evaluate Ms. Palmer for signs and symptoms of dehydration and hyponatremia. Discuss the assessment you would make. Identify which of these signs and symptoms might be difficult to evaluate considering the patient's age.*

● *Review Questions*

1. When evaluating the effectiveness of acetazolamide (Diamox) given for acute glaucoma, the nurse questions the patient about _____.

A. the amount of urine each time the patient voids
B. the relief of eye pain
C. the amount of fluid being taken
D. occipital headaches

2. When a patient taking mannitol for increased intracranial pressure is being assessed, which of the following findings would be most important for the nurse to report?

A. A serum potassium of 3.5 mEq/mL
B. Urine output of 20 mL for the last 2 hours
C. A blood pressure of 140/80 mm Hg
D. A heart rate of 72 bpm

3. When administering spironolactone (Aldactone), the nurse monitors the patient closely for which of the following electrolyte imbalances?

A. Hypernatremia
B. Hyponatremia
C. Hyperkalemia
D. Hypokalemia

4. When a diuretic is being administered for heart failure, which of the following would be most indicative of an effective response of diuretic therapy?

A. Output of 30 mL/h
B. Daily weight loss of 2 lb
C. An increase in blood pressure
D. Increasing edema of the lower extremities

5. Which electrolyte imbalance would the patient receiving a loop or thiazide diuretic most likely develop?

A. Hypernatremia
B. Hyponatremia
C. Hyperkalemia
D. Hypokalemia

6. Which of the following foods would the nurse most likely recommend the patient include in the daily diet to prevent hypokalemia?

A. Green beans
B. Apples
C. Bananas
D. Corn

● *Medication Dosage Problems*

1. The primary care provider prescribes spironolactone (Aldactone) 100 mg PO. The drug is available in 50-mg tablets. The nurse administers _____.

2. Furosemide (Lasix) 20 mg oral solution is prescribed. The oral solution is available in a concentration of 40 mg/5 mL. The nurse administers _____.

Urinary Anti-infectives and Miscellaneous Urinary Drugs

Key Terms

anti-infectives
bactericidal
bacteriostatic
cystitis
dysuria
neurogenic bladder

overactive bladder
prostatitis
pyelonephritis
urge incontinence
urinary tract infections
urinary urgency

Chapter Objectives

On completion of this chapter, the student will:

- Discuss the uses, general drug actions, adverse reactions, contraindications, precautions, and interactions of the drugs used to treat infections and symptoms associated with urinary tract infections or an overactive bladder.
- Discuss important preadministration and ongoing assessment activities the nurse should perform on the patient taking a drug for a urinary tract infection or an overactive bladder.
- List some nursing diagnoses particular to a patient taking a drug for a urinary tract infection or an overactive bladder.
- Discuss ways to promote an optimal response to therapy, how to manage adverse reactions, and important points to keep in mind when educating patients about the use of drugs used to treat a urinary tract infection or symptoms associated with an overactive bladder.

This chapter discusses drugs used to treat urinary tract infections (UTIs) and certain miscellaneous drugs used to relieve the symptoms associated with an **overactive bladder** (involuntary contractions of the detrusor or bladder muscle). Structures of the urinary system that may be affected include the bladder (**cystitis**), prostate gland (**prostatitis**), the kidney, or the urethra (see Fig. 47-1). These drugs also help control the discomfort associated with irritation of the lower urinary tract mucosa caused by infection, trauma, surgery, and endoscopic procedures.

Urinary tract infection (UTI) is an infection caused by pathogenic microorganisms of one or more structures of the urinary tract. The most common structure affected is the bladder, with the urethra, prostate, and kidney also affected (see Fig. 47-1). Display 47-1 identifies the disorder most frequently associated with each of these structures within the urinary system. Clinical manifestations of a UTI of the bladder (cystitis) include urgency, frequency, burning and pain on urination, and pain caused by spasm in the region of the bladder and the suprapubic area.

Some drugs used in the treatment of UTIs do not belong to the antibiotic or sulfonamide groups of drugs. The drugs discussed in this chapter are **anti-infectives** (against infection) used in the treatment of UTIs, which have an effect on bacteria in the urinary tract. Although administered systemically, that is, by the oral or parenteral route, they do not achieve significant levels in the bloodstream and are of no value in the treatment of systemic infections. They are primarily excreted by the kidneys and exert their major antibacterial effects in the urine. (See Summary Drug Table: Urinary Anti-infectives for a listing of these and other drugs used to treat problems associated with the urinary system.)

DISPLAY 47-1 ● Common Disorders Associated With the Urinary System

Cystitis—inflammation of the bladder
Urethritis—inflammation of the urethra
Prostatitis—inflammation of the male prostate gland
Pyelonephritis—inflammation of the kidney and renal pelvis

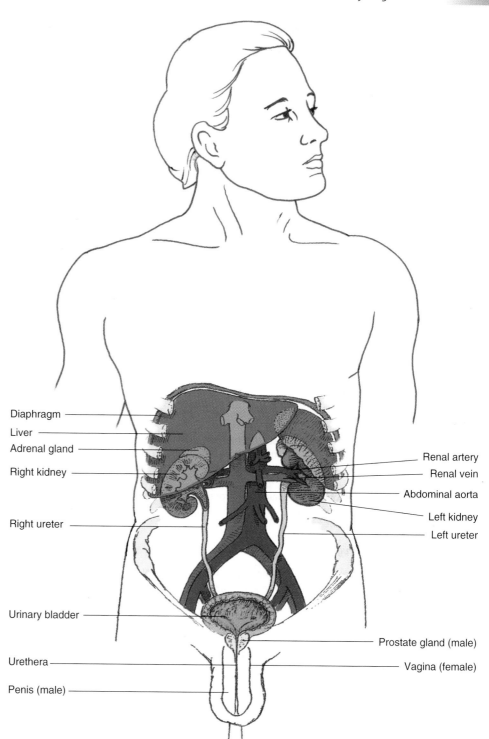

Diaphragm
Liver
Adrenal gland
Right kidney

Renal artery
Renal vein
Abdominal aorta
Left kidney
Left ureter

Right ureter

Urinary bladder

Prostate gland (male)

Urethera
Vagina (female)
Penis (male)

FIGURE 47-1. The normal urinary system, male and female. (Source: Wynsbergke, D., Noback, C. & Carola, R. [1995]. *Human anatomy & physiology* [3rd ed., p. 889]. New York: McGraw-Hill.)

Examples of urinary anti-infectives include cinoxacin (Cinobac), fosfomycin (Monurol), methenamine mandelate (Mandelamine), nalidixic acid (NegGram), and nitrofurantoin (Furadantin).

Additional drugs can be used in the treatment of UTIs. Examples of these drugs include ampicillin (see Chap. 7), the cephalosporins (see Chap. 8), sulfonamides (see Chap. 6), and norfloxacin (see Chap. 10). Combination drugs are also available. The Summary Drug Table: Urinary Anti-infectives gives examples of the combination drugs used for UTIs.

Trimethoprim

Trimethoprim (Trimpex) interferes with the ability of bacteria to metabolize folinic acid, thereby exerting bacteriostatic activity. Trimethoprim is used for UTIs that are caused by susceptible microorganisms. Trimethoprim administration may result in rash, pruritus, epigastric distress, nausea, and vomiting. When trimethoprim is combined with sulfamethoxazole (Septra), the adverse effects associated with a sulfonamide may also occur. The adverse reactions seen with other anti-infectives, such as ampicillin, the sulfonamides, and cephalosporins, are given in their appropriate chapters.

Flavoxate

Flavoxate (Urispas) counteracts smooth muscle spasm of the urinary tract by relaxing the detrusor and other muscles through action at the parasympathetic receptors. Flavoxate is used to relieve symptoms of **dysuria** (painful or difficult urination), urinary urgency (a strong and sudden desire to urinate), nocturia (excessive urination during the night), suprapubic pain and frequency, and **urge incontinence** (accidental loss of urine caused by a sudden and unstoppable urge to void). Flavoxate can cause blurred vision, drowsiness, nausea and vomiting, nervousness, vertigo, headache, and mental confusion (particularly in the elderly).

Oxybutynin

Oxybutynin (Ditropan) acts by relaxing the bladder muscle and reducing spasm. Oxybutynin is used to treat bladder instability (ie, urgency, frequency, leakage, incontinence, and painful or difficult urination) caused by a **neurogenic bladder** (altered bladder function caused by a nervous system abnormality). Adverse reactions observed in patients taking oxybutynin include dry mouth, constipation or diarrhea, decreased production of tears, decreased sweating, gastrointestinal disturbances, dim vision, and urinary hesistancy.

Phenazopyridine

Phenazopyridine (Pyridium) is a dye that exerts a topical analgesic effect on the lining of the urinary tract. It has no anti-infective activity. Phenazopyridine, a urinary analgesic, is available as a separate drug but is also included in some urinary anti-infective combination drugs. This drug is a urinary tract analgesic used to relieve the pain, burning, urgency, frequency, and irritation caused by infection, trauma, catheters, or surgical procedures of the urinary tract. Adverse reactions associated with phenazopyridine include headache, rash, and gastrointestinal upset.

Tolterodine

Tolerodine (Detrol) is an anticholinergic drug that is able to inhibit bladder contractions and delay the urge to void. Tolerodine tartrate is used to treat symptoms of overactive bladder, such as urinary frequency, urgency, or urge incontinence. Tolterodine is associated with anticholinergic adverse reactions such as dry mouth (the most commonly reported adverse reaction), drowsiness, decreased sweating, blurred vision, nausea, vomiting, dizziness, and abdominal pain. The adverse reactions of tolterodine, compared with other anticholinergic drugs, are less problematic because tolterodine is more specific for the bladder.

CONTRAINDICATIONS, PRECAUTIONS, AND INTERACTIONS

Cinoxacin

Cinoxacin is contraindicated in patients with known hypersensitivity to the individual drug and in patients with anuria. Cinoxacin is a Pregnancy Category B drug and should be used with caution during pregnancy and lactation. Cinoxacin is used with caution in patients with hepatic impairment. When cinoxacin is administered with probenecid, there is a risk for lowered urine concentration of cinoxacin.

Methenamine and Methenamine Salts

Methenamine is contraindicated in patients with a hypersensitivity to the drug, those with hepatic impairment, and during pregnancy (Pregnancy Category C) and lactation. Patients who are allergic to tartrazine should not take methenamine hippurate (Hiprex). The drug is used cautiously in patients with renal or hepatic impairment or gout (may cause crystals to form in the urine). No serious interactions have been reported.

Nalidixic Acid

Nalidixic acid is contraindicated in patients who are hypersensitive to the drug or any of its components, those who have convulsive disorders, and during pregnancy (Pregnancy Category C) and lactation. Nalidixic acid is used cautiously in patients with renal and hepatic impairment, cerebral arteriosclerosis, and in patients with glucose-6-phosphate dehydrogenase (G6PD) deficiency. When nalidixic acid is administered with the oral anticoagulants there is an increased risk of bleeding.

Nitrofurantoin

Nitrofurantoin is contraindicated in patients with renal impairment, those with hypersensitivity to the drug, and in lactating women. Nitrofurantoin is classified as a Pregnancy Category B drug and is used with caution during pregnancy. The drug is also used with caution in patients with a G6PD deficiency (see Chap. 1), anemia, or diabetes. There is a decreased absorption of nitrofurantoin when the drug is administered with magnesium trisilicate or magaldrate. When nitrofurantoin is administered with anticholinergics, there is a delay in gastric emptying, increasing the absorption of nitrofurantoin.

Fosfomycin

Fosfomycin is contraindicated in patients with a hypersensitivity to the drug. Fosfomycin is used cautiously during pregnancy (Pregnancy Category B) and lactation. There is a lowered plasma concentration and urinary tract excretion when fosfomycin is administered with metoclopramide.

Trimethoprim

Trimethoprim is contraindicated in patients with a hypersensitivity to the drug and in those with a creatine clearance of less than 15 mL/min. The drug is used cautiously in patients with hepatic or renal impairment and in patients with megaloblastic anemia caused by folate deficiency. Trimethoprim is classified as a Pregnancy Category C drug, and its use is not recommended during pregnancy and lactation.

No significant interactions have been reported.

There is an increased risk for hypoglycemia when products containing sulfamethoxazole are administered with oral antidiabetic drugs such as tolbutamide, tolazamide, and glipizide and an increased risk of hemorrhage when given with oral anticoagulants. An increased urinary pH decreases the effectiveness of methenamine. Therefore, to avoid raising the urine pH when taking methenamine, the patient should not use antacids containing sodium bicarbonate or sodium carbonate. Nalidixic acid may increase the effects of the anticoagulants.

Flavoxate

This drug is contraindicated in patients with intestinal or gastric blockage, abdominal bleeding, or urinary tract blockage. The drug is used cautiously in patients with glaucoma and during pregnancy (Pregnancy Category C) and lactation. No significant interactions have been reported.

Oxybutynin

Oxybutynin is contraindicated in patients with a hypersensitivity to the drug, those with glaucoma, partial or complete blockage of the gastrointestinal tract, myasthenia gravis, or urinary tract obstruction. The drug is used cautiously in patients with kidney or liver disease, heart failure, irregular or rapid heart rate, hypertension, or enlarged prostate and during pregnancy (Pregnancy Category C) and lactation. There is a decreased effectiveness of the phenothiazines when these drugs are administered with oxybutynin. A decreased response and increased risk of tardive dyskinesia may occur when haloperidol is administered with oxybutynin.

Phenazopyridine

Phenazopyridine is contraindicated in patients with renal impairment and in undiagnosed urinary tract pain. Phenazopyridine is used cautiously during pregnancy (Pregnancy Category C) and lactation.

 Nursing Alert

Phenazopyridine is not administered for more than 2 days when used in combination with an antibacterial drug to treat a UTI. When used more than 2 days, the drug may mask the symptoms of a more serious disorder.

Phenazopyridine treats the symptom of pain but does not treat the cause of the disorder. No significant interactions have been reported.

Tolterodine

Tolterodine is contraindicated in patients with urinary retention (inability to urinate), gastric retention, uncontrolled narrow-angle glaucoma, and in patients with hypersensitivity to the drug. Tolterodine is used with caution in patients with significant bladder outflow blockage or slow urinary stream because of the risk of urinary retention, pyloric stenosis (a narrowing of the opening where the stomach contents are emptied into the small intestine), and liver or kidney disease. This drug is classified as a Pregnancy Category C drug and should not be used during pregnancy or lactation. No significant interactions have been reported.

Miscellaneous Drugs

The miscellaneous drugs are used to relieve the symptoms associated with an overactive bladder (involuntary contractions of the detrusor or bladder muscle) that sometimes occur due to disorders such as cystitis, prostatitis, or other affected structures such as the kidney or the urethra. Overactive bladder is estimated to affect more than 16 million individuals in the United States. Symptoms of an overactive bladder include **urinary urgency,** frequent urination day and night, and **urge incontinence,** accidental loss of urine caused by a sudden and unstoppable need to urinate. These drugs also help control the discomfort associated with irritation of the lower urinary tract mucosa caused by infection, trauma, surgery, and endoscopic procedures. Other miscellaneous drugs are used to relieve the pain associated with irritation of the lower genitourinary tract (eg, phenazopyridine) caused by infection, trauma, surgery, and endoscopic procedures.

 Health Supplement Alert: Cranberry

Cranberry juice has long been recommended for use in treating and preventing urinary tract infections (UTIs). Clinical studies have confirmed that cranberry juice is beneficial to individuals with frequent UTIs. Cranberries inhibit bacteria from attaching to the walls of the urinary tract and prevent certain bacteria from forming dental plaque in the mouth. Cranberry juice is safe for use as a food and for urinary tract health. Cranberry juice and capsules have no contraindications, no known adverse reactions, and no drug interactions. The recommended dosage is 9 to 15 capsules a day (400–500 mg/d) or 4 to 8 ounces of juice per day. (See Chap. 6 for more information.)

NURSING PROCESS

● **The Patient Receiving a Urinary Anti-infective or a Miscellaneous Urinary Drug**

ASSESSMENT

Preadministration Assessment

When a UTI has been diagnosed, sensitivity tests are performed to determine bacterial sensitivity to the drugs (antibiotics and urinary anti-infectives) that will control the infection. The nurse questions the patient regarding symptoms of the infection before instituting therapy. The nurse records the color and appearance of the urine. The nurse takes and records the vital signs. A urine sample for culture and sensitivity is obtained before the first dose of the drug is given.

When the miscellaneous drugs are administered, the nurse documents the symptoms the patient is experiencing to provide a baseline for future assessment. The nurse assesses for and documents pain, urinary frequency, bladder distension, or other symptoms associated with the urinary system.

Ongoing Assessment

Many UTIs are treated on an outpatient basis because hospitalization usually is not required. UTIs may be seen in the hospitalized or nursing home patient with an indwelling urethral catheter or a disorder such as a stone in the urinary tract.

When caring for a hospitalized patient with a UTI, the nurse monitors the vital signs every 4 hours or as ordered by the primary health care provider. Any significant rise in temperature is reported to the primary health care provider because methods of reducing the fever or repeat culture and sensitivity tests may be necessary.

The nurse monitors the patient's response to therapy daily. If after several days the symptoms of the UTI have not improved or if they become worse, the nurse notifies the primary health care provider as soon as possible. Periodic urinalysis and urine culture and sensitivity tests may be ordered to monitor the effects of drug therapy.

When the nurse is administering any of the miscellaneous drugs, the nurse monitors the patient for a reduction in the symptoms obtained in the preadministration assessment such as dysuria, urinary frequency, urgency, nocturia, and relief of any pain associated with irritation of the lower genitourinary tract.

NURSING DIAGNOSES

Drug-specific nursing diagnoses are highlighted in the Nursing Diagnoses Checklist. Other nursing diagnoses applicable to these drugs are discussed in depth in Chapter 4.

PLANNING

The expected outcomes for the patient may include an optimal response to drug therapy, management of common adverse drug reactions, and an understanding of and compliance with the prescribed therapeutic regimen.

IMPLEMENTATION

Promoting an Optimal Response to Therapy

URINARY ANTI-INFECTIVES. To promote an optimal response to therapy, the nurse gives these drugs with food to prevent gastrointestinal upset. The nurse

---

Nursing Diagnoses Checklist

☑ **Impaired Urinary Elimination** related to urinary tract infection

☑ **Impaired Nutrition: Less than Body Requirements** related to adverse drug effects (eg, nausea, vomiting)

☑ **Pain** or discomfort related to infectious process

Patient and Family Teaching Checklist

Using Fluids to Prevent and Treat UTIs

The nurse:

✓ Discusses UTIs, their causes, and the need for fluids and drug therapy.

✓ Reviews the drug therapy regimen, including prescribed drug, dose, and frequency of administration.

✓ Stresses the importance of continued therapy even if patient feels better after a few doses.

✓ Instructs to continue therapy until all of drug is finished or prescriber discontinues therapy.

✓ Explains the rationale for increasing fluid intake to at least 2000 mL/d (unless contraindicated) to aid in physical removal of bacteria.

✓ Urges patient to drink fluids every hour.

✓ Offers suggestions for fluids to drink based on patient's likes and dislikes.

✓ Demonstrates procedure for measuring intake and output using household measures.

✓ Informs about urine appearance when intake is increased.

✓ Encourages continued increased fluid intake even if symptoms subside.

✓ Instructs to notify primary health care provider if urine output is low, urine appears dark or concentrated during the daytime, or symptoms do not improve after 3 to 4 days.

✓ Reviews signs and symptoms of possible adverse reactions and of new infection or worsening infection, both verbally and in writing.

✓ Emphasizes the importance of follow-up visits and laboratory tests to determine the effectiveness of therapy.

administers nitrofurantoin with food, meals, or milk because this drug is particularly irritating to the stomach. Fosfomycin comes in a 3-g one-dose packet that must be dissolved in 90 to 120 mL water (not hot water). It can be administered with food to prevent gastric upset. The nurse administers the drug immediately after dissolving it in water.

The nurse advises the patient to drink at least 2000 mL or more of fluids each day unless the primary health care provider orders otherwise. Drinking extra fluids aids in the physical removal of bacteria from the genitourinary tract and is an important part of the treatment of UTIs (see Patient and Family Teaching Checklist: Using Fluids to Prevent and Treat UTIs). The nurse offers fluids, preferably water, to the patient at hourly intervals. Cranberry or prune juice is usually given rather than orange juice, other citrus juices, or vegetable juices.

The nurse notifies the primary health care provider if the patient fails to drink extra fluids, if the urine output is low, or if the urine appears concentrated during daytime hours. The urine of those drinking 2000 mL or more per day will appear dilute and light in color.

Elderly patients often have a decreased thirst sensation and must receive encouragement to increase fluid intake. The nurse offers fluids at regular intervals to elderly patients or those who seem unable to increase their fluid intake without supervision.

The nurse measures the fluid intake and output, especially when the primary health care provider orders an increase in fluid intake or when a kidney infection is being treated. The primary health care provider may also order daily urinary pH levels when methenamine or nitrofurantoin is administered. These drugs work best in acid urine; failure of the urine to remain acidic may require administration of a urinary acidifier, such as ascorbic acid.

MISCELLANEOUS URINARY DRUGS. Flavoxate is administered orally three to four times daily. The dosage may be reduced when the patient's symptoms improve. Phenazopyridine is administered after meals to prevent GI upset. This drug is not administered for more than 2 days to patients receiving antibiotics for treatment of a UTI. Continued use may mask the symptoms of a urinary tract infection that is not responding to treatment with an antibiotic. When administering these drugs, the nurse monitors the fluid intake and urinary output for volume and frequency. The patient is encouraged to drink at least 2000 mL of fluid daily (if condition permits) to dilute urine and decrease pain on voiding.

Monitoring and Managing Adverse Drug Reactions

URINARY ANTI-INFECTIVES. The nurse observes the patient for adverse drug reactions. If an adverse reaction occurs, the nurse contacts the primary health care provider before the next dose of the drug is due. However, serious drug reactions, such as a pulmonary reaction, are reported immediately.

Pulmonary reactions have been reported with the use of nitrofurantoin and may be seen within hours and up to 3 weeks after therapy with this drug is initiated. Signs and symptoms of an acute pulmonary reaction include dyspnea, chest pain, cough, fever, and chills. If these reactions occur, the nurse immediately notifies the primary health care provider and withholds the next dose of the drug until the patient is seen by a primary health care provider. Signs and symptoms of chronic pulmonary reactions, which may be seen during prolonged therapy, include dyspnea, nonproductive cough, and malaise.

MISCELLANEOUS URINARY DRUGS. Common adverse reactions with flavoxate, oxybutynin, and tolterodine include dry mouth, dizziness, blurred vision, and constipation.

For patients with dry mouth the nurse suggests that the patient suck on hard candy, sugarless lozenges, or small pieces of ice and performs frequent mouth care. This effect sometimes lessens with continued use of the drug. Hospitalized patients experiencing drowsiness or blurred vision may require assistance when ambulating. For patients with constipation, the nurse encourages fluids, provides a high-fiber diet, and provides times for ambulation or exercise (if the patient's condition allows). If constipation persists, the primary health care provider may prescribe a mild laxative or stool softener.

The nurse informs the patient that phenazopyridine may cause a reddish orange discoloration of the urine and may stain fabrics or contact lenses. The nurse assures the patient that this is normal and will subside when use of the drug is discontinued.

Educating the Patient and Family

The nurse stresses the importance of increasing fluid intake to at least 2000 mL/d (unless contraindicated) to help remove bacteria from the genitourinary tract (see Patient and Family Teaching Checklist: Using Fluids to Prevent and Treat UTIs). In many cases, symptoms are relieved after several days of drug therapy. To ensure compliance with the prescribed drug regimen, the nurse stresses the importance of completing the full course of drug therapy even though symptoms have been relieved. A full course of therapy is necessary to ensure all bacteria have been eliminated from the urinary tract. The nurse should include the following points in a patient and family teaching plan:

- Take the drug with food or meals (nitrofurantoin must be taken with food or milk). If gastrointestinal upset occurs despite taking the drug with food, contact the primary health care provider.
- Take the drug at the prescribed intervals and complete the full course of therapy. Do not discontinue taking the drug even though the symptoms have disappeared, unless directed to do so by the primary health care provider.
- If drowsiness or dizziness occurs, avoid driving and performing tasks that require alertness.
- During therapy with this drug, avoid alcoholic beverages and do not take any nonprescription drug unless its use has been approved by the primary health care provider.
- Notify the primary health care provider immediately if symptoms do not improve after 3 or 4 days.
- Nitrofurantoin: Take this drug with food or milk to improve absorption. Continue therapy for at least 1 week or for 3 days after the urine shows no signs of infection. Notify the primary health care provider immediately if any of the following occur: fever, chills, cough, shortness of breath, chest pain, or difficulty breathing. Do not take the next dose of the drug until the primary health care provider has been contacted. The urine may appear brown during therapy with this drug; this is not abnormal.
- Nalidixic acid: Take this drug with food to prevent GI upset. Avoid prolonged exposure to sunlight or ultraviolet light (tanning beds or lamps) because an exaggerated sunburn may occur.
- Methenamine, methenamine salts: Avoid excessive intake of citrus products, milk, and milk products.
- Fosfomycin comes in dry form as a one-dose packet to be dissolved in 90 to 120 mL water (not hot water). Drink immediately after mixing and take with food to prevent gastric upset.

MISCELLANEOUS DRUGS

- For dry mouth, suck on hard candy, sugarless lozenges, or small pieces of ice and perform frequent mouth care.
- These drugs may cause drowsiness or blurred vision. Do not drive or operate dangerous machinery or participate in any activity that requires full mental alertness until you know how this medication affects you.
- If you experience constipation, drink plenty of fluids, eat a high-fiber diet, and exercise (if your condition allows). If constipation persists, the primary health care provider may prescribe a mild laxative or stool softener.
- Flavoxate: Take this drug three to four times daily as prescribed. This drug is used to treat symptoms; other drugs are given to treat the cause.
- Oxybutynin: Take this drug with food or without food. Oxybutynin (Ditropan XL) contains an outer coating that may not disintegrate and may be observed on occasion in the stool. This is not a cause for concern. This drug can cause heat prostration (fever and heat stroke caused by decreased sweating) in high temperatures. If you live in hot climates or will be exposed to high temperatures, take appropriate precautions.
- Phenazopyridine: This drug may cause a reddish-orange discoloration of the urine and may stain fabrics or contact lenses. This is normal. Take the drug after meals. Do not take this drug for more than 2 days if you are also taking an antibiotic for the treatment of a UTI.
- Tolterodine: If you experience difficulty voiding, take the drug immediately after voiding. If dysuria persists, notify the primary health care provider.

EVALUATION

- The therapeutic effect is achieved.
- Adverse reactions are identified, reported to the primary health care provider, and managed successfully through appropriate nursing interventions.

- The patient and family demonstrate an understanding of the drug regimen.
- The patient verbalizes the importance of complying with the prescribed therapeutic regimen.

● *Critical Thinking Exercises*

1. *Mr. Elliott, age 42 years, had a UTI 8 weeks ago. He failed to see his primary health care provider for a follow-up urine sample 2 weeks after completing his course of drug therapy. Mr. Elliot is in to see his primary health care provider because his symptoms of a UTI have recurred. The primary health care provider suspects that Mr. Elliott may not have followed instructions regarding treatment for his UTI. Analyze the situation to determine what points you would stress in a teaching plan for this patient.*

2. *Ms. Howard, age 86 years, has Alzheimer's disease and is a resident in a nursing home. She has a UTI and is prescribed cinoxacin (Cinobac). Discuss specific nursing tasks to include in a nursing care plan for this patient. What potential problems could be anticipated because of the Alzheimer's disease? What drugs might the primary care provider prescribe for the Alzheimer's disease?*

● *Review Questions*

1. The nurse correctly administers nitrofurantoin (Macrodantin) _____.

   A. with food
   B. no longer than 7 days
   C. without regard to food
   D. no longer than 2 days

2. To avoid raising the pH when taking methenamine (Mandelamine), the nurse advises the patient to _____.

   A. use an antacid before taking the drug
   B. take an antacid immediately after taking the drug
   C. avoid antacids containing sodium bicarbonate or sodium carbonate
   D. avoid the use of antacids 1 hour before or 2 hours after taking the drug

3. What instruction would be most important to give a patient prescribed fosfomycin (Monurol)?

   A. Drink one to two glasses of cranberry juice daily to promote healing of the urinary tract.
   B. You may take the drug without regard to meals.
   C. This drug comes in a one-dose packet that must be dissolved in 90 mL or more of fluids.
   D. This drug may cause mental confusion.

4. What statement(s) would be included in a teaching plan for a patient prescribed phenazopyridine (Pyridium)?

   A. There is a danger of heat prostration or heat stroke when taking phenazopyridine in a hot climate.
   B. This drug may turn the urine dark brown. This is an indication of a serious condition and should be reported immediately.
   C. This drug may cause photosensitivity. Take precautions when out in the sun by wearing sunscreen, a hat, and long-sleeved shirts for protection.
   D. This drug may turn the urine reddish-orange. This is a normal occurrence that will disappear when use of the drug is discontinued.

● *Medication Dosage Problems*

1. Cinoxacin 500 mg is prescribed. The drug is available in 250-mg tablets. The nurse administers _____.

2. Nitrofurantoin oral suspension 50 mg is prescribed. The oral suspension contains 25 mg/5 mL. The nurse administers _____.

chapter 48

Drugs That Affect the Gastrointestinal System

The gastrointestinal (GI) tract is subject to more diseases and disorders than any other system of the body. Some drugs used for GI disorders are available as nonprescription drugs, thereby creating the potential problems of misuse and overuse of the drugs and the disguising of more serious medical problems.

The drugs presented in this chapter include the antacids, anticholinergics, GI stimulants, proton pump inhibitors, histamine H_2 antagonists, antidiarrheals, antiflatulents, digestive enzymes, emetics, gallstone-solubilizing drugs, laxatives, and miscellaneous drugs. Some of the more common preparations are listed in the Summary Drug Table: Drugs Used in the Management of Gastrointestinal Disorders.

ANTACIDS

ACTIONS

Some of the cells of the stomach secrete **hydrochloric acid,** a substance that aids in the initial digestive process.

Antacids (against acids) are drugs that neutralize or reduce the acidity of stomach and duodenal contents by combining with hydrochloric acid and producing salt and water. Examples of antacids include aluminum hydroxide gel (Amphojel), magaldrate (Riopan), and magnesia or magnesium hydroxide (Milk of Magnesia).

USES

Antacids are used in the treatment of hyperacidity, such as heartburn, gastroesophageal reflux, sour stomach, acid indigestion, and in the medical treatment of peptic ulcer. Many antacid preparations contain more than one ingredient. An additional use for aluminum carbonate is in the treatment of hyperphosphatemia or for use with a low phosphate diet to prevent formation of phosphate urinary stones. Calcium carbonate may be used in treating calcium deficiency states such as menopausal osteoporosis. Magnesium oxide may be used in the treatment of magnesium deficiencies or magnesium depletion from malnutrition, restricted diet, or alcoholism.

(text continues on page 471)

SUMMARY DRUG TABLE DRUGS USED IN THE MANAGEMENT OF GASTROINTESTINAL DISORDERS

GENERIC NAME	TRADE NAME*	USES	DOSAGE RANGES
Proton Pump Inhibitors			
esomeprazole magnesium *ess-oh-me´-pra-zol*	Nexium	Erosive esophagitis, gastroesophageal reflux disease (GERD), long-term treatment of pathologic hypersecretory conditions	20–40 mg/d PO
lansoprazole *lan-soe´-pra-zole*	Prevacid	Duodenal ulcer, *H. pylori* eradication in patients with duodenal ulcer, gastric ulcer, erosive esophagitis, GERD, hypersecretory conditions	15–30 mg/d PO
omeprazole *oh-me´-pra-zol*	Prilosec	Duodenal ulcer, *H. pylori* eradication, hypersecretory conditions, gastric ulcer, erosive esophagitis, GERD, hypersecretory conditions	20–40 mg/d PO; 60 mg/d up to 120 mg TID
pantoprazole sodium *pan-toe´-pray-zol*	Protonix, Protonix IV	GERD	40 mg PO daily to BID up to 120 mg/d; IV, 80 mg; maximum dosage 240 mg/d
rabeprazole sodium *rah-beh´-pray-zol*	Aciphex	Duodenal ulcer, GERD, hypersecretory conditions	2–60 mg/d
Miscellaneous Gastrointestinal Drugs			
bismuth subsalicylate	Bismatrol Pepto-Bismol, Pink Bismuth	Nausea, diarrhea, abdominal cramps, *H. pylori* with duodenal ulcer	2 tablets or 30 mL PO q 30 min–1 h up to 8 doses in 24 h
balsalazide disodium *bal-sal´-a-zyde*	Colazal	Ulcerative colitis	3 750-mg capsules PO TID for 8 wk
infliximab *in-flicks´-ih-mab*	Remicade	Crohn's disease, rheumatoid arthritis	RA: 3 mg/kg IV; Crohn's: 5 mg/kg IV
mesalamine *me-sal´-a-meen*	Asacol, Rowasa, *generic*	Treatment of active to moderate ulcerative colitis, proctosigmoiditis, or proctitis	Suspension enema: 4 g once daily in 60 mL; rectal suppository: 500 mg (1 suppository) BID; oral: 800 mg TID PO
misoprostol *mye-soe-prost´-ole*	Cytotec	Prevention of gastric ulcers caused by aspirin or NSAID use (unlabeled use)	100–200 μg QID PO
olsalazine *ole-sal´-a-zeen*	Dipentum	Maintenance of remission of ulcerative colitis in patients intolerant of sulfasalazine	1 g/d in two divided doses PO
sucralfate *soo-kral´-fate*	Carafate, *generic*	Active duodenal ulcer	1 g/d PO in divided doses
sulfasalazine *sul-fa-sal´-a-zeen*	Azulfidine, *generic*	Ulcerative colitis, rheumatoid arthritis	I g QID PO
Antacids			
aluminum carbonate gel, basic *a-loo´-mi-num*	Basaljel		2 tablets or capsules or 10 mL of regular suspension (in water or fruit juice) or 5 mL of extra strength suspension as often as every 2 h, up to 12 times daily

(continued)

SUMMARY DRUG TABLE DRUGS USED IN THE MANAGEMENT OF GASTROINTESTINAL DISORDERS (Continued)

GENERIC NAME	TRADE NAME*	USES	DOSAGE RANGES
aluminum hydroxide gel	Alu-Tab, Amphojel, Dialume, *generic*		Tablets or capsules: 500–1500 mg 3–6 times daily PO between meals and HS; suspension: 5–15 mL as needed between meals and HS PO
calcium carbonate *kal´-see-um*	Chooz, Tums, *generic*		0.5–12 g PO as needed
magaldrate (hydroxymagnesium aluminate) *mag´-al-drate*	Riopan, *generic*		980–1080 mg PO 1 and 3 hours after meals and HS
magnesia (magnesium hydroxide) *mag-nee´-zee-ah*	Milk of Magnesia, Phillips' Chewable		Liquid: 5–15 mL PO QID with water; tablets: 650 mg–1.3 g QID PO; laxative: 15–60 mL PO taken with liquid
magnesium oxide *mag-nee´-zee-um*	Mag-Ox 400, Maox 420, Uro-mag, *generic*		Capsules: 280 mg–1.5 g QID PO; tablets: 400–820 mg/d PO
sodium bicarbonate *sow-dee´-um*	Bell/ans, *generic*		0.3–2 g 1–4 times daily PO
Anticholinergics			
belladonna	*Generic*		Tincture: 0.6–1 mL TID–QID
clindinium bromide *klin-din´-ee-um*	Quarzan		2.5–5 mg PO TID–QID AC and HS geriatric or debilitated patients: 2.5 mg TID AC
dicyclomine HCl *dye-sye-klo´-meen*	Bentyl, Di-Spasz, *generic*		Oral: 80–160 mg/d in 4 doses PO; parenteral: 80 mg/d IM
glycopyrrolate *gly-ko-pie´-roll-ate*	Robinul, Robinul Forte, *generic*		Oral: 1 mg TID or 2 mg BID–TID PO; parenteral: 0.1–0.2 mg IM or IV TID–QID
1-hyoscyamine sulfate *el-hi´-o-si-ah-meen*	Anaspaz, Donnamar, Levbid, Levsin		Oral: 0.125–0.25 mg PO TID–QID PO or sublingually; sustained release: 0.375–0.75 mg q12h PO; parenteral: 0.25–0.5 mg SC, IM, IV BID–QID
mepenzolate bromide *me-pin-zo´-late*	Cantil		25–50 mg QID with meals and HS
methantheline bromide *meth-an´-tha-leen*	Banthine, *generic*		Adult: 50–100 mg PO q6h
methscopolamine bromide *meth-sco-pol´-a-meen*	Pamine		2.5 mg 30 min AC and 2.5–5 mg HS PO
propantheline bromide *proe-pan´-the-leen*	Pro-Banthine, *generic*		15 mg PO 30 min AC and HS
tridihexethyl chloride *tri-di-hex´-eth-l*	Pathilon		25–50 mg TID–QID AC and 50 mg HS PO

SUMMARY DRUG TABLE DRUGS USED IN THE MANAGEMENT OF GASTROINTESTINAL DISORDERS (*Continued*)

GENERIC NAME	TRADE NAME*	USES	DOSAGE RANGES
Gastrointestinal Stimulants			
dexpanthenol *dex-pan´-the-nole*	Ilopan, generic		250–500 mg IM, IV

metoclopramide
met-oh-kloe-pra´-mide
	Reglan,
	  generic
			10–15 mg PO 30 min AC
			  and HS; 10–20 mg IM, IV

Histamine H₂ Antagonists			

cimetidine
sye-met´-i-deen
	Tagamet, Tagamet
	  HB, *generic*
			300–2400 mg/d PO;
			  300 mg q6h IM, IV;
			  50 mg/h continuous IV
			  infusion

famotidine
fa-moe´-ti-deen
	Pepcid, Pepcid IV,
	  generic
			20–40 mg PO, IV as
			  one dose or BID

nizatidine
ni-za´-ti-deen
	Axid Pulvules		Gastric or duodenal ulcer:
			  300 mg/d PO HS or
			  150 mg BID PO;
			  maintenance of healed
			  ulcer: 150 mg/d PO HS;
			  heartburn: 75 mg
			  PO ½–1 h before food or
			  beverages that cause the
			  problem, taken with water

ranitidine
ra-nye´-te-deen
	Zantac		150 mg PO BID or 300 mg
			  PO HS; 50 mg q6–8h IM,
			  IV (do not exceed
			  400 mg/d)

Antidiarrheals			

difenoxin HCl
  with atropine
*dye-fen-ox´-in
  a´-troe-peen*
	Motofen		Initial dose 2 tablets PO,
			  then 1 tablet after each
			  loose stool (no more than
			  8 mg/d for no more
			  than 2 days)

diphenoxylate HCl
  with atropine
di-fen-ox´-i´-late
	Lomotil, Lonox, *generic*		Initial dose 5 mg PO
			  TID–QID as needed

loperamide HCl
loe-per´-a-mide
	Imodium A-D,
	  Kaopectate II,
	  Maalox Anti-Diarrheal
	  caplets, *generic*
			Initial dose 4 mg PO then
			  2 mg after each loose
			  stool (no more than
			  16 mg/d)

Antiflatulents			

charcoal
char´-kole
	Liqui-Char,
	  generic
			520 mg PO after meals or
			  at the first sign of
			  discomfort (up to 4.16 g/d)

simethicone
sigh-meth´-ih-kohn
	Gas-X, Mylicon,
	  generic
			Capsules: 125 mg PO QID
			  PC and HS; tablets:
			  40–125 mg PO QID PC
			  and HS; drops: 40–80 mg
			  PO QID PC and HS
			  (up to 500 mg/d)

(continued)

SUMMARY DRUG TABLE DRUGS USED IN THE MANAGEMENT OF GASTROINTESTINAL DISORDERS (*Continued*)

GENERIC NAME	TRADE NAME*	USES	DOSAGE RANGES
Digestive Enzymes			
pancreatin *pan-kre-at´-in*	Creon, Digepepsin, Donnazyme		1–2 tablets PO with meals or snacks
pancrelipase *pan-kre-li´-pase*	Cotazym Capsules, Viokase Powder, Ilozyme tablets		4000–48,000 lipase PO with meals and snacks; usually 1–3 capsules or tablets before or with meals and snacks
Emetics			
apomorphine HCl *a-po-mor´-feen*	Generic		2–10 mg SC; do not repeat
ipecac syrup *ip´-e-kak*	Generic		15–30 mL PO, followed by 3–4 glasses of water; children's dosage based on age: 5–15 mL PO followed by ½–3 glasses of water
Gallstone-Solubilizing Agent			
ursodiol *ur-soe-dye´-ole*	Actigall, *generic*		8–10 mg/kg/d PO in 2–3 divided doses
Laxatives			
Saline Laxatives			
magnesium preparations *mag-nez´-e-um*	Epsom Salt, Milk of Magnesia		Follow directions given on the container
Irritant or Stimulant Laxatives			
cascara sagrada *kas-kar´-a-sa-grad´-a*	Auromatic Cascara, *generic*		Follow directions given on the container
sennosides *sen-oh-sides*	Agoral, Ex-Lax, Senexon, Senna-Gel, Senokot		Follow directions given on the container
bisacodyl *bis-a-koe´-dill*	Bisca-Evac, Dulcolax, Modane		Tablets: 10–15 mg daily PO Suppositories: 10 mg once daily
Bulk-Producing Laxatives			
psyllium *sill´-i-um*	Fiberall Tropical Fruit Flavor, Genfiber, Hydrocil Instant, Konsyl, Metamucil, Serutan		Follow directions on the container
polycarbophil *pol-i-kar´-boe-fil*	Equalactin, FiberCon, Mitrolan		1250 mg one to four times daily or as needed (do not exceed 5 g in 24 h)
Emollients			
mineral oil	Kondremul Plain, Milkinol, *generic*		15–45 mL PO at HS
Fecal Softeners/Surfactants			
docusate sodium (dioctyl sodium sulfosuccinate: DDS) *dok´-yoo-sate*	Colace, D-S-S, Ex-Lax Stool Softener, Modane Soft, *generic*		Follow directions on the container
docusate calcium (dioctyl calcium sulfosuccinate) *dok´-yoo-sate*	Surfak Liquigels, *generic*		240 mg/d until bowel movements are normal

SUMMARY DRUG TABLE DRUGS USED IN THE MANAGEMENT OF GASTROINTESTINAL DISORDERS (*Continued*)

GENERIC NAME	TRADE NAME*	USES	DOSAGE RANGES
Hyperosmotic Agents			
glycerin *gli´-ser-in*	Colace Suppositories, Sani-Supp, *generic*		Suppositories: insert 1 high in the rectum and retain 15 min; rectal liquid: insert all the liquid into rectum toward the navel
lactulose *lak-tyoo-los*	Chronulac, Constilac, Duphalac, *generic*		10–60 mL/d PO
Bowel Evacuants			
polyethylene glycol-electrolyte solution (PEG-ES) *pol-e-eth-i-leen*	CoLyte, GoLYTELY, NuLytely, OCL, *generic*		4 L oral solution before GI exam (do not give solid foods within 2 h before administration)
polyethylene glycol (PEG) solution	MiraLax		17 g of powder/d in 8 oz of water (48–72 h may be required to produce a bowel movement)

*The term *generic* indicates the drug is available in generic form.

ADVERSE REACTIONS

The magnesium- and sodium-containing antacids may have a laxative effect and produce diarrhea. Aluminum- and calcium-containing products tend to produce constipation. Some of the less common but more serious adverse reactions include:

- Aluminum-containing antacids—constipation, intestinal impaction, anorexia, weakness, tremors, and bone pain
- Magnesium-containing antacids—severe diarrhea, dehydration, and hypermagnesemia (nausea, vomiting, hypotension, decreased respirations)
- Calcium-containing antacids—rebound hyperacidity, metabolic alkalosis, hypercalcemia, vomiting, confusion, headache, renal calculi, and neurologic impairment
- Sodium bicarbonate—systemic alkalosis and rebound hypersecretion

Although the antacids have the potential for serious adverse reactions, they have a wide margin of safety, especially when used as prescribed.

CONTRAINDICATIONS, PRECAUTIONS, AND INTERACTIONS

The antacids are contraindicated in patients with severe abdominal pain of unknown cause and during lactation. Sodium-containing antacids are contraindicated in patients with cardiovascular problems, such as hypertension or congestive heart failure, and those on sodium-restricted diets. Calcium-containing antacids are contraindicated in patients with renal calculi or hypercalcemia.

Aluminum-containing antacids are used cautiously in patients with gastric outlet obstruction. Magnesium- and aluminum-containing antacids are used cautiously in patients with decreased kidney function. The calcium-containing antacids are used cautiously in patients with respiratory insufficiency, renal impairment, or cardiac disease. Antacids are classified as Pregnancy Category C drugs and should be used with caution during pregnancy.

Antacids may interfere with other drugs in three ways:

1. Increasing the gastric pH, which causes a decrease in absorption of weakly acidic drugs and results in a decreased drug effect (eg, digoxin, phenytoin, chlorpromazine, and isoniazid)
2. Absorbing or binding drugs to their surface, resulting in decreased bioavailability (eg, tetracycline)
3. Affecting the rate of drug elimination by increasing urinary pH (eg, the excretion of salicylates is increased, whereas excretion of quinidine and amphetamines is decreased)

The following drugs have a decreased pharmacologic effect when administered with an antacid: corticosteroids, digoxin, chlorpromazine, oral iron products, isoniazid, phenothiazines, ranitidine, phenytoin, valproic acid, and the tetracyclines.

ANTICHOLINERGICS

ACTIONS

Anticholinergics (cholinergic blocking drugs) reduce gastric motility and decrease the amount of acid secreted by the stomach (see Chap. 25). Examples of anticholinergics used for GI disorders include propantheline (Pro-Banthine) and glycopyrrolate (Robinul).

USES

Specific anticholinergic drugs are occasionally used in the medical treatment of peptic ulcer. These drugs have been largely replaced by histamine H_2 antagonists, which appear to be more effective and have fewer adverse drug reactions.

ADVERSE REACTIONS

Dry mouth, blurred vision, urinary hesitancy, urinary retention, nausea, vomiting, palpitations, and headache are some of the adverse reactions that may be seen with the use of anticholinergic drugs (see Chap. 25).

Contraindications, precautions, and interactions of the anticholinergic drugs are discussed in Chapter 25.

GASTROINTESTINAL STIMULANTS

ACTIONS

Metoclopramide (Reglan) and dexpanthenol (Ilopan) increase the motility of the upper GI tract. The exact mode of action of these drugs is unclear.

USES

Oral preparations of metoclopramide are used in the treatment of symptomatic **gastroesophageal reflux disease** (GERD; a reflux or backup of gastric contents into the esophagus) and **gastric stasis** (failure to normally move food out of the stomach) in patients with diabetes. This drug is given intravenously (IV) to prevent nausea and vomiting associated with cancer chemotherapy and to prevent nausea and vomiting during the immediate postoperative period. Dexpanthenol may be given IV immediately after major abdominal surgery to reduce the risk of **paralytic ileus** (lack of peristalsis or movement of the intestines).

ADVERSE REACTIONS

The adverse reactions associated with metoclopramide are usually mild. Higher doses or prolonged administration may produce central nervous system (CNS) symptoms, such as drowsiness, dizziness, Parkinson-like symptoms (tremor, mask-like facial expression, muscle rigidity), depression, facial grimacing, motor restlessness, and involuntary movements of the eyes, face, or limbs. Dexpanthenol administration may cause itching, difficulty breathing, and urticaria.

CONTRAINDICATIONS, PRECAUTIONS, AND INTERACTIONS

The GI stimulants are contraindicated in patients with known hypersensitivity to the drugs, GI obstruction, gastric perforation or hemorrhage, or epilepsy. These drugs are secreted in breast milk and should not be used during lactation.

These drugs are used cautiously in patients with diabetes and cardiovascular disease. Metoclopramide is a Pregnancy Category B drug; dexpanthenol is a Pregnancy Category C drug.

The effects of metoclopramide are antagonized by concurrent administration of anticholinergics or narcotic analgesics. Metoclopramide may decrease the absorption of digoxin and cimetidine and increase absorption of acetaminophen, tetracyclines, and levodopa. Metoclopramide may alter the body's insulin requirements.

HISTAMINE H_2 ANTAGONISTS

ACTIONS

These drugs inhibit the action of histamine at histamine H_2 receptor cells of the stomach, which then reduces the secretion of gastric acid and reduces total pepsin output. The decrease in acid allows the ulcerated areas to heal. Examples of histamine H_2 antagonists include cimetidine (Tagamet), famotidine (Pepcid), nizatidine (Axid Pulvules), ranitidine (Zantac).

USES

These drugs are used for the medical treatment of a gastric or duodenal ulcer, gastric **hypersecretory** (excessive gastric secretion of hydrochloric acid) conditions, and GERD. These drugs may also be used as prophylaxis of stress-related ulcers and acute upper GI bleeding in critically ill patients.

ADVERSE REACTIONS

Adverse reactions of the histamine H_2 antagonists include dizziness, somnolence, headache, confusion, hallucinations, diarrhea, and impotence (that is reversible when the drug is discontinued). Adverse reactions are usually mild and transient.

CONTRAINDICATIONS, PRECAUTIONS, AND INTERACTIONS

The histamine H_2 antagonists are contraindicated in patients with a known hypersensitivity to the drugs.

These drugs are used cautiously in patients with renal or hepatic impairment and in the severely ill or debilitated patient. Cimetidine is used cautiously in patients with diabetes. The histamine H_2 antagonists are used cautiously in the older adult (causes confusion). A dosage reduction may be required. Histamine antagonists are Pregnancy Category B (cimetidine, famotidine, and ranitidine) drugs and C (nizatidine) drugs and should be used with caution during pregnancy and lactation.

There are many drug–drug interactions with the histamine H_2 antagonists. The following discussion does not cover all drugs that may interact with the H_2 antagonists but represents some of the more common interactions. Antacids and metoclopramide may decrease absorption of the H_2 antagonists if administered concurrently. Concurrent use of cimetidine and digoxin may decrease serum digoxin levels. There may be a decrease in white blood cell count when the H_2 antagonists are administered with the alkylating drugs or the antimetabolites. There is an increased risk of toxicity of oral anticoagulants, phenytoin, quinidine, lidocaine, or theophylline when administered with H_2 antagonists. Concurrent use of cimetidine and morphine increases the risk of respiratory depression.

ANTIDIARRHEALS

ACTIONS

Antidiarrheals decrease intestinal peristalsis, which is usually increased when the patient has diarrhea. Examples of these drugs include difenoxin with atropine (Motofen), diphenoxylate with atropine (Lomotil), and loperamide (Imodium).

USES

Antidiarrheals are used in the treatment of diarrhea.

ADVERSE REACTIONS

Diphenoxylate use may result in anorexia, nausea, vomiting, constipation, rash, dizziness, drowsiness, sedation, euphoria, and headache. This drug is a narcotic-related drug that has no analgesic activity but has sedative and euphoric effects and drug dependence potential. To discourage abuse, it is combined with atropine (an anticholinergic or cholinergic blocking drug), which causes dry mouth and other mild adverse effects. Loperamide is not a narcotic-related drug, and minimal adverse reactions are associated with its use. Occasionally, abdominal discomfort, pain, and distention have been seen, but these symptoms also occur with severe diarrhea and are difficult to distinguish from an adverse drug reaction.

CONTRAINDICATIONS, PRECAUTIONS, AND INTERACTIONS

These drugs are contraindicated in patients whose diarrhea is associated with organisms that can harm the intestinal mucosa (*Escherichia coli*, *Salmonella*, *Shigella*) and in patients with pseudomembranous colitis, abdominal pain of unknown origin, and obstructive jaundice. The antidiarrheal drugs are contraindicated in children younger than 2 years.

The antidiarrheal drugs are used cautiously in patients with severe hepatic impairment or inflammatory bowel disease. Antidiarrheals are classified as Pregnancy Category B drugs and should be used cautiously during pregnancy and lactation.

The antidiarrheal drugs cause an additive CNS depression when administered with alcohol, antihistamines, narcotics, and sedatives or hypnotics. There are additive cholinergic effects when administered with other drugs having anticholinergic activity, such as antidepressants or antihistamines. Concurrent use of the antidiarrheals with a monoamine oxidase inhibitor increases the risk of a hypertensive crisis.

ANTIFLATULENTS

ACTIONS

Simethicone (Mylicon) and charcoal are used as **antiflatulents** (against flatus or gas in the intestinal tract). Simethicone has a defoaming action that disperses and prevents the formation of mucus-surrounded gas pockets in the intestine. Charcoal is an absorbent that reduces the amount of intestinal gas.

USES

Antiflatulents are used for the relief of painful symptoms of excess gas in the digestive tract. These drugs are useful as adjunctive treatment of any condition in which gas retention may be a problem (ie, postoperative gaseous distention, air swallowing, dyspepsia, peptic ulcer, irritable colon, or diverticulosis). In addition to its use for the relief of intestinal gas, charcoal may be used in the prevention of nonspecific pruritus associated with kidney dialysis treatment and as an antidote in poisoning. Simethicone is in some antacid products, such as Mylanta Liquid and Di-Gel Liquid.

ADVERSE REACTIONS

No adverse reactions have been reported with the use of antiflatulents.

CONTRAINDICATIONS, PRECAUTIONS, AND INTERACTIONS

The antiflatulents are contraindicated in patients with known hypersensitivity to any components of the drug. The pregnancy category of simethicone is unknown; charcoal is a Pregnancy Category C drug. There may be a decreased effectiveness of other drugs because of adsorption by charcoal, which can also adsorb other drugs in the GI tract. There are no known interactions with simethicone.

DIGESTIVE ENZYMES

ACTIONS

The enzymes pancreatin and pancrelipase, which are manufactured and secreted by the pancreas, are responsible for the breakdown of fats, starches, and proteins. These enzymes are necessary for the breakdown and digestion of food. Both enzymes are available as oral supplements.

USES

These drugs are prescribed as replacement therapy for those with pancreatic enzyme insufficiency. Conditions or diseases that may cause a decrease in or absence of pancreatic digestive enzymes include cystic fibrosis, chronic pancreatitis, cancer of the pancreas, the malabsorption syndrome, surgical removal of all or part of the stomach, and surgical removal of all or part of the pancreas.

ADVERSE REACTIONS

No adverse reactions have been reported with the use of digestive enzymes; however, high doses may cause nausea and diarrhea.

CONTRAINDICATIONS, PRECAUTIONS, AND INTERACTIONS

The digestive enzymes are contraindicated in patients with a hypersensitivity to hog or cow proteins and in patients with acute pancreatitis. The digestive enzymes are used cautiously in patients with asthma (an acute asthmatic attack can occur), hyperuricemia, and during pregnancy and lactation. These drugs are Pregnancy Category C drugs, and safe use in pregnancy has not been established.

Calcium carbonate or magnesium hydroxide antacids may decrease the effectiveness of the digestive enzymes. When administered concurrently with an iron preparation, the digestive enzymes decrease the absorption of oral iron preparations.

EMETICS

ACTIONS

The **emetic** (a drug that induces vomiting) ipecac causes vomiting because of its local irritating effect on the stomach and by stimulation of the vomiting center in the medulla.

USES

Emetics are used to cause vomiting to empty the stomach rapidly when an individual has accidentally or intentionally ingested a poison or drug overdose. Not all poison ingestions or drug overdoses are treated with emetics.

ADVERSE REACTIONS

There are no apparent adverse reactions to ipecac. Although not an adverse reaction, a danger associated with any emetic is the aspiration of vomitus.

CONTRAINDICATIONS, PRECAUTIONS, AND INTERACTIONS

Emetics are contraindicated in patients who are unconscious, semiconscious, or convulsing and in poisoning caused by corrosive substances, such as strong acids or petroleum products. Ipecac is a Pregnancy Category C drug, and safe use in pregnancy has not been established. Activated charcoal may absorb ipecac, negating its effects.

GALLSTONE-SOLUBILIZING DRUGS

ACTIONS

Gallstone-solubilizing (gallstone-dissolving) drugs, such as ursodiol (Actigall), suppress the manufacture of cholesterol and cholic acid by the liver. The suppression of the manufacture of cholesterol and cholic acid may ultimately result in a decrease in the size of radiolucent gallstones.

USES

These drugs are used in the nonsurgical treatment of radiolucent gallstones. They are not effective for all types of gallstones and require many months of usage to produce results. Because of the potential toxic effects associated with long-term use, these drugs are recommended for only carefully selected and closely monitored patients.

ADVERSE REACTIONS

Diarrhea, cramps, nausea, and vomiting are the more common adverse drug reactions. A reduction in the dose may reduce or eliminate these problems. Prolonged use of these drugs may result in hepatotoxicity (toxic to the liver).

CONTRAINDICATIONS, PRECAUTIONS, AND INTERACTIONS

Ursodiol is used cautiously in patients with a hypersensitivity to the drug or bile salts and in patients with liver impairment, calcified stones, radiopaque stones or radiolucent bile pigment stones, severe acute cholecystitis, biliary obstruction, and gallstone pancreatitis. Ursodiol is used cautiously during pregnancy (Pregnancy Category B) and lactation. Absorption of ursodiol is decreased if the agent is taken with bile acid sequestering drugs or aluminum-containing antacids. Clofibrate, estrogens, and oral contraceptives increase hepatic cholesterol secretion and encourage cholesterol gallstone formation and may counteract the effectiveness of ursodiol.

LAXATIVES

ACTIONS

There are various types of laxatives (see the Summary Drug Table: Drugs Used in the Management of Gastrointestinal Disorders). The action of each laxative is somewhat different, yet they produce the same result—the relief of constipation (Display 48-1).

USES

A laxative is most often prescribed for the short-term relief or prevention of constipation. Certain stimulant, emollient, and saline laxatives are used to evacuate the colon for rectal and bowel examinations. Fecal softeners or mineral oil are used prophylactically in patients who should not strain during defecation, such as after anorectal surgery or a myocardial infarction. Psyllium may be used in patients with irritable bowel syndrome and diverticular disease. Polycarbophil may be prescribed for constipation or diarrhea associated with irritable bowel syndrome and diverticulosis. Mineral oil is

---

DISPLAY 48-1 ● Actions of Different Types of Laxatives

- Bulk-producing laxatives are not digested by the body and therefore add bulk and water to the contents of the intestines. The added bulk in the intestines stimulates peristalsis, moves the products of digestion through the intestine, and encourages evacuation of the stool. Examples of bulk-forming laxatives are psyllium (Metamucil) and polycarbophil (FiberCon).
- Emollient laxatives lubricate the intestinal walls and soften the stool, thereby enhancing passage of fecal material. Mineral oil is an emollient laxative.
- Fecal softeners promote water retention in the fecal mass and soften the stool. One difference between emollient laxatives and fecal softeners is that the emollient laxatives do not promote the retention of water in the stool. Examples of fecal softeners include docusate sodium (Colace) and docusate calcium (Surfak).
- Hyperosmolar drugs dehydrate local tissues, which causes irritation and increased peristalsis, with consequent evacuation of the fecal mass. Glycerin is a hyperosmolar drug.
- Irritant or stimulant laxatives increase peristalsis by direct action on the intestine. An example of an irritant laxative is cascara sagrada and senna (Senokot).
- Saline laxatives attract or pull water into the intestine, thereby increasing pressure in the intestine, followed by an increase in peristalsis. Magnesium hydroxide (Milk of Magnesia) is a saline laxative.

useful for the relief of fecal impaction. Docusate is used to prevent dry, hard stools.

Constipation may occur as an adverse drug reaction. When the patient has constipation as an adverse reaction to another drug, the primary care provider may prescribe a stool softener or another laxative to prevent constipation during the drug therapy. Display 48-2 lists the names of some drugs and drug classifications that may cause constipation.

ADVERSE REACTIONS

Laxative use, especially high doses or use over a long time, can cause diarrhea and a loss of water and electrolytes. For some patients, this may be a serious adverse effect. Laxatives may also cause abdominal pain or discomfort, nausea, vomiting, perianal irritation, fainting, bloating, flatulence, cramps, and weakness. Prolonged use of a laxative can result in serious electrolyte imbalances, as well as the "laxative habit," that is, a dependency on a laxative to have a bowel movement. Some of these products contain tartrazine, which may cause allergic-type reactions (including bronchial asthma) in susceptible individuals.

Obstruction of the esophagus, stomach, small intestine, and colon has occurred when bulk-forming laxatives are administered without adequate fluid intake or in patients with intestinal stenosis.

CONTRAINDICATIONS, PRECAUTIONS, AND INTERACTIONS

Laxatives are contraindicated in patients with known hypersensitivity and those with persistent abdominal pain, nausea, or vomiting of unknown cause or signs of acute appendicitis, fecal impaction, intestinal obstruction, or acute hepatitis. These drugs are used only as directed because excessive or prolonged use may cause dependence. Magnesium hydroxide is used cautiously in patients with any degree of renal impairment. Laxatives

are used cautiously in patients with rectal bleeding, in pregnant women, and during lactation. The following laxatives are Pregnancy Category C drugs: cascara, sagrada, docusate, glycerin, phenolphthalein, magnesium hydroxide, and senna. These drugs are used during pregnancy only when the benefits clearly outweigh the risks to the fetus.

Mineral oil may impair the GI absorption of fat-soluble vitamins (A, D, E, and K). Laxatives may reduce absorption of other drugs present in the GI tract, by combining with them chemically or hastening their passage through the intestinal tract. When surfactants are administered with mineral oil, surfactants may increase mineral oil absorption. Milk, antacids, H_2 antagonists, and proton pump inhibitors should not be administered 1 to 2 hours before bisacodyl tablets because the enteric coating may dissolve early (before reaching the intestinal tract), resulting in gastric lining irritation or dyspepsia and decreasing the laxative effect of the drug.

PROTON PUMP INHIBITORS

Proton pump inhibitors, such as lansoprazole, omeprazole, pantoprazole and rabeprazole, belong to a group of drugs with antisecretory properties. These drugs suppress gastric acid secretion by inhibition of the hydrogen-potassium adenosine triphosphatase (ATPase) enzyme system at the secretory surface of the gastric parietal cells. They block the last step of acid production.

The proton pump inhibitors are particularly important in the treatment of *Helicobacter pylori* in patients with active duodenal ulcers. ***Helicobacter pylori*** (*H. pylori*) has been implicated as a causative organism in a type of chronic gastritis and in a large number of cases of peptic and duodenal ulcers.

ACTIONS

The proton pump inhibitors suppress gastric acid secretion by blocking the final step in the production of gastric acid by the gastric mucosa.

USES

The proton pump inhibitors are used for treatment or symptomatic relief of various gastric disorders, including gastric and duodenal ulcers, GERD, or pathological hypersecretory conditions. Painful, persistent heartburn 2 or more days a week may indicate acid reflux disease, which can erode the delicate lining of the esophagus, causing erosive esophagitis. Esomeprazole (Nexium) or Omeprazole (Prilosec) may provide 24-hour relief from the heartburn associated with GERD or erosive esophagitis while healing occurs.

An important use of these drugs is combination therapy for the treatment of *H. pylori* in patients with duodenal ulcers. One treatment regimen used to treat infection with *H. pylori* is a triple-drug treatment regimen, such as one of the proton pump inhibitors (eg, omeprazole or lansoprazole) and two anti-infectives (eg, amoxicillin and clarithromycin). Another treatment regimen includes bismuth subsalicylate plus two anti-infective drugs. Helidac, a treatment regimen of three drugs (bismuth subsalicylate, metronidazole, and tetracycline) may be given along with a histamine H$_2$ antagonist to treat disorders of the GI tract infected with *H. pylori*. Table 48-1 provides a listing of the various combinations used in the treatment of *H. pylori*. Additional information concerning the anti-infectives listed is found in Chapters 6 through 11. The Summary Drug Table: Drugs Used in the Management of Gastrointestinal Disorders provide information on the drugs used in the treatment of *H. pylori*.

ADVERSE REACTIONS

The most common adverse reactions seen with the proton pump inhibitors include headache, diarrhea, and abdominal pain. Other less common adverse reactions include nausea, flatulence, constipation, and dry mouth.

CONTRAINDICATIONS, PRECAUTIONS, AND INTERACTIONS

The proton pump inhibitors are contraindicated in patients who have hypersensitivity to any of the drugs. Omeprazole (Pregnancy Category C) and lansoprazole, rabeprazole, and pantoprazole (Pregnancy Category B) are contraindicated during pregnancy and lactation. The proton pump inhibitors are used cautiously in older adults and in patients with hepatic impairment.

There is a decreased absorption of lansoprazole when it is administered with sucralfate. Lansoprazole may decrease the effects of ketoconazole, iron salts, and digoxin. When lansoprazole is administered with theophylline, there is an

TABLE 48-1	Agents Used to Treat *H. Pylori* in Patients With Duodenal Ulcers	
DRUG	**USE FOR ERADICATION OF *H. PYLORI* IN PATIENTS WITH DUODENAL ULCER**	**DOSAGE RANGE**
amoxicillin *a-mocks´-ih-sill-in*	In combination with lansoprazole and clarithromycin or lansoprazole alone	1 g BID for 14 d (triple therapy) or 1 g TID (double therapy)
bismuth *bis´-muth*	In combination with other products	525 mg QID in combination with other products
bismuth subsalicylate (Bismatrol) *bis´-muth sub-sa-li´-si-late*	*H. pylori* eradication in patients with duodenal ulcer	525-mg chewable tablets QID in combination with at least two anti-infectives
bismuth subsalicylate, metronidazole *me-troe-ni´-da-zole* Tetracycline *tet-ra-sye´-cleen* (Helidac)	*H. pylori* eradication in patients with duodenal ulcer	525-mg chewable tablets, 250 mg metronidazole, 500 mg tetracycline QID PO
clarithromycin (Biaxin) *clair-ith´-row-my-sin*	In combination with amoxicillin	500 mg TID
lansoprazole (Prevacid) *lan-sew-prah´-zoll*	In combination with clarithromycin and/or amoxicillin	30 mg BID for 14 d (triple therapy) or 30 mg TID for 14 d (double therapy)
metronidazole (Flagyl) *meh-trow-nye´-dah-zoll*	In combination with other products	250 mg QID
omeprazole (Prilosec) *oh-mep´-rah-zole*	In combination with clarithromycin	40 mg BID for 4 wk and 20 mg/d for 15–28 d
ranitidine bismuth citrate (Tritec) *rah-nih´-tih-deen*	In combination with clarithromycin	400 mg BID for 4 wk in combination with clarithromycin
tetracycline *tet-rah-si´-cleen*	In combination with other products	500 mg QID

increase in theophylline clearance requiring dosage changes of the theophylline. When omeprazole is administered with clarithromycin, there is a risk for an increase in plasma levels of both drugs. Omeprazole may prolong the elimination of warfarin when the two drugs are administered together. Increased serum levels and the risk for toxicity of benzodiazepines, phenytoin, and warfarin may occur if any of these drugs are used with omeprazole.

MISCELLANEOUS DRUGS

The miscellaneous GI drugs include bismuth subsalicylate, mesalamine, misoprostol, olsalazine, sucralfate, and sulfasalazine.

ACTIONS

Bismuth disrupts the integrity of the bacterial cell wall. Misoprostol (Cytotec) inhibits gastric acid secretion and increases the protective property of the mucosal lining of the GI tract by increasing the production of mucus by the lining of the GI tract. Sucralfate (Carafate) exerts a local action on the lining of the stomach. The drug forms a complex with the exudate of the stomach lining. This complex forms a protective layer over a duodenal ulcer, thus aiding in healing of the ulcer. Mesalamine (Asacol), olsalazine (Dipentum), and sulfasalazine (Azulfidine) exert a topical anti-inflammatory effect in the bowel. The exact mechanism of action of these drugs is unknown.

USES

Bismuth subsalicylate is used in combination with other drugs to treat gastric and duodenal ulcers caused by *H. pylori* bacteria. Mesalamine is used in the treatment of chronic inflammatory bowel disease. Misoprostol is used to prevent gastric ulcers in those taking aspirin or nonsteroidal anti-inflammatory drugs in high doses for a prolonged time. Olsalazine is used in the treatment of ulcerative colitis in those allergic to sulfasalazine. Sulfasalazine is used in the treatment of Crohn's disease and ulcerative colitis. Sucralfate is used in the treatment of duodenal ulcer.

ADVERSE REACTIONS

Adverse reactions of bismuth subsalicylate, include a temporary and harmless darkening of the tongue and stool and constipation. Salicylate toxicity (eg, tinnitus, rapid respirations, see Chap. 17) may also occur, particularly when the drug is used for an extended period of time.

Oral administration of mesalamine may cause abdominal pain, nausea, headache, dizziness, fever, and weakness. The adverse reactions associated with rectal administration are less than those seen with oral administration, but headache, abdominal discomfort, flu-like syndrome, and weakness may still occur. Olsalazine administration may result in diarrhea, abdominal discomfort, and nausea. Sulfasalazine is a sulfonamide with adverse reactions the same as for the sulfonamide drugs (see Chap. 6).

The adverse reactions seen with the administration of sucralfate are usually mild, but constipation may be seen in a small number of patients. Misoprostol administration may result in diarrhea, abdominal pain, nausea, GI distress, and vomiting.

CONTRAINDICATIONS, PRECAUTIONS, AND INTERACTIONS

The miscellaneous GI drugs are given with caution to patients with a known hypersensitivity to the drugs. In addition mesalamine, olsalazine, and sulfasalazine are contraindicated in patients who have hypersensitivity to the sulfonamides and salicylates or intestinal obstruction, and in children younger than 2 years. There is a possible cross-sensitivity of mesalamine, olsalazine, and sulfasalazine with furosemide, sulfonylurea antidiabetic drugs, and carbonic anhydrase inhibitors. Misoprostol is contraindicated in those with an allergy to the prostaglandins and during pregnancy (Pregnancy Category X) and lactation.

Misoprostol is used cautiously in women of childbearing age. Mesalamine, olsalazine, sucralfate, and sulfasalazine are Pregnancy Category B drugs; all are used with caution during pregnancy (safety has not been established) and lactation.

There is an increased risk of diarrhea in patients taking misoprostol with the magnesium-containing antacids. Sulfasalazine may increase the risk of toxicity of oral hypoglycemic drugs, zidovudine, methotrexate, and phenytoin. There is an increased risk of crystalluria when sulfasalazine is administered with methenamine. A decrease in the absorption of iron and folic acid may occur when these agents are administered with sulfasalazine. When bismuth subsalicylate is administered with aspirin-containing drugs, there is an increased risk of salicylate toxicity. There is an increased risk of toxicity of valproic acid and methotrexate and decreased effectiveness of the corticosteroids when these agents are administered with bismuth subsalicylate.

Herbal Alert: Ginger

Ginger is a pungent herb used primarily for GI problems such as motion sickness, nausea, vomiting, and digestion. In addition, it is recommended for the pain and inflammation of arthritis and may help lower cholesterol. The dosage of the dried form of ginger is 1 g (1000 mg) per day. Adverse reactions are rare, although heartburn has been reported by some individuals. The herb should be used cautiously in patients with hypertension or gallstones and during pregnancy or lactation. As with all herbs, a primary care provider should be consulted before any herbal remedy is taken. Ginger, like many herbs, has been used safely as a food by millions of individuals for hundreds of years.

Herbal Alert: Chamomile

Chamomile has several uses in traditional herbal therapy, such as a mild sedative, digestive upsets, menstrual cramps, and stomach ulcers. It has been used topically for skin irritation and inflammation. Chamomile is on the US Food and Drug Administration list of herbs generally recognized as safe (GRAS). It is one of the most popular teas in Europe. When used as a tea, it appears to produce an antispasmodic effect on the smooth muscle of the gastrointestinal (GI) tract and to protect against the development of stomach ulcers. Although the herb is generally safe and nontoxic, the tea is prepared from the pollen-filled flower heads and has resulted in mild symptoms of contact dermatitis to severe anaphylactic reactions in individuals hypersensitive to ragweed, asters, and chrysanthemums.

Nursing Diagnoses Checklist

- ☑ **Deficient Fluid Volume** related to uncontrolled vomiting or diarrhea
- ☑ **Constipation** related to adverse drug effects (aluminum- or calcium-containing antacids)
- ☑ **Diarrhea** related to adverse reactions of magnesium- or sodium-containing antacids or other digestive system drugs
- ☑ **Risk for Imbalanced Nutrition: Less than Body Requirements** related to inability to eat, digest food, anorexia
- ☑ **Risk for Injury** related to adverse drug effects (eg, weakness, dizziness)

NURSING PROCESS

● The Patient Receiving a Drug for a Gastrointestinal Disorder

ASSESSMENT

Preadministration Assessment

During the preadministration assessment, the nurse reviews the patient's chart for the medical diagnosis and reason for administration of the prescribed drug. The nurse questions the patient regarding the type and intensity of symptoms (such as pain, discomfort, diarrhea, or constipation) to provide a baseline for evaluation of the effectiveness of drug therapy.

Ongoing Assessment

The nurse assesses the patient receiving one of these drugs for relief of symptoms (such as diarrhea, pain, or constipation). The primary health care provider is notified if the drug fails to relieve symptoms. The nurse monitors vital signs daily or more frequently if the patient has a bleeding peptic ulcer, severe diarrhea, or other condition that may warrant more frequent observation. The nurse observes the patient for adverse drug reactions associated with the specific GI drug being administered and reports any adverse reactions to the primary health care provider before the next dose is due. The nurse evaluates the effectiveness of drug therapy by a daily comparison of symptoms with those experienced before the initiation of therapy. In some instances, frequent evaluation of the patient's response to therapy may be necessary.

NURSING DIAGNOSES

Drug-specific nursing diagnoses are highlighted in the Nursing Diagnoses Checklist. Other nursing diagnoses applicable to these drugs are discussed in depth in Chapter 4.

PLANNING

The expected outcomes for the patient depend on the reason for administration of the drug but may include an optimal response to drug therapy, management of common adverse reactions, and an understanding of and compliance with the prescribed therapeutic regimen.

IMPLEMENTATION

Promoting an Optimal Response to Therapy

Ways in which the nurse can help promote an optimal response to therapy when administering GI drugs are listed in the following sections.

ANTACIDS. The nurse should not give antacids within 2 hours before or after administration of other oral drugs. Liquid antacid preparations must be shaken thoroughly immediately before administration. If tablets are given, the nurse instructs the patient to chew the tablets thoroughly before swallowing and then drink a full glass of water or milk. Liquid antacids are followed by a small amount of water. If the patient expresses a dislike for the taste of the antacid or has difficulty chewing the tablet form, the nurse informs the primary health care provider. A flavored antacid may be ordered if the taste is a problem. A liquid form may be ordered if the patient has a problem chewing a tablet. The primary health care provider may order that the antacid be left at the patient's bedside for self-administration. The nurse makes certain an adequate supply of water and cups for measuring the dose are available. The antacid may be administered hourly for the first 2 weeks when used to treat acute peptic ulcer. After the first 2 weeks, the drug is administered 1 to 2 hours after meals and at bedtime.

> ### ☀ Nursing Alert
>
> *Because of the possibility of an antacid interfering with the activity of other oral drugs, no oral drug should be administered within 1 to 2 hours of an antacid.*

GASTROINTESTINAL STIMULANTS. The nurse carefully times the administration of oral metoclopramide for 30 minutes before each meal. Dexpanthenol is administered intramuscularly or IV. The nurse tells the patient that intestinal colic may occur within 30 minutes of administration and that this is not abnormal and will pass within a short time.

HISTAMINE H$_2$ ANTAGONISTS. The nurse administers ranitidine and oral cimetidine before or with meals and at bedtime. Nizatidine and famotidine are given at bedtime or, if twice-a-day dosing is prescribed, in the morning and at bedtime. These drugs are usually given concurrently with an antacid to relieve the pain. In certain situations or disorders, cimetidine and ranitidine may also be given by intermittent IV infusion or direct IV injection.

> ### ☀ Nursing Alert
>
> *When one of these drugs is given IV, the nurse monitors the rate of infusion at frequent intervals. Too rapid an infusion may result in cardiac arrhythmias.*

Cimetidine and ranitidine may be administered by the intramuscular (IM) route. When administered via the IM route the nurse gives the drug deep into a large muscle group.

ANTIDIARRHEALS. These drugs may be ordered to be given after each loose bowel movement. The nurse inspects each bowel movement before making a decision to administer the drug.

DIGESTIVE ENZYMES. When digestive enzymes are given in capsule or enteric-coated tablet form, the nurse instructs the patient not to bite or chew the capsule or tablet. If the patient experiences difficulty swallowing the capsule form, the nurse opens the capsule and sprinkles the contents on a small amount of soft food, such as applesauce or flavored gelatin, which is at room temperature.

EMETICS. Because treatment of poison ingestion is an emergency, the nurse immediately obtains equipment for treatment. The nurse obtains the drug, an emesis basin, towels, specimen containers for sending contents of the stomach to the laboratory for analysis, and a suction machine and places them near the patient. The nurse obtains the patient's blood pressure, pulse, and respiratory rate and performs a brief physical examination to determine what other damages or injuries, if any, may have occurred.

> ### ☀ Nursing Alert
>
> *Before an emetic is given, it is extremely important to know the chemicals or substances that have been ingested, the time they were ingested, and what symptoms were noted before seeking medical treatment. This information will probably be obtained from a family member or friend, but the adult patient may also contribute to the history. The primary health care provider or nurse may also contact the local poison control center to obtain information regarding treatment.*

The nurse must not give an emetic when a corrosive substance (such as lye) or a petroleum distillate (paint thinner, kerosene) has been ingested. In many cases of poisoning, it is preferable to insert a nasogastric tube to empty stomach contents. Emetics are used with great caution, if at all, when the substance ingested is unknown or in question. An emetic is never given to a patient who is unconscious or semiconscious because aspiration of vomitus may occur.

The nurse positions the patient on his or her side before or immediately after the drug is given. When emesis occurs, the nurse suctions the patient as needed and observes closely for the possible aspiration of vomitus. The nurse monitors vital signs every 5 to 10 minutes until signs are stable.

LAXATIVES. The nurse gives bulk-producing or fecal-softening laxatives with a full glass of water or juice. The administration of a bulk-producing laxative is followed by an additional full glass of water. Mineral oil is preferably given to the patient with an empty stomach in the evening. Immediately before administration, the nurse thoroughly mixes and stirs laxatives that are in powder, flake, or granule form. If the laxative has an unpleasant or salty taste, the nurse explains this to the patient. The taste of some of these preparations may be disguised by chilling, adding to juice, or pouring over cracked ice.

ANTIFLATULENTS. Activated charcoal can adsorb drugs while they are in the GI tract. The nurse administers charcoal 2 hours before or 1 hour after other medications. If diarrhea persists or lasts longer than 2 days or is accompanied by fever, the nurse notifies the primary care provider. Simethicone is administered after each meal and at bedtime.

PROTON PUMP INHIBITORS. The nurse administers omeprazole before meals. The drug should be swallowed whole and not chewed or crushed. Esomeprazole magnesium must be swallowed whole and is administered at least 1 hour before meals. For patients who have difficulty swallowing, the nurse may open the capsule and place the granules onto a small amount of applesauce. The granules are mixed lightly with the applesauce and administered immediately. The patient is instructed to swallow the mixture without chewing. Likewise, lansoprazole may be sprinkled on approximately 1 tablespoon of applesauce, cottage cheese, Ensure pudding, yogurt, or strained pears. The drug may also be administered through a nasogastric tube (NG). The granules are mixed with 40 mL of apple juice and injected through a tube. The tube is flushed with fluid afterward.

Monitoring and Managing Adverse Drug Reactions

ANTACIDS. When antacids are given, the nurse keeps a record of the patient's bowel movements because these drugs may cause constipation or diarrhea. If the patient experiences diarrhea, the nurse keeps an accurate record of fluid intake and output along with a description of the diarrhea stool. Changing to a different antacid usually alleviates the problem. Diarrhea may be controlled by combining a magnesium antacid with an antacid containing aluminum or calcium.

ANTICHOLINERGICS. Urinary retention or hesitancy may be seen during therapy with these drugs. This can be avoided by instructing the patient to void before taking the drug. If urinary retention is suspected, the nurse monitors fluid intake and output. These drugs also may cause drowsiness, dizziness, and blurred vision, which may interfere with activities such as reading or watching television. If dizziness occurs, the patient will require assistance with ambulatory activities. If **photophobia** (aversion to bright light) occurs, the room may be kept semidark.

GASTROINTESTINAL STIMULANTS. If drowsiness or dizziness occurs with the administration of metoclopramide, the patient will require assistance with ambulatory activities. The nurse observes patients receiving high or prolonged doses of this drug for adverse reactions related to the CNS (extrapyramidal reactions or tardive dyskinesia, see Chap. 32). The nurse reports any

sign of extrapyramidal reaction or tardive dyskinesia to the primary health care provider before the next dose of metoclopramide is administered because the drug therapy may be discontinued. These reactions are irreversible if therapy is continued.

Dexpanthenol is administered to prevent paralytic ileus (intestinal atony) during the immediate postoperative period. The drug also may be given if a paralytic ileus has occurred, in which case bowel sounds will be diminished or absent. During the administration of the drug, the abdomen is frequently auscultated for the presence or absence of bowel sounds and the primary health care provider notified of the results of these assessments. The nurse observes the patient taking dexpanthenol for adverse reactions, such as nausea, vomiting, and diarrhea. The nurse checks the blood pressure at frequent intervals because a slight drop in blood pressure may occur. A common adverse reaction is intestinal colic that may occur within 30 minutes after administration of the drug.

HISTAMINE H_2 ANTAGONISTS. During early therapy with these drugs, the patient may experience dizziness or drowsiness. The patient may require assistance with ambulation. These reactions usually must be tolerated, but the nurse reassures the patient that they will disappear after several days of therapy.

The nurse immediately reports adverse reactions, such as skin rash, sore throat, fever, unusual bleeding, or hallucinations because the primary health care provider may want to discontinue the drug therapy.

 Gerontologic Alert

The older adult is particularly sensitive to the effects of the histamine H_2 antagonists. The nurse must closely monitor older adults for confusion and dizziness. Dizziness increases the risk for falls in the older adult.

Assistance is needed for ambulatory activities. The environment is made safe by removing throw rugs or small pieces of furniture and so forth. The nurse reports any change in orientation to the primary health care provider.

ANTIDIARRHEALS. The nurse notifies the primary health care provider if an elevation in temperature occurs or if severe abdominal pain or abdominal rigidity or distention occurs because this may indicate a complication of the disorder, such as infection or intestinal perforation. If diarrhea is severe, additional treatment measures, such as IV fluids and electrolyte replacement, may be necessary.

Drowsiness or dizziness may occur with these drugs. The patient may require assistance with ambulatory activities. If diarrhea is chronic, the nurse encourages the patient to drink extra fluids. Fluids such as weak tea, water, bouillon, or a commercial electrolyte preparation may be used. The nurse closely monitors fluid intake and output. In some instances, the primary health care provider may prescribe an oral electrolyte supplement to replace electrolytes lost by frequent loose stools. For perianal irritation caused by loose stools, the nurse cleanses the area with mild soap and water after each bowel movement, dries the area with a soft cloth, and applies an emollient, such as petrolatum.

DIGESTIVE ENZYMES. The nurse observes the patient for nausea and diarrhea. If these occur, the nurse notifies the primary health care provider before the next dose is due because the dosage may need to be reduced. Digestive enzymes come in regular capsule form or as delayed-released capsules. The capsules are taken before or with meals. If necessary the capsules may be opened and sprinkled over soft foods (eg, Jello, applesauce, ice cream) that can be swallowed without chewing. It is particularly important that enteric-coated beads from the time-released capsules be swallowed and not chewed. If the drug is sprinkled over certain foods, it is important that the nurse check the patient's tray after each meal to determine if the foods sprinkled with the drug are eaten. If these foods are not eaten, the nurse notifies the primary health care provider. The nurse weighs the patient weekly (or as ordered) and alerts the primary health care provider if there is any significant or steady weight loss.

The nurse notes and records the appearance of each stool. Periodic stool examinations, as well as ongoing descriptions of the appearance of the stools, help the primary health care provider determine the effectiveness of therapy.

EMETICS. After the administration of an emetic, the nurse closely observes the patient for signs of shock, respiratory depression, or other signs and symptoms that may be part of the clinical picture of the specific poison or drug that was accidentally or purposely taken.

LAXATIVES. The nurse records the results of administration on the patient's chart. If excessive bowel movements or severe prolonged diarrhea occur or if the laxative is ineffective, the nurse notifies the primary health care provider. If a laxative is ordered for constipation, the nurse encourages a liberal fluid intake and an increase in foods high in fiber to prevent a repeat of this problem.

PROTON PUMP INHIBITORS. The adverse reactions of the proton pump inhibitors are usually mild. The most common adverse reactions associated with the proton

pump inhibitors are headache, diarrhea, and abdominal pain. Headache may be treated with analgesics. The nurse notes the number, color, and consistency of the stools. The nurse reports any excessive diarrhea or severe headache.

Educating the Patient and Family

When a GI drug must be taken for a long time, there is a possibility that the patient may begin to skip doses or stop taking the drug. The nurse encourages patients to take the prescribed drug as directed by the primary health care provider and emphasizes the importance of not omitting doses or stopping the therapy unless advised to do so by the primary health care provider.

The nurse includes the following information in a patient and family teaching plan:

ANTACIDS

- Do not use the drug indiscriminately. Check with a primary health care provider before using an antacid if other medical problems, such as a cardiac condition (some laxatives contain sodium), exist.
- Chew tablets thoroughly before swallowing and then drink a full glass of water.
- Effervescent tablets: allow to completely dissolve in water. Allow most of the bubbling to stop before drinking.
- Adhere to the dosage schedule recommended by the primary health care provider. Do not increase the frequency of use or the dose if symptoms become worse; instead, see the primary health care provider as soon as possible.
- Antacids impair the absorption of some drugs. Do not take other drugs within 2 hours before or after taking the antacid unless use of an antacid with a drug is recommended by the primary health care provider.
- If pain or discomfort remains the same or becomes worse, if the stools turn black or coffee ground vomitus occurs, contact the primary health care provider as soon as possible.
- Antacids may change the color of the stool (white, white streaks); this is normal.
- Magnesium-containing products may produce a laxative effect and may cause diarrhea; aluminum- or calcium-containing antacids may cause constipation; magnesium-containing antacids are used to avoid bowel dysfunction.
- Taking too much antacid may cause the stomach to secrete excess stomach acid. Consult the primary care provider or pharmacist about appropriate dose. Do not use the maximum dose for more than 2 weeks, except under the supervision of a primary care provider.

ANTICHOLINERGICS

● If an aversion to light occurs, wear sunglasses when outside, keep rooms dimly lit, and schedule outdoor activities (when necessary) before the first dose of the drug is taken, such as early in the morning.
● If a dry mouth occurs, take frequent sips of cool water during the day, several sips of water before taking oral drugs, and frequent sips of water during meals.
● Constipation may be avoided by drinking plenty of fluids during the day.
● Drowsiness may occur with these drugs. Schedule tasks requiring alertness during times when drowsiness does not occur, such as early in the morning before the first dose of the drug is taken.

GASTROINTESTINAL STIMULANTS. Metoclopramide—Take 30 minutes before meals. If drowsiness or dizziness occurs, observe caution while driving or performing hazardous tasks. Immediately report any of the following signs: difficulty speaking or swallowing; mask-like face; shuffling gait; rigidity; tremors; uncontrolled movements of the mouth, face, or extremities; and uncontrolled chewing or unusual movements of the tongue.

HISTAMINE H₂ ANTAGONISTS

● Keep the primary health care provider informed of the results of therapy, that is, relief of pain or discomfort.
● Take as directed (eg, with meals, at bedtime) on the prescription container.
● Follow the primary health care provider's recommendations regarding additional treatment, such as eliminating certain foods, avoiding the use of alcohol, and using additional drugs, such as an antacid.
● If drowsiness occurs, avoid driving or performing other hazardous tasks.
● Notify the primary health care provider of the following adverse reactions: sore throat, rash, fever, unusual bleeding, black or tarry stools, easy bruising, or confusion.
● Regular follow-up appointments are required while taking these drugs. These drugs may need to be taken for 4 to 6 weeks or longer.
● Cimetidine—Inform the primary health care provider if you smoke. Cigarette smoking may decrease the effectiveness of the drug.

ANTIDIARRHEALS

● Do not exceed the recommended dosage.
● The drug may cause drowsiness. Observe caution when driving or performing other hazardous tasks.

● Avoid the use of alcohol or other CNS depressants (tranquilizers, sleeping pills) and other nonprescription drugs unless use has been approved by the primary health care provider.
● Notify the primary health care provider if diarrhea persists or becomes more severe.

ANTIFLATULENTS

● Take simethicone after each meal and at bedtime. Thoroughly chew tablets because complete particle dispersion enhances antiflatulent action.
● Take charcoal 2 hours before or 1 hour after meals.
● Notify the health care provider if symptoms are not relieved within several days.

DIGESTIVE ENZYMES

● Take the drugs as directed by the primary health care provider. Do not exceed the recommended dose.
● Do not chew tablets or capsules. Swallow the whole form of the drug quickly, while sitting upright to enhance swallowing and prevent mouth and throat irritation. Eat immediately after taking the drug.
● If capsules are difficult to swallow, they may be opened and their contents sprinkled over small quantities of food. Avoid sprinkling the drug over hot foods. All the food sprinkled with the powder must be eaten.
● Do not change brands without consulting with the primary care provider or the pharmacist.
● Do not inhale the powder dosage form or powder from capsules because it may irritate the skin or mucous membranes.

EMETICS (IPECAC SYRUP)

● Ipecac is available without a prescription for use in the home. The instructions for use and the recommended dose are printed on the label.
● Read the directions on the label after the drug is purchased and be familiar with these instructions before an emergency occurs.
● In case of accidental or intentional poisoning, contact the nearest poison control center before using or giving this drug. Not all poisoning can be treated with this drug.
● Do not give this drug to semiconscious, unconscious, or convulsing individuals.
● Vomiting should occur in 20 to 30 minutes. Seek medical attention immediately after contacting the poison control center and giving this drug.

GALLSTONE-SOLUBILIZING DRUGS

● Periodic laboratory tests (liver function studies) and ultrasound or radiologic examinations of the gallbladder may be scheduled by the primary health care provider.

- If diarrhea occurs, contact the primary health care provider. If symptoms of gallbladder disease (pain, nausea, or vomiting) occur, immediately contact the primary health care provider.
- Never take these drugs with aluminum-containing antacids. If antacids are required, take them 2 to 3 hours after ursodiol.

LAXATIVES

- Avoid long-term use of these products unless use of the product has been recommended by the primary health care provider. Long-term use may result in the "laxative habit," which is a dependence on a laxative to have a bowel movement. Constipation may also occur with overuse of these drugs. Read and follow the directions on the label.
- Avoid long-term use of mineral oil. Daily use of this product may interfere with the absorption of some vitamins (vitamins A, D, E, K). Take with the stomach empty, preferably at bedtime.
- Do not use these products in the presence of abdominal pain, nausea, or vomiting.
- Notify the primary health care provider if constipation is not relieved or if rectal bleeding or other symptoms occur.
- To avoid constipation, drink plenty of fluids, get exercise, and eat foods high in bulk or roughage.
- Bulk-producing or fecal-softening laxatives—Drink a full glass of water or juice, followed by more glasses of fluid in the next few hours.
- Bisacodyl (Dulcolax)—Do not chew the tablets or take them within 1 hour of taking antacids or milk.
- Cascara sagrada or senna—Pink-red, red-violet, red-brown, yellow-brown, or black discoloration of urine may occur.

PROTON PUMP INHIBITORS

- Esomeprazole—Swallow whole at least 1 hour before eating. If you have difficulty swallowing, the capsule may be opened and the granules sprinkled on a small amount of applesauce.
- Omeprazole—Swallow tablets whole; do not chew them. This drug will be taken for up to 8 weeks or for a prolonged period. Regular medical check-ups are required.
- Lansoprazole—Take the drug before meals. Swallow the capsules whole. Do not chew, open, or crush. If you have difficulty swallowing the capsule, open and sprinkle granules on Jell-O or applesauce. You will need regular medical check-ups while taking this drug.

H. PYLORI COMBINATION DRUGS

- Helidac—Each dose includes four tablets: two round, chewable pink tablets (bismuth), one white

tablet (metronidazole), and one pale orange and white capsule (tetracycline). Take each dose four times a day with meals and at bedtime for 14 days. Chew and swallow the bismuth subsalicylate tablets; swallow the metronidazole tablet and tetracycline capsule with a full glass of water. Take concomitantly prescribed H_2 antagonist therapy, as directed. Drink an adequate amount of fluid to reduce the risk of esophageal irritation and ulceration. Missed doses may be made up by continuing the formal dosing schedule until the medication is gone. Do not take double doses. If more than four doses are missed, contact the primary care provider.
- Bismuth subsalicylate—Immediately report any symptoms of salicylate toxicity (ringing in the ears, rapid respirations). Chew tablets thoroughly or dissolve them in the mouth. Do not swallow tablets whole. Stools may become dark. This is normal and will disappear when the drug therapy is discontinued. Do not take this drug with aspirin or aspirin products.

MISCELLANEOUS DRUGS

- Olsalazine—If diarrhea develops, contact the primary health care provider as soon as possible.
- Mesalamine—Swallow tablets whole; do not chew them. For the suppository, remove foil wrapper and immediately insert the pointed end into the rectum without using force. For the suspension form, instructions are included with the product. Shake well, remove the protective sheath from the applicator tip, and gently insert the tip into the rectum. Partially intact tablets may be found in the stool; if this occurs, notify the primary health care provider.
- Misoprostol—Take this drug four times a day with meals and at bedtime. Continue to take the NSAID during this drug therapy. Take the drug with meals to decrease the severity of diarrhea. The administration of antacids before or after misoprostol may decrease the pain. Magnesium-containing antacids are avoided because of the risk of increasing the diarrhea.

This drug may cause spontaneous abortion. Women of childbearing age must use a reliable contraceptive. If pregnancy is suspected, discontinue use of the drug and notify the primary health care provider. Report severe menstrual pain, bleeding, or spotting.

- Sucralfate—Take on an empty stomach 1 hour before meals. Antacids may be taken for pain but not within 1/2 hour before or after sucralfate. Therapy will continue for 4 to 8 weeks. Keep all follow-up appointments with the primary health care provider.

EVALUATION

- The therapeutic drug effect is achieved.
- Adverse reactions are identified and reported to the primary health care provider.
- The patient and family demonstrate an understanding of the drug regimen.
- The patient verbalizes the importance of complying with the prescribed treatment regimen.
- The patient verbalizes an understanding of treatment modalities and the importance of continued follow-up care.

● Critical Thinking Exercises

1. *Ms. Harris, age 76 years, tells you that she has been using various laxatives for constipation. She states that a laxative did help, but now she is more constipated than she was before she began taking a laxative. Discuss what advice or suggestions you would give this patient.*
2. *James is prescribed 0.7 g of powdered pancrelipase with meals. Discuss the preparation and administration of this drug.*
3. *Mr. Gates, your neighbor, has been given a prescription for diphenoxylate with atropine (Lomotil) to be taken if he should experience diarrhea while he is traveling in a foreign country. Describe the warnings you would give to your neighbor regarding this drug.*
4. *The primary health care provider has prescribed cimetidine for the treatment of a duodenal ulcer in Mr. Talley, who is 68 years old. A drug history by the nurse reveals that Mr. Talley is also taking the following drugs: Lanoxin 0.5 mg orally each day and a daily aspirin tablet. Analyze this situation. Discuss what you would tell Mr. Talley.*
5. *Ms. Jerkins has four children and wants to keep syrup of ipecac available in case of accidental poisoning. Discuss the information you feel that Ms. Jerkins should know before she administers this drug.*

● Review Questions

1. When would the nurse most correctly administer an antacid to a patient taking other oral medications?
   A. With the other drugs
   B. 30 minutes before or after administration of other drugs
   C. 2 hours before or after administration of other drugs
   D. In early morning and at bedtime

2. The patient asks how fecal softeners relieve constipation. Which of the following would be the best response by the nurse? Fecal softeners relieve constipation by _____.

A. stimulating the walls of the intestine
B. promoting the retention of sodium in the fecal mass
C. promoting water retention in the fecal mass
D. lubricating the intestinal walls

3. When an anticholinergic drug is prescribed for the treatment of a peptic ulcer, the nurse observes the patient for which of the following adverse effects?
   A. Dry mouth, urinary retention
   B. Edema, tachycardia
   C. Weight gain, increased respiratory rate
   D. Diarrhea, anorexia

4. The nurse administers antidiarrheal drugs _____.
   A. hourly until diarrhea ceases
   B. after each loose bowel movement
   C. with food
   D. twice a day, in the morning and at bedtime

5. When an emetic is administered, the nurse must be alert to the possibility that the patient may _____.
   A. become violent
   B. experience severe diarrhea
   C. retain fluid
   D. aspirate vomitus

6. A nurse is to administer nizatidine once daily. When would the nurse most correctly administer the once-daily dose of nizatidine?
   A. At bedtime
   B. With the noon meal
   C. In the morning before eating
   D. Any time of the day with 4 ounces of orange juice

● Medication Dosage Problems

1. The patient is to receive 800 mg cimetidine PO. Available for use is the cimetidine shown below. The nurse administers _____.

Store between 15° and 30°C (59° and 86°F)
Dispense in a tight, light-resistant container.
Each Tiltab™ tablet contains cimetidine, 400 mg
Dosage: See accompanying prescribing information
Important: Use safety closures when dispensing this product unless otherwise directed by physician or requested by purchaser.
GlaxoSmithKline
Research Triangle Park, NC 27709

400mg NDC 0108-5026-18
TAGAMET®
CIMETIDINE TABLETS
60 TILTAB® Tablets
GlaxoSmithKline R only

2. Prescribed is 15 mL of 1.5% ipecac syrup. Available is 30 mL ipecac 1.5% syrup. The nurse administers _____.

c h a p t e r **49**

Antidiabetic Drugs

Key Terms

diabetes mellitus
diabetic ketoacidosis
Escherichia coli
glucagon
glucometer
glycosylated
 hemoglobin

hyperglycemia
hypoglycemia
insulin
lipodystrophy
secondary failure

Chapter Objectives

On completion of this chapter, the student will:

● Describe the two types of diabetes mellitus.
● Discuss the types, uses, general drug actions, adverse reactions, contraindications, precautions, and interactions of the antidiabetic drugs.
● Discuss important preadministration and ongoing assessment activities the nurse should perform on the patient taking an antidiabetic drug.
● List some nursing diagnoses particular to a patient taking an antidiabetic drug.
● Discuss ways to promote an optimal response to therapy, how to manage common adverse reactions, and important points to keep in mind when educating patients about the use of the antidiabetic drugs.

Insulin, a hormone produced by the pancreas, acts to maintain blood glucose levels within normal limits (60–120 mg/dL). This is accomplished by the release of small amounts of insulin into the bloodstream throughout the day in response to changes in blood glucose levels. Insulin is essential for the utilization of glucose in cellular metabolism and for the proper metabolism of protein and fat.

Diabetes mellitus is a complicated, chronic disorder characterized by either insufficient insulin production by the beta cells of the pancreas or by cellular resistance to insulin. Insulin insufficiency results in elevated blood glucose levels, or hyperglycemia. As a result of the disease, individuals with diabetes are at greater risk for a number of disorders, including myocardial infarction, cerebrovascular accident (stroke), blindness, kidney disease, and lower limb amputations.

Insulin and the oral antidiabetic drugs, along with diet and exercise, are the cornerstones of treatment for diabetes mellitus. They are used to prevent episodes of hypoglycemia and to normalize carbohydrate metabolism.

There are two major types of diabetes mellitus:

● Type 1—Insulin-dependent diabetes mellitus (IDDM). Former names of this type of diabetes mellitus include juvenile diabetes, juvenile-onset diabetes, and brittle diabetes.
● Type 2—Noninsulin-dependent diabetes mellitus (NIDDM). Former names of this type of diabetes mellitus include maturity-onset diabetes, adult-onset diabetes, and stable diabetes.

Those with type 1 diabetes mellitus produce insulin in insufficient amounts and therefore must have insulin supplementation to survive. Type 1 diabetes usually has a rapid onset, occurs before the age of 20 years, produces more severe symptoms than type 2 diabetes, and is more difficult to control. Major symptoms of type 1 diabetes include hyperglycemia, polydipsia (increased thirst), polyphagia (increased appetite), polyuria (increased urination), and weight loss. Treatment of type 1 diabetes is particularly difficult to control because of the lack of insulin production by the pancreas. Treatment requires a strict regimen that typically includes a carefully calculated diet, planned physical activity, home glucose testing several times a day, and multiple daily insulin injections.

Type 2 diabetes mellitus affects about 90% to 95% of individuals with diabetes. Those with type 2 diabetes mellitus either have a decreased production of insulin by the beta cells of the pancreas or a decreased sensitivity of the cells to insulin, making the cells insulin resistant. Although type 2 diabetes mellitus may occur at any age, the disorder occurs most often after the age of 40 years. The onset of type 2 diabetes is usually insidious, symptoms are less severe than in type 1 diabetes mellitus, and because it tends to be more stable, it is easier to control than type 1 diabetes. Risk factors for type 2 diabetes include:

- Obesity
- Older age
- Family history of diabetes
- History of gestational diabetes (diabetes that develops during pregnancy but disappears when pregnancy is over)
- Impaired glucose tolerance
- Minimal or no physical activity
- Race/ethnicity (African Americans, Hispanic/Latino Americans, American Indians, and some Asian Americans)

Obesity is thought to contribute to type 2 diabetes by placing additional stress on the pancreas, which makes it less able to respond and produce adequate insulin to meet the body's metabolic needs.

Many individuals with type 2 diabetes are able to control the disorder with diet, exercise, and oral antidiabetic drugs. However, about 40% of those with type 2 diabetes do not have a good response to the oral antidiabetic drugs and require the addition of insulin to control the diabetes.

INSULIN

Insulin is a hormone manufactured by the beta cells of the pancreas. It is the principal hormone required for the proper use of glucose (carbohydrate) by the body. Insulin also controls the storage and utilization of amino acids and fatty acids. Insulin lowers blood glucose levels by inhibiting glucose production by the liver.

Insulin is available as purified extracts from beef and pork pancreas and is biologically similar to human insulin. However, these animal source insulins are used less frequently today than in years past. They are being replaced by synthetic insulins, including human insulin or insulin analogs.

Human insulin is derived from a biosynthetic process using strains of ***Escherichia coli*** (recombinant DNA, rDNA). Human insulin appears to cause fewer allergic reactions than does insulin obtained from animal sources. Insulin analogs, insulin lispro, and insulin aspart are newer forms of human insulin made by using recombinant DNA technology and are structurally similar to human insulin.

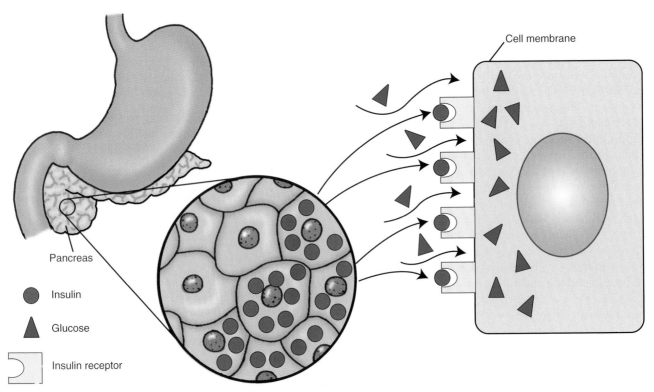

FIGURE 49-1. Normal glucose metabolism. Once insulin binds with receptors on the cell membrane, glucose can move into the cell, promoting cellular metabolism and energy production.

ACTIONS

Insulin appears to activate a process that helps glucose molecules enter the cells of striated muscle and adipose tissue. Figure 49-1 depicts normal glucose metabolism. Insulin also stimulates the synthesis of glycogen by the liver. In addition, insulin promotes protein synthesis and helps the body store fat by preventing its breakdown for energy.

Onset, Peak, and Duration of Action

Onset, peak, and duration are three properties of insulin that are of clinical importance.

- Onset—when insulin first begins to act in the body

- Peak—when the insulin is exerting maximum action
- Duration—the length of time the insulin remains in effect

To meet the needs of those with diabetes mellitus, various insulin preparations have been developed to delay the onset and prolong the duration of action of insulin. When insulin is combined with protamine (a protein), the absorption of insulin from the injection site is slowed and the duration of action is prolonged. The addition of zinc also modifies the onset and duration of action of insulin. Insulin preparations are classified as rapid-acting, intermediate-acting, or long-acting. The Summary Drug Table: Insulin Preparations gives information concerning the onset, peak, and duration of various insulins.

SUMMARY DRUG TABLE INSULIN PREPARATIONS

		ACTIVITY		
TYPES OF INSULIN	**TRADE NAME**	**Onset**	**Peak**	**Duration**
Rapid-Acting Insulins				
insulin injection (regular)	Humulin R, Iletin II Regular, Novolin R, Novolin R PenFill, Novolin R Prefilled, Velosulin BR	30–60 min	2–4 h	6–8 h
insulin lispro (insulin analog)	Humalog, Humalog Mix 50/50, Humalog Mix 75/25	45 min 30–60 min then 1–2 h	.1 h 2–4 h then 6–12 h	3.5–4.5 h 6–8 h then 8–24 h
insulin aspart solution (insulin analog)	Novolog	5–10 min	30–60 min	2–3 h
Intermediate-Acting Insulin				
isophane insulin suspension (NPH)	Humulin N, Novolin N, Novolin N PenFill, Novolin N Prefilled, NPH Iletin II	1–2 h	6–12 h	18–24 h
insulin zinc suspension (Lente)	Humulin L, Lente Iletin II, Novolin L	1–2.5 h	6–12 h	18–24 h
Long-Acting Insulins				
Insulin glargine solution	Lantus	30–60 min	none	8 h
extended insulin zinc suspension (Ultralente)	Humulin U	4–8 h	8–20 h	24–48 h
Mixed Insulins				
isophane insulin suspension and insulin injections (NPH)	Humulin 70/30, Novolin 70/30, Novolin 70/30 PenFill, Novolin 70/30 Prefilled	30–60 min then 1–2 h	2–4 h then 6–12 h	6–8 h then 18–24 h
isophane insulin suspension and insulin injection	Humulin 50/50	30–60 min then 1–2 h	2–4 h then 6–12 h	6–8 h then 18–24 h
High-Potency Insulin				
insulin injection concentrated	Humulin R Regular U-500			24 h

USES

Insulin is necessary for controlling type 1 diabetes mellitus that is caused by a marked decrease in the amount of insulin produced by the pancreas. Insulin is also used to control the more severe and complicated forms of type 2 diabetes mellitus. However, many patients can control type 2 diabetes with diet and exercise alone or with diet, exercise, and an oral antidiabetic drug (see section "Oral Antidiabetic Drugs"). Insulin may also be used in the treatment of severe diabetic ketoacidosis (DKA) or diabetic coma. Insulin is also used in combination with glucose to treat hypokalemia by producing a shift of potassium from the blood and into the cells.

ADVERSE REACTIONS

The two major adverse reactions seen with insulin administration are **hypoglycemia** (low blood glucose or sugar) and **hyperglycemia** (elevated blood glucose or sugar). The symptoms of hypoglycemia and hyperglycemia are listed in Table 49-1.

Hypoglycemia may occur when there is too much insulin in the bloodstream in relation to the available glucose (hyperinsulinism). Hypoglycemia may occur:

- When the patient eats too little food
- When the insulin dose is incorrectly measured and is greater than that prescribed
- When the patient drastically increases physical activity

Hyperglycemia may occur if there is too little insulin in the bloodstream in relation to the available glucose (hypoinsulinism). Hyperglycemia may occur:

- When the patient eats too much food
- When too little or no insulin is given
- When the patient experiences emotional stress, infection, surgery, pregnancy, or an acute illness

Another potential adverse reaction may be if the patient has an allergy to the animal (pig or cow) from which the insulin is obtained or to the protein or zinc added to insulin. To minimize the possibility of an allergic reaction, some health care providers prescribe human insulin or purified insulin. However, on rare occasions, some individuals become allergic to the human and purified insulins.

An individual can also become insulin resistant because of the development of antibodies against insulin. These patients have impaired receptor function and become so unresponsive to insulin that the daily dose requirement may be in excess of 500 units per day (U/d), rather than the usual 40 to 60 U/d. High-potency insulin in a concentrated form (U500; see the Summary Drug Table: Insulin Preparations) is used for patients requiring more than 200 U/d.

CONTRAINDICATIONS

Insulin is contraindicated in patients with hypersensitivity to any ingredient of the product (eg, beef or pork) and when the patient is hypoglycemic.

PRECAUTIONS

Insulin is used cautiously in patients with renal and hepatic impairment and during pregnancy (Pregnancy Category B and Category C, insulin glargine and insulin

TABLE 49-1	Hypoglycemia Versus Hyperglycemia	
SYMPTOMS	**HYPOGLYCEMIA (INSULIN REACTION)**	**HYPERGLYCEMIA (DIABETIC COMA, KETOACIDOSIS)**
Onset	Sudden	Gradual (hours or days)
Blood glucose	<60 mg/dL	>200 mg/dL
Central nervous system	Fatigue, weakness, nervousness, agitation, confusion, headache, diplopia, convulsions, dizziness, unconsciousness	Drowsiness, dim vision
Respirations	Normal to rapid, shallow	Deep, rapid (air hunger)
Gastrointestinal	Hunger, nausea	Thirst, nausea, vomiting, abdominal pain, loss of appetite, excessive urination
Skin	Pale, moist, cool, diaphoretic	Dry, flushed, warm
Pulse	Normal or uncharacteristic	Rapid, weak
Miscellaneous	Numbness, tingling of the lips or tongue	Acetone breath

aspart) and lactation (may inhibit milk formation with large doses of insulin). Insulin appears to inhibit milk production in lactating women and could interfere with breastfeeding. Lactating women may require adjustment in insulin dose and diet.

> ## ☀ Nursing Alert
>
> *Pregnancy makes diabetes more difficult to manage. Insulin requirements usually decrease in the first trimester, increase during the second and third trimester, and decrease rapidly after delivery. The patient with diabetes or a history of gestational diabetes must be encouraged to maintain good metabolic control before conception and throughout pregnancy. Frequent monitoring is necessary.*

INTERACTIONS

When certain drugs are administered with insulin, a resultant decrease or increase in hypoglycemic effect can occur. Display 49-1 identifies selected drugs that decrease the hypoglycemic effect of insulin.

Display 49-2 identifies select drugs which, when administered with insulin, may increase the hypoglycemic effect of insulin.

NURSING PROCESS

● The Patient Receiving Insulin

ASSESSMENT

Preadministration Assessment

If the patient has recently received a diagnosis of diabetes mellitus and has not received insulin or if the patient is known to have diabetes, the initial physical

---

DISPLAY 49-1 ● Select Drugs That Decrease the Hypoglycemic Effect of Insulin

- AIDS antivirals
- albuterol
- contraceptives, oral
- corticosteroids
- diltiazem
- diuretics
- dobutamine
- epinephrine
- estrogens
- lithium
- morphine sulfate
- niacin
- phenothiazines
- thyroid hormones

DISPLAY 49-2 ● Drugs That Increase the Hypoglycemic Effect of Insulin

- alcohol
- angiotensin-converting enzyme (ACE) inhibitors
- antidiabetic drugs, oral
- beta blocking drugs
- calcium
- clonidine
- disopyramide
- lithium
- monoamine oxidase inhibitors (MAOIs)
- salicylates
- sulfonamides
- tetracycline

---

assessment before administering the first dose of insulin includes taking the blood pressure, pulse, and respiratory rate, and weighing the patient. The nurse makes a general assessment of the skin, mucous membranes, and extremities, with special attention given to any sores or cuts that appear to be infected or healing poorly, as well as any ulcerations or other skin or mucous membrane changes. The nurse obtains the following information and includes it in the patient's chart:

- Dietary habits
- Family history of diabetes (if any)
- Type and duration of symptoms experienced

The nurse reviews the patient's chart for recent laboratory and diagnostic tests. If the patient has diabetes and has been receiving insulin, the nurse includes the type and dosage of insulin used, the type of diabetic diet, and the average results of glucose testing in the patient's chart. The nurse evaluates the patient's past compliance to the prescribed therapeutic regimen, such as diet, weight control, and periodic evaluation by a health care provider.

Ongoing Assessment

The number and amount of daily insulin doses, times of administration, and diet and exercise requirements require continual assessment. Dosage adjustments may be necessary when changing types of insulin, particularly when changing from the single-peak to the more pure Humulin insulins.

The nurse must assess the patient for signs and symptoms of hypoglycemia and hyperglycemia (see Table 49-1) throughout insulin therapy. The patient is particularly prone to hypoglycemic reactions at the time of peak insulin action (see the Summary Drug Table: Insulin Preparations) or when the patient has not eaten for some time or has skipped a meal. In acute care settings, frequent blood glucose monitoring is routinely done to help detect abnormalities of blood glucose.

Testing usually occurs before meals and at bedtime (see section on "Managing Hypoglycemia").

> ### ✴ Nursing Alert
>
> *The nurse must closely observe the patient after administering any insulin, but particularly U500 insulin, because secondary hypoglycemic reactions may occur as long as 24 hours after the administration.*

Blood glucose levels are monitored frequently in patients with diabetes. Patients in the acute care setting are monitored closely for hyperglycemia. Insulin needs increase in times of stress or illness. The health care provider may order regular insulin as a supplement to the drug regimen to "cover" any episodes of hyperglycemia. For example, blood glucose levels are monitored every 6 hours or before meals and at bedtime, with insulin prescribed to cover any hyperglycemia detected. This coverage is sometimes referred to as a sliding scale or insulin coverage. Table 49-2 provides an example of a sliding scale by which regular insulin may be administered.

The nurse administers supplemental insulin based on blood glucose readings and the amount of insulin prescribed by the health care provider in the sliding scale. The nurse must notify the health care provider if the blood glucose level is greater than 400 mg/dL.

The primary care provider may prescribe use of a sliding scale at various times, such as every 4 hours, every 6 hours, or at specified times (eg, 7:00 AM, 11:00 AM, 4 PM, and 11 PM), depending on the patient's individual needs.

NURSING DIAGNOSES

Drug-specific nursing diagnoses are highlighted in the Nursing Diagnoses Checklist. Other nursing diagnoses applicable to these drugs are discussed in depth in Chapter 4.

TABLE 49-2	Example of Insulin Administration Using a Sliding Scale

Administer regular humulin insulin subcutaneously 30 minutes before meals and at bedtime according to the following blood glucose levels.

BLOOD GLUCOSE LEVEL	REGULAR HUMULIN INSULIN TO BE ADMINISTERED
150–200 mg/dL	2 U
201–250 mg/dL	4 U
251–300 mg/dL	6 U
301–350 mg/dL	8 U
351–400 mg/dL	10 U
> 400 mg/dL	Call physician

> ### Nursing Diagnoses Checklist ━━━━━━●
>
> ☑ **Confusion** related to adverse drug reaction (hypoglycemia)
>
> ☑ **Anxiety** related to diagnosis, fear of giving own injections, dietary restrictions, other factors (specify)
>
> ☑ **Ineffective Coping** related to inability to accept diagnosis, other factors (specify)
>
> ☑ **Fear** related to diagnosis, consequences of diabetes
>
> ☑ **Ineffective Health Maintenance** related to inability to comprehend drug regimen, lack of equipment to monitor drug effects, lack of knowledge
>
> ☑ **Risk for Ineffective Therapeutic Regimen Management** related to lack of knowledge, misunderstanding, or complexity of prescribed treatment program, other factors (specify)

PLANNING

The expected outcomes of the patient may include an optimal response to therapy, management of common adverse drug reactions, a reduction in anxiety and fear, improved ability to cope with the diagnosis, and an understanding of and compliance with the prescribed therapeutic regimen.

IMPLEMENTATION

Nursing management of a patient with diabetes requires diligent, skillful, and comprehensive nursing care.

Promoting an Optimal Response to Therapy

There is no standard dose of insulin as there is for most other drugs. Insulin dosage is highly individualized. Sometimes the health care provider finds that the patient achieves best control with one injection of insulin per day; sometimes the patient requires two or more injections per day. In addition, two different types of insulin may be combined, such as a rapid-acting and a long-acting preparation. The number of insulin injections, dosage, times of administration, and type of insulin are determined by the health care provider after careful evaluation of the patient's metabolic needs and response to therapy. The dosage prescribed for the patient may require changes until the dosage is found that best meets the patient's needs.

> ### ✴ Nursing Alert
>
> *Insulin requirements may change when the patient experiences any form of stress and with any illness, particularly illnesses resulting in nausea and vomiting.*

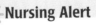

Insulin is ordered by the generic name (insulin zinc suspension, extended) or the trade (brand) name (Humulin U) (see the Summary Drug Table: Insulin Preparations). The nurse must never substitute one brand of insulin for another unless the substitution is approved by the health care provider because some patients may be sensitive to changes in brands of insulin. In addition, it is important never to substitute one type of insulin for another. For example, do not use insulin zinc suspension instead of the prescribed protamine zinc insulin.

Care must be taken when giving insulin to use the correct insulin. Names and packaging are similar and can easily be confused. The nurse carefully reads all drug labels before preparing any insulin preparation. For example, Humalog (insulin lispro) and Humulin R (regular human insulin) are easily confused because of the similar names.

Insulin must be administered via the parenteral route, usually the subcutaneous (SC) route. Insulin cannot be administered orally because it is a protein and readily destroyed in the gastrointestinal tract. Regular insulin is the only insulin preparation given intravenously (IV). Regular insulin is given 30 to 60 minutes before a meal to achieve optimal results.

Insulin aspart is given immediately before a meal (within 5 to 10 minutes of beginning a meal). Insulin lispro is given 15 minutes before a meal or immediately after a meal. Insulin aspart and lispro make insulin administration more convenient for many patients who find taking a drug 30 to 60 minutes before meals bothersome. In addition, insulin lispro (Humalog) appears to lower the blood sugar level 1 to 2 hours after meals

better than does regular human insulin because it more closely mimics the body's natural insulin. It also lowers the risk of low blood sugar reactions from midnight to 6 AM in patients with type 1 diabetes. The longer acting insulins are given before breakfast or at bedtime (depending on the health care provider's instructions). Many patients are maintained on a single dose of intermediate-acting insulin administered SC in the morning.

Insulin glargine is given SC once daily at bedtime. This type of insulin is used in the treatment of adults and children with type 1 diabetes mellitus and in adults with type 2 diabetes who need long-acting insulin for the control of hyperglycemia.

Insulin is available in concentrations of U100 and U500. The nurse must read the label of the insulin bottle carefully for the name, source of insulin (eg, human, beef, pork, beef and pork, purified beef), and the number of units per milliliter (U/mL). The dose of insulin is measured in units (U). U100 insulin has 100 units in each milliliter; U500 has 500 units in each milliliter. Most people with diabetes use the U100 concentration. Patients who are resistant to insulin and require large insulin doses require the U500 concentration.

MIXING INSULINS. If the patient is to receive regular insulin and NPH insulin, or regular and Lente insulin, the nurse must clarify with the health care provider whether two separate injections are to be given or if the insulins may be mixed in the same syringe. If the two insulins are to be given in the same syringe, the short-acting insulin (regular or lispro) is drawn into the syringe first (see Fig. 49-2). Even small amounts of

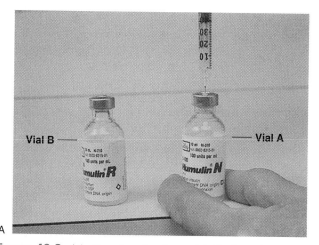
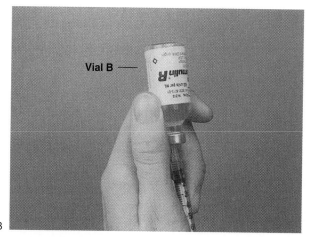

FIGURE 49-2. **(A)** After cleansing tops of both the Humulin R (Regular) insulin and Humulin N (intermediate acting insulin), the nurse injects air into the Humulin N insulin equal to the prescribed dosage of Humulin N. The nurse then injects the amount of air into the prescribed dosage of the regular insulin and withdraws the prescribed dosage of regular insulin into the syringe. **(B)** After removing any air bubbles and determining what the total combined volume of the two insulins would measure, the nurse inverts the vial with the NPH insulin and carefully withdraws the correct volume of medication. *Note*: The nurse must be sure to check medication and dosage again before returning or discarding vials or administering the insulin.

intermediate- or long-acting insulin, if mixed with the short-acting insulin, can bind with the short-acting insulin and delay its onset. (Hint: Regular insulin is clear, whereas intermediate- and long-acting insulins are cloudy. The clear insulin should be drawn up first.) When insulin lispro is mixed with a longer-acting insulin, the insulin lispro is drawn up first.

An unexpected response may be obtained when changing from mixed injections to separate injections or vice versa. If the patient had been using insulin mixtures before admission, the nurse asks whether the insulins were given separately or together.

Several types of premixed insulins are currently available. These insulins combine regular insulin with the longer-acting NPH insulin. The mixtures are available in ratios of 70/30 and 50/50 of NPH to regular. Although these premixed insulins are helpful for patients who have difficulty drawing up their insulin or seeing the markings on the syringe, they prohibit individualizing the dosage. For patients who have difficulty controlling their diabetes, these premixed insulins may not be effective.

> ### ☀ Nursing Alert
>
> *Do not mix or dilute insulin glargine with any other insulin or solution because glucose control will be lost and the insulin will not be effective.*

PREPARING INSULIN FOR ADMINISTRATION. The nurse always checks the expiration date printed on the label of the insulin bottle before withdrawing the insulin. An insulin syringe that matches the concentration of insulin to be given is always used. For example, a syringe labeled as U100 is used only with insulin labeled U100. U500 insulin is given only via the SC route or the intramuscular (IM) route, and may be administered using a tuberculin syringe if necessary.

When insulin is in a suspension (this can be seen when looking at a vial that has been untouched for about 1 hour), the nurse gently rotates the vial between the palms of the hands and tilts it gently end-to-end immediately before withdrawing the insulin. This ensures even distribution of the suspended particles. Care is taken not to shake the insulin vigorously.

The nurse carefully checks the health care provider's order for the type and dosage of insulin immediately before withdrawing the insulin from the vial. All air bubbles must be eliminated from the syringe barrel and hub of the needle before withdrawing the syringe from the insulin vial.

> ### ☀ Nursing Alert
>
> *Accuracy is of the utmost importance when measuring any insulin preparation because of the potential danger of administering an incorrect dosage. If possible, the nurse should check and compare with another nurse for accuracy of the insulin dosage by comparing the insulin container, the syringe, and the primary health care provider's order before administration.*

When regular insulin and another insulin are mixed in the same syringe, the nurse must administer the insulin within 5 minutes of withdrawing the two insulins from the two vials.

ROTATING INJECTION SITES. Insulin may be injected into the arms, thighs, abdomen, or buttocks (see Home Care Checklist: Rotating Insulin Injection Sites). Sites of insulin injection are rotated to prevent **lipodystrophy** (atrophy of SC fat), a problem that can interfere with the absorption of insulin from the injection site. Lipodystrophy appears as a slight dimpling or pitting of the SC fat. Because absorption rates vary at the different sites, with the abdomen having the most rapid rate of absorption, followed by the upper arm, thigh, and buttocks, some health care providers recommend rotating the injection sites within one specific area, rather than rotating areas. For example, all available sites within the abdomen would be used before moving to the thigh.

The nurse carefully plans the pattern of rotation of the injection sites and writes this plan in the patient's chart. Before each dose of insulin is given, the nurse checks the patient's chart for the site of the previous injection and uses the next site (according to the rotation plan) for injection. After giving the injection, the nurse records the site used for injection. Each time insulin is given, previous injection sites are inspected for inflammation, which may indicate a localized allergic reaction. The nurse notes any inflammation or other skin reactions. The nurse reports localized allergic reactions, signs of inflammation, or other skin changes to the health care provider as soon as possible because a different type of insulin may be necessary.

METHODS OF ADMINISTERING INSULIN. Several methods can be used to administer insulin. The most common method is the use of a needle and syringe. Use of microfine needles has reduced the discomfort associated with an injection. Another method is the jet injection system, which uses pressure to deliver a fine stream of insulin below the skin. Another method uses a disposable needle and special syringe. The syringe uses a cartridge that is prefilled with a specific type of insulin (eg, regular human insulin, isophane [NPH] insulin, or a mixture of isophane and regular insulin).

Home Care Checklist

ROTATING INSULIN INJECTION SITES

If your patient must self-administer insulin at home, be sure he or she knows where to inject the insulin and how to rotate the site. Site rotation is crucial to prevent injury to the skin and fatty tissue. Review with the patient appropriate sites, including:

✓ Upper arms, outer aspect

✓ Stomach, except for a 2-inch margin around the umbilicus

✓ Back, right, and left sides just below the waist

✓ Upper thighs, both front and side

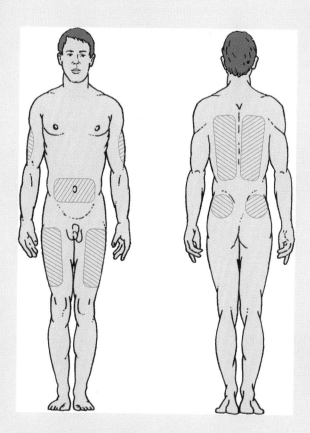

To rotate sites, teach the patient to do the following:

✓ Note the site of the last injection

✓ Place the side of his or her thumb at the old site and measure across its width—about 1 inch

✓ Select a site on the other side of the thumb for the next injection

✓ Repeat the procedure for each subsequent injection

✓ Use the same area for a total of about 10 to 15 injections and then move to another area

The desired units are selected by turning a dial and the locking ring.

Another method of insulin delivery is the insulin pump, which is intended for a select group of individuals, such as the pregnant woman with diabetes with early long-term complications and those with, or candidates for, renal transplantation. This system attempts to mimic the body's normal pancreatic function, uses only regular insulin, is battery powered, and requires insertion of a needle into SC tissue. The needle is changed every 1 to 3 days. The amount of insulin injected can be adjusted according to blood glucose monitoring, which is usually done four to eight times per day.

The insulin dosage pattern that most closely follows normal insulin production is a multiple-dose plan sometimes called intensive insulin therapy. In this regimen, a single dose of intermediate- or long-acting insulin is taken in the morning or at bedtime. Small doses of regular insulin are taken before meals based on the patient's blood glucose levels. This allows for greater flexibility in the patient's life-style, but can also be an inconvenience to the patient (eg, the need to always have supplies with them, the lack of privacy, inconvenient schedules).

BLOOD AND URINE TESTING. Blood glucose levels are monitored often in the patient with diabetes. The health care provider may order blood glucose levels to be tested before meals, after meals, and at bedtime. Less frequent monitoring may be performed if the patient's glucose levels are well controlled. The **glucometer** is a device used by the patient with diabetes or the nursing personnel to monitor blood glucose levels. Nursing personnel or the laboratory is responsible for obtaining blood glucose levels during hospitalization, but the patient must be taught to monitor blood glucose levels after dismissal from the acute care setting (see Patient and Family Teaching Checklist: Obtaining a Blood Glucose Reading Using a Glucometer).

Urine testing has been widely used to monitor glucose levels in the past, but this method has largely been replaced with blood glucose monitoring.

Urine testing can play a role in identifying ketone excretion in patients prone to ketoacidosis. If urine testing is done, it is usually recommended that the nurse use the second voided specimen (ie, fresh urine collected 30 minutes after the initial voiding) to check glucose or acetone levels, rather than the first specimen obtained.

Glycosylated hemoglobin (HbA$_{1c}$) is a blood test used to monitor the patient's average blood glucose level throughout a 3- to 4-month period. When blood glucose levels are high, glucose molecules attach to hemoglobin in the red blood cell. The longer hyperglycemia occurs in the blood, the more glucose binds

Patient and Family Teaching Checklist

Obtaining a Blood Glucose Reading Using a Glucometer

The nurse teaches the patient to:

✓ Carefully follow manufacturer's instructions because blood glucose monitoring devices vary greatly.

✓ Read all of the manufacturer's instructions before using the glucometer.

✓ Prepare the finger using an alcohol wipe to cleanse the area. Wear gloves to comply with the guidelines of the Centers for Disease Control and Prevention (Standard Precautions).

✓ Most glucometers require a small sample of capillary blood that is obtained from the fingertip using a spring-loaded lancet.

✓ Using the lancet device, perform a finger stick on the side of a finger where there are fewer nerve endings and more capillaries. Milk the finger to produce a large, hanging drop of blood. Use of this technique to obtain a blood sample will help prevent inaccurate readings. Note: Do not smear the blood or try to obtain an extra drop.

✓ Drop the blood sample on a reagent test strip, wait 45 to 60 seconds, and then wipe off the excess blood with a cotton ball (some newer glucometers have eliminated the step of excess blood removal from the strip). With these devices, the reagent strip is placed in the glucometer first, allowing all of the blood to remain on the strip for the entire test. Another type of monitoring device uses a sensor cartridge instead of strips to obtain blood glucose levels. The blood is placed on the sensor, and automatic timers provide readings in shorter periods of time than the traditional glucometer.

✓ Place the test strip in a glucometer that automatically uses the sample to determine a numerical reading representing the current blood glucose level.

✓ The blood glucose level reading should be between 70 and 120 mg/dL.

to the red blood cell and the higher the glycosylated hemoglobin. This binding lasts for the life of the red blood cell (about 4 months). When the patient's diabetes is well controlled with normal or near normal blood glucose levels, the overall HbA$_{1c}$ level will not be greatly elevated. However, if blood glucose levels are consistently high, the HbA$_{1c}$ level will be elevated. The test result (expressed in percentage) refers to the average amount of glucose that has been in the blood throughout the last 4 months. Normal levels vary with the laboratory method used for analysis, but generally levels between 2.5% and 6% indicate good control of the diabetes. Results of 10% or greater indicate poor blood glucose control for the last several months. HbA$_{1c}$ is useful in evaluating the success of treatment of diabetes, comparing new treatment regimens with past regimens used, and in individualizing treatment.

Monitoring and Managing Adverse Reactions

MANAGING HYPOGLYCEMIC REACTIONS. Close observation of the patient with diabetes is important, especially when diabetes is newly diagnosed in the patient, the insulin dosage is changed, the patient is pregnant, the patient has a medical illness or has had surgery, or the patient haïs failed to adhere to the prescribed diet. Episodes of hypoglycemia are corrected as soon as the symptoms are recognized.

> ### Nursing Alert
>
> *The nurse should check the patient for hypoglycemia (see Table 49-1) at the peak time of action of the insulin (see Summary Drug Table: Insulin Preparations). Hypoglycemia, which can develop suddenly, may indicate a need for an adjustment in the insulin dosage or other changes in treatment, such as a change in diet. Hypoglycemic reactions can occur at any time but are most likely to occur when insulin is at its peak activity.*

Methods of terminating a hypoglycemic reaction include the administration of one or more of the following:

- Orange juice or other fruit juice
- Hard candy or honey
- Commercial glucose products
- Glucagon by the SC, IM, or IV route
- Glucose 10% or 50% IV

Selection of any one or more of the above methods for terminating a hypoglycemic reaction, as well as other procedures to be followed, such as drawing blood for glucose levels, depends on the written order of the health care provider or hospital policy. The nurse should never give oral fluids or substances (such as candy) used to terminate a hypoglycemic reaction to a patient unless the swallowing and gag reflexes are present. Absence of these reflexes may result in aspiration of the oral fluid or substance into the lungs, which can result in extremely serious consequences and even death. If swallowing and gag reflexes are absent, or if the patient is unconscious, glucose or glucagon is given by the parenteral route.

Glucagon is a hormone produced by the alpha cells of the pancreas; it acts to increase blood sugar by stimulating the conversion of glycogen to glucose in the liver. A return of consciousness is observed within 5 to 20 minutes after parenteral administration of glucagon. Glucagon is effective in treating hypoglycemia only if liver glycogen is available.

The nurse notifies the health care provider of any hypoglycemic reaction, the substance and amount used to terminate the reaction, blood samples drawn (if any), the length of time required for the symptoms of hypoglycemia to disappear, and the current status of the patient. After termination of a hypoglycemic reaction, the nurse closely observes the patient for additional hypoglycemic reactions. The length of time close observation is required depends on the peak and duration of the insulin administered.

> ### Nursing Alert
>
> *Hypoglycemic symptoms are more pronounced in patients taking animal-based products than in patients taking human insulin.*

MANAGING DIABETIC KETOACIDOSIS. **Diabetic ketoacidosis** (DKA) is a potentially life-threatening deficiency of insulin (hypoinsulinism), resulting in severe hyperglycemia and requiring prompt diagnosis and treatment. Because insulin is unavailable to allow glucose to enter the cell, dangerously high levels of glucose build up in the blood (hyperglycemia). The body, needing energy, begins to break down fat for energy. As fats are broken down, ketones are produced by the liver. As more and more fat is used for energy, higher levels of ketones accumulate in the blood. This increase in ketones disrupts the acid–base balance within the body, leading to DKA. DKA is treated with fluids, correction of acidosis and hypotension, and low-doses of regular insulin.

> ### Nursing Alert
>
> *The nurse immediately reports any of the following symptoms of hyperglycemia: elevated blood glucose levels (>200 mg/mL); headache; increased thirst; epigastric pain; nausea; vomiting; hot, dry, flushed skin; restlessness; and diaphoresis (sweating).*

Relieving Anxiety and Fear

The patient with newly diagnosed diabetes often has many concerns regarding the diagnosis. For some, initially coping with diabetes and the methods required for controlling the disorder creates many problems. Some of the fears and concerns of these patients may include having to give themselves an injection, having to follow a diet, weight control, the complications associated with diabetes, and changes in eating times and habits. An effective teaching program helps relieve some of this anxiety. The patient in this situation needs time to talk about the disorder, express concerns, and ask questions.

Assisting the Patient With Impaired Adjustment, Coping, and Altered Health Maintenance

The patient with newly diagnosed diabetes may have difficulty accepting the diagnosis, and the complexity of the therapeutic regimen can seem overwhelming. Before patients can be expected to carry out treatment, they must accept that they have diabetes and deal with their feelings about having the disorder. The nurse has an important role in helping these patients gradually accept the diagnosis and begin to understand their feelings. Understanding diabetes may help patients work with health care providers and other medical personnel in managing their diabetes.

Educating the Patient and Family

Noncompliance is a problem with some patients with diabetes, making patient and family teaching vital to the proper management of diabetes. Patients may occasionally lapse in their adherence to the prescribed diet, such as around holidays or other special occasions. This slip may not cause a problem if it is brief and not excessive and if the patient immediately returns to the prescribed regimen. However, some patients frequently stray from the prescribed regimen, take extra insulin to cover dietary indiscretions, fast for several days before follow-up blood glucose determinations, and engage in other dangerous behaviors. Although some patients can be convinced that failure to adhere to the prescribed therapeutic regimen is detrimental to their health, others continue to deviate from the prescribed regimen until serious complications develop. Every effort is made to stress the importance of adherence to the prescribed treatment during the initial teaching session and during follow-up office or clinic visits.

The nurse establishes a thorough teaching plan for all patients with newly diagnosed diabetes, for those who have had any change in the management of their diabetes (eg, diet, insulin type, insulin dosage), and for those whose management has changed because of an illness or disability, such as loss of sight or disabling arthritis. The newly diagnosed patient with diabetes and the family must have an explanation of the disease and methods of treatment as soon as the health care provider has revealed the diagnosis to the patient. The nurse should always individualize the teaching plan because the needs of each patient are different.

Self-monitoring of blood glucose is an important component in the management of diabetes (see Patient and Family Teaching Checklist: Obtaining a Blood Glucose Reading Using a Glucometer). It is the preferred method for monitoring glucose by most health care providers for all patients with diabetes, with variations only in the suggested frequency of testing. If the patient is to use a blood glucose moni-

toring device, the nurse reviews the method of obtaining a small sample of blood from the finger and the use of the device with the patient. Printed instructions and illustrations are supplied with the device and must be reviewed with the patient. The nurse encourages the patient to purchase the brand recommended by the health care provider. Time is allowed for supervised practice. The nurse includes the following information in the teaching plan for a patient with diabetes:

- Blood glucose or urine testing—the testing material recommended by the health care provider; a review of the instructions included with the glucometer or the materials used for urine testing; the technique of collecting the specimen; interpreting test results; number of times a day or week the blood or urine is tested (as recommended by the health care provider); a record of test results.
- Insulin—types; how dosage is expressed; calculating the insulin dosage; importance of using only the type, source, and brand name recommended by the health care provider; importance of not changing brands unless the health care provider approves; keeping a spare vial on hand; prescription for insulin purchase not required.
- Storage of insulin—insulin is kept at room temperature away from heat and direct sunlight if used within 1 month (and up to 3 months if refrigerated); vials not in use are stored in the refrigerator; prefilled insulin in glass or plastic syringes is stable for 1 week under refrigeration. Keep filled syringes in a vertical or oblique position with the needle pointing upward to avoid plugging the needle. Before injection, pull back the plunger and tip the syringe back and forth slightly to agitate and remix the insulins.
- Needle and syringe—purchase the same brand and needle size each time; parts of the syringe; reading the syringe scale.
- Preparation for administration—principles of aseptic technique; how to hold the syringe; how to withdraw insulin from the vial; measurement of insulin in the syringe using the syringe scale; mixing insulin in the same syringe (when appropriate); elimination of air in the syringe and needle; what to do if the syringe or needle is contaminated.
- Administration of insulin—sites to be used; rotation of injection sites (see Home Care Checklist: Rotating Insulin Injection Sites); angle of injection; administration at the time of day prescribed by the health care provider; disposal of the needle and syringe.
- Insulin needs may change in patients who become ill, especially with vomiting or fever and during

periods of stress or emotional disturbances. Contact the primary health care provider if these situations occur.

- Diet—importance of following the prescribed diet; calories allowed; food exchanges; planning daily menus; establishing meal schedules; selecting food from a restaurant menu; reading food labels; use of artificial sweeteners.
- Traveling—importance of carrying an extra supply of insulin and a prescription for needles and syringes; storage of insulin when traveling; protecting needles and syringes from theft; importance of discussing travel plans (especially foreign travel) with the health care provider.
- Hypoglycemia/hyperglycemia—signs and symptoms of hypoglycemia and hyperglycemia; food or fluid used to terminate a hypoglycemic reaction; importance of notifying the health care provider immediately if either reaction occurs.
- Personal hygiene—importance of good skin and foot care, personal cleanliness, frequent dental checkups, and routine eye examinations.
- Exercise—importance of following the health care provider's recommendations regarding physical activity.
- When to notify the health care provider—increase in blood glucose levels; urine positive for ketones; if pregnancy occurs; occurrence of antidiabetic or hyperglycemic episodes; occurrence of illness, infection, or diarrhea (insulin dosage may require adjustment); appearance of new problems (eg, leg ulcers, numbness of the extremities, significant weight gain or loss).
- Identification—wear identification, such as a medical alert tag, to inform medical personnel and others of the use of insulin to control the disease.

EVALUATION

- The therapeutic effect is achieved and normal or near-normal blood glucose levels are maintained.
- Adverse reactions are identified, reported to the health care provider, and managed successfully through appropriate nursing interventions.
- Anxiety and fear are reduced.
- The patient demonstrates a beginning ability to cope with the disorder and its required treatment.
- The patient demonstrates a positive outlook and adjustment to the diagnosis.
- The patient verbalizes a willingness to comply with the prescribed therapeutic regimen.
- The patient and family demonstrate an understanding of the drug regimen.

- The patient is able to test blood glucose levels using a glucometer.
- The patient administers insulin correctly.

ORAL ANTIDIABETIC DRUGS

The oral antidiabetic drugs are used to treat patients with type 2 diabetes that is not controlled by diet and exercise alone. These drugs are not effective for treating type 1 diabetes. Five types of oral antidiabetic drugs are currently in use:

- Sulfonylureas (glimepiride, glyburide)
- Biguanides (metformin)
- Alpha (α)-glucosidase inhibitors (acarbose, miglitol)
- Meglitinides (nateglinide, repaglinide)
- Thiazolidinediones (pioglitazone, rosiglitazone)

Additional drugs are listed in the Summary Drug Table: Antidiabetic Drugs.

USES OF THE ANTIDIABETIC DRUGS

The oral antidiabetic drugs are of value only in the treatment of patients with type 2 (NIDDM) diabetes mellitus whose condition cannot be controlled by diet alone. These drugs may also be used with insulin in the management of some patients with diabetes mellitus. Use of an oral antidiabetic drug with insulin may decrease the insulin dosage in some individuals. Two oral antidiabetic drugs (eg, a sulfonylurea and metformin) may also be used together when one antidiabetic drug and diet do not control blood glucose levels in type 2 diabetes mellitus. Figure 49-3 is a pharmacological algorithm indicating the appropriate medication regimen for type 2 diabetes mellitus.

ACTIONS

Sulfonylureas

The sulfonylureas appear to lower blood glucose by stimulating the beta cells of the pancreas to release insulin. The sulfonylureas are not effective if the beta cells of the pancreas are unable to release a sufficient amount of insulin to meet the individual's needs. The first generation sulfonylureas (eg, chlorpropamide, tolazamide, and tolbutamide) are not commonly used today because they have a long duration of action and a higher incidence of adverse

SUMMARY DRUG TABLE ANTIDIABETIC DRUGS

GENERIC NAME	TRADE NAME*	USES	ADVERSE REACTIONS	DOSAGE RANGES
Sulfonylureas				
acetohexamide *a-set-oh-hex´-a-mide*	Dymelor, *generic*	Adjunct to diet to lower blood glucose in type 2 diabetes; adjunct to insulin therapy in certain patients with type 1 diabetes	Anorexia, nausea, vomiting, epigastric discomfort, heartburn, hypoglycemia	250 mg–1.5 g/d PO
chlorpropamide *klor-proe´-pa-mide*	Diabinese, *generic*	Adjunct to diet in type 2 diabetes	Anorexia, nausea, vomiting, epigastric discomfort, heartburn, hypoglycemia	100–500 mg/d PO
glimepiride *glye-meh´-per-ide*	Amaryl	Adjunct to diet to lower blood glucose in type 2 diabetes; adjunct to insulin therapy in certain patients with type 1 diabetes	Anorexia, nausea, vomiting, epigastric discomfort, heartburn, diarrhea, hypoglycemia, allergic skin reactions	1–4 mg/d PO (do not exceed 8 mg/d)
glipizide *glip´-i-zide*	Glucotrol, Glucotrol XL, *generic*	Type 2 diabetes; adjunct to insulin therapy in the stabilization of certain cases of insulin-dependent diabetes (type 1)	Anorexia, nausea, vomiting, epigastric discomfort, heartburn, diarrhea, hypoglycemia, allergic skin reactions	5–40 mg/d PO
glyburide (glibenclamide) *glye-byoor-ide*	DiaBeta, Micronase, *generic*	Type 2 diabetes; adjunct to metformin when adequate results are not achieved with either drug alone; adjunct to insulin in stabilization of certain individuals with type 1 diabetes	Anorexia, nausea, vomiting, epigastric discomfort, heartburn, hypoglycemia	1.25–20 mg/d PO
tolazamide *tole-az´-a-mide*	Tolinase, *generic*	Type 2 diabetes; adjunct to insulin therapy in the stabilization of certain cases of insulin-dependent diabetes (type 1)	Anorexia, nausea, vomiting, epigastric discomfort, heartburn, hypoglycemia	100–1000 mg/d PO
tolbutamide *tole-byoo´-ta-mide*	Orinase, *generic*	Type 2 diabetes; adunct to insulin therapy in the stabilization of certain cases of insulin-dependent diabetes (type 1)	Anorexia, nausea, vomiting, epigastric discomfort, heartburn, hypoglycemia	0.25–3 g/d PO
α-Glucosidase Inhibitors				
acarbose *aye-kar´-bose*	Precose	Type 2 diabetes; combination therapy with a sulfonylurea to enhance glycemic control	Flatulence, diarrhea, abdominal pain	25–100 mg TID PO
miglitol *mi´-gli-tole*	Glyset	Type 2 diabetes; combination therapy with a sulfonylurea to enhance glycemic control	Skin rash, flatulence, diarrhea, abdominal pain	25–100 mg TID PO

SUMMARY DRUG TABLE ANTIDIABETIC DRUGS (*Continued*)

GENERIC NAME	TRADE NAME*	USES	ADVERSE REACTIONS	DOSAGE RANGES
Biguanide				
metformin *met-for´-min*	Glucophage, Glucophage XR, *generic*	Type 2 diabetes; with a sulfonylurea or insulin to improve glycemic control	Anorexia, nausea, vomiting, epigastric pain, heartburn, diarrhea, hypoglycemia, allergic skin reactions	500−3000 mg/d PO; XR (extended release): 500−2000 mg/d
Meglitinides				
nateglinide *nah-teg´-lah-nyde*	Starlix	Type 2 diabetes; in combination with metformin to improve glycemic control	Headache, upper respiratory tract infection, back pain, flu symptoms, bronchitis	60−120 mg TID before meals
repaglinide *re-pag´-lah-nyd*	Prandin	Type 2 diabetes; in combination with metformin to improve glycemic control	Hyperglycemia, hypoglycemia, nausea, diarrhea, upper respiratory tract infection, sinusitis, headache, arthralgia, back pain	0.5−4 mg before meals PO (maximum dose is 16 mg/d)
Thiazolidinediones				
pioglitazone HCl *pie-oh-glit´-ah-zohn*	Actos	Type 2 diabetes; with sulfonylurea, metformin, or insulin to improve glycemic control	Headache, pain, myalgia, aggravated diabetes, infections, fatigue	15−45 mg/d PO
rosiglitazone maleate *roh-zee-glit´-ah-zohn*	Avandia	Type 2 diabetes; in combination with metformin to improve glycemic control	Headache, pain, diarrhea, hypoglycemia, hyperglycemia, fatigue, infections	4−8 mg/d PO
Antidiabetic Combination Drugs				
glyburide/ metformin HCl	Glucovance	Type 2 diabetes	See individual drugs	Starting dose: 1.25 mg/250 mg PO once or twice daily with meals, second- line therapy: 2.5 mg/500 mg−5 mg/ 500 mg PO BID with meals; maximum daily dosage: 20 mg/2500 mg
Glucose-Elevating Agents				
diazoxide, oral *die-aze-ox´-ide*	Proglycem	Hypoglycemia due to hyperinsulinism	Sodium and fluid retention, hyperglycemia, glycosuria, tachycardia, congestive heart failure	3−8 mg/kg/d PO in 2 or 3 equal doses every 8 or 12 h
glucagon *glue-kuh-gahn*	Glucagon Emergency Kit	Hypoglycemia	Nausea, vomiting, generalized allergic reactions	See instructions on the product

*The term *generic* indicates the drug is available in generic form.

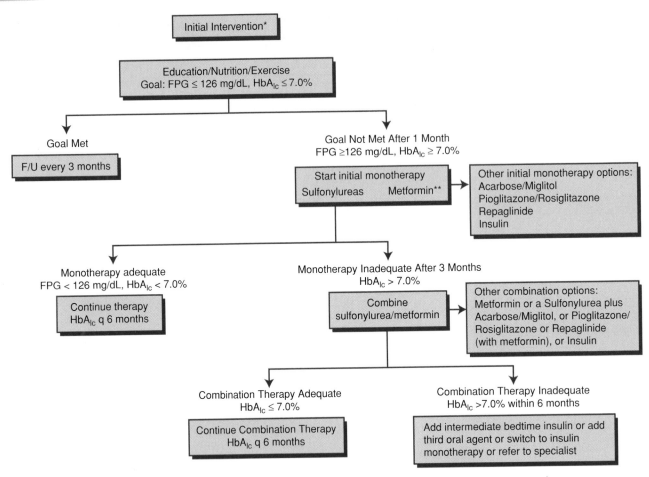

*If initial presentation with fasting glucose ≥ 260 mg/dL is a symptomatic patient, consider insulin as initial intervention.
**Preferred in obese or dyslipidemic patients
–Normal HbA$_{Ic}$ = 4-6.1%
–Normal FPG: < 126 mg/dL
–Goals and therapies must be individualized.

FIGURE 49-3. Pharmacological algorithm for treating type 2 diabetes.

reactions, and are more likely to react with other drugs. More commonly used sulfonylureas are the second and third generation drugs, such as glimepiride (Amaryl), glipizide (Glucotrol), and glyburide (DiaBeta, Micronase).

Biguanides

Metformin (Glucophage), currently the only biguanide, acts by reducing hepatic glucose production and increasing insulin sensitivity in muscle and fat cells. The liver normally releases glucose by detecting the level of circulating insulin. When insulin levels are high, glucose is available in the blood, and the liver produces little or no glucose. When insulin levels are low, there is little circulating glucose, so the liver produces more glucose. In type 2 diabetes, the liver may not detect levels of glucose in the blood and, instead of regulating glucose production, releases glucose despite blood sugar levels.

Metformin sensitizes the liver to circulating insulin levels and reduces hepatic glucose production.

α-Glucosidase Inhibitors

The α-glucosidase inhibitors, acarbose (Precose) and miglitol (Glyset), lower blood sugar by delaying the digestion of carbohydrates and absorption of carbohydrates in the intestine.

Meglitinides

Like the sulfonylureas, the meglitinides act to lower blood glucose levels by stimulating the release of insulin from the pancreas. This action is dependent on the ability of the beta cell in the pancreas to produce some insulin. However, the action of the meglitinides is more rapid than that of the sulfonylureas and their duration of action much shorter. Because of this they must be taken three times a day. Examples of the meglitinides include nateglinide (Starlix) and repaglinide (Prandin).

Thiazolidinediones

The thiazolidinediones, also called glitazones, decrease insulin resistance and increase insulin sensitivity by modifying several processes, with the end result being decreasing hepatic glucogenesis (formation of glucose from glycogen) and increasing insulin-dependent muscle glucose uptake. Examples of the thiazolidinediones are rosiglitazone (Avandia) and pioglitazone (Actos).

ADVERSE REACTIONS

Sulfonylureas

Adverse reactions seen with the sulfonylureas include hypoglycemia, anorexia, nausea, vomiting, epigastric discomfort, weight gain, heartburn, and various vague neurologic symptoms, such as weakness and numbness of the extremities. Often, these can be eliminated by reducing the dosage or giving the drug in divided doses. If these reactions become severe, the health care provider may try another oral antidiabetic drug or discontinue the use of these drugs. If the drug therapy is discontinued, it may be necessary to control the diabetes with insulin.

Biguanides

Adverse reactions associated with the biguanide (metformin) include gastrointestinal upsets (such as abdominal bloating, nausea, cramping, diarrhea) and metallic taste (usually self-limiting). These adverse reactions are self-limiting and can be reduced if the patients are started on a low dose with dosage increased slowly and if the drug is taken with meals. Hypoglycemia rarely occurs when metformin is used alone.

Lactic acidosis (buildup of lactic acid in the blood) may also occur with the administration of metformin. Although lactic acidosis is a rare adverse reaction, its occurrence is serious and can be fatal. Lactic acidosis occurs mainly in patients with kidney dysfunction. Symptoms of lactic acidosis include malaise (vague feeling of bodily discomfort), abdominal pain, rapid respirations, shortness of breath, and muscular pain. In some patients vitamin B_{12} levels are decreased. This can be reversed with vitamin B_{12} supplements or with discontinuation of the drug therapy. Because

weight loss can occur, metformin is sometimes recommended for obese patients or patients with insulin-resistant diabetes.

α-Glucosidase Inhibitors

Because the α-glucosidase inhibitors, acarbose or miglitol, increase the transit time of food in the digestive tract, gastrointestinal disturbances may occur. The most common adverse reactions are bloating and flatulence. Other adverse reactions, such as abdominal pain, and diarrhea can occur. While most oral antidiabetic drugs produce hypoglycemia, acarbose and miglitol, when used alone, do not cause hypoglycemia.

Meglitinides

Adverse reactions associated with the administration of the meglitinides include upper respiratory infection, headache, rhinitis, bronchitis, headache, back pain, and hypoglycemia.

Thiazolidinediones

Adverse reactions associated with the administration of the thiazolidinediones include aggravated diabetes mellitus, upper respiratory infections, sinusitis, headache, pharyngitis, myalgia, diarrhea, and back pain. When used alone, rosiglitazone and pioglitazone rarely cause hypoglycemia. However, patients receiving these drugs in combination with insulin or other oral hypoglycemics (eg, the sulfonylureas) are at greater risk for hypoglycemia. A reduction in the dosage of insulin or the sulfonylurea may be required to prevent episodes of hypoglycemia.

CONTRAINDICATIONS, PRECAUTIONS, AND INTERACTIONS

Sulfonylureas

The oral antidiabetic drugs are contraindicated in patients with known hypersensitivity to the drugs, DKA, severe infection, or severe endocrine disease. The first generation sulfonylureas (chlorpropamide, tolazamide, and tolbutamide) are contraindicated in patients with coronary artery disease or liver or renal dysfunction. Other sulfonylureas are used cautiously in patients with impaired liver function because liver dysfunction can prolong the drug's effect. In addition, the sulfonylureas are used cautiously in patients with renal impairment and severe cardiovascular disease. There is a risk for cross-sensitivity with the sulfonylureas and the sulfonamides.

Many drugs may affect the action of the sulfonylureas; the nurse must monitor blood glucose carefully when beginning therapy, discontinuing therapy, and any time any change is made in the drug regimen with these drugs. The sulfonylureas may have an increased hypoglycemic effect when administered with the anti-coagulants, chloramphenicol, clofibrate, fluconazole, histamine H_2 antagonists, methyldopa, monoamine oxidase inhibitors (MAOIs), salicylates, sulfonamides, and tricyclic antidepressants. The hypoglycemic effect of the sulfonylureas may be decreased when the agents are administered with beta blockers, calcium channel blockers, cholestyramine, corticosteroids, estrogens, hydantoins, isoniazid, oral contraceptives, phenothiazines, thiazide diuretics, and thyroid agents.

Biguanides

Metformin is contraindicated in patients with heart failure, renal disease, hypersensitivity to metformin, and acute or chronic metabolic acidosis, including ketoacidosis. The drug is also contraindicated in patients older than 80 years and during pregnancy (Pregnancy Category B) and lactation.

The drug is used cautiously during surgery. Metformin use is temporarily discontinued for surgical procedures. The drug therapy is restarted when the patient's oral intake has been resumed and renal function is normal.

There is a risk of acute renal failure when iodinated contrast material that is used for radiological studies is administered with metformin. Metformin therapy is stopped for 48 hours before and after radiological studies using iodinated material. Alcohol, amiloride, digoxin, morphine, procainamide, quinidine, quinine, ranitidine, triamterene, trimethoprim, vancomycin, cimetidine, and furosemide all increase the risk of hypoglycemia. There is an increased risk of lactic acidosis when metformin is administered with the glucocorticoids.

α-Glucosidase Inhibitors

The α-glucosidase inhibitors are contraindicated in patients with a hypersensitivity to the drug, diabetic ketoacidosis, cirrhosis, inflammatory bowel disease, colonic ulceration, partial intestinal obstruction or predisposition to intestinal obstruction, or chronic intestinal diseases. Acarbose and miglitol are used cautiously in patients with renal impairment or pre-existing gastrointestinal (GI) problems such as irritable

bowel syndrome and Crohn's disease. These drugs are Pregnancy Category B drugs and safety for use during pregnancy has not been established. Digestive enzymes may reduce the effect of miglitol. The effects of acarbose may increase when the agent is administered with the loop or thiazide diuretics, glucocorticoids, oral contraceptives, calcium channel blockers, phenytoin, thyroid drugs, or the phenothiazines. Miglitol may decrease absorption of ranitidine and propranolol.

Meglitinides

Theses drugs are contraindicated in patients with hypersensitivity to the drug, type I diabetes, and diabetic ketoacidosis. Both repaglinide and nateglinide are Pregnancy Category C drugs and are not recommended for use during pregnancy and lactation. These drugs are used cautiously in patients with renal or hepatic impairment. Certain drugs, such as NSAIDs, salicylates, MAOIs, and beta adrenergic blocking drugs, may potentiate the hypoglycemic action of the meglitinides. Drugs such as the thiazides, corticosteroids, thyroid drugs, and sympathomimetics may decrease the hypoglycemic action of these drugs. The nurse must closely observe the patient receiving one or more of these drugs along with an oral antidiabetic drug.

Thiazolidinediones

The thiazolidinediones are contraindicated in patients with a hypersensitivity to the drug or any component of the drug and severe heart failure. These drugs are Pregnancy Category C drugs and should not be used during pregnancy unless the potential benefit of therapy outweighs the potential risk to the fetus. The thiazolidinediones are used cautiously in patients with edema, cardiovascular disease, and liver or kidney disease. These drugs may alter the effects of oral contraceptives.

NURSING PROCESS

● The Patient Receiving an Oral Antidiabetic Drug

ASSESSMENT

Preadministration Assessment

If the patient has recently received a diagnosis of diabetes mellitus and has not received an oral antidiabetic drug, or if the patient is known to have diabetes and has been taking one of these drugs, the nurse should include weight, blood pressure, pulse, and respiratory rate in the initial assessment. The nurse makes a general assessment of the skin, mucous membranes, and extremities, with special attention given to sores or cuts that appear to be healing poorly and ulcerations or other skin or mucous membrane changes. Dietary habits, a family history of diabetes (if any), and an inquiry into the type and duration of symptoms experienced are included in the history. The nurse reviews the patient's chart for recent laboratory and diagnostic tests. If the patient has diabetes and has been receiving an oral antidiabetic drug, the nurse includes the name of the drug and the dosage, the type of diabetic diet, the results of blood glucose testing, and an inquiry into adherence to the dietary and weight control regimen prescribed by the health care provider.

Ongoing Assessment

The most important aspect of the ongoing assessment is observation of the patient every 2 to 4 hours for symptoms of hypoglycemia (see Table 49-1), particularly during initial therapy or after a change in dosage. If both an oral antidiabetic drug and insulin are given, the nurse observes the patient more frequently for hypoglycemic episodes during the initial period of combination therapy. If the patient is receiving only an oral antidiabetic drug and a hypoglycemic reaction occurs, it is often (but not always) less intense than one seen with insulin administration.

The nurse conducts daily ongoing assessments, including monitoring vital signs and observing for adverse drug reactions. The health care provider may also order the patient be weighed daily or weekly. The nurse notifies the health care provider if an adverse reaction occurs or if there is a significant weight gain or loss.

The best way to monitor long-term glycemic control and response to treatment is with HbA_{1c} levels measured at 3-month intervals. If the first HbA_{1c} indicates that glycemic control during the last 3 months was inadequate, the dosage may be increased for better control.

NURSING DIAGNOSES

Drug-specific nursing diagnoses are highlighted in the Nursing Diagnoses Checklist. Other nursing diagnoses applicable to these drugs are discussed in depth in Chapter 4.

PLANNING

The expected outcomes of the patient may include an optimal response to therapy, management of common adverse reactions, a reduction in anxiety, improved abil-

---

Nursing Diagnoses Checklist

☑ **Confusion** related to adverse drug reaction (hypoglycemia)

☑ **Imbalanced Nutrition: More Than Body Requirements** related to disease process or adverse drug reactions

☑ **Anxiety** related to diagnosis, dietary restrictions, other factors (specify)

☑ **Ineffective Coping** related to inability to accept diagnosis

☑ **Ineffective Health Maintenance** related to inability to comprehend drug regimen, lack of knowledge

☑ **Risk of Ineffective Therapeutic Regimen Management** related to lack of knowledge, misunderstanding, or complexity of prescribed treatment program, other factors (specify)

---

ity in coping with the diagnosis, and an understanding of and compliance with the prescribed therapeutic regimen.

IMPLEMENTATION

Promoting an Optimal Response to Therapy

There is no fixed dosage for the treatment of diabetes. The drug regimen is individualized on the basis of the effectiveness and tolerance of the drug(s) used and the maximum recommended dose of the drug(s). Glycemic control can often be improved when a second oral medication is added to the drug regimen. The choice of a second medication will vary from patient to patient and is prescribed by the health care provider. Glucovance, a combination drug, is a mixture of glyburide and metformin. The drug is useful for individuals needing dual therapy and those who are forgetful (only once-daily dosing is required) or mildly confused.

☀ Nursing Alert

Exposure to stress, such as infection, fever, surgery, or trauma, may cause a loss of control of blood glucose levels in patients who have been stabilized with oral antidiabetic drugs. Should this occur, the health care provider may discontinue use of the oral drug and administer insulin.

Oral antidiabetic drugs are given as a single daily dose or in divided doses. The following sections provide specific information for each group of oral antidiabetic drugs.

SULFONYLUREAS. Acetohexamide (Dymelor), chlorpropamide (Diabinese), tolazamide (Tolinase), and tolbutamide (Orinase) are given with food to prevent gastrointestinal upset. However, because food delays absorption, the nurse gives glipizide (Glucotrol) 30 minutes before a meal. Glyburide (Micronase) is administered with breakfast or with the first main meal of the day. The health care provider orders the meal with which glyburide is given. Glimepiride is give once daily with breakfast or the first main meal of the day.

❄ Gerontologic Alert

Older adults have an increased sensitivity to the sulfonylureas and may require a dosage reduction.

After the patient has been taking sulfonylureas for a period of time, a condition called secondary failure may occur. **Secondary failure** occurs when the sulfonylurea loses its effectiveness. When the nurse notes that a normally compliant patient has a gradual increase in blood sugar levels, secondary failure may be the cause. This increase in blood glucose levels can be caused by an increase in the severity of the diabetes or a decreased response to the drug. When secondary failure occurs, the health care provider may prescribe another sulfonylurea or add an oral antidiabetic drug such as metformin to the drug regimen. See the Summary Drug Table: Antidiabetic Drugs for additional drugs that can be used in combination with the sulfonylureas.

α-GLUCOSIDASE INHIBITORS. Acarbose and miglitol are given three times as day with the first bite of the meal because food increases absorption. Some patients begin therapy with a lower dose once daily to minimize gastrointestinal effects, such as abdominal discomfort, flatulence, and diarrhea. The dose is then gradually increased to three times daily. The nurse monitors the response to these drugs by periodic testing. Dosage adjustments are made at 4- to 16-week intervals based on 1-hour postprandial glucose levels.

BIGUANIDES. The nurse gives metformin two or three times a day with meals. If the patient has not experienced a response in 4 weeks using the maximum dose of metformin, the primary care giver may add an oral sulfonylurea while continuing metformin at the maximum dose. Glucophage XR (metformin extended release) is administered once daily with the evening meal.

MEGLITINIDES. The nurse usually gives repaglinide 15 minutes before meals but can give it immediately, or up to 30 minutes, before the meal. Nateglinide is taken up to 30 minutes before meals.

THIAZOLIDINEDIONES. The thiazolidinediones, pioglitazone and rosiglitazone, are given with or without meals. If the dose is missed at the usual meal, the drug is taken at the next meal. If the dose is missed on one day, do not double the dose the following day. If the drug is taken, do not delay the meal. Delay of a meal for as little as ½ hour can cause hypoglycemia.

Monitoring and Managing Adverse Reactions

MANAGING HYPOGLYCEMIA. The nurse must immediately terminate a hypoglycemic reaction. The method of terminating a hypoglycemic reaction is the same as for a hypoglycemic reaction occurring with insulin administration, with the following exception: The nurse notifies the health care provider as soon as possible if episodes of hypoglycemia occur because the dosage of the oral antidiabetic drug (or insulin, when both insulin and an oral antidiabetic drug are given) may need to be changed.

❋ Nursing Alert

When hypoglycemia occurs in a patient taking an α-glucosidase inhibitor (eg, acarbose or miglitol), the nurse gives the patient an oral form of glucose, such as glucose tablets or dextrose, rather than sugar (sucrose). Absorption of sugar is blocked by acarbose or miglitol.

When oral antidiabetic drugs are combined with other antidiabetic drugs (eg, sulfonylureas) or insulin, the hypoglycemic effect may be enhanced. Elderly, debilitated, or malnourished patients are more likely to experience hypoglycemia.

❄ Gerontologic Alert

Although elderly patients taking the oral antidiabetic drugs are particularly susceptible to hypoglycemic reactions, these reactions may be difficult to detect in the elderly. The nurse notifies the health care provider if blood sugar levels are elevated (consistently > 200 mg/dL) or if ketones are present in the urine.

MANAGING HYPERGLYCEMIA AND KETOACIDOSIS. Capillary blood specimens are obtained and tested in the same manner as for insulin (see Patient and Family Teaching Checklist, p. 497). The nurse notifies the health care provider if blood sugar levels are elevated (consistently > 200 mg/dL) or if ketones are present in the urine.

MANAGING ANXIETY AND PROMOTING COPING SKILLS.

The patient with newly diagnosed diabetes often has many concerns about the management of the disease. Some patients, when learning that management of their diabetes can be achieved by diet and an oral drug, may have a tendency to discount the seriousness of the disorder. Without creating additional anxiety, the nurse emphasizes the importance of following the prescribed treatment regimen.

The nurse encourages the patient to talk about the disorder, express concerns, and ask questions. Allowing these patients time to talk may help them begin to cope with their diabetes.

The patient receiving an oral antidiabetic drug may also express concern about the possibility of having to take insulin in the future. The nurse encourages the patient to discuss this and other concerns with the health care provider.

MANAGING LACTIC ACIDOSIS.

When taking metformin, the patient is at risk for lactic acidosis. The nurse monitors the patient for symptoms of lactic acidosis, which include unexplained hyperventilation, myalgia, malaise, gastrointestinal symptoms, or unusual somnolence. If the patient experiences these symptoms, the nurse should contact the primary care provider at once. Elevated blood lactate levels of greater than 5 mmol/L are associated with lactic acidosis and should be reported immediately. Once a patient's diabetes is stabilized on metformin therapy, the adverse GI reactions that often occur at the beginning of such therapy are unlikely to be related to the drug therapy. A later occurrence of GI symptoms is more likely to be related to lactic acidosis or other serious disease.

Educating the Patient and Family

Failing to comply with the prescribed treatment regimen may be a problem with patients taking an oral antidiabetic drug because of the erroneous belief that not having to take insulin means that their disease is not serious and therefore does not require strict adherence to the recommended dietary plan. The nurse informs these patients that control of their diabetes is just as important as for patients requiring insulin and that control is achieved only when they adhere to the treatment regimen prescribed by the health care provider.

If the diagnosis of diabetes mellitus is new, the nurse discusses the disease and methods of control with the patient and family after the health care provider has revealed the diagnosis to the patient. Although taking an oral antidiabetic drug is less complicated than self-administration of insulin, the patient with diabetes taking one of these drugs needs a thorough explanation of the management of the disease. The teaching plan is individualized because the needs of each patient are different. The nurse includes the following information in a teaching plan:

- Take the drug exactly as directed on the container (eg, with food, 30 minutes before a meal).
- To control diabetes, follow the diet and drug regimen prescribed by the health care provider exactly.
- This drug is not oral insulin and cannot be substituted for insulin.
- Never stop taking this drug or increase or decrease the dose unless told to do so by the health care provider.
- Take the drug at the same time or times each day.
- Eat meals at about the same time each day. Erratic meal hours or skipped meals may result in difficulty in controlling diabetes with this drug.
- Avoid alcohol, dieting, commercial weight-loss products, and strenuous exercise programs unless use or participation has been approved by the health care provider.
- Test blood for glucose and urine for ketones as directed by the health care provider. Keep a record of test results and bring this record to each visit to the health care provider or clinic.
- Maintain good foot and skin care and routine eye and dental examinations for the early detection of the complications that may occur.
- Exercise should be moderate; avoid strenuous exercise and erratic periods of exercise.
- Wear identification, such as a medical alert tag, to inform medical personnel and others of diabetes and the drug or drugs currently being used to treat the disease.
- Notify the health care provider if any of the following occur: episodes of hypoglycemia, apparent symptoms of hyperglycemia, elevated blood glucose levels, positive results of urine tests for glucose or ketone bodies, or pregnancy. Also notify the health care provider of any serious illness not requiring hospitalization.
- Know the symptoms of hypoglycemia and hyperglycemia and the health care provider's method for terminating a hypoglycemic reaction.

- Metformin—there is a risk of lactic acidosis when using this drug. Discontinue the drug therapy and notify the health care provider immediately if any of the following should occur: respiratory distress, muscular aches, unusual somnolence, unexplained malaise, or nonspecific abdominal distress.
- α-Glucosidase Inhibitors—these drugs do not generally cause hypoglycemia. However, if sulfonylureas or insulin are used in combination with acarbose or miglitol, blood sugar levels can be lowered enough to cause symptoms or even life-threatening hypoglycemia. Have a ready source of glucose to treat symptoms of low blood sugar when taking insulin or a sulfonylurea with these drugs. Adverse reactions generally develop during the first few weeks of therapy and usually involve the gastrointestinal tract: flatulence, diarrhea, or abdominal discomfort.
- Meglitinides—if a meal is skipped, do not take the drug. Similarly, if a meal is added, add a dose of the drug for that meal.

EVALUATION

- The therapeutic drug effect is achieved and normal or near-normal blood glucose levels are maintained.
- Hypoglycemic reactions are identified, reported to the health care provider, and managed successfully.
- Anxiety is reduced.
- The patient begins to demonstrate the ability to cope with the disorder and its required treatment.
- The patient demonstrates a positive outlook and adjustment to the diagnosis.
- The patient verbalizes a willingness to comply with the prescribed treatment regimen.
- The patient demonstrates an understanding of the drug regimen.
- The patient demonstrates an understanding of the information presented in teaching sessions.
- The patient is able to use the glucometer correctly to monitor blood sugar or test urine for glucose and ketones.

● *Critical Thinking Exercises*

1. *Ms. Baxter, age 37 years, has been taking insulin for the past 6 years for type 1 diabetes mellitus. An assessment at the outpatient clinic reveals a blood sugar of 110 mg/dL. In examining Ms. Baxter's skin, the nurse notices several areas on the thighs that appear scarred and other areas that appear as dimples or pitting in the skin. Analyze this problem. Discuss suggestions you would make to Ms. Baxter for better care.*

2. *Mr. Goddard, age 78 years, recently has received a diagnosis of type 2 diabetes mellitus, and the health care provider has ordered an oral antidiabetic drug. Mr. Goddard says his friend with diabetes takes insulin and he wonders why insulin was not prescribed for him. How would you help Mr. Goddard understand why he is taking an oral drug and not insulin? What other information does Mr. Goddard, as a patient with newly diagnosed diabetes, need to have?*

3. *When assessing Jerry Jones, age 24 years, a patient with recently diagnosed diabetes, you note that he is confused and agitated. His skin is cool and clammy, and he is complaining of hunger. Discuss other assessments you could make and what action, if any, you feel should be taken for Jerry.*

● *Review Questions*

1. Which of the following would the nurse mostly likely choose to terminate a hypoglycemic reaction?

   A. Regular insulin
   B. NPH insulin
   C. Orange juice
   D. Crackers and milk

2. Which of the following would be the correct method of administering insulin glargine?

   A. Within 10 minutes of meals
   B. Immediately before meals
   C. Anytime within 30 minutes before or 30 minutes after a meal
   D. At bedtime

3. Which of the following symptoms would alert the nurse to a possible hyperglycemic reaction?

   A. Fatigue, weakness, confusion
   B. Pale skin, elevated temperature
   C. Thirst, abdominal pain, nausea
   D. Rapid, shallow respirations, headache, nervousness

4. A patient with diabetes received a glycosylated hemoglobin test result of 10%. This indicates _____.

   A. the diabetes is well controlled
   B. poor blood glucose control
   C. the need for an increase in the insulin dosage
   D. the patient is at increased risk for hypoglycemia

5. In patients receiving oral hypoglycemic drugs, the nurse must be aware that hypoglycemic reactions _____.

 A. will most likely occur 1 to 2 hours after a meal
 B. may be more intense than reactions seen with insulin administration
 C. may be less intense than reactions seen with insulin administration
 D. may occur more frequently in patients receiving oral hypoglycemic drugs.

● *Medication Dosage Problems*

1. A patient is prescribed 40 units NPH insulin mixed with 5 units of regular insulin. What is the total insulin dosage? Draw a line on the syringe below showing the total insulin dosage. Describe how you would prepare the insulins.

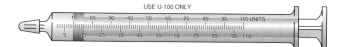

2. A patient is prescribed metformin (Glucophage) 1000 mg BID PO. The drug is available in 500-mg tablets. The nurse administers_____.What is the total daily dosage of metformin?_____.

3. A patient is prescribed rosiglitazone (Avandia) 8 mg PO daily. Available are 2-mg tablets. The nurse would administer ____.

4. A patient is prescribed insulin Humulin L 32 U. Choose the correct label for the insulin.

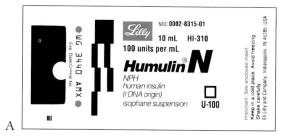

Pituitary and Adrenocortical Hormones

The pituitary gland lies deep within the cranial vault, connected to the brain by the infundibular stalk (a downward extension of the floor of the third ventricle) and protected by an indentation of the sphenoid bone called the sella turcica (see Fig. 50-1). The pituitary gland, a small, gray rounded structure, has two parts:

- Anterior pituitary (adenohypophysis)
- Posterior pituitary (neurohypophysis)

The gland secretes a number of pituitary hormones that regulate growth, metabolism, the reproductive cycle, electrolyte balance, and water retention or loss. Because the pituitary gland secretes so many hormones that regulate numerous vital processes, the gland is often referred to as the "master gland." The hormones secreted by the anterior and posterior pituitary and the organs influenced by these hormones are shown in Figure 50-2.

ANTERIOR PITUITARY HORMONES

The hormones of the anterior pituitary include:

- Follicle-stimulating hormone (FSH)
- Luteinizing hormone (LH)

- Growth hormone (GH)
- Adrenocorticotropic hormone (ACTH)
- Thyroid-stimulating hormone (TSH), and prolactin

This section of the chapter discusses FSH, LH, GH, and ACTH. FSH and LH are called **gonadotropins** because they influence the **gonads** (the organs of reproduction). GH, also called somatotropin, contributes to the growth of the body during childhood, especially the growth of muscles and bones. ACTH is produced by the anterior pituitary and stimulates the adrenal cortex to secrete the corticosteroids. The anterior pituitary hormone, TSH, is discussed in Chapter 51. Prolactin, which is also secreted by the anterior pituitary, stimulates the production of breast milk in the postpartum patient. Additional functions of prolactin are not well understood. Prolactin is the only anterior pituitary hormone that is not used medically.

GONADOTROPINS: FSH AND LH

The gonadotropins (FSH and LH) influence the secretion of sex hormones, development of secondary sex characteristics, and the reproductive cycle in both men and

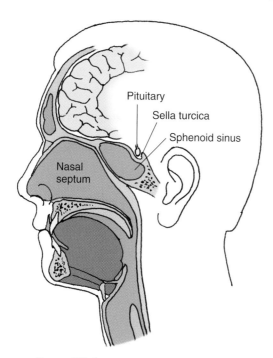

FIGURE 50-1. Location of the pituitary gland.

women. The gonadotropins discussed in this chapter include menotropins, urofollitropin, clomiphene, and chorionic gonadotropin.

ACTION AND USES

Menotropins and Urofollitropin

Menotropins (Pergonal) and urofollitropin (Metrodin) are purified preparations of the gonadotropins (FSH and LH) extracted from the urine of postmenopausal women. Menotropins are used to induce ovulation and pregnancy in anovulatory (failure to produce an ovum or failure to ovulate) women. Menotropins are also used with human chorionic gonadotropin in women to stimulate multiple follicles for in vitro fertilization. In men, menotropins are used to induce the production of sperm (spermatogenesis). Urofollitropin is used to induce ovulation in women with polycystic ovarian disease and to stimulate multiple follicular development in ovulatory women for in vitro fertilization. See the Summary Drug Table: Anterior and Posterior Pituitary Hormones for additional information on the gonadotropins.

Clomiphene and Chorionic Gonadotropin

Clomiphene (Clomid) is a synthetic nonsteroidal compound that binds to estrogen receptors, decreasing the amount of available estrogen receptors and causing the anterior pituitary to increase secretion of FSH and LH. It is used to induce ovulation in anovulatory (nonovulating) women.

Chorionic gonadotropin (HCG) is extracted from human placentas. The actions of HCG are identical to those of the pituitary LH. The hormone is used to induce ovulation in anovulatory women. This drug is also used for the treatment of prepubertal **cryptorchism** (failure of the testes to descend into the scrotum) and in men to treat selected cases of hypogonadotropic hypogonadism.

ADVERSE REACTIONS

Menotropins and Urofollitropin

The adverse reactions associated with the menotropins include ovarian enlargement, hemoperitoneum (blood in the peritoneal cavity), abdominal discomfort, and febrile reactions. Urofollitropin administration may result in mild to moderate ovarian enlargement, abdominal discomfort, nausea, vomiting, breast tenderness, and irritation at the injection site. Multiple births and birth defects have been reported with the use of both menotropins and urofollitropin.

Clomiphene and HCG

Administration of clomiphene may result in vasomotor flushes (which are like the hot flashes of menopause), abdominal discomfort, ovarian enlargement, blurred vision, nausea, vomiting, and nervousness. HCG administration may result in headache, irritability, restlessness, fatigue, edema, and precocious puberty (when given for cryptorchism).

CONTRAINDICATIONS, PRECAUTIONS, AND INTERACTIONS

Menotropins and Urofollitropin

These drugs are contraindicated in patients who have hypersensitivity to the drug or any component of the drug. Menotropins are contraindicated in patients with high gonadotropin levels, thyroid dysfunction, adrenal dysfunction, abnormal bleeding, ovarian cysts, or those with an organic intracranial lesion. Urofollitropin is contraindicated during pregnancy (Pregnancy Category X). Menotropins are Pregnancy Category C drugs and also are contraindicated for use during pregnancy.

Clomiphene and HCG

These drugs are contraindicated in patients with known hypersensitivity to the drugs. Clomiphene is contraindicated in patients with liver disease, abnormal bleeding of undetermined origin, or ovarian cysts, and during

NURSING DIAGNOSES

Drug-specific nursing diagnoses are highlighted in the Nursing Diagnoses Checklist. Other nursing diagnoses applicable to these drugs are discussed in depth in Chapter 4.

PLANNING

The expected outcomes of the patient may include an optimal response to drug therapy, identification of adverse reactions, reduction in anxiety, and an understanding of the therapeutic regimen.

IMPLEMENTATION

Promoting an Optimal Response to Therapy

CLOMIPHENE. Clomiphene is an oral tablet prescribed for 5 days and is self-administered in the outpatient setting.

> ### Nursing Alert
>
> *If the patient complains of visual disturbances, the drug therapy is discontinued and the physician notified. An examination by an ophthalmologist is usually indicated.*

The patient is observed for symptoms of ovarian stimulation (abdominal pain, distension, sudden ovarian enlargement, ascites). Use of the drug is discontinued and the primary care provider notified if symptoms occur.

Menotropins, urofollitropin, and HCG injections are given in the primary health care provider's office or clinic. These drugs are administered intramuscularly (IM) because they are destroyed in the gastrointestinal (GI) tract. Urofollitropin may cause pain and irritation at the injection site. The nurse should rotate sites and examine previous sites for redness and irritation. Female patients taking these drugs are usually examined by the primary health care provider every other day during treatment and at 2-week intervals to detect excessive ovarian stimulation, called **hyperstimulation syndrome** (sudden ovarian enlargement with ascites). The patient may or may not report pain. This syndrome usually develops quickly, during a period of 3 to 4 days, and requires hospitalization of the patient and discontinuation of the drug therapy. Abdominal pain and distention are indicators that hyperstimulation syndrome may be developing.

Managing Anxiety

Patients wishing to become pregnant often experience a great deal of anxiety. In addition, when taking these drugs there is the possibility of multiple births. The success rate of these drugs varies and depends on many factors. The primary health care provider usually discusses the value of this, as well as other approaches, with the patient and her sexual partner. The nurse allows the patient time to talk about her problems or concerns about the proposed treatment program.

Educating the Patient and Family

The nurse should instruct the patient taking the gonadotropins to keep all primary health care provider appointments. Adverse reactions should be reported to the nurse or primary health care provider. The nurse includes the following information when a gonadotropin is prescribed:

MENOTROPINS AND UROFOLLITROPIN

- Before beginning therapy, be aware of the possibility of multiple births and birth defects.
- It is a good idea to use a calendar to track the treatment schedule and ovulation.
- Report bloating, abdominal pain, flushing, breast tenderness, and pain at the injection site.

CLOMIPHENE

- Take the drug as prescribed (5 days) and do not stop taking the drug before the course of therapy is finished unless told to do so by the primary health care provider.
- Notify the primary health care provider if bloating, stomach or pelvic pain, jaundice, blurred vision, hot flashes, breast discomfort, headache, nausea, or vomiting occurs.
- If ovulation has not occurred after the first course, a second or third course of therapy may be used. If the drug is not successful after three regimens, the therapy is considered unsuccessful and use of the drug is discontinued.

EVALUATION

- The therapeutic effect is achieved.
- Adverse reactions are identified and reported to the primary health care provider.
- Anxiety is reduced.
- The patient demonstrates knowledge of treatment and dosage regimen, adverse drug reactions, risks of treatment, and importance of complying with the primary health care provider's recommendations.

● Growth Hormone

Growth hormone, also called **somatotropic hormone,** is secreted by the anterior pituitary. This hormone regulates the growth of the individual until somewhere around early adulthood or the time when the person no longer gains height.

ACTION AND USES

Growth hormone is available as the synthetic products somatrem (Protropin) and somatropin (Humatrope). Both are of recombinant DNA origin and are identical to human GH and produce skeletal growth in children. These drugs are administered to children who have not grown because of a deficiency of pituitary GH and must be used before closure of bone epiphyses. Bone epiphyses are the ends of bones, separated from the main bone but joined to its cartilage, that allow for growth or lengthening of the bone. GH is ineffective in patients with closed epiphyses because when the epiphyses close, growth (in height) can no longer occur.

ADVERSE REACTIONS

These hormones cause few adverse reactions when administered as directed. Antibodies to somatropin may develop in a small number of patients, resulting in a failure to experience response to therapy, namely, failure of the drug to produce growth in the child. Some patients may experience hypothyroidism or insulin resistance. Swelling, joint pain, and muscle pain may also occur.

CONTRAINDICATIONS, PRECAUTIONS, AND INTERACTIONS

Somatrem and somatropin are contraindicated in patients with known hypersensitivity to somatropin or sensitivity to benzyl alcohol, and those with epiphyseal closure or underlying cranial lesions. The drug is used cautiously in patients with thyroid disease or diabetes, and during pregnancy (Pregnancy Category C) and lactation. Excessive amounts of glucocorticoids may decrease response to somatropin.

NURSING PROCESS

● **The Patient Receiving a Growth Hormone**

ASSESSMENT

Preadministration Assessment

A thorough physical examination and laboratory and diagnostic tests are performed before a child is accepted into a growth program. Before therapy is started, the nurse takes and records the patient's vital signs, height, and weight.

Ongoing Assessment

Children may increase their growth rate from 3.5 to 4 cm/year before treatment to 8 to 10 cm/year during

---

> **Nursing Diagnoses Checklist**
>
> ✓ **Body Image Disturbance** related to changes in appearance, physical size, other (specify)
> ✓ **Anxiety** related to failure to grow (parents and child)

the first year of treatment. Each time the child visits the primary health care provider's office or clinic (usually every 3–6 months), the nurse measures and records the child's height and weight to evaluate the response to therapy. Bone age is monitored periodically. The bone age monitors bone growth and detects epiphyseal closure, at which time therapy must be stopped.

NURSING DIAGNOSES

Drug-specific nursing diagnoses are highlighted in the Nursing Diagnoses Checklist. Other nursing diagnoses applicable to these drugs are discussed in depth in Chapter 4.

PLANNING

The expected outcomes of the patient may include an optimal response to drug therapy, management of common adverse drug reactions, reduction in anxiety, and an understanding of the therapeutic regimen.

IMPLEMENTATION

Promoting an Optimal Response to Therapy

Growth hormone is given either IM or subcutaneously (SC). The vial is not shaken but swirled to mix. The solution is clear, and the nurse should not give it if it is cloudy. These drugs are administered IM or SC. The weekly dosage is divided and given in three to seven doses throughout the week. The drug may (if possible) be given at bedtime to most closely adhere to the body's natural release of the hormone.

Periodic testing of growth hormone levels, glucose tolerance, and thyroid functioning may be done at intervals during treatment.

Managing Anxiety and Body Image Disturbance

The parents, and sometimes the children, may be concerned about the success or possible failure of treatment with GH. The child is provided with the opportunity to share fears, concerns, or anger. The nurse acknowledges these feelings as normal and corrects any misconceptions the child or parents may have concerning treatment. Time is allowed for the parents and children to ask questions not only before therapy is started but also during the months of treatment.

Educating the Patient and Family

When the patient is receiving GH, the primary health care provider discusses in detail the therapeutic regimen for increasing growth (height) with the child's parents or guardians. If the drug is to be given at bedtime and not in the outpatient clinic, the nurse instructs the parents on the proper technique to administer the injections. The parents are encouraged to keep all clinic or office visits. The nurse explains that the child may experience sudden growth and increase in appetite. The nurse instructs the parents to report lack of growth, symptoms of diabetes (eg, increased hunger, increased thirst, or frequent voiding) or symptoms of hypothyroidism (eg, fatigue, dry skin, intolerance to cold).

EVALUATION

- The therapeutic effect is achieved and the child grows in height.
- Adverse reactions are identified and reported to the primary health care provider.
- Anxiety is reduced.
- The parents verbalize understanding of the treatment program.
- The child maintains a positive body image.

● Adrenocorticotropic Hormone: Corticotropin

ACTIONS AND USES ●

Corticotropin (ACTH) is an anterior pituitary hormone that stimulates the adrenal cortex to produce and secrete adrenocortical hormones, primarily the glucocorticoids.

Corticotropin is used for diagnostic testing of adrenocortical function. This drug may also be used for the management of acute exacerbations of multiple sclerosis, nonsuppurative thyroiditis, and hypercalcemia associated with cancer. It is also used as an anti-inflammatory and immunosuppressant drug when conventional glucocorticoid therapy has not been effective (see Display 50-1).

ADVERSE REACTIONS ●

Because ACTH stimulates the release of glucocorticoids from the adrenal gland, adverse reactions seen with the administration of this hormone are similar to those seen with the glucocorticoids (see Display 50-2) and affect many body systems. The most common adverse reactions include:

- Central nervous system—mental depression, mood swings, insomnia, psychosis, euphoria, nervousness, and headaches;
- Cardiovascular system—hypertension, edema, congestive heart failure, and thromboembolism;

DISPLAY 50-1 ● Uses of Glucocorticoids

ENDOCRINE DISORDERS
Primary or secondary adrenal cortical insufficiency, congenital adrenal hyperplasia, nonsuppressive thyroiditis, hypercalcemia associated with cancer

RHEUMATIC DISORDERS
Short-term management of acute ankylosing spondylitis, acute and subacute bursitis, acute nonspecific tenosynovitis, acute gouty arthritis, psoriatic arthritis, rheumatoid arthritis, post-traumatic osteoarthritis, synovitis of osteoarthritis, epicondylitis

COLLAGEN DISEASES
Lupus erythematosus, acute rheumatic carditis, systemic dermatomyositis

DERMATOLOGIC DISEASES
Pemphigus, bullous dermatitis herpetiformis, severe erythema multiforme (Stevens-Johnson syndrome), exfoliative dermatitis, mycosis fungoides, severe psoriasis, severe seborrheic dermatitis, angioedema, urticaria, various skin disorders, such as lichen planus or keloids

ALLERGIC STATES
Control of severe or incapacitating allergic conditions not controlled by other methods, bronchial asthma (including status asthmaticus), contact dermatitis, atopic dermatitis, serum sickness, drug hypersensitivity reactions

OPHTHALMIC DISEASES
Severe acute and chronic allergic and inflammatory processes, keratitis, allergic corneal marginal ulcers, herpes zoster of the eye, iritis, iridocyclitis, chorioretinitis, diffuse posterior uveitis, optic neuritis, sympathetic ophthalmia, anterior segment inflammation

RESPIRATORY DISEASES
Sarcoidosis, berylliosis, fulminating or disseminating pulmonary tuberculosis, aspiration pneumonia

HEMATOLOGIC DISORDERS
Idiopathic or secondary thrombocytopenic purpura, hemolytic anemia, red blood cell anemia, congenital hypoplastic anemia

NEOPLASTIC DISEASES
Leukemia, lymphomas

EDEMATOUS STATES
To induce diuresis or remission of proteinuria in the nephrotic state

GASTROINTESTINAL DISEASES
During critical period of ulcerative colitis, regional enteritis, intractable sprue

NERVOUS SYSTEM
Acute exacerbations of multiple sclerosis

- Gastrointestinal system—nausea, vomiting, increased appetite, weight gain, and peptic ulcer;
- Genitourinary system—amenorrhea and irregular menses;
- Integumentary system—petechiae, ecchymosis, decreased wound healing, hirsutism (excessive growth of body hair), and acne;
- Musculoskeletal system—weakness and osteoporosis;
- Endocrine system—menstrual irregularities, hyperglycemia, and decreased growth in children; and

---

DISPLAY 50-2 ● **Adverse Reactions Associated With Glucocorticoids**

FLUID AND ELECTROLYTE DISTURBANCES
Sodium and fluid retention, congestive heart failure in susceptible patients, potassium loss, hypokalemic alkalosis, hypertension, hypocalcemia, hypotension or shocklike reactions

MUSCULOSKELETAL
Muscle weakness, loss of muscle mass, tendon rupture, osteoporosis, aseptic necrosis of femoral and humoral heads, spontaneous fractures

CARDIOVASCULAR
Thromboembolism or fat embolism, thrombophlebitis, necrotizing angiitis, syncopal episodes, cardiac arrhythmias, aggravation of hypertension

GASTROINTESTINAL
Pancreatitis, abdominal distention, ulcerative esophagitis, nausea, increased appetite and weight gain, possible peptic ulcer with perforation, hemorrhage

DERMATOLOGIC
Impaired wound healing, thin fragile skin, petechiae, ecchymoses, erythema, increased sweating, suppression of skin test reactions, subcutaneous fat atrophy purpura, striae, hyperpigmentation, hirsutism, acneiform eruptions, urticaria, angioneurotic edema

NEUROLOGIC
Convulsions, steroid-induced catatonia, increased intracranial pressure with papilledema (usually after treatment is discontinued), vertigo, headache, neuritis or paresthesia, steroid psychosis, insomnia

ENDOCRINE
Amenorrhea, other menstrual irregularities, development of cushingoid state, suppression of growth in children, secondary adrenocortical and pituitary unresponsive (particularly in times of stress), decreased carbohydrate tolerance, manifestation of latent diabetes mellitus, increased requirements for insulin or oral hypoglycemic agents (in diabetics)

OPHTHALMIC
Posterior subcapsular cataracts, increased intraocular pressure, glaucoma, exophthalmos

METABOLIC
Negative nitrogen balance (due to protein catabolism)

OTHER
Anaphylactoid or hypersensitivity reactions, aggravation of existing infections, malaise, increase or decrease in sperm motility and number

---

- Miscellaneous—hypersensitivity reactions, hypokalemia, hypernatremia, increased susceptibility to infection, cushingoid appearance (eg, moon face, "buffalo hump," hirsutism), cataracts, and increased intraocular pressure.

CONTRAINDICATIONS, PRECAUTIONS, AND INTERACTIONS

ACTH is contraindicated in patients with adrenocortical insufficiency or hyperfunction, allergy to pork or pork products (corticotropin is obtained from porcine pituitaries), systemic fungal infections, ocular herpes simplex, scleroderma, osteoporosis, and hypertension. Patients taking ACTH also should avoid any vaccinations with live virus.

ACTH is used cautiously in patients with diabetes, diverticulosis, renal insufficiencies, myasthenia gravis, tuberculosis (may reactivate the disease), hypothyroidism, cirrhosis, nonspecific ulcerative colitis, heart failure, seizures, or febrile infections. The drug is classified as a Pregnancy Category C drug and is used cautiously during pregnancy and lactation. ACTH is used cautiously in children because it can inhibit skeletal growth.

When amphotericin B or diuretics are administered with ACTH, the potential for hypokalemia is increased. There may be an increased need for insulin or oral antidiabetic drugs in the patient with diabetes who is taking ACTH. There is a decreased effect of ACTH when the agent is administered with the barbiturates. Profound muscular depression is possible when ACTH is administered with the anticholinesterase drugs. Live virus vaccines taken while taking ACTH may potentiate virus replication, increase vaccine adverse reaction, and decrease the patient's antibody response to the vaccine.

NURSING PROCESS

● **The Patient Receiving Corticotropin (ACTH)**

ASSESSMENT

Preadministration Assessment
Before administering ACTH, the nurse reviews the patient's chart for the diagnosis, laboratory tests, and other pertinent information. The nurse obtains the patient's weight and assesses skin integrity, lungs, and mental status. The nurse takes and records vital signs. Additional assessments depend on the patient's condition and diagnosis. The primary health care provider may order baseline diagnostic tests, such as chest x-rays, upper GI x-ray, serum electrolytes, complete blood count, or urinalysis.

Ongoing Assessment
The nurse monitors the patient's weight and fluid intake and output daily during therapy. The nurse observes for and reports any evidence of edema, such as weight gain, rales, increased pulse or dyspnea, or swollen extremities. The nurse monitors blood glucose levels for a rise in blood glucose concentration. In addition, the nurse checks stools for evidence of bleeding (dark or tarry in color, positive guaiac). Patients receiving prolonged therapy should have periodic hematologic, serum electrolytes, and serum glucose studies.

NURSING DIAGNOSES

Drug-specific nursing diagnoses are highlighted in the Nursing Diagnoses Checklist. Other nursing diagnoses applicable to these drugs are discussed in depth in Chapter 4.

PLANNING

The expected outcomes of the patient may include an optimal response to therapy, identification and management of adverse reactions (see section "Monitoring and Managing Adverse Reactions"), and an understanding of the therapeutic regimen.

IMPLEMENTATION

Promoting an Optimal Response to Therapy

Nursing management depends on the patient's diagnosis, physical status, and the reason for use of the drug. The nurse may need to assess vital signs every 4 hours and observe for the adverse reactions seen with glucocorticoid administration.

This drug may be given by the intravenous (IV), SC, or IM route. During parenteral administration of ACTH, the nurse observes the patient for hypersensitivity reactions. Symptoms of hypersensitivity include a rash, urticaria, hypotension, tachycardia, or difficulty breathing. If the drug is given IM or SC, the nurse observes the patient for hypersensitivity reactions immediately and for about 2 hours after the drug is given. If a hypersensitivity reaction occurs, the nurse notifies the primary health care provider immediately. Long-term use increases the risk of hypersensitivity.

Monitoring and Managing Adverse Reactions

Corticotropin may mask signs of infection, including fungal or viral eye infections.

> ### ✳ Nursing Alert
>
> *The nurse reports any complaints of sore throat, cough, fever, malaise, sores that do not heal, or redness or irritation of the eyes in the patient taking ACTH.*

There may be a decreased resistance and inability to localize infection. The nurse observes the skin daily for localized signs of infection, especially at injection sites or IV access sites. Visitors are monitored to protect the patient against those with infectious illness.

Corticotropin can also cause alterations in the psyche. The nurse must report any evidence of behavior change, such as mental depression, insomnia, euphoria, mood swings, or nervousness. Should alterations in the psyche occur, the nurse encourages communication with the staff and family members, provides a quiet nonthreatening environment, and spends time actively listening as the patient talks. It is important to encourage verbalization of fears and concerns. Anxiety is decreased with understanding of the therapeutic regimen. The nurse allows time for a thorough explanation of the drug regimen and answering of questions.

Educating the Patient and Family

The nurse includes the following in a teaching plan for the patient receiving ACTH.

- Report any adverse reactions.
- Avoid contact with those who have an infection because resistance to infection may be decreased.
- Report any symptoms of infection immediately (eg, sore throat, fever, cough, or sores that do not heal).
- Patients with diabetes—Monitor blood glucose (if self-monitoring is being done) or urine closely and notify the primary health care provider if glucose appears in the urine or the blood glucose level increases significantly. An increase in the dosage of the oral antidiabetic drug or insulin may be needed.
- Notify the primary health care provider of a marked weight gain, swelling in the extremities, muscle weakness, persistent headache, visual disturbances, or behavior change.

EVALUATION

- The therapeutic effect is achieved.
- Adverse reactions are identified, reported to the primary health care provider, and managed using appropriate nursing interventions.
- The patient verbalizes an understanding of the therapeutic regimen and adverse effects requiring notification of the primary health care provider.

POSTERIOR PITUITARY HORMONES

The posterior pituitary gland produces two hormones: vasopressin (antidiuretic hormone) and oxytocin (see Chap. 53). Posterior pituitary hormones are summarized in the Summary Drug Table: Anterior and Posterior Pituitary Hormones.

● Vasopressin

ACTIONS AND USES

Vasopressin (Pitressin Synthetic) and its derivatives, namely lypressin (Diapid) and desmopressin (DDAVP), regulate the reabsorption of water by the kidneys. Vasopressin is secreted by the pituitary when body fluids must be conserved. An example of this mechanism may be seen when an individual has severe vomiting and diarrhea with little or no fluid intake. When this and similar conditions are present, the posterior pituitary releases the hormone vasopressin, water in the kidneys is reabsorbed into the blood (ie, conserved), and the urine becomes concentrated. Vasopressin exhibits its greatest activity on the renal tubular epithelium, where it promotes water resorption and smooth muscle contraction throughout the vascular bed. Vasopressin has some vasopressor activity.

Vasopressin and its derivatives are used in the treatment of **diabetes insipidus**, a disease resulting from the failure of the pituitary to secrete vasopressin or from surgical removal of the pituitary. Diabetes insipidus is characterized by marked increase in urination (as much as 10 L in 24 hours) and excessive thirst by inadequate secretion of the antidiuretic hormone or vasopressin. Treatment with vasopressin therapy replaces the hormone in the body and restores normal urination and thirst. Vasopressin may also be used for the prevention and treatment of postoperative abdominal distention and to dispel gas interfering with abdominal roentgenography.

ADVERSE REACTIONS

Local or systemic hypersensitivity reactions may occur in some patients receiving vasopressin. Tremor, sweating, vertigo, nausea, vomiting, abdominal cramps, and water intoxication (overdosage, toxicity) may also be seen.

CONTRAINDICATIONS, PRECAUTIONS, AND INTERACTIONS

Vasopressin is contraindicated in patients with chronic renal failure, increased blood urea nitrogen, and those with allergy to beef or pork proteins.

Vasopressin is used cautiously in patients with a history of seizures, migraine headaches, asthma, congestive heart failure, or vascular disease (may precipitate angina or myocardial infarction) and in those with perioperative polyuria. The drug is classified as a Pregnancy Category C drug and must be used cautiously during pregnancy and lactation.

The antidiuretic effects of vasopressin may be decreased when the agent is taken with the following drugs: lithium, heparin, norepinephrine, or alcohol. Antidiuretic effect may be increased when the drug is used with carbamazepine, clofibrate, or fludrocortisone.

NURSING PROCESS

● The Patient Receiving Vasopressin

ASSESSMENT

Preadministration Assessment

Before administering the first dose of vasopressin for the management of diabetes insipidus, the nurse takes the patient's blood pressure, pulse, and respiratory rate. The nurse weighs the patient to obtain a baseline weight for future comparison. Serum electrolyte levels and other laboratory tests may be ordered by the primary health care provider.

Before administering vasopressin to relieve abdominal distention, the nurse takes the patient's blood pressure, pulse, and respiratory rate. The nurse auscultates the abdomen and records the findings. The nurse measures and records the patient's abdominal girth.

Ongoing Assessment

During the ongoing assessment the nurse monitors the blood pressure, pulse, and respiratory rate every 4 hours or as ordered by the primary health care provider. The primary health care provider is notified if there are any significant changes in these vital signs because a dosage adjustment may be necessary.

The dosage of vasopressin or its derivatives may require periodic adjustments. After administration of the drug, the nurse observes the patient every 10 to 15 minutes for signs of an excessive dosage (eg, blanching of the skin, abdominal cramps, and nausea). If these occur, the nurse reassures the patient that recovery from these effects will occur in a few minutes.

 Gerontologic Alert

Older adults are particularly sensitive to the effects of vasopressin and should be monitored closely during administration of the drug.

NURSING DIAGNOSES

Drug-specific nursing diagnoses are highlighted in the Nursing Diagnoses Checklist. Other nursing diagnoses applicable to these drugs are discussed in depth in Chapter 4.

Nursing Diagnoses Checklist

✓ **Deficient Fluid Volume** related to inadequate fluid intake, need to increase dose of drug, failure to recognize symptoms of dehydration (diabetes insipidus)

✓ **Excess Fluid Volume** related to adverse reactions (water intoxication)

PLANNING

The expected outcomes of the patient may include an optimal response to therapy, identification of adverse reactions, and an understanding of the therapeutic regimen.

IMPLEMENTATION

Promoting an Optimal Response to Therapy

Vasopressin may be given IM or SC to treat diabetes insipidus. The injection solution may also be administered intranasally on cotton pledgets, by nasal spray, or dropper. When given parenterally 5 to 10 units administered two to three times daily is usually sufficient. To prevent or relieve abdominal distension, 5 units of the drug is administered initially and may increase to 10 units every 3 or 4 hours IM. When the drug is administered before abdominal roentgenography, the nurse administers 2 injections of 10 units each. The first dose is given 2 hours before x-ray examination and the second dose ½ hour before the testing. An enema may be given before the first dose.

Lypressin is administered intranasally by spraying 1 or 2 sprays in one or both nostrils usually four times per day or when the frequency of urination increases or significant thirst develops. Dosages greater than 10 sprays in each nostril every 3 to 4 hours are not recommended. Patients learn to regulate their dosage based on the frequency of urination and increase of thirst. The nurse instructs the patient to hold the bottle upright with the head in a vertical position when administering the drug.

Desmopressin may be given orally, intranasally, SC, or IV. The oral dose must be determined for each individual patient and adjusted according to the patient's response to therapy. When the drug is administered nasally, a nasal tube is used for administration. The nasal tube delivery system comes with a flexible calibrated plastic tube called a **rhinyle**. The solution is drawn into the rhinyle. One end is inserted into the nostril and the patient (if condition allows) blows the other end to deposit solution deep into the nasal cavity. A nasal spray pump may also be used. Most adults require 0.2 mL daily in two divided doses to control diabetes insipidus. The drug may also be administered via the SC route or direct IV injection.

Monitoring and Managing Adverse Reactions

The adverse reactions associated with vasopressin, such as skin blanching, abdominal cramps, and nausea, may be decreased by administering the agent with one or two glasses of water. Should these adverse reactions occur, the nurse informs the patient that these reactions are not serious and should disappear within a few minutes.

Nursing Alert

Excessive dosage is manifested as water intoxication (fluid overload). Symptoms of water intoxication include drowsiness, listlessness, confusion, and headache (which may precede convulsions and coma). If signs of excessive dosage occur, the nurse should notify the primary health care provider before the next dose of the drug is due because a change in the dosage, the restriction of oral or IV fluids, and the administration of a diuretic may be necessary.

MANAGING FLUID VOLUME. The symptoms of diabetes insipidus include the voiding of a large volume of urine at frequent intervals during the day and throughout the night. Accompanied by frequent urination is the need to drink large volumes of fluid because these patients are continually thirsty. Patients must be supplied with large amounts of drinking water. The nurse is careful to refill the water container at frequent intervals. This is especially important when the patient has limited ambulatory activities. Until controlled by a drug, the symptoms of frequent urination and excessive thirst may cause a great deal of anxiety. The nurse reassures the patient that with the proper drug therapy, these symptoms will most likely be reduced or eliminated.

When the patient has diabetes insipidus, the nurse measures the fluid intake and output accurately and observes the patient for signs of dehydration (dry mucous membranes, concentrated urine, poor skin turgor, flushed dry skin, confusion). This is especially important early in treatment and until such time as the optimum dosage is determined and symptoms have diminished. If the patient's output greatly exceeds intake, the nurse notifies the primary health care provider. In some instances, the primary health care provider may order specific gravity and volume measurements of each voiding or at hourly intervals. The nurse records these results in the chart to aid the primary health care provider in adjusting the dosage to the patient's needs.

MANAGING ABDOMINAL DISTENTION. If the patient is receiving vasopressin for abdominal distention, the nurse explains in detail the method of treating this problem and the necessity of monitoring drug effectiveness (ie, auscultation of the abdomen for bowel sounds, insertion of a rectal tube, measurement of the abdomen).

After administration of vasopressin for abdominal distention, a rectal tube may be ordered. The lubricated end of the tube is inserted past the anal sphincter and taped in place. The tube is left in place for 1 hour or as prescribed by the primary health care provider. The nurse auscultates the abdomen every 15 to 30 minutes and measures the abdominal girth every hour, or as ordered by the primary health care provider.

Educating the Patient and Family

If lypressin or desmopressin is to be used in the form of a nasal spray or is to be instilled intranasally using the nasal tube delivery system, the nurse demonstrates the technique of instillation (see Patient and Family Teaching Checklist: Self-Administering Nasal Vasopressin). The nurse includes illustrated patient instructions with the drug and reviews them with the patient. If possible, the nurse has the patient demonstrate the technique of administration. The nurse should discuss the need to take the drug only as directed by the primary health care provider. The patient should not increase the dosage (ie, the number or frequency of sprays) unless advised to do so by the primary health care provider.

On occasion, a patient may need to self-administer vasopressin by the parenteral route. If so, the nurse instructs the patient or a family member in the preparation and administration of the drug and measurement of the specific gravity of the urine.

The nurse stresses the importance of adhering to the prescribed treatment program to control symptoms. In addition to instruction in administration, the nurse includes the following in a patient and family teaching plan:

- Drink one or two glasses of water immediately before taking the drug.
- Measure the amount of fluids taken each day.
- Measure the amount of urine passed at each voiding and then total the amount for each 24-hour period.
- Avoid the use of alcohol while taking these drugs.
- Rotate injection sites for parenteral administration.
- Contact the primary health care provider immediately if any of the following occur: a significant increase or decrease in urinary output, abdominal cramps, blanching of the skin, nausea, signs of inflammation or infection at the injection sites, confusion, headache, or drowsiness.
- Wear a medical alert tag identifying the disease (diabetes insipidus) and the drug regimen.

EVALUATION

- The therapeutic effect is achieved.
- Anxiety is reduced.
- Signs of a fluid volume deficit are absent (diabetes insipidus).

Patient and Family Teaching Checklist

Self-Administering Nasal Vasopressin

The nurse:

✓ Explains the reason for the drug and prescribed therapy, including drug name, correct dose (number of sprays), and frequency of administration.

✓ Describes equipment to be used for intranasal administration.

✓ Reviews schedule of administration and prescribed number of sprays to each nostril based on signs and symptoms of disease (diabetes insipidus), such as frequency of urination and increased thirst.

✓ Demonstrates step-by-step procedure for instillation and care, with patient performing a return demonstration of procedure.

✓ Provides written instructions for procedure.

✓ Reassures that symptoms of the disorder will most likely be reduced or eliminated with drug therapy.

✓ Instructs in signs and symptoms of fluid overload and the need to notify health care provider should any occur.

✓ Emphasizes importance of wearing medical alert tag identifying the disorder and drug therapy.

✓ Reinforces the need for continued follow-up to evaluate therapy.

Lypressin

✓ Instructs to hold bottle upright with head in vertical position.

✓ Discusses importance of taking drug exactly as prescribed (usually 1–2 sprays to one or both nostrils 4 times a day) and not to increase the number of sprays unless directed to do so by prescriber.

✓ Warns that dosages greater than 10 sprays in each nostril every 3 to 4 hours are not recommended.

Desmopressin

✓ When administering nasally, a nasal tube is used for administration. The nasal tube delivery system comes with a flexible calibrated plastic tube called a rhinyle.

✓ The prescribed amount of solution is drawn into the rhinyle. One end is inserted into the nostril, and the patient blows the other end to deposit solution deep into the nasal cavity.

✓ A nasal spray pump may also be used.

- The patient verbalizes an understanding of the treatment modalities and the importance of continued follow-up care (diabetes insipidus).
- The patient and family demonstrate an understanding of the drug regimen.

- Adverse reactions are identified and reported to the primary health care provider (diabetes insipidus).
- The patient verbalizes the importance of complying with the prescribed therapeutic regimen (diabetes insipidus).

ADRENOCORTICAL HORMONES

The adrenal gland lies on the superior surface of each kidney. It is a double organ composed of an outer cortex and an inner medulla. In response to ACTH secreted by the anterior pituitary, the adrenal cortex secretes several hormones (the glucocorticoids, the mineralocorticoids, and small amounts of sex hormones).

This section of the chapter discusses the hormones produced by the adrenal cortex or the adrenocortical hormones, which are the glucocorticoids and mineralocorticoids. These hormones are essential to life and influence many organs and structures of the body. The **glucocorticoids** and **mineralocorticoids** are collectively called **corticosteroids.**

● GLUCOCORTICOIDS

The glucocorticoids influence or regulate functions such as the immune response system, the regulation of glucose, fat and protein metabolism, and control of the anti-inflammatory response. Table 50-1 describes the activity of the glucocorticoids within the body.

ACTIONS AND USES

The glucocorticoids enter target cells and bind to receptors, initiating many complex reactions in the body. Some of these actions are considered undesirable, depending on the indication for which these drugs are being used. Examples of the glucocorticoids include cortisone, hydrocortisone, prednisone, prednisolone, and triamcinolone. The Summary Drug Table: Adrenocortical Hormones: Glucocorticoids and Mineralocorticoids provides information concerning these hormones.

The glucocorticoids are used as replacement therapy for adrenocortical insufficiency, to treat allergic reactions, collagen diseases (eg, systemic lupus erythematosus), dermatologic conditions, rheumatic disorders, shock, and other conditions (see Display 50-1). The anti-inflammatory activity of these hormones make them valuable as anti-inflammatories and as immunosuppressants to suppress inflammation and modify the immune response.

ADVERSE REACTIONS

The adverse reactions that may be seen with the administration of the glucocorticoids are given in Display 50-2. Long- or short-term high-dose therapy may also produce many of the signs and symptoms seen with **Cushing's syndrome,** a disease caused by the overproduction of endogenous glucocorticoids. Some of the signs and symptoms of this Cushing-like (or cushingoid) state include a "buffalo" hump (a hump on the back of

TABLE 50-1	Activity of Glucocorticoids in the Body
FUNCTION WITHIN THE BODY	**DESCRIPTION OF BODILY ACTIVITY**
Anti-inflammatory	Stabilizes lysosomal membrane and prevents the release of proteolytic enzymes released during the inflammatory process
Regulation of blood pressure	Potentiates vasoconstrictor action of norepinephrine. Without glucocorticoids the vasoconstricting action is decreased, and blood pressure falls.
Metabolism of carbohydrates and protein	Facilitates the breakdown of protein in the muscle, leading to increased plasma amino acid levels. Increases activity of enzymes necessary for glucogenesis producing hyperglycemia, which can aggravate diabetes, precipitate latent diabetes, and cause insulin resistance
Metabolism of fat	A complex phenomena that promotes the use of fat for energy (a positive effect) and permits fat stores to accumulate in the body, causing buffalo hump and moon- or round-shaped face (a negative effect).
Interference with the immune response	Decreases the production of lymphocytes and eosinophils in the blood by causing atrophy of the thymus gland; blocks the release of cytokines, resulting in a decreased performance of T and B monocytes in the immune response. (This action, coupled with the anti-inflammatory action, makes the corticosteroids useful in delaying organ rejection in patients with transplants.)
Stress	As a protective mechanism, the corticosteroids are released during periods of stress (eg, injury or surgery). The release of epinephrine or norepinephrine by the adrenal medulla during stress has a synergistic effect along with the corticosteroids.
Central nervous system disturbances	Affects mood and possibly causes neuronal or brain excitability, causing euphoria, anxiety, depression, psychosis, and an increase in motor activity in some individuals

SUMMARY DRUG TABLE ADRENOCORTICAL HORMONES: CORTICOSTEROIDS AND MINERALOCORTICOIDS

GENERIC NAME	TRADE NAME*	USES	ADVERSE REACTIONS	DOSAGE RANGES
Glucocorticoids				
betamethasone *bay-ta-meth'-a-zone*	Celestone	See Display 50-1	See Display 50-2	Individualize dosage: 0.6–7.2 mg/d PO
betamethasone sodium phosphate *bay-ta-meth'-a-zone*	Celestone Phosphate	See Display 50-1	See Display 50-2	Up to 9 mg/d IM, IV
budesonide *bue-des'-oh-nide*	Entocort EC	Crohn's disease	See Display 50-2	9 mg once daily in AM for 8 wk
cortisone *kor'-ti-sone*	*Generic*	See Display 50-1	See Display 50-2	25–300 mg/day PO
dexamethasone *dex-a-meth'-a-sone*	Decadron, Dexameth, Dexone, Hexadrol, *generic*	Acute self-limited allergic disorder or acute exacerbations of chronic allergic disorders	See Display 50-2	Individualize dosage based on severity of condition and response; give daily dose before 9 AM to minimize adrenal suppression; after long-term therapy, reduce slowly to avoid adrenal insufficiency
dexamethasone acetate *dex-a-meth'-a-sone*	Cortastat-LA, Dalalone-LA, Decadron-LA, Dexasone-LA, Dalalone DP, *generic*	See Display 50-1	See Display 50-2	0.5–9 mg/d 10 mg IV, then 4 mg IM q6h; intra-articular: large joints 4–16 mg; soft tissue: 0.8–1.6 mg
hydrocortisone (cortisol) *hye-droe-kor'-ti-zone*	Cortef, *generic*	See Display 50-1	See Display 50-2	20–240 mg PO in single or divided doses
hydrocortisone sodium phosphate *hye-droe-kor'-ti-zone*	*Generic*	See Display 50-1	See Display 50-2	20–240 mg/d q12h
hydrocortisone sodium succinate *hye-droe-kor'-ti-zone*	A-hydroCort, Solu-Cortef	See Display 50-1	See Display 50-2	Reduce dose based on condition and response but give no less than 25 mg/d
methylprednisolone *meth-ill-pred-niss'-oh-lone*	Medrol, *generic*	See Display 50-1	See Display 50-2	Initial dose: 4–48 mg/d PO; Dosepak 21 day therapy: follow manufacturer's directions; alternate day therapy: twice the usual dose is administered every other morning
methylprednisolone acetate *meth-ill-pred-niss'-oh-lone*	Depoject, DepoMedrol, Depopred, *generic*	See Display 50-1	See Display 50-2	40–120 mg IM; 4–80 mg intra-articular and soft tissue injections
methylprednisolone sodium succinate *meth-ill-pred-niss'-oh-lone*	A-Methapred, Solu-Medrol, *generic*	See Display 50-1	See Display 50-2	10–40 mg IV, IM
prednisolone *pred-niss'-oh-lone*	Prelone, *generic*	See Display 50-1	See Display 50-2	5–60 mg/d PO; acute exacerbations in MS: 200 mg/d for 1 wk, followed by 80 mg every other day for 1 month PO

(continued)

SUMMARY DRUG TABLE ADRENOCORTICAL HORMONES: CORTICOSTEROIDS AND MINERALOCORTICOIDS (*Continued*)

GENERIC NAME	TRADE NAME*	USES	ADVERSE REACTIONS	DOSAGE RANGES
prednisolone acetate *pred-niss'-oh-lone*	Key-Pred 50, Predcor-50, *generic*	See Display 50-1	See Display 50-2	4–60 mg/d IM (not for IV use); MS: 200 mg/d for 1 wk, followed by 80 mg/d every other day for 1 month IM
prednisone *pred'-ni-sone*	Deltasone, Meticorten, Orasone, *generic*	See Display 50-1	See Display 50-2	Individualize dosage: initial dose usually between 5 and 60 mg/d PO
triamcinolone *trye-am-sin'-oh-lone*	Aristocort, Atolone, Kenacort *generic*	See Display 50-1	See Display 50-2	4–48 mg/d PO
triamcinolone acetonide *trye-am-sin'-oh-lone*	Kenalog-10, Tac-3, Triam-A, *generic*	See Display 50-1	See Display 50-2	Systemic: 2.5–60 mg/d IM; Intra-articular: 2.5–15 mg
Corticosteroid Retention Enemas				
Corticosteroid intrarectal foam, hydrocortisone acetate intrarectal foam	Cortifoam	Adjunctive therapy in treatment of ulcerative proctitis of the distal portion of the rectum	Local pain or burning, rectal bleeding, apparent exacerbations or sensitivity reactions	1 applicatorful once or twice daily for 2 wk and every second day thereafter
Mineralocorticoid				
fludrocortisone acetate *floo-droe-kor'-te-sone*	Florinef Acetate	Partial replacement therapy for Addison's disease, salt-losing adrenogenital syndrome	See Display 50-2	0.1 mg 3 times a week to 0.2 mg/d PO

*The term *generic* indicates the drug is available in generic form.

the neck), moon face, oily skin and acne, osteoporosis, purple striae on the abdomen and hips, skin pigmentation, and weight gain. When a serious disease or disorder is being treated, it is often necessary to allow these effects to occur because therapy with these drugs is absolutely necessary.

CONTRAINDICATIONS, PRECAUTIONS, AND INTERACTIONS

The glucocorticoids are contraindicated in patients with serious infections, such as tuberculosis and fungal and antibiotic-resistant infections.

The glucocorticoids are administered with caution to patients with renal or hepatic disease, hypothyroidism, ulcerative colitis, diverticulitis, peptic ulcer disease, inflammatory bowel disease, hypertension, osteoporosis, convulsive disorders, or diabetes. The glucocorticoids

are classified as Pregnancy Category C drugs and should be used with caution during pregnancy and lactation.

Multiple drug interactions may occur with the glucocorticoids. Table 50-2 identifies select clinically significant interactions.

● Mineralocorticoids

ACTIONS AND USES

The mineralocorticoids consist of aldosterone and desoxycorticosterone and play an important role in conserving sodium and increasing the excretion of potassium. Because of these activities, the mineralocorticoids are important in controlling salt and water balance. Aldosterone is the more potent of these two hormones. Deficiencies of the mineralocorticoids result in a loss of sodium and water and a retention of potassium.

TABLE 50-2	Select Drug Interactions of Glucocorticoids	
PRECIPITANT DRUG	**OBJECT DRUG**	**DESCRIPTION**
Barbiturates	Corticosteroids	Decreased pharmacologic effects of the corticosteroid may be observed.
Cholestyramine	Hydrocortisone	The effects of hydrocortisone may be decreased.
Contraceptives, oral	Corticosteroids	Corticosteroid concentration may be increased and clearance decreased.
Estrogens	Corticosteroids	Corticosteroid clearance may be decreased.
Hydantoins	Corticosteroids	Corticosteroid clearance may be increased, resulting in reduced therapeutic effects.
Ketoconazole	Corticosteroids	Corticosteroid clearance may be decreased.
Rifampin	Corticosteroids	Corticosteroid clearance may be increased, resulting in decreased therapeutic effects.
Corticosteroids	Anticholinesterases	Anticholinesterase effects may be antagonized in myasthenia gravis.
Corticosteroids	Anticoagulants, oral	Anticoagulant dose requirements may be reduced. Corticosteroids may decrease the anticoagulant action.
Corticosteroids	Digitalis glycosides	Co-administration may enhance the possibility of digitalis toxicity associated with hypokalemia.
Corticosteroids	Isoniazid	Isoniazid serum concentrations may be decreased.
Corticosteroids	Potassium-depleting diuretics	Hypokalemia may occur.
Corticosteroids	Salicylates	Corticosteroids will reduce serum salicylate levels and may decrease their effectiveness.
Corticosteroids	Somatrem	Growth-promoting effect of somatrem may be inhibited.
Corticosteroids	Theophyllines	Alterations in the pharmacologic activity of either agent may occur.

Fludrocortisone (Florinef) is a drug that has both glucocorticoid and mineralocorticoid activity and is the only currently available mineralocorticoid drug.

Fludrocortisone is used for replacement therapy for primary and secondary adrenocortical deficiency. Even though this drug has both mineralocorticoid and glucocorticoid activity, it is used only for its mineralocorticoid effects.

ADVERSE REACTIONS

Adverse reactions may occur if the dosage is too high or prolonged, or if withdrawal is too rapid. Administration of fludrocortisone may cause edema, hypertension, congestive heart failure, enlargement of the heart, increased sweating, or allergic skin rash. Additional adverse reactions include hypokalemia, muscular weakness, headache, and hypersensitivity reactions. Because this drug has glucocorticoid and mineralocorticoid activity and is often given with the glucocorticoids, adverse reactions of the glucocorticoids must be closely monitored as well (see Display 50-2).

CONTRAINDICATIONS, PRECAUTIONS, AND INTERACTIONS

Fludrocortisone is contraindicated in patients with hypersensitivity to fludrocortisone and those with systemic fungal infections. Fludrocortisone is used cautiously in patients with Addison's disease, infection, and during pregnancy (Pregnancy Category C) and lactation. Fludrocortisone decreases the effects of the barbiturates, hydantoins, and rifampin. There is a decrease in serum levels of the salicylates when those agents are administered with fludrocortisone.

N U R S I N G   P R O C E S S

● **The Patient Receiving a Glucocorticoid or Mineralocorticoid**

ASSESSMENT

Preadministration Assessment

Before administering a glucocorticoid or mineralocorticoid, the nurse takes and records the patient's blood pressure, pulse, and respiratory rate. Additional physical assessments depend on the reason for use and the general condition of the patient. When feasible, the nurse performs an assessment of the area of disease involvement, such as the respiratory tract or skin, and records the findings in the patient's record. These findings provide baseline data for the evaluation of the patient's response to drug therapy. The nurse weighs patients who are acutely ill and those with a serious systemic disease before starting therapy.

Ongoing Assessment

Ongoing assessments of the patient receiving a glucocorticoid, and the frequency of these assessments, depend largely on the disease being treated. The nurse should take and record vital signs every 4 to 8 hours. The nurse weighs the patient daily to weekly, depending on the diagnosis and the primary health care provider's orders. The patient's response to the drug is assessed by daily evaluations. More frequent assessment may be necessary if a glucocorticoid is used for emergency situations. Because these drugs are used to treat a great many diseases and conditions, an evaluation of drug response is based on the patient's diagnosis and the signs and symptoms of disease.

The nurse assesses for signs of adverse effects of the mineralocorticoid or glucocorticoid, particularly signs of electrolyte imbalance, such as hypocalcemia, hypokalemia, and hypernatremia (see Chap. 58). The nurse assesses the patient's mental status for any change, especially if there is a history of depression or other psychiatric problems or if high doses of the drug are being given. The nurse also monitors for signs of an infection, which may be masked by glucocorticoid therapy. The blood of the patient without diabetes is checked weekly for glucose levels because glucocorticoids may aggravate latent diabetes. Those with diabetes must be checked more frequently.

When administering fludrocortisone, the nurse monitors the patient's blood pressure at frequent intervals. Hypotension may indicate insufficient dosage. The nurse weighs the patient daily and assesses for edema, particularly swelling of the feet and hands. The lungs are auscultated for adventitious sounds (eg, rales/crackles).

NURSING DIAGNOSES

Drug-specific nursing diagnoses are highlighted in the Nursing Diagnoses Checklist. Other nursing diagnoses applicable to these drugs are discussed in depth in Chapter 4.

PLANNING

The expected outcomes of the patient include an optimal response to therapy, identification and management

---

> ### Nursing Diagnoses Checklist
>
> ✓ **Risk for Infection** related to adverse drug reactions (impaired wound healing, aggravation of existing infections)
>
> ✓ **Risk for Injury** related to adverse reactions (muscle atrophy, osteoporosis, spontaneous fractures)
>
> ✓ **Excess Fluid Volume** related to adverse reactions (sodium and water retention)
>
> ✓ **Disturbed Body Image** related to adverse reactions (cushingoid appearance)
>
> ✓ **Disturbed Thought Processes** related to adverse reactions (depression, psychosis, other changes in mental status)

of adverse drug effects, and an understanding of the therapeutic regimen.

IMPLEMENTATION

Promoting an Optimal Response to Therapy

The glucocorticoids may be administered orally, IM, SC, IV, topically, or as an inhalant. The primary health care provider may also inject the drug into a joint (intra-articular), a lesion (intralesional), soft tissue, or bursa. The dosage of the drug is individualized and based on the severity of the condition and the patient's response.

 Nursing Alert

The nurse must never omit the dose of a glucocorticoid. If the patient cannot take the drug orally because of nausea or vomiting, the nurse must notify the primary health care provider immediately because the drug needs to be ordered given by the parenteral route. Patients who are receiving nothing by mouth for any reason must have the glucocorticoid given by the parenteral route.

Daily oral doses are generally given before 9:00 AM to minimize adrenal suppression and to coincide with normal adrenal function. However, alternate-day therapy may be prescribed for patients receiving long-term therapy (see below). Fludrocortisone is given orally and is well tolerated in the GI tract.

 Gerontologic Alert

The corticosteroids are administered with caution in older adults because they are more likely to have preexisting conditions, such as congestive heart failure, hypertension, osteoporosis, and arthritis, which may be worsened by the use of such agents. The nurse monitors older adults for exacerbation of existing conditions during corticosteroid therapy. In addition, lower dosages may be needed because of the effects of aging, such as decreased muscle mass, renal function, and plasma volume.

ALTERNATE-DAY THERAPY. The alternate-day therapy approach to glucocorticoid administration is used in the treatment of diseases and disorders requiring long-term therapy, especially the arthritic disorders. This regimen involves giving twice the daily dose of the glucocorticoid every other day. The drug is given only once on the alternate day and before 9 AM. The purpose of alternate-day administration is to provide the patient requiring long-term glucocorticoid therapy with the beneficial effects of the drug while minimizing certain undesirable reactions (see Display 50-2).

Plasma levels of the endogenous adrenocortical hormones vary throughout the day and nighttime hours. They are normally higher between 2 AM and about 8 AM, and lower between 4 PM and midnight. When plasma levels are lower, the anterior pituitary releases ACTH, which in turn stimulates the adrenal cortex to manufacture and release glucocorticoids. When plasma levels are high, the pituitary gland does not release ACTH. The response of the pituitary to high or low plasma levels of glucocorticoids and the resulting release or nonrelease of ACTH is an example of the feedback mechanism, which may also be seen in other glands of the body, such as the thyroid gland. The **feedback mechanism** (also called the feedback control) is the method by which the body maintains most hormones at relatively constant levels within the bloodstream. When the hormone concentration falls, the rate of production of that hormone increases. Likewise, when the hormone level becomes too high, the body decreases production of that hormone.

Administration of a short-acting glucocorticoid on alternate days and before 9 AM, when glucocorticoid plasma levels are still relatively high, does not affect the release of ACTH later in the day, yet it gives the patient the benefit of exogenous glucocorticoid therapy.

THE PATIENT WITH DIABETES. Patients with diabetes who are receiving a glucocorticoid may require frequent adjustment of their insulin or oral hypoglycemic drug dosage. The nurse monitors blood glucose levels several times daily or as prescribed by the primary health care provider. If the blood glucose levels increase or urine is positive for glucose or ketones, the nurse notifies the primary health care provider. Some patients may have latent (hidden) diabetes. In these cases the corticosteroid may precipitate hyperglycemia. Therefore all patients, those with diabetes and those without, should have frequent checks of blood glucose levels.

Monitoring and Managing Adverse Reactions

ADRENAL INSUFFICIENCY. Administration of the glucocorticoids poses the threat of adrenal gland insufficiency (particularly if the alternate-day therapy is not prescribed). Administration of glucocorticoids several times a day and during a short time (as little as 5–10 days) results in shutting off the pituitary release of ACTH

because there are always high levels of the glucocorticoids in the plasma (caused by the body's own glucocorticoid production plus the administration of a glucocorticoid drug). Ultimately, the pituitary atrophies and ceases to release ACTH. Without ACTH, the adrenals fail to manufacture and release (endogenous) glucocorticoids. When this happens, the patient has acute adrenal insufficiency, which is a life-threatening situation until corrected with the administration of an exogenous glucocorticoid.

Adrenal insufficiency is a critical deficiency of the mineralocorticoids and the glucocorticoids that requires immediate treatment. Symptoms of adrenal insufficiency include fever, myalgia, arthralgia, malaise, anorexia, nausea, orthostatic hypotension, dizziness, fainting, dyspnea, and hypoglycemia. Death due to circulatory collapse will result unless the condition is treated promptly. Situations producing stress (eg, trauma, surgery, severe illness) may precipitate the need for an increase in dosage of the corticosteroids until the crisis situation or stressful situation is resolved.

> ### ☀ Nursing Alert
>
> *At no time must glucocorticoid therapy be discontinued suddenly. When administration of a glucocorticoid extends beyond 5 days and the drug therapy is to be discontinued, the dosage must be tapered over several days. In some instances, it may be necessary to taper the dose over 7 to 10 or more days. Abrupt discontinuation of glucocorticoid therapy usually results in acute adrenal insufficiency, which, if not recognized in time, can result in death. Tapering the dosage allows normal adrenal function to return gradually, preventing adrenal insufficiency.*

MANAGING INFECTION. The nurse should report any slight rise in temperature, sore throat, or other signs of infection to the primary health care provider as soon as possible because of a possible decreased resistance to infection during glucocorticoid therapy. Nursing personnel and visitors with any type of infection or recent exposure to an infectious disease should avoid patient contact.

MANAGING MENTAL AND EMOTIONAL CHANGES. Mental and emotional changes may occur when the glucocorticoids are administered. The nurse accurately documents mental changes and informs the primary health care provider of their occurrence. Patients who appear extremely depressed must be closely observed. The nurse evaluates mental status, memory, and impaired thinking (eg, changes in orientation, impaired judgment, thoughts of hopelessness, guilt). The nurse allows time for the patient to express feeling and concerns.

MANAGING FLUID AND ELECTROLYTE IMBALANCES. Fluid and electrolyte imbalances, particularly excess fluid volume, are common with corticosteroid therapy. The nurse checks the patient for visible edema, keeps an accurate fluid intake and output record, obtains a daily weight, and restricts sodium if indicated by the primary health care provider. Edematous extremities are elevated and the patient's position is changed frequently. The nurse informs the primary health care provider if signs of electrolyte imbalance or glucocorticoid drug effects are noted. Dietary adjustments are made for the increased loss of potassium and the retention of sodium if necessary. Consultation with a dietitian may be indicated.

MANAGING FRACTURES. The nurse observes patients receiving long-term glucocorticoid therapy, especially those allowed limited activity, for signs of compression fractures of the vertebrae and pathologic fractures of the long bones. If the patient reports back or bone pain, the nurse notifies the primary health care provider. Extra care is also necessary to prevent falls and other injuries when the patient is confused or is allowed out of bed. If the patient is weak, the nurse assists the patient to the bathroom or when ambulating. Edematous extremities are handled with care to prevent trauma.

MANAGING ULCERS. Peptic ulcer has been associated with glucocorticoid therapy. The nurse reports to the primary care provider any patient complaints of epigastric burning or pain, bloody or coffee-ground emesis, or the passing of tarry stools. Giving oral corticosteroids with food or a full glass of water may minimize gastric irritation.

MANAGING BODY IMAGE DISTURBANCE. A body image disturbance may occur, especially if the patient experiences cushingoid appearance (buffalo hump, moon face), acne, or hirsutism. If continuation of the drug therapy is necessary, the nurse thoroughly explains the cushingoid appearance reaction and emphasizes the necessity of continuing the drug regimen. The nurse assesses the patient's emotional state and helps the patient to express feelings and concerns. The nurse offers positive reinforcement, when possible. The nurse instructs the patient with acne to keep the affected areas clean and use over-the-counter acne drugs and water-based cosmetics or creams.

Educating the Patient and Family

To prevent noncompliance, the nurse must provide the patient and family with thorough instructions and warnings about the drug regimen.

- These drugs may cause GI upset. To decrease GI effects, take the oral drug with meals or snacks.
- Take antacids between meals to help prevent peptic ulcer.

SHORT-TERM GLUCOCORTICOID THERAPY

- Take the drug exactly as directed in the prescription container. Do not increase, decrease, or omit a dose

unless advised to do so by the primary health care provider.
- Take single daily doses before 9:00 AM.
- Follow the instructions for tapering the dose because they are extremely important.
- If the problem does not improve, contact the primary health care provider.

ALTERNATE-DAY GLUCOCORTICOID THERAPY (ORAL)

- Take this drug before 9 AM once every other day. Use a calendar or some other method to identify the days of each week the drug is taken.
- Do not stop taking the drug unless advised to do so by the primary health care provider.
- If the problem becomes worse, especially on the days the drug is not taken, contact the primary health care provider.

Most of the teaching points given below may also apply to alternate-day therapy, especially when higher doses are used and therapy extends over many months.

LONG-TERM OR HIGH-DOSE GLUCOCORTICOID THERAPY

- Do not omit this drug or increase or decrease the dosage except on the advice of the primary health care provider.
- Inform other primary health care providers, dentists, and all medical personnel of therapy with this drug. Wear a medical alert tag or other form of identification to alert medical personnel of long-term therapy with a glucocorticoid.
- Do not take any nonprescription drug unless its use has been approved by the primary health care provider.
- Do not take live virus vaccinations (eg, smallpox) because of the risk of a lack of antibody response. This does not include patients receiving the corticosteroids as replacement therapy.
- Whenever possible, avoid exposure to infections. Contact the primary health care provider if minor cuts or abrasions fail to heal, persistent joint swelling or tenderness is noted, or fever, sore throat, upper respiratory infection, or other signs of infection occur.
- If the drug cannot be taken orally for any reason or if diarrhea occurs, contact the primary health care provider immediately. If you are unable to contact the primary health care provider before the next dose is due, go to the nearest hospital emergency department (preferably where the original treatment was started or where the primary health care provider is on the hospital staff) because the drug has to be given by injection.
- Weigh yourself weekly. If significant weight gain or swelling of the extremities is noted, contact the primary health care provider.
- Remember that dietary recommendations made by the primary health care provider are an important part of therapy and must be followed.

● Follow the primary health care provider's recommendations regarding periodic eye examinations and laboratory tests.

INTRA-ARTICULAR OR INTRALESIONAL ADMINISTRATION

● Do not overuse the injected joint, even if the pain is gone.
● Follow the primary care provider's instructions concerning rest and exercise.

MINERALOCORTICOID (FLUDROCORTISONE) THERAPY

● Take the drug as directed. Do not increase or decrease the dosage except as instructed to do so by the primary health care provider.
● Do not discontinue use of the drug abruptly.
● Inform the primary health care provider if the following adverse reactions occur: edema, muscle weakness, weight gain, anorexia, swelling of the extremities, dizziness, severe headache, or shortness of breath.
● Carry patient identification, such as a medical alert tag, so that drug therapy will be known to medical personnel during an emergency situation.
● Keep follow-up appointments to determine if a dosage adjustment is necessary.

EVALUATION

● The therapeutic effect is achieved.
● Adverse reactions are identified, reported to the primary health care provider, and managed appropriately.
● The patient verbalizes an understanding of the dosage regimen.
● The patient verbalizes the importance of complying with the prescribed therapeutic regimen and importance of continued follow-up care.
● The patient and family demonstrate an understanding of the drug regimen.
● The patient demonstrates an understanding of the importance of not suddenly discontinuing therapy (long-term or high-dose therapy).

● *Critical Thinking Exercises*

1. *Judy Cowan, age 28 years, has been prescribed clomiphene to induce ovulation and pregnancy. Judy is very anxious and wants desperately to become pregnant. Her husband, Jim, has come to the clinic with her. Discuss assessments the nurse would consider important before initiating treatment with clomiphene. Discuss information the nurse would include in a teaching plan for Jim and Judy.*

2. *Plan a team conference to discuss the administration of ACTH (corticotropin). Identify three critical points*

that would be essential to discuss. Explain your rationale for choosing each point.

3. *Discuss the rationale for administering oral prednisone at 7 AM every other day.*

● *Review Questions*

1. Which of the following adverse reactions would the nurse expect with the administration of clomiphene?
   A. Edema
   B. Vasomotor flushes
   C. Sedation
   D. Hypertension

2. Which of the following assessments would be most important for the nurse to make when a child receiving the growth hormone comes to the primary care provider's office?
   A. Blood pressure, pulse, and respiration
   B. Diet history
   C. Height and weight
   D. Measurement of abdominal girth

3. Which of the following adverse reactions would lead the nurse to suspect cushingoid appearance in a patient taking a corticosteroid?
   A. Moon face, hirsutism
   B. Kyphosis, periorbital edema
   C. Pallor of the skin, acne
   D. Exophthalmos

4. Which of the following statements, if made by the patient, would indicate a possible adverse reaction seen with the administration of vasopressin?
   A. "I am unable to see well at night."
   B. "My stomach is cramping."
   C. "I have a sore throat."
   D. "I am hungry all the time."

5. Adverse reactions seen with the administration of fludrocortisone include: _____.
   A. hyperactivity and headache
   B. sedation, lethargy
   C. edema, hypertension
   D. dyspnea, confusion

● *Medication Dosage Problems*

1. Methylprednisolone 40 mg IM is prescribed. The drug is available in a suspension for injections in a solution of 20 mg/mL. The nurse prepares to administer _____.

2. Prednisolone 60 mg PO is prescribed. The drug is available as a syrup with 15 mg/5 mL. The nurse administers _____.

chapter 51

Thyroid and Antithyroid Drugs

Key Terms

euthyroid
goiter
hyperthyroidism
hypothyroidism
iodine
iodism

myxedema
thyroid gland
thyroid storm
thyrotoxicosis
thyroxine
triiodothyronine

Chapter Objectives

On completion of this chapter, the student will:

- Identify the hormones produced by the thyroid gland.
- Discuss the uses, general drug actions, adverse reactions, contraindications, precautions, and interactions of thyroid and antithyroid drugs.
- Discuss important preadministration and ongoing assessment activities the nurse should perform on the patient taking thyroid and antithyroid drugs.
- List the signs and symptoms of iodism and iodine allergy.
- Discuss ways to promote an optimal response to therapy, how to manage adverse reactions, and important points to keep in mind when educating patients about the use of thyroid and antithyroid drugs.

The **thyroid gland** is located in the neck in front of the trachea. This highly vascular gland manufactures and secretes two hormones: **thyroxine** (T_4) and **triiodothyronine** (T_3). **Iodine** is an essential element for the manufacture of both of these hormones. The activity of the thyroid gland is regulated by thyroid-stimulating hormone, produced by the anterior pituitary gland (see Fig. 50-1). When the level of circulating thyroid hormones decreases, the anterior pituitary secretes thyroid-stimulating hormone, which then activates the cells of the thyroid to release stored thyroid hormones. This is an example of the feedback mechanism (see Chap. 50).

Two diseases are related to the hormone-producing activity of the thyroid gland:

- **Hypothyroidism**—a decrease in the amount of thyroid hormones manufactured and secreted.
- **Hyperthyroidism**—an increase in the amount of thyroid hormones manufactured and secreted.

The symptoms of hypothyroidism and hyperthyroidism are given in Table 51-1. A severe form of hyperthyroidism, called **thyrotoxicosis** or thyroid **storm**, is characterized by high fever, extreme tachycardia, and altered mental status. Thyroid hormones are used to treat hypothyroidism and antithyroid drugs and radioactive iodine are used to treat hyperthyroidism.

THYROID HORMONES

Thyroid hormones used in medicine include both the natural and synthetic hormones. The synthetic hormones are generally preferred because they are more uniform in potency than are the natural hormones obtained from animals. Thyroid hormones are listed in the Summary Drug Table: Thyroid and Antithyroid Drugs.

ACTIONS

The thyroid hormones influence every organ and tissue of the body. These hormones are principally concerned with increasing the metabolic rate of tissues, which results in increases in the heart and respiratory rate, body temperature, cardiac output, oxygen consumption, and the metabolism of fats, proteins, and carbohydrates. The exact mechanisms by which the thyroid hormones exert their influence on body organs and tissues are not well understood.

TABLE 51-1	Signs and Symptoms of Thyroid Dysfunction	
BODY SYSTEM OR FUNCTION	**HYPOTHYROIDISM**	**HYPERTHYROIDISM**
Metabolism	Decreased with anorexia, intolerance to cold, low body temperature, weight gain despite anorexia	Increased with increased appetite, intolerance to heat, elevated body temperature, weight loss despite increased appetite
Cardiovascular	Bradycardia, moderate hypotension	Tachycardia, moderate hypertension
Central nervous system	Lethargy, sleepiness	Nervousness, anxiety, insomnia, tremors
Skin, skin structures	Pale, cool, dry skin; face appears puffy; hair coarse; nails thick and hard	Flushed, warm, moist skin
Ovarian function	Heavy menses, may be unable to conceive, loss of fetus possible	Irregular or scant menses
Testicular function	Low sperm count	

USES

Thyroid hormones are used as replacement therapy when the patient is hypothyroid. By supplementing the decreased endogenous thyroid production and secretion with exogenous thyroid hormones, an attempt is made to create a **euthyroid** (normal thyroid) state. Levothyroxine (Synthroid) is the drug of choice for hypothyroidism because it is relatively inexpensive, requires once-a-day dosages, and has a more uniform potency than do other thyroid hormone replacement drugs.

Myxedema is a severe hypothyroidism manifested by lethargy, apathy, memory impairment, emotional changes, slow speech, deep coarse voice, thick dry skin, cold intolerance, slow pulse, constipation, weight gain, and absence of menses.

Thyroid hormones are also used in the treatment or prevention of various types of euthyroid **goiters** (enlargement of the thyroid gland), including thyroid nodules, subacute or chronic lymphocytic thyroiditis (Hashimoto's), and multinodular goiter and in the management of thyroid cancer. The hormone may be used with the antithyroid drugs to treat thyrotoxicosis. Thyroid hormones also may be used as a diagnostic measure to differentiate suspected hyperthyroidism from euthyroidism.

ADVERSE REACTIONS

During initial therapy, the most common adverse reactions seen are signs of overdose and hyperthyroidism (see Table 51-1). Adverse reactions other than symptoms of hyperthyroidism are rare.

CONTRAINDICATIONS

These drugs are contraindicated in patients with known hypersensitivity to the drug or to any constituents of the drug, after a recent myocardial infarction (heart attack), or in patients with thyrotoxicosis. When hypothyroidism is a cause or contributing factor to a myocardial infarction or heart disease, the physician may prescribe small doses of thyroid hormone.

PRECAUTIONS

These drugs are used cautiously in patients with Addison's disease and during lactation. The thyroid hormones are classified as Pregnancy Category A and are considered safe to use during pregnancy.

INTERACTIONS

When administered with cholestyramine or colestipol there is a decreased absorption of the oral thyroid preparations. These drugs should not be administered within 4 of 6 hours of the thyroid hormones. When administered with the oral anticoagulants there is an increased risk of bleeding. It may be advantageous to decrease the dosage of the anticoagulant when a thyroid preparation is prescribed. There is a decreased effectiveness of the digitalis preparation if taken with a thyroid preparation.

SUMMARY DRUG TABLE THYROID AND ANTITHYROID DRUGS

GENERIC NAME	TRADE NAME*	USES	ADVERSE REACTIONS	DOSAGE RANGES
Thyroid Hormones				
levothyroxine sodium (T$_4$) *lee-voe-thye-rox'-een*	Eltroxin, Levo-T Levothroid, Levoxyl, Synthroid, *generic*	Hypothyroidism, thyrotoxicosis	Palpitations, tachycardia, headache, nervousness, insomnia, diarrhea, vomiting, weight loss, sweating, heat intolerance	0.025–0.3 mg/d PO; 0.05–0.1 mg IV; 0.05 mg initially, increase by 0.025 mg PO q2–3 wk; maintenance dose, 0.2 mg/d, may subsitute IV IM
liothyronine sodium (T$_3$) *lye'-oh-thye'-roe-neen*	Cytomel, *generic* Trio stat	Hypothyroidism, thyrotoxicosis	Same as levothyroxine	5–75 mcg/d PO, 25–50 µg IV q4–12h
liotrix (T$_2$, T$_4$) *lye'-oh-trix*	Thyrolar	Hypothyroidism, thyrotoxicosis	Same as levothyroxine	15–120 mg/d PO
thyroid desiccated *thye'-roid*	Armour Thyroid, *generic*	Hypothyroidism, thyrotoxicosis	Same as levothyroxine	65–195 mg/d PO
Antithyroid Preparations				
methimazole *meth-im-a-zole*	Tapazole, *generic*	Hyperthyroidism	Agranulocytosis, headache, exfoliative dermatitis, granulocytopenia, thrombocytopenia, hepatitis, hypoprothrombinemia, jaundice, loss of hair, nausea, vomiting	15–60 mg/d
propylthiouracil (PTU) *proe-pill-thye-oh-yoor'-a-sill*	PTU *generic*	Same as methimazole	Same as methimazole	300–900 mg/d PO, usually in divided doses at about 8-h intervals
Iodine Products				
strong iodine solution *eye'-oh-dine*	Lugol's Solution, Thyro-Block, *generic*	To prepare hyperthyroid patients for thyroid surgery, thyrotoxic crisis, thyroid blocking in radiation therapy	Rash, swelling of salivary glands, "iodism" (metallic taste, burning mouth and throat, sore teeth and gums, symptoms of a head cold, diarrhea, nausea), allergic reactions (fever, joint pains, swelling of parts of face and body)	2–6 drops PO TID for 10 d before surgery; 130 mg/d PO
Sodium iodine (^{131}I) *so'-de-um,* *eye'-oh-dide*	Iodotope, *generic*	Thyrotoxicosis, selected cases of thyroid cancer	Bone marrow depression, anemia, blood dyscrasias, nausea, vomiting, tachycardia, itching, rash, hives, tenderness and swelling of the neck, sore throat, and cough	Measured by a radioactivity calibration system before administering PO 4–10 mCi; thyroid cancer: 50–150 mCi

*The term *generic* indicates the drug is available in generic form.

● **The Patient Receiving a Thyroid Hormone**

ASSESSMENT

Preadministration Assessment

After a patient receives a diagnosis of hypothyroidism and before therapy starts, the nurse takes vital signs and weighs the patient. A history of the patient's signs and symptoms is obtained. The nurse performs a general physical assessment to determine outward signs of hypothyroidism.

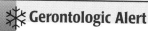
❄ Gerontologic Alert

The symptoms of hypothyroidism may be confused with symptoms associated with aging, such as depression, cold intolerance, weight gain, confusion, or unsteady gait. The presence of these symptoms should be thoroughly evaluated and documented in the preadministration assessment and periodically throughout therapy.

Ongoing Assessment

The full effects of thyroid hormone replacement therapy may not be apparent for several weeks or more, but early effects may be apparent in as little as 48 hours. During the ongoing assessment, the nurse monitors the vital signs daily or as ordered and observes the patient for signs of hyperthyroidism, which is a sign of excessive drug dosage. Signs of a therapeutic response include weight loss, mild diuresis, a sense of well-being, increased appetite, an increased pulse rate, an increase in mental activity, and decreased puffiness of the face, hands, and feet.

NURSING DIAGNOSES

Drug-specific nursing diagnoses are highlighted in the Nursing Diagnoses Checklist. Other nursing diagnoses applicable to these drugs are discussed in depth in Chapter 4.

PLANNING

The expected outcomes of the patient may include an optimal response to therapy, identification of adverse reactions, and an understanding of and compliance with the prescribed therapeutic regimen.

Nursing Diagnoses Checklist

✓ **Decreased Cardiac** output related to adverse reactions

✓ **Anxiety** related to symptoms, adverse reactions, treatment regimen, other (specify)

IMPLEMENTATION

Promoting an Optimal Response to Therapy

Thyroid hormones are administered once a day, early in the morning and preferably before breakfast. An empty stomach increases the absorption of the oral preparation. Levothyroxine (Synthroid) also can be given intravenously and is prepared for administration immediately before use.

The dosage is individualized to the needs of the patient. The dose of thyroid hormones must be carefully adjusted according to the patient's hormone requirements. At times, several upward or downward dosage adjustments must be made until the optimal therapeutic dosage is reached and the patient becomes euthyroid.

Some patients may exhibit anxiety related to the symptoms of their disorder, as well as concern about relief of their symptoms. The patient should be reassured that although relief may not be immediate, symptoms should begin to decrease or even disappear in a few weeks.

Monitoring and Managing Adverse Reactions

The nurse monitors the patient for any adverse reactions, especially during the initial stages of dosage adjustment. The nurse notifies the primary health care provider if the patient experiences these or any adverse drug reactions. If the dosage is inadequate the patient will continue to experience signs of hypothyroidism (see Table 51-1). If the dosage is excessive, the patient will exhibit signs of hyperthyroidism.

❊ Nursing Alert

If signs of hyperthyroidism (eg, nervousness, anxiety, increased appetite, elevated body temperature, tachycardia, moderate hypertension or flushed, warm, moist skin) are apparent, the nurse reports these to the primary health care provider before the next dose is due because it may be necessary to decrease the daily dosage.

Thyroid hormone replacement therapy in patients with diabetes may increase the intensity of the symptoms or the diabetes. The nurse closely monitors the patient with diabetes during thyroid hormone replacement therapy for signs of hyperglycemia (see Chap. 49) and notifies the primary health care provider if this problem occurs.

The nurse carefully observes patients with cardiovascular disease taking the thyroid hormones. The development of chest pain or worsening of cardiovascular disease should be reported to the primary health care provider immediately because the patient may require a reduction in the dosage of the thyroid hormone.

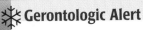
❄ Gerontologic Alert

Older adults are more sensitive to thyroid hormone replace-ment therapy and are more likely to experience adverse reac-tions when taking the thyroid hormones. In addition, the eld-erly are at increased risk for adverse cardiovascular reactions when taking thyroid drugs. The initial dosage is smaller for an older adult, and increases, if necessary, are made in smaller increments during a period of about 8 weeks. Periodic thyroid function tests are necessary to monitor drug therapy. Dosage may need to be reduced with age. If the pulse rate is 100 bpm or more, the nurse notifies the primary health care provider before the drug is administered.

Educating the Patient and Family

Thyroid hormones are usually given on an outpatient basis. The nurse emphasizes the importance of taking the drug exactly as directed and not stopping the drug even though symptoms have improved. The nurse provides the following information to the patient and family when thyroid hormone replacement therapy is prescribed:

- Replacement therapy is for life, with the exception of transient hypothyroidism seen in those with thy-roiditis.
- Do not increase, decrease, or skip a dose unless advised to do so by the primary health care provider.
- Take this drug in the morning, preferably before breakfast, unless advised by the primary health care provider to take it at a different time of day.
- Notify the primary health care provider if any of the following occur: headache, nervousness, palpita-tions, diarrhea, excessive sweating, heat intolerance, chest pain, increased pulse rate, or any unusual physical change or event.
- The dosage of this drug may require periodic adjust-ments; this is normal. Dosage changes are based on a response to therapy and thyroid function tests.
- Therapy needs to be evaluated at periodic intervals, which may vary from every 2 weeks during the beginning of therapy to every 6 to 12 months once symptoms are controlled. Periodic thyroid function tests will be needed.
- Weigh yourself weekly and report any significant weight gain or loss to the primary health care provider.
- Do not change from one brand of this drug to another without consulting the primary health care provider.

EVALUATION

- The therapeutic effect is achieved.
- Adverse reactions are identified and reported to the primary health care provider.
- The patient verbalizes the importance of complying with the prescribed treatment regimen.
- The patient verbalizes an understanding of the treatment modalities and importance of continued follow-up care.
- The patient and family demonstrate an understand-ing of the drug regimen.

ANTITHYROID DRUGS

Antithyroid drugs or thyroid antagonists are used to treat hyperthyroidism. In addition to the antithyroid drugs, hyperthyroidism may be treated by the adminis-tration of strong iodine solutions, use of radioactive iodine (^{131}I), or by surgical removal of some or almost all of the thyroid gland (subtotal thyroidectomy).

ACTIONS

Antithyroid drugs inhibit the manufacture of thyroid hormones. They do not affect existing thyroid hor-mones that are circulating in the blood or stored in the thyroid gland. For this reason, therapeutic effects of the antithyroid drugs may not be observed for 3 to 4 weeks. Antithyroid drugs are listed in the Summary Drug Table: Thyroid and Antithyroid Drugs.

Strong iodide solutions act by decreasing the vascu-larity of the thyroid gland by rapidly inhibiting the release of the thyroid hormones. Radioactive iodine is distributed within the cellular fluid and excreted. The radioactive isotope accumulates in the cells of the thy-roid gland, where destruction of thyroid cells occurs without damaging other cells throughout the body.

USES

Methimazole (Tapazole) and propylthiouracil (PTU) are used for the medical management of hyperthyroidism. Not all patients respond adequately to antithyroid drugs; therefore, a thyroidectomy may be necessary. Antithyroid drugs may be administered before surgery to temporarily return the patient to a euthyroid state. When used for this reason, the vascularity of the thyroid gland is reduced and the tendency to bleed excessively during and immediately after surgery is decreased.

Strong iodine solution, also known as Lugol's solution, may be given orally with methimazole or propylthiouracil to prepare for thyroid surgery. Iodine solutions are also used for rapid treatment of hyperthyroidism because they can decrease symptoms in 2 to 7 days. Radioactive iodine (^{131}I) may be used for treatment of hyperthyroidism and selected cases of cancer of the thyroid. The drug is given orally either as a solution or in a gelatin capsule.

ADVERSE REACTIONS

Methimazole and Propylthiouracil

The most serious adverse reaction associated with these drugs is agranulocytosis (decrease in the number of white blood cells [eg, neutrophils, basophils, and eosinophils]). Reactions observed with agranulocytosis include hay fever, sore throat, skin rash, fever, or headache. Other major reactions include exfoliative dermatitis, granulocytopenia, aplastic anemia, hypoprothrombinemia, and hepatitis. Minor reactions, such as nausea, vomiting, and paresthesias, also may be seen.

Strong Iodine Solutions

Reactions that may be seen with strong iodine solution include symptoms of **iodism** (excessive amounts of iodine in the body), which are a metallic taste in the mouth, swelling and soreness of the parotid glands, burning of the mouth and throat, sore teeth and gums, symptoms of a head cold, and occasionally gastrointestinal upset. Allergy to iodine may also be seen and can be serious. Symptoms of iodine allergy include swelling of parts of the face and body, fever, joint pains, and sometimes difficulty in breathing. Difficulty breathing requires immediate medical attention.

Radioactive Iodine (¹³¹I)

Reactions after administration of ¹³¹I include sore throat, swelling in the neck, nausea, vomiting, cough, and pain on swallowing. Other reactions include bone marrow depression, anemia, leukopenia, thrombocytopenia, and tachycardia.

CONTRAINDICATIONS

The antithyroid drugs are contraindicated in patients with hypersensitivity to the drug or any constituent of the drug. Methimazole and propylthiouracil are contraindicated during pregnancy and lactation. Radioactive iodine is contraindicated during pregnancy (Pregnancy Category X) and lactation.

PRECAUTIONS

Methimazole and propylthiouracil are used with extreme caution during pregnancy (Pregnancy Category D) because they can cause hypothyroidism in the fetus. However, if an antithyroid drug is necessary during pregnancy or lactation, propylthiouracil is the drug most often prescribed. In many pregnant women thyroid dysfunction diminishes as the pregnancy proceeds, making a dosage reduction possible. Methimazole and propylthiouracil are used cautiously in patients older than 40 years because there is an increased risk of agranulocytosis and in patients with a decrease in bone marrow reserve (eg, after radiation therapy for cancer). Strong iodine preparations (except ¹³¹I) are classified as Pregnancy Category D and are used cautiously during pregnancy.

INTERACTIONS

There is an additive bone marrow depression when methimazole or propylthiouracil is administered with other bone marrow depressants, such as the antineoplastic drugs, or with radiation therapy. When methimazole is administered with digitalis, there is an increased effectiveness of the digitalis and increased risk of toxicity. There is an additive effect of propylthiouracil when the drug is administered with lithium, potassium iodide, or sodium iodide. When iodine products are administered with lithium products, synergistic hypothyroid activity is likely to occur.

NURSING PROCESS

● The Patient Receiving an Antithyroid Drug

ASSESSMENT

Preadministration Assessment

Before a patient starts therapy with an antithyroid drug, the nurse obtains a history of the symptoms of hyperthyroidism. It is important to include vital signs, weight, and a notation regarding the outward symptoms of the hyperthyroidism (see Table 51-1) in the physical assessment. If the patient is prescribed an iodine solution, it is essential that the nurse take a careful allergy history, particularly to iodine or seafood (which contains iodine).

Ongoing Assessment

During the ongoing assessment, the nurse observes the patient for adverse drug effects. During short-term therapy before surgery, adverse drug reactions are usually minimal. Long-term therapy is usually on an outpatient basis. The nurse questions the patient regarding relief of symptoms, as well as signs or symptoms indicating an adverse reaction related to the blood cells, such as fever, sore throat, easy bruising or bleeding, fever, cough, or any other signs of infection. As the patient becomes euthyroid, signs and symptoms of hyperthyroidism become less obvious. The nurse observes the patient for signs of **thyroid storm** (high fever, extreme tachycardia, and altered mental status), which can occur in patients whose hyperthyroidism is inadequately treated.

NURSING DIAGNOSES

Drug-specific nursing diagnoses are highlighted in the Nursing Diagnoses Checklist. Other nursing diagnoses applicable to these drugs are discussed in depth in Chapter 4.

PLANNING

The expected outcomes of the patient may include an optimal response to therapy, identification and management of adverse reactions, and an understanding of and compliance with the prescribed drug regimen.

IMPLEMENTATION

Promoting an Optimal Response to Therapy

The patient with an enlarged thyroid gland may have difficulty swallowing the tablet. If this occurs, the nurse discusses the problem with the primary health care provider. Strong iodine solution is measured in drops, which are added to water or fruit juice. This drug has a strong, salty taste. The patient is allowed to experiment with various types of fruit juices to determine which one best disguises the taste of the drug. Iodine solutions should be drunk through a straw because they may cause tooth discoloration.

Radioactive iodine is given by the primary health care provider, orally as a single dose. The effects of iodides are evident within 24 hours, with maximum effects attained after 10 to 15 days of continuous therapy. If the patient is hospitalized, radiation safety precautions identified by the hospital's department of nuclear medicine are followed.

Once a euthyroid state is achieved, the primary health care provider may add a thyroid hormone to the therapeutic regimen to prevent or treat hypothyroidism, which may develop slowly during long-term antithyroid drug therapy or after administration of [131]I.

The patient with hyperthyroidism is likely to have cardiac symptoms such as tachycardia or palpitations. Propranolol, a adrenergic blocking drug (see Chap. 21), may be prescribed by the primary health care provider as adjunctive treatment for several weeks until the therapeutic effects of the antithyroid drug are obtained.

The patient with hyperthyroidism may be concerned with the results of medical treatment and with the problem of taking the drug at regular intervals around the clock (usually every 8 hours). Whereas some patients may be awake early in the morning and retire late at night, others may experience difficulty in an 8-hour dosage schedule. Another concern may be a tendency to forget the first dose early in the morning, thus causing a problem with the two following doses.

If the patient expresses a concern about the dosage schedule, the nurse may be able to offer suggestions. For example, the nurse suggests the following 8-hour interval schedule: 7 AM, 3 PM, and 11 PM. The nurse may also suggest posting a notice on a bathroom mirror to remind the individual that the first dose is due immediately after rising. After a week or more of therapy, most patients remember to take their morning dose on time. If the first or last dose interferes with sleep, the nurse should suggest the patient discuss this with the primary health care provider.

Monitoring and Managing Adverse Drug Reactions

The nurse monitors the patient throughout therapy for adverse drug reactions. The nurse monitors the patient frequently for signs of agranulocytosis. It is important that the patient be protected from individuals with infectious disease because if agranulocytosis is present, the patient is at increased risk of contracting any infection, particularly an upper respiratory infection. The nurse monitors for signs of infection, particularly upper respiratory infection in visitors and other health care personnel.

> **Nursing Alert**
>
> *Agranulocytosis is potentially the most serious adverse reaction to methimazole and propylthiouracil. The nurse notifies the primary health care provider if fever, sore throat, rash, headache, hay fever, yellow discoloration of the skin, or vomiting occurs.*

If the patient experiences a rash while taking methimazole or propylthiouracil, the nurse carefully documents the affected areas, noting size, texture, and extent of the rash, and reports the occurrence of the rash to the primary health care provider. Soothing creams or lubricants may be applied, and soap is used sparingly, if at all, until the rash subsides.

When iodine solutions are administered, the nurse observes the patient closely for symptoms of iodism and iodine allergy (see Adverse Reactions). If these occur, the nurse withholds the drug and immediately notifies the primary health care provider. This is especially important if swelling around or in the mouth or difficulty in breathing occurs.

Educating the Patient and Family

The nurse reviews with the patient and family the dosage and times the drug is to be taken. The following additional teaching points are included in a teaching plan.

METHIMAZOLE AND PROPYLTHIOURACIL

- Take these drugs at regular intervals around the clock (eg, every 8 hours) unless directed otherwise by the primary health care provider.
- Do not take these drugs in larger doses or more frequently than as directed on the prescription container.
- Notify the primary health care provider promptly if any of the following occur: sore throat, fever, cough, easy bleeding or bruising, headache, or a general feeling of malaise.
- Record weight twice a week and notify the primary health care provider if there is any sudden weight gain or loss. (Note: the primary health care provider may also want the patient to monitor pulse rate. If this is recommended, the patient needs instruction in the proper technique and a recommendation to record the pulse rate and bring the record to the primary health care provider's office or clinic.)
- Avoid the use of nonprescription drugs unless the primary health care provider has approved the use of a specific drug.

STRONG IODINE SOLUTION

- Dilute the solution with water or fruit juice. Fruit juice often disguises the taste more than water does. Experiment with the types of fruit juice that best reduce the unpleasant taste of this drug.
- Discontinue the use of this drug and notify the primary health care provider if any of the following occur: skin rash, metallic taste in the mouth, swelling and soreness in front of the ears, sore teeth and gums, severe gastrointestinal distress, or symptoms of a head cold.

RADIOACTIVE IODINE

- Follow the directions of the department of nuclear medicine regarding precautions to be taken. (Note: In some instances, the dosage is small and no special precautions may be necessary.)
- Thyroid hormone replacement therapy may be necessary if hypothyroidism develops.
- Follow-up evaluations of the thyroid gland and the effectiveness of treatment with this drug are necessary.

EVALUATION

- The therapeutic effect is achieved.
- Adverse reactions are identified and reported to the primary health care provider.
- Anxiety is reduced.
- The patient verbalizes an understanding of the dosage regimen.
- The patient verbalizes the importance of complying with the prescribed treatment regimen.
- The patient and family demonstrate an understanding of the drug regimen.

● *Critical Thinking Exercises*

1. Ms. Hartman, age 47 years, has been prescribed levothyroxine (Synthroid) for hypothyroidism. Develop a teaching plan for Ms. Hartman that would provide her with the knowledge she needs to maintain a therapeutic treatment regimen.
2. Mr. Conrad will receive a dose of radioactive iodine from the primary health care provider. Discuss how you would prepare Mr. Conrad before the drug is administered. In preparation for dismissal, analyze the most important points to stress to Mr. Conrad about radioactive iodine.
3. Ms. Coker, age 38 years, is prescribed methimazole for hyperthyroidism. Discuss important preadministration assessments for Ms. Coker.

● *Review Questions*

1. What adverse reaction is most likely to occur in the early days of therapy in a patient taking a thyroid hormone?
   A. Congestive heart failure
   B. Hyperthyroidism
   C. Hypothyroidism
   D. Euthyroidism

2. The nurse informs the patient that therapy with a thyroid hormone may not produce a therapeutic response for _____.
   A. 24 to 48 days
   B. 1 to 3 days
   C. several weeks or more
   D. 8 to 12 months

3. Which of the following symptoms best indicates that serious adverse reactions are developing in a patient receiving methimazole (Tapazole)?
   A. Fever, sore throat, bleeding from an injection site
   B. Cough, periorbital edema, constipation
   C. Constipation, anorexia, blurred vision
   D. Unsteady gait, blurred vision, insomnia

4. Which of the following statements made by a patient would indicate to the nurse that the patient is experiencing an adverse reaction to radioactive iodine?
   A. "I am sleepy most of the day."
   B. "I am unable to sleep at night."
   C. "My throat hurts when I swallow."
   D. "My body aches all over."

● *Medication Dosage Problems*

1. Methimazole 60 mg is prescribed. The drug is available in 10-mg tablets. The nurse administers _____.
2. Levothyroxine 0.2 mg PO is prescribed. Available are 0.1-mg tablets. The nurse administers _____.

TABLE 52-1	Oral and Implantable Contraceptives

GENERIC NAME	TRADE NAME
Monophasic Oral Contraceptives	
50 mcg ethinyl estradiol acetate 1mg norethindrone	Necon 1/50, Norinyl 1+50, Ortho-Novum 1/50
50 mcg ethinyl estradiol, 1 mg ethynodiol diacetate	Demulen 1/50, Zovia 1/50E
50 mcg ethinyl estradiol, 0.5 mg norgestrel	Orgestrel, Ovral
35 mg ethinyl estradiol, 1 mg norethindrone	Necon 1/35, Norinyl 1+35, Ortho Novum 1/35
35 mcg ethinyl estradiol, 0.5 mg norethindrone	Brevicon, Modicon, Necon 0.5/35, Notrel
35 mcg ethinyl estradiol, 0.4 mg norethindrone	Ovcon-35
35 mcg ethinyl estradiol, 0.25 mg norgestimate	Ortho-Cyclen, Sprintex
35 mcg ethinyl estradiol, 1 mg ethynodiol diacetate	Demulen 1/35, Zovia 1/35 E
30 mcg ethinyl estradiol, 1.5 mg norethindrone acetate	Loestrin, 21 1.5/30, Loestrin Fe 1.5/30, Microgestin Fe 1.5/30
30 mcg ethinyl estradiol, 0.3 mg norgestrel	Lo/Ovral, Low-Ogestrel, Cryselle
30 mcg ethinyl estradiol, 0.15 mg desogestrel	Apri, Desogen, Ortho-Cept
30 mcg ethinyl estradiol, 0.15 mg levonorgestrel	Levler, Levora, Nordette, Portia
20 mcg ethinyl estradiol, 1 mg norethindrone acetate	Loestrin 21 1/20, Loestrin Fe 1/20, Microgestin Fe 1/20
20 mcg ethinyl estradiol, 0.1 mg levonorgestrel	Alesse, Aviane, Levlite
Biphasic Oral Contraceptives	
Phase one: 35 mcg ethinyl estradiol, 0.5 mg norethindrone Phase two: 35 mcg ethinyl estradiol, 1 mg norethindrone	Necon 10/11, Ortho-Novum 10/11
Triphasic Oral Contraceptives	
Phase one: 35 mcg ethinyl estradiol, 0.5 mg norethindrone Phase two: 35 mcg ethinyl estradiol, 1 mg norethindrone Phase three: 35 mcg ethinyl estradiol, 0.5 mg norethindrone	Tri-Norinyl
Phase one: 35 mcg ethinyl estradiol, 0.5 mg norethindrone Phase two: 35 mcg ethinyl estradiol, 0.75 mg norethindrone Phase three: 35 mcg ethinyl estradiol, 1 mg norethindrone	Ortho-Novum 7/7/7, Necon 7/7/7
Phase one: 30 mcg ethinyl estradiol, 0.05 mg levonorgestrel Phase two: 40 mcg ethinyl estradiol, 0.075 mg levonorgestrel Phase three: 30 mcg ethinyl estradiol, 0.125 mg levonorgestrel	Tri-Levlen, Triphasil, Trivora, Enpresse
Phase one: 35 mcg ethinyl estradiol, 0.18 mg norgestimate Phase two: 35 mcg ethinyl estradiol, 0.215 mg norgestimate Phase three: 35 mcg ethinyl estradiol, 0.25 mg norgestimate	Ortho Tri-Cyclen
Phase one: 25 mcg ethinyl estradiol, 0.18 mg norgestimate Phase two: 25 mcg ethinyl estradiol, 0.215 mg norgestimate Phase three: 25 mcg ethinyl estradiol, 0.25 mg norgestimate	Ortho Tri-Cyclen Lo
Phase one: 1 mg norethindrone acetate, 20 mcg ethinyl estradiol Phase two: 30 mcg ethinyl estradiol, 1 mg norethindrone acetate Phase three: 35 mcg ethinyl estradiol, 1 mg norethindrone acetate	Estrostep 21, Estrostep Fe
Phase one: 25 mcg ethinyl estradiol, 0.1 mg desogestrel Phase two: 25 mcg ethinyl estradiol, 0.125 mg desogestrel Phase three: 25 mcg ethinyl estradiol, 0.15 mg desogestrel	Cyclessa
Progestin Only Contraceptives	
0.35 mg norethindrone	Camila, Errin, Nor-QD, Nora-BE, Ortho Micronor
0.075 norgestrel	Ovrette
Implant Contraceptive Systems (Progestins)	
levonorgestrel: 6 capsules, each containing 36 mg levonorgestrel for subdermal implantation	Norplant System
progesterone: T-shaped unit containing 38 mg progesterone for insertion in the uterine cavity	Progestasert

combinations found in Ortho Tri-Cyclen have been shown to help reduce moderate acne and maintain clear skin in women 15 years of age or older (who menstruate, want contraception, and have no response to topical anti-acne medications).

ADVERSE REACTIONS

Estrogens

Administration of estrogens by any route may result in many adverse reactions, although the incidence and intensity of these reactions vary. Some of the adverse reactions seen with the administration of estrogens include:

- Central nervous system—headache, migraine, dizziness, mental depression
- Dermatologic—chloasma (pigmentation of the skin) or melasma (discoloration of the skin), which may continue when use of the drug is discontinued
- Gastrointestinal—nausea, vomiting, abdominal cramps, dermatitis, pruritus
- Genitourinary—breakthrough bleeding, withdrawal bleeding, spotting, change in menstrual flow, dysmenorrheal, premenstrual-like syndrome, amenorrhea, vaginal candidiasis, cervical erosion, vaginitis
- Local—pain at injection site, sterile abscess, redness and irritation at the application site with transdermal system
- Ophthalmic—steepening of corneal curvature, intolerance to contact lenses
- Miscellaneous—edema; changes in libido; breast pain, enlargement, and tenderness; reduced carbohydrate tolerance; venous thromboembolism; pulmonary embolism; increase or decrease in weight; skeletal pain

Warnings associated with the administration of estrogen include an increased risk of endometrial cancer, gallbladder disease, hypertension, hepatic adenoma (a benign tumor of the liver), cardiovascular disease, increased risk of thromboembolic disease, and hypercalcemia in those with breast cancer and bone metastases.

Progestins

Administration of the progestins by any route may result in many adverse reactions, although the incidence and intensity of these reactions varies. Progestin administration may result in breakthrough bleeding, spotting, change in the menstrual flow, amenorrhea, breast tenderness, edema, weight increase or decrease, acne, chloasma or melasma, and mental depression. In addition to the adverse reactions seen with progestins, the use of a levonorgestrel implant system may result in bruising after insertion, scar tissue formation at the site of insertion, and hyperpigmentation at the implant site. The use of medroxyprogesterone acetate contraceptive injection may result in the same adverse reactions as those associated with administration of any progestin.

Contraceptive Hormones

When estrogen/progestin combinations are used as oral contraceptives, the adverse reactions associated with the estrogens and the progestins must be considered. Because these drugs may exhibit adverse reactions that vary depending on their estrogen or progestin content, the adverse reactions of each must be considered. Table 52-2 identifies the symptoms of estrogen and progestin

TABLE 52-2	Estrogen and Progestin: Excess and Deficiency	
HORMONE*	**SIGNS OF EXCESS**	**SIGNS OF DEFICIENCY**
estrogen	Nausea, bloating, cervical mucorrhea (increased cervical discharge), polyposis (numerous ployps), melasma (discoloration of the skin), hypertension, migraine headache, breast fullness or tenderness, edema	Early or midcycle breakthrough bleeding, increased spotting, hypomenorrhea
progestin	Increased appetite, weight gain, tiredness, fatigue, hypomenorrhea, acne, oily scalp, hair loss, hirsutism (excessive growth of hair), depression, monilial vaginitis, breast regression	Late breakthrough bleeding, amenorrhea, hypermenorrhea

*Hormonal balance is achieved by adjusting the estrogen/progestin dosage. Oral contraceptives have different amounts of progestin and estrogen varying the estrogenic and progestational activity in each product.

excess or deficiency. The adverse effects are minimized by adjusting the estrogen progestin balance or dosage.

CONTRAINDICATIONS, PRECAUTIONS, AND INTERACTIONS

Estrogens

Estrogen therapy is contraindicated in patients with known hypersensitivity to the drugs, breast cancer (except for metastatic disease), estrogen-dependent neoplasms, undiagnosed abnormal genital bleeding, known or suspected pregnancy (Pregnancy Category X), and thromboembolic disorders.

The estrogens are used cautiously in patients with gallbladder disease, hypercalcemia (may lead to severe hypercalcemia in patients with breast cancer and bone metastasis), cardiovascular disease, and liver impairment.

The effects of the oral anticoagulants may be decreased when administered with the estrogens. When the estrogens are combined with the tricyclic antidepressants there is an increased risk of toxicity of the antidepressant. Barbiturates or rifampin may decrease estrogen blood levels, increasing the risk for breakthrough bleeding. When estrogens are administered concurrently with the hydantoins, breakthrough bleeding, spotting, and pregnancy have occurred. A loss of seizure control has also been reported. Cigarette smoking increases the risk for cardiovascular complications.

Progestins

The progestins are contraindicated in patients with known hypersensitivity to the drugs, thromboembolic disorders, cerebral hemorrhage, impaired liver function, and cancer of the breast or genital organs. Both the estrogens and progestins are classified as Pregnancy Category X drugs and are contraindicated during pregnancy. The progestins are used cautiously in patients with a history of migraine headaches, epilepsy, asthma, and cardiac or renal impairment.

The effects of the progestins are decreased when administered with anticonvulsants, barbiturates, or rifampin. Administration of the penicillins or tetracyclines with the oral contraceptives decreases the effects of the oral contraceptives.

Contraceptive Hormones

See the "Contraindications, Precautions, and Interactions" section regarding estrogens and progestins in this chapter for information regarding the combination oral contraceptives. The warnings associated with the use of oral contraceptives are the same as those for the estrogens and progestins and include cigarette smoking, which increases the risk of cardiovascular side effects,

such as venous and arterial thromboembolism, myocardial infarction, and thrombotic and hemorrhagic stroke. Also reported with oral contraceptive use are hepatic adenomas and tumors, visual disturbances, gallbladder disease, hypertension, and fetal abnormalities.

❀ Herbal Alert: Black Cohosh

Black cohosh, a herb reported to be beneficial in managing symptoms of menopause, is generally regarded as safe when used as directed. Black cohosh is a member of the buttercup flower family. The dosage of standardized extract is 2 tablets twice a day, or 40 drops of standardized tincture twice a day or one 500- to 600-mg tablet or capsule three times daily. Black cohosh tea is not considered as effective as other forms. Boiling of the root releases only a portion of the therapeutic constituents.

The benefits of black cohosh (not to be confused with blue cohosh) include:

- *Reduction in physical symptoms of menopause: hot flushes, night sweats, headaches, heart palpitations, dizziness, vaginal atrophy, and tinnitus (ringing in the ears)*
- *Decrease in psychological symptoms of menopause: insomnia, nervousness, irritability, and depression*
- *Improvement in menstrual cycles by balancing the hormones and reducing uterine spasms*

Adverse reactions are rare when using the recommended dosage. The most common adverse reaction is nausea. Black cohosh is contraindicated during pregnancy. Toxic effects include dizziness, headache, nausea, impaired vision, and vomiting. This herb is purported to be an alternative to hormone alternative replacement therapy (HART). Women who choose HART may increase their risk for endometrial cancer (cancer of the membrane lining the uterus), along with gallbladder disease, breast tenderness, high blood pressure, depression, and weight gain. Patients desiring to use any herbal remedy should consult with the primary health care provider before beginning therapy. Although no specific drug interactions have been reported, it is important that women taking HART should consult with their primary health care provider. In addition to its popularity as an herb for women's hormonal balance, black cohosh has been used for muscular and arthritic pain, headache, and eyestrain.

❀ Herbal Alert: Saw Palmetto

Saw palmetto is used to relieve the symptoms of benign prostatic hypertrophy. The herb reduces urinary frequency, increases the flow of urine, and decreases the incidence of nocturia. Saw palmetto may delay the need for prostate surgery. The dosage of the herb is:

- *160 mg twice daily of standardized extract*
- *One 585-mg capsule or tablet up to three times/day*
- *20 to 30 drops up to four times a day tincture (1:2 liquid extract)*

It is not recommended to take saw palmetto as a tea because the active constituents are not water soluble. Improvement can be seen after 1 to 3 months of therapy. It is usually recommended that the herb be taken for 6 months, followed by evaluation by a primary health care provider.

● **The Patient Receiving a Female Hormone**

ASSESSMENT

Preadministration Assessment

Before administering an estrogen or progestin, the nurse obtains a complete patient health history, including a menstrual history, which includes the **menarche** (age of onset of first menstruation), menstrual pattern, and any changes in the menstrual pattern (including a menopause history when applicable). In patients prescribed an estrogen (including oral contraceptives), the nurse obtains a history of thrombophlebitis or other vascular disorders, a smoking history, and a history of liver diseases. Blood pressure, pulse, and respiratory rate are taken and recorded. The primary health care provider usually performs a breast and pelvic examination and obtains a Pap smear before starting therapy. He or she may also order hepatic function tests.

If the male or female patient is being treated for a malignancy, the nurse enters in the patient's record a general evaluation of the patient's physical and mental status. The primary health care provider may also order laboratory tests, such as serum electrolytes and liver function tests.

Ongoing Assessments

ASSESSMENT OF THE OUTPATIENT. At the time of each office or clinic visit, the nurse obtains the blood pressure, pulse, respiratory rate, and weight. The nurse questions the patient regarding any adverse drug effects, as well as the result of drug therapy. For example, if the patient is receiving an estrogen for the symptoms of menopause, the nurse asks her to compare her original symptoms with the symptoms she is currently experiencing, if any. The nurse weighs the patient and reports a steady weight gain or loss. A periodic (usually annual) physical examination is performed by the primary health care provider and may include a pelvic examination, breast examination, Pap smear, and laboratory tests. The patient with a prostatic or breast carcinoma usually requires more frequent evaluations of response to drug therapy.

ASSESSMENT OF THE HOSPITALIZED PATIENT. The hospitalized patient receiving a female hormone requires careful monitoring. The nurse takes the vital signs daily or more often, depending on the patient's physical condition and the reason for drug use. The nurse observes the patient for adverse drug reactions, especially those related to the liver (the development of jaundice) or the cardiovascular system (thromboembolism). The nurse weighs the patient weekly or as ordered by the primary health care provider. The nurse

reports any significant weight gain or loss to the primary health care provider.

In patients with breast carcinoma or prostatic carcinoma, the nurse observes for and evaluates signs indicating a response to therapy, for example, a relief of pain, an increase in appetite, a feeling of well-being. In prostatic carcinoma, the response to therapy may be rapid, but in breast carcinoma the response is usually slow.

NURSING DIAGNOSES

Drug-specific nursing diagnoses are highlighted in the Nursing Diagnoses Checklist. Other nursing diagnoses applicable to these drugs are discussed in depth in Chapter 4.

PLANNING

The expected outcomes of the patient may include an optimal response to therapy, identification and management of adverse reactions, a reduction in anxiety, and an understanding of and compliance with the prescribed therapeutic regimen.

IMPLEMENTATION

Promoting an Optimal Response to Therapy

ESTROGENS. Estrogens may be administered orally, IM, IV, or intravaginally. Oral estrogens are administered with food or immediately after eating to reduce gastrointestinal upset. When estrogens are given vaginally for atrophic vaginitis, the nurse gives the patient instructions on proper use.

CONTRACEPTIVE HORMONES. The monophasic oral contraceptives are administered on a 21-day regimen, with the first tablet taken on the first Sunday after the menses begins or on the day the menses begin if the menses begin on Sunday. After the 21-day regimen, the next 7 days are skipped, then the cycle is begun again. With the biphasic oral contraceptives, the first phase is 10 days of a smaller dosage of progestin, and the second phase is a larger amount of progestin.

Nursing Diagnoses Checklist

☑ **Ineffective Tissue Perfusion** related to adverse reactions (thromboembolic effects)

☑ **Excess Fluid Volume** related to adverse reactions (sodium and water retention)

☑ **Imbalanced Nutrition: More or Less than Body Requirements** related to adverse reactions (weight gain or loss)

☑ **Anxiety** related to diagnosis, use of estrogen replacement therapy, other factors

The estrogen dosage remains constant for 21 days, followed by no estrogen for 7 days. Some regimens contain seven placebo tablets for easier management of the therapeutic regimen. With the triphasic oral contraceptives, the estrogen amount stays the same or may vary and the progestin amount varies throughout the 21-day cycle. Progestin-only oral contraceptives are taken daily and continuously.

IMPLANT CONTRACEPTIVE SYSTEM. Levonorgestrel, a progestin, is available as an implant contraceptive system (Norplant System). Six capsules, each containing levonorgestrel, are implanted under local anesthesia in the subdermal (below the skin) tissues of the mid-portion of the upper arm. The capsules provide contraceptive protection for 5 years but may be removed at any time at the request of the patient. See Table 52-3 for more information on ways to promote an optimal response when taking the contraceptive hormones.

MEDROXYPROGESTERONE ACETATE CONTRACEPTIVE INJECTION. Medroxyprogesterone acetate (Depo-Provera), a synthetic progestin used in the treatment of abnormal uterine bleeding and secondary amenorrhea, is also used as a contraceptive. This drug is given IM every 3 months, and the initial dosage is given within the first 5 days of menstruation or within 5 days postpartum. When this drug is given IM, the solution must be shaken vigorously before use to ensure uniform suspension, and the drug is given deep IM into the gluteal or deltoid muscle.

> ### ☀ Nursing Alert
>
> *If the interval is greater than 14 weeks between the IM injections, the nurse must be certain that the patient is not pregnant before administering the next injection.*

Monitoring and Managing Adverse Reactions

The patient prescribed the female hormones usually takes them for several months or years. Throughout that time, the patient must be monitored for adverse reactions (see "Ongoing Assessment"). These drugs are self-administered at home. This makes patient education an important avenue for detecting and managing adverse reactions.

With the estrogens it is important to monitor for breakthrough bleeding. If breakthrough bleeding occurs with either the estrogens or progestin, the patient notifies the primary health care provider. A dosage change may be necessary.

Gastrointestinal upsets, such as nausea, vomiting, abdominal cramps, and bloating may also occur. Nausea usually decreases or subsides within 1 to 2 months of therapy. However, until that time the discomfort may lessen if the drug is taken with food. If nausea is continual, frequent small meals may help. If nausea and vomiting persist, an antiemetic may be prescribed. Bloating may be lessened with light to moderate exercise or by limiting fluid intake with meals.

The nurse carefully monitors the patient with diabetes who is taking female hormones. The primary health care provider is notified if blood glucose levels are elevated or the urine is positive for glucose or ketone bodies because a change in the dosage of insulin or the oral hypoglycemic drug may be required. See Chapter 49 for how to manage hypo- and hyperglycemic episodes.

MANAGING SODIUM AND WATER RETENTION. Sodium and water retention may occur during female hormone therapy. In addition to reporting any swelling of the hands, ankles, or feet to the primary health care provider, the nurse weighs the hospitalized patient daily, keeps an accurate record of the intake and output, encourages ambulation (if not on bed rest), and helps the patient to eat a diet low in sodium (if prescribed by the primary health care provider).

MANAGING THROMBOEMBOLIC EFFECTS. The nurse monitors the patient for signs of thromboembolic effects, such as pain, swelling, tenderness in the extremities, headache, chest pain, and blurred vision. These adverse effects are reported to the primary health care provider. Patients with previous venous insufficiency, who are on bed rest for other medical reasons, or who smoke are at increased risk for thromboembolic effects. The nurse encourages the patient to elevate the lower extremities when sitting, if possible, and to exercise the lower extremities by walking.

> ### ☀ Nursing Alert
>
> *There is an increased risk of post-operative thromboembolic complications in women taking oral contraceptives. If possible, use of the drug is discontinued at least 4 weeks before a surgical procedure associated with thromboembolism or during prolonged immobilization.*

MANAGING ALTERATIONS IN NUTRITION. Alterations in nutrition can occur, resulting in significant weight gain or loss. Weight gain occurs more frequently than weight loss. The nurse encourages a daily diet that includes adequate amounts of protein and carbohydrates and that is low in fats. A variety of nutritious foods (fruits, vegetables, grains, cereals, meats, and poultry) should be included in the daily diet, with portion sizes decreased to meet individual needs. A dietitian may be consulted if necessary. An exercise program is helpful in both losing weight and maintaining weight loss.

TABLE 52-3	Contraceptive Hormones

GENERIC AND TRADE NAME*	PROMOTING AN OPTIMAL RESPONSE
emergency contraceptives (Plan B, Preven)	Used for emergency contraception after unprotected intercourse. When using Plan B take one tablet within 72 h after unprotected intercourse. The second dose of Plan B is taken 12 h later. When using Preven take 2 tablets within 72 h of unprotected intercourse and the last 2 tablets 12 h after the first dose. These drugs can be used anytime during the menstrual cycle. If vomiting occurs within 1 hour after taking either dose, notify the primary health care provider. Emergency contraceptives are not effective in terminating an existing pregnancy. Should not be used as a routine form of contraception.
etonogestrel/ethinyl estradiol vaginal ring (Nuvaring, *generic*)	The woman inserts vaginal ring in the vagina, where it remains continuously for 3 weeks. Remove for 1 week, during which bleeding usually occurs (usually 2–3 days after removal). Insert new ring 1 week after the last ring removed on the same day of the week as it was inserted in the previous cycle. Do this even if bleeding is not finished. Insertion: Position for insertion by the woman may be standing with one leg up, squatting, or lying down. Compress the ring and insert into the vagina. (The exact position of the vaginal ring inside the vagina is not critical to its effectiveness.) The vaginal ring is removed after 3 weeks on the same day of the week as it was started. Removal is accomplished by hooking the index finger under the forward rim or by grasping the rim between the index finger and pulling it out. Discard the used ring in the foil pouch in a waste receptacle out of the reach of children or pets. (Do not flush the ring down the toilet.) Consider the menstrual cycle, ovulation, and the possibility of pregnancy before beginning treatment. The vaginal ring may be accidentally expelled (eg, when it was not inserted properly, during straining for defecation, removing a tampon, or with severe constipation). If this occurs, rinse the vaginal ring with lukewarm water and reinsert promptly. (If the ring has been out of the vagina for more than 3 h, contraceptive effectiveness may be reduced and an alternate contraceptive must be used for the next 7 days. The most common adverse reactions leading to discontinuation include: device-related problems (eg, foreign body sensations, coital problems, device expulsion). Other adverse reactions include vaginitis, headache, upper respiratory tract infection, leukorrhea, sinusitis, weight gain, and nausea.
intrauterine progesterone contraceptive system (Progestasert)	Intrauterine contraception device (IUD) for women who have had at least one child, are in a stable monogamous relationship, and have no history of pelvic inflammatory disease (PID). There is an increased risk of PID associated with IUD use, most often occurring within the first 4 months of use. The device prevents uterine pregnancy but it does not prevent ovulation or ectopic (implantation of the fertilized egg outside of the uterus) pregnancy. Before insertion, a complete medical and social history is performed, including Pap smear, gonorrhea, and *Chlamydia* culture, and tests for other sexually transmitted diseases. The patient is reexamined shortly after the first menses after insertion or within the first 3 months and at any time the patient exhibits symptoms. The device is removed for the following reasons: pelvic infection, endometritis, genital actinomycosis (a noncontagious bacterial infection), intractable pelvic pain, pregnancy, endometrial or cervical malignancy, increase in length of the threads extending from the cervix or any other indication of partial expulsion. Retrieval threads should be visible. If they are not visible, they may have retracted into the uterus or have been broken. After menstrual period, determine if the threads still protrude from the cervix. If threads are not found, the system is considered displaced and removed. Caution the patient not to pull the threads. If partial expulsion occurs, removal is indicated and a new system inserted. For the first few weeks after insertion, bleeding and cramping may occur. If symptoms continue or become severe, the health care provider is contacted.

(continued)

TABLE 52-3	Contraceptive Hormones (*Continued*)

GENERIC AND TRADE NAME*	PROMOTING AN OPTIMAL RESPONSE
	Prophylactic antibiotics may be prescribed before IUD insertion to decrease the risk of PID.
	Patient package insert and instructions are available with the product. The primary health care provider should be notified if any of the following occurs: abnormal or excessive bleeding, severe cramping, abnormal or odorous vaginal discharge, fever or flu-like symptoms, pain, genital lesions, or missed periods.
	The device is replaced every 12 months.
levonorgestrel implants *lev'-oh-nor-jes-trel* (Norplant System)	An informed consent may be required in some institutions before this procedure. A surgical incision is required to insert six capsules. Removal also requires surgical Intervention. The capsules are inserted during the first 7 days of the cycle or immediately after an abortion. Irregular menstrual bleeding, spotting, prolonged episodes of bleeding, and amenorrhea may occur. These symptoms diminish with continued use.
levonorgestrel-releasing intrauterine system (LRIS) *lev'-oh-nor-jes-trel* (Mirena)	Before insertion, provide the patient with the patient package insert. LRIS is an intrauterine contraception device for use of not more than 5 years. Inserted with the provided inserter into the uterine cavity within 7 days of the onset of menstruation or immediately after the first trimester abortion. Teach the patient to check after each menstrual period to make certain that the thread still protrudes from the cervix and caution her not to pull the thread. If pregnancy occurs with the LRIS in place, the LRIS should be removed. If the LRIS is not removed there is an increase in the risk of miscarriage, sepsis, premature labor, and premature delivery. Monitor the woman for flu-like symptoms, fever, chills, cramping, pain, bleeding, vaginal discharge, or leakage of fluid. Before insertion a complete medical and social history, including that of the partner, is obtained to determine conditions that might influence the use of an IUD. Initial insertion is done by the physician within 7 days of the onset of a menstrual period. Re-examination and evaluation is done shortly after the first menses or within the first 3 months after insertion. Menstrual flow usually decreases after the first 3–6 months of LRIS use; therefore, an increase of menstrual flow may indicate expulsion of the device. Symptoms of partial or complete expulsion include pain and bleeding. However, the LRIS can be expelled without any noticeable effects.
medroxyprogesterone acetate/estradiol cypionate (MPA/E2C) (Lunelle) *me-drox'-ee-proe-jess'-te-rone*	The first injection is given during the first 5 days of a normal menstrual period and is administered no earlier than 4 weeks after delivery if not breastfeeding or 6 weeks if breastfeeding. Second and subsequent injections given monthly (28–30 days) after the previous injection, not to exceed 33 days. Give patient a copy of the patient labeling before administration of the drug. The injection schedules are indicated according to the number of days and not bleeding episodes. If any patient misses 2 consecutive menstrual periods, the possibility of pregnancy should be considered. Another form of contraception should be used if the monthly dosage is late (more than 33 days since the last injection). Menstrual bleeding patterns are usually disrupted but should normalize. Irregular bleeding, amenorrhea, and excessive or prolonged bleeding should be reported to the health care provider.
medroxyprogesterone contraceptive injection (Depo-Provera) *me-drox'-ee-proe-jess'-te-rone*	Long-term injectable contraceptive administered IM every 3 months. The injection is given only during the first 5 days after the onset of a normal menstrual period, within 5 days postpartum if not breastfeeding, or at 6 weeks postpartum. Bleeding irregularities may occur (ie, irregular or unpredictable bleeding or spotting, or heavy continuous bleeding). Bleeding usually decreases to amenorrhea as the treatment continues. The drug is not readministered if there is a sudden partial or complete loss of vision or if the patient experiences ptosis, diplopia, or migraine.
norelgestromin/ethinyl estradiol transdermal system (Ortho Evra) *nor-el-jes'-tro-min*	A 28-day cycle, with a new patch applied each week for 3 weeks. Week 4 is patch free. Apply new patch on the same day each week (note patch change day on the calendar).

TABLE 52-3	Contraceptive Hormones (*Continued*)

GENERIC AND TRADE NAME*	PROMOTING AN OPTIMAL RESPONSE
	Discard used patch (only wear one patch at a time).
	Patch is applied to clean, dry, intact, healthy skin on the buttock, abdomen, upper outer arm, or upper torso in a place where the patch will not be rubbed by clothing.
	Patch should not be placed on the breast or on areas that are red or irritated.
	Beginning treatment: First day start (apply first patch on the first day of the menstrual cycle) or Sunday start (apply first patch on the first Sunday after the menstrual period begins).
	Use no creams or lotions on area where patch is to be applied.
	A backup contraceptive should be used for the first week of the **first** treatment cycle.
	Patch partially or completely detached for no longer that 24 hours: reapply to the same place or replace with a new patch immediately (no backup contraception needed).
	Patch detached for more than 24 hours: apply new patch immediately (new patch change day). Backup contraception needed for the first week (7 days).
	Forgets to change patch: begin again immediately with new patch change day (backup contraception needed for the first 7 days).
	If breakthrough bleeding continues longer than a few cycles, a cause other than the patch should be considered.
	Bleeding should occur during the patch-free week. If no bleeding occurs, consider the possibility of pregnancy.
	If pregnancy is confirmed, discontinue treatment.

*The term *generic* indicates that the drug is available in generic form.

Weight loss is often as difficult to manage as weight gain. When a patient taking the female hormones has a decrease in appetite and loses weight, the nurse encourages the individual to increase protein, carbohydrates, and calories in the diet. Small feedings with several daily snacks are usually better tolerated in those with a loss of appetite than are three larger meals. Patients are encouraged to eat foods that they like. Dietary supplements may be necessary if a significant weight loss occurs. A dietitian may be consulted if necessary. Weights are usually taken on a weekly, rather than daily, basis.

Managing Anxiety

The woman taking female hormones may have many concerns about therapy with these drugs. Some concerns may be based on inaccurate knowledge; for example, the woman who hears incorrect facts about certain dangers associated with female hormones. Although there are dangers associated with long-term use of female hormones, many of these adverse reactions occur in a small number of patients. When the patient is closely followed up by the primary health care provider, the dangers associated with long-term use are often minimized.

Some women may be anxious because of a fear of experiencing uterine cancer as the result of taking ERT. The nurse explains that taking progestin, which counteracts the negative effect of estrogen, can prevent estrogen-induced cancer of the uterus. Other women may fear the development of breast cancer. Most research studies find that there is little risk for breast cancer developing and that the benefits of ERT often outweigh the risk of breast cancer.

The nurse encourages the patient to ask questions about her therapy. Information that is inaccurate is clarified before therapy is started. The nurse refers to the primary health care provider questions that cannot or should not be answered by a nurse.

The male patient with inoperable prostatic carcinoma also may have concerns about taking a female hormone. The nurse assures the patient that the dosage is carefully regulated and that feminizing effects, if they occur, are usually minimal.

Educating the Patient and Family

The instructions for starting oral contraceptive therapy vary with the product used. Each product has detailed patient instruction sheets regarding starting oral contraceptive therapy, and the nurse reviews them with the patient. The instructions for missed doses also are included in the package insert and are reviewed with the patient.

The nurse gives the patient a thorough explanation of the dose regimen and adverse reactions that may be seen with the prescribed drug. The nurse advises those taking oral contraceptives that skipping a dose could result in pregnancy. See Table 52-3 for more information to include in a teaching plan for a woman taking the contraceptive hormones.

In most instances, the primary health care provider performs periodic examinations, for example, laboratory tests, a pelvic examination, or a Pap smear. The patient is encouraged to keep all appointments for follow-up evaluation of therapy. The nurse includes several points in a teaching plan.

Estrogens and Progestins

- A patient package insert is available with the drug. Read the information carefully. If there are any questions about this information, discuss them with the primary health care provider.
- If gastrointestinal upset occurs, take the drug with food.
- Notify the primary health care provider if any of the following occurs: pain in the legs or groin area, sharp chest pain or sudden shortness of breath, lumps in the breast, sudden severe headache, dizziness or fainting, vision or speech disturbances, weakness or numbness in the arms or legs, severe abdominal pain, depression, or yellowing of the skin or eyes.
- Female patient: If pregnancy is suspected or abnormal vaginal bleeding occurs, stop taking the drug and contact the primary health care provider immediately.
- Patient with diabetes: Check the blood glucose or urine daily, or more often. Contact the primary health care provider if the blood glucose is elevated or if the urine is positive for glucose or ketones. An elevated blood glucose level or urine positive for glucose or ketones may require a change in diabetic therapy (insulin, oral hypoglycemic drug) or diet; these changes must be made by the primary health care provider.

Oral Contraceptives

- A patient package insert is available with the drug. Read the information carefully. Begin the first dose as directed in the package insert or as directed by the primary health care provider. If there are any questions about this information, discuss them with the primary health care provider.
- To obtain a maximum effect, take this drug as prescribed and at intervals not exceeding once every 24 hours. An oral contraceptive is best taken with the evening meal or at bedtime. The effectiveness of this drug depends on following the prescribed dosage schedule. Failure to comply with the dosage schedule may result in a pregnancy.
- Use an additional method of birth control (as recommended by the primary health care provider) until after the first week in the initial cycle.
- If one day's dose is missed, take the missed dose as soon as remembered or take 2 tablets the next day. If 2 days are missed, take 2 tablets for the next 2 days and continue on with the normal dosing schedule. However, another form of birth control must be used until the cycle is completed and a new cycle is begun. If 3 days in a row or more are missed, discontinue use of the drug and use another form of birth control until a new cycle can begin. Before restarting the dosage regimen, make sure a pregnancy did not result from the break in the dosage regimen.
- If there are any questions regarding what to do about a missed dose, discuss the procedure with the primary health care provider.
- Avoid smoking or excessive exposure to secondhand smoke while taking these drugs; cigarette smoking during estrogen therapy may increase the risk of cardiovascular effects.
- Report adverse reactions such as fluid retention or edema to the extremities; weight gain; pain, swelling, or tenderness in the legs; blurred vision; chest pain; yellowed skin or eyes; dark urine; or abnormal vaginal bleeding.
- While taking these drugs, periodic examinations by the primary health care provider and laboratory tests are necessary.

Estradiol Transdermal System

- Alora, Estraderm, Esclim, and Vivelle are applied twice a week; Climara and FemPatch are applied every 7 days.
- Apply the system immediately after opening the pouch, with the adhesive side down (Fig. 52-1). Apply to clean, dry skin of the trunk (not breast or waistline), buttocks, abdomen, upper inner thigh, or upper arm. (Do not apply to breasts or a site exposed to sunlight.) The area should not be oily or irritated.
- Press the system firmly in place with the palm of the hand for about 10 seconds. The application site is rotated with at least 1-week intervals between applications to a particular site.
- Avoid areas that may be exposed to rubbing or where clothing may rub the system off or loosen the edges.
- Remove the old system before applying a new system unless the primary health care provider directs

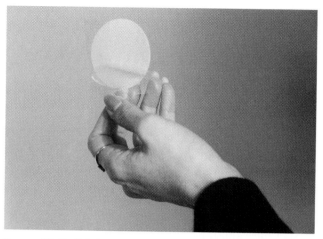

FIGURE 52-1. This low-dose estrogen transdermal patch, available as the trade name Estraderm (Estradiol Transdermal System), is transparent and about the size of a silver dollar. It releases small amounts of estrogen directly into the bloodstream at a constant and controlled rate to a female requiring estrogen replacement therapy for postmenopausal symptoms.

otherwise. Rotate application sites to prevent skin irritation.

- Follow the directions of the primary health care provider regarding application of the system (eg, continuous, 3 weeks use followed by 1 week off, changed weekly, or applied twice weekly).
- If the system falls off, reapply it or apply a new system. Continue the original treatment schedule.

Intravaginal Application

- Use the applicator correctly. Refer to the package insert for correct procedure. The applicator is marked with the correct dosage and accompanies the drug when purchased.
- Wash the applicator after each use in warm water with a mild soap and rinse well.
- Maintain a recumbent position for at least 30 minutes after instillation.
- Use a sanitary napkin or panty liner to protect clothing if necessary.
- Do not double the dosage if a dose is missed. Instead, skip the dose and resume treatment the next day (see Patient and Family Teaching Checklist: Self-Administering Intravaginal Estrogen).
- When using the vaginal ring, press the ring into an oval and insert into the upper third of the vaginal vault.

EVALUATION

- The therapeutic effect is achieved.
- Adverse reactions are identified, reported to the primary health care provider, and managed using appropriate nursing interventions.

Patient and Family Teaching Checklist

Self-Administering Intravaginal Estrogen

The nurse:

✔ Explains the reason for the drug and prescribed therapy, including drug name, correct dosage, and frequency of administration.
✔ Describes the equipment to be used.
✔ Reinforces the need to empty the bladder and wash hands before administration.
✔ Demonstrates step-by-step procedure for filling applicator with drug and administration.
✔ Recommends a supine position with knees flexed and legs spread.
✔ Instructs patient to insert applicator into vagina, angling it toward the tailbone and advancing it about 2 inches.
✔ Warns that drug may feel cold when inserted.
✔ Urges patient to remain recumbent for about 30 minutes after inserting drug.
✔ Suggests use of sanitary pad or napkin to prevent staining of clothes.
✔ Advises patient to wash applicator with mild soap and warm water, rinse well, and dry with paper towel after use.
✔ Cautions not to double dose if dose is missed but to skip dose and resume treatment the next day.
✔ Encourages daily inspection of perineal area for irritation or signs of allergic reaction.

- Anxiety is reduced.
- The patient verbalizes an understanding of the dosage regimen and the importance of continued follow-up care.
- The patient verbalizes the importance of complying with the prescribed therapeutic regimen.

● Critical Thinking Exercises

1. *Ms. Burton is receiving methyltestosterone (Oreton Methyl) for treatment of metastatic breast cancer. The drug has caused changes in her appearance, namely deepening of her voice, some male pattern baldness, and facial hair. Analyze the situation and decide what suggestions you could give this patient who has a limited income and may be unable to afford extensive cosmetic and wardrobe changes.*
2. *John, a friend of your brother, has started to use anabolic steroids to increase his strength and muscle mass*

to improve his chances of getting a football scholarship. Your brother tells you that this is acceptable because his friend wants an education. Discuss what you would tell your brother.

3. *Susan Parker, a mother of three young children, calls the health clinic where you work stating that she has missed 3 days of oral contraceptives when she was ill. She wants to know if she can continue with the oral contraceptive. Discuss what information Susan needs to know to protect herself from becoming pregnant.*

● Review Questions

1. The nurse monitors the patient taking an anabolic steroid for the more severe adverse reactions, which include _____.

   A. anorexia
   B. nausea and vomiting
   C. severe mental changes
   D. acne

2. The nurse must be aware that older men taking the androgens are _____.

   A. prone to urinary problems
   B. at greater risk for hypertension
   C. at increased risk for confusion
   D. at increased risk for prostate cancer

3. When monitoring a patient taking an oral contraceptive, the nurse would observe the patient for signs of excess progestin. Which of the following reactions would indicate to the nurse that a patient has an excess of progestin?

   A. Increased appetite, hair loss
   B. Virilization, constipation
   C. Nausea, early breakthrough bleeding
   D. Deepening of the voice, light-headedness

4. A patient calls the outpatient clinic and says that she missed one day's dose of her "birth control pills." Which of the following statements would be most appropriate for the nurse to make to the patient?

   A. Do not take an additional tablet but resume the regular schedule today.
   B. Discontinue use of the drug and use another type of contraceptive until after your next menstrual period.
   C. Take 2 tablets today; then resume the regular daily schedule.
   D. Come into the office immediately for a pregnancy test.

5. When teaching the patient taking an oral contraceptive for the first time, the nurse emphasizes the importance of taking _____.

   A. two tablets per day at the first sign of ovulation
   B. the drug at the same time each day
   C. the drug early in the morning before arising
   D. the drug each day for 20 days beginning on the first of the month

● Medication Dosage Problems

1. Medroxyprogesterone 650 mg IM is prescribed. The drug is available in a solution of 400 mg/mL. The nurse administers _____.

2. The physician prescribes estrone 0.5 mg IM for a postmenopausal woman with vasomotor symptoms. On hand is a vial of estrone with a solution containing 0.5 mg/mL. The nurse administers _____.

Drugs Acting on the Uterus

Key Terms

ergotism
oxytocic
oxytocin

uterine atony
uterine relaxants
water intoxication

Chapter Objectives

On completion of this chapter, the student will:

- Discuss the actions, uses, adverse reactions, contraindications, precautions, and interactions of drugs acting on the uterus.
- Discuss important preadministration and ongoing assessment activities the nurse should perform on the patient taking an oxytocic drug or uterine relaxant.
- List some nursing diagnoses particular to a patient taking an oxytocic drug or uterine relaxant.
- Discuss ways to promote an optimal response to therapy, how to manage adverse reactions, and important points to keep in mind when educating patients about the use of an oxytocic drug or uterine relaxant.

Drug therapy is beneficial for use in labor and delivery to promote the well-being of the woman and fetus. Depending on the patient's need, drugs may be used to stimulate, intensify, or inhibit uterine contractions. The two types of drugs discussed in this chapter for their effect on the uterus are the oxytocics and the uterine relaxants. Drugs acting on the uterus are listed in the Summary Drug Table: Drugs Acting on the Uterus.

OXYTOCIC DRUGS

Oxytocic drugs are drugs that are used in antepartum (before birth of the neonate) to induce uterine contractions similar to those of normal labor. These drugs are desirable when early vaginal delivery is in the best interest of the woman and the fetus.

An oxytocic drug is one that stimulates the uterus. Included in this group of drugs are ergonovine (Ergotrate), methylergonovine (Methergine), and oxytocin (Pitocin).

ACTION AND USES

Ergonovine and Methylergonovine

Ergonovine and methylergonovine both increase the strength, duration, and frequency of uterine contractions and decrease the incidence of uterine bleeding. They are given after the delivery of the placenta and are used to prevent postpartum and postabortal hemorrhage caused by **uterine atony** (marked relaxation of the uterine muscle).

Oxytocin

Oxytocin is an endogenous hormone produced by the posterior pituitary gland (see Chap. 50). This hormone has uterine-stimulating properties, especially on the pregnant uterus. As pregnancy progresses, the sensitivity of the uterus to oxytocin increases, reaching peak sensitivity immediately before the birth of the infant. This sensitivity enables oxytocic drugs to exert their full therapeutic effect on the uterus and produce the desired results. Oxytocin also has antidiuretic and vasopressor effects. The exact role of oxytocin in normal labor and medically induced labor is not well understood.

SUMMARY DRUG TABLE DRUGS ACTING ON THE UTERUS

GENERIC NAME	TRADE NAME*	USES	ADVERSE REACTIONS	DOSAGE RANGES
Oxytocics				
ergonovine maleate *er-goe-noe'-veen*	Ergotrate, *generic*	Uterine atony and hemorrhage	Nausea, vomiting, elevated blood pressure, temporary chest pain, dizziness, headache	0.2 mg IM, IV q2–4h
methylergonovine maleate *meth-ill-er-goe-noe'-veen*	Methergine	Routine management after delivery of the placenta, uterine atony, and hemorrhage	Nausea, vomiting, elevated blood pressure, transient chest pain, dizziness, headache	0.2 mg IM, IV after delivery of the placenta; 0.2 mg PO TID, QID
oxytocin (parenteral) *ox-i-toe'-sin*	Pitocin, Syntocinon, *generic*	Antepartum: to initiate or improve uterine contractions; postpartum: to produce uterine contractions in third stage of labor, control of postpartum bleeding and hemorrhage	Nausea, vomiting, uterine hypertonicity or rupture, fetal bradycardia, water intoxication, cardiac arrhythmias, anaphylactic reactions	Induction of labor: 1–2 mU/min IV infusion, gradually increase dosage by 1–2 mU/min with maximum dosage 20 mU/min; postpartum bleeding: IV infusion of 10–40 U in 1000 mL; 10 U IM
Uterine Relaxants				
ritodrine hydrochloride *ri'-toe-dreen*	Yutopar, *generic*	Preterm labor	Alterations in fetal and maternal heart rates and maternal blood pressure, palpitations, headache, nausea, vomiting	IV: 0.05–0.35 mg/min depending on patient response
terbutaline *ter-byoo'-ta-leen*	Brethaire, Brethine, *generic*	Preterm labor	Nervousness, restlessness, tremor, headache, anxiety, hypertension, palpitations, arrhythmias, hypokalemia, pulmonary edema	Preterm labor: IV 10 mcg/min q10 min up to 80 mcg/min; SQ: 250 mcg qh until contractions stop; PO: 2.5 mg q4–6h until delivery

*The term *generic* indicates the drug is available in generic form.

Oxytocin is administered intravenously (IV) for starting or improving labor contractions to obtain an early vaginal delivery of the fetus. An early vaginal delivery may be indicated when there are fetal or maternal problems, for example, a woman with diabetes and a large fetus, Rh problems, premature rupture of the membranes, uterine inertia, and eclampsia or preeclampsia (also called pregnancy-induced hypertension). Preeclampsia is a condition of pregnancy characterized by hypertension, headaches, albuminuria, and edema of the lower extremities occurring at or near term. The condition may progressively worsen until eclampsia (a serious condition occurring between the 20th week of pregnancy and the end of the first week postpartum and characterized by convulsive seizures and coma) occurs. Oxytocin may also be used in the management of inevitable or incomplete abortion. Oxytocin is given intramuscularly (IM) during the third stage of labor (period from the time the neonate is expelled until the placenta is expelled) to produce uterine contractions and control postpartum bleeding and hemorrhage. It may also be used intranasally to stimulate the milk ejection (milk letdown) reflex.

ADVERSE REACTIONS

Ergonovine and Methylergonovine

The adverse reactions associated with ergonovine and methylergonovine include nausea, vomiting, elevated blood pressure, temporary chest pain, dizziness, water intoxication, and headache. Allergic reactions may also be seen. In some instances hypertension associated with seizure or headache may occur. **Ergotism** (overdosage of ergonovine) is manifested by nausea, vomiting, abdominal pain, numbness, tingling of the extremities, and an increase in blood pressure. In severe cases, these symptoms are followed by hypotension, respiratory depression, hypothermia, gangrene of the fingers and toes, convulsions, hallucinations, and coma.

Oxytocin

Administration of oxytocin may result in fetal brady-cardia, uterine rupture, uterine hypertonicity, nausea, vomiting, cardiac arrhythmias, and anaphylactic reactions. Serious **water intoxication** (fluid overload, fluid volume excess) may occur, particularly when the drug is administered by continuous infusion and the patient is receiving fluids by mouth. When used as a nasal spray, adverse reactions are rare.

CONTRAINDICATIONS, PRECAUTIONS, AND INTERACTIONS

Ergonovine and Methylergonovine

Ergonovine is contraindicated in those with known hypersensitivity to the drug, hypertension, and before the delivery of the placenta. Ergonovine is used cautiously in patients with heart disease, obliterative vascular disease, renal or hepatic disease, and during lactation.

Methylergonovine is contraindicated in patients with a known hypersensitivity to the drug, hypertension, and preeclampsia and should not be used to induce labor (Pregnancy Category C). Methylergonovine is used cautiously in patients with renal or hepatic impairment. When methylergonovine is administered concurrently with vasopressors or to patients who are heavy cigarette smokers, excessive vasoconstriction may occur.

Oxytocin

Oxytocin is contraindicated in patients with known hypersensitivity to the drug, cephalopelvic disproportion, unfavorable fetal position or presentation, in obstetric emergencies, situations of fetal distress when delivery is not imminent, severe toxemia (preeclampsia, eclampsia), hypertonic uterus, during pregnancy (intranasal administration), when there is total placenta previa, or to induce labor when vaginal delivery is contraindicated. Oxytocin is not expected to be a risk to the fetus when administered as indicated. When oxytocin is administered with vasopressors, severe hypertension may occur.

NURSING PROCESS

● **The Patient Receiving an Oxytocic Drug**

ASSESSMENT

Preadministration Assessment

Before starting an IV infusion of oxytocin for the induction of labor, the nurse obtains an obstetric history (parity, gravidity, previous obstetric problems, type of labor, stillbirths, abortions, live birth infant abnormalities)

and a general health history. Immediately before starting the IV infusion of oxytocin, the nurse assesses the fetal heart rate (FHR) and the patient's blood pressure, pulse, and respiratory rate.

In addition, the nurse assesses and records the activity of the uterus (strength, duration, and frequency of contractions, if any). Monitoring of the uterine contractions for strength and length of the contractions can be done with the use of an external monitor or by an internal uterine catheter with an electronic monitor. A fetal monitor is placed to assess the FHR.

Ergonovine and methylergonovine may be given orally during the postpartum period to reduce the possibility of postpartum hemorrhage and to prevent relaxation of the uterus. When the patient is to receive either of these drugs after delivery, it is important to take the blood pressure, pulse, and respiratory rate before administration.

Ongoing Assessment

After injection of an oxytocic drug, the nurse monitors the blood pressure, pulse, and respiratory rate at the intervals ordered by the primary health care provider.

Nursing Alert

All patients receiving IV oxytocin must be under constant observation to identify complications. A one-to-one nurse–patient ratio is recommended when monitoring a patient receiving an oxytocin infusion. In addition, the primary health care provider should be immediately available at all times.

The nurse assesses the patient's blood pressure, pulse, and respiratory rate every 30 minutes. The FHR and uterine contractions are assessed every 15 minutes or as ordered by the primary health care provider. Three to four firm uterine contractions should occur every 10 minutes, followed by a palpable relaxation of the uterus.

Nursing Alert

Hyperstimulation of the uterus during labor may lead to uterine tetany with marked impairment of the uteroplacental blood flow, uterine rupture, cervical rupture, amniotic fluid embolism, and trauma to the infant. Overstimulation of the uterus is dangerous to both the fetus and the mother and may occur even when the drug is administered properly in a uterus that is hypersensitive to oxytocin.

When monitoring uterine contractions, the nurse notifies the primary health care provider immediately if any of the following occurs:

● Any significant change in the FHR or rhythm
● Any marked change in the frequency, rate, or rhythm of uterine contractions: uterine contractions

lasting more than 60 seconds or contractions occurring more frequently than every 2 to 3 minutes or there is no palpable relaxation of the uterus

● A marked increase or decrease in the patient's blood pressure or pulse or any significant change in the patient's general condition

If any of these are noted, the nurse should immediately discontinue the oxytocin infusion and run the primary IV line at the rate prescribed by the primary health care provider until the primary health care provider examines the patient.

The nurse immediately reports any signs of water intoxication or fluid overload (eg, drowsiness, confusion, headache, listlessness, and wheezing, coughing, rapid breathing) to the primary health care provider.

Oxytocin may be given IM after delivery of the placenta. The nurse obtains the blood pressure, pulse, and respiratory rate every 5 to 10 minutes after the drug is administered. The nurse palpates the patient's uterine fundus for firmness and position. The nurse immediately reports any excess bleeding to the primary health care provider.

When administering ergonovine and methylergonovine after delivery, the nurse monitors vital signs every 4 hours. In addition, the nurse notes the character and amount of vaginal bleeding. The patient may report abdominal cramping with the administration of these drugs. If cramping is moderately severe to severe, the nurse notifies the primary health care provider because it may be necessary to discontinue use of the drug.

NURSING DIAGNOSES

Drug-specific nursing diagnoses are highlighted in the Nursing Diagnoses Checklist. Other nursing diagnoses applicable to these drugs are discussed in depth in Chapter 4.

PLANNING

The expected outcomes of the patient may include an optimal response to drug therapy (ie, initiation of the normal labor process), adverse reactions identified and reported to the primary health care provider (eg,

Nursing Diagnoses Checklist

- ✓ **Anxiety** related to labor and delivery
- ✓ **Excess Fluid Volume** related to administration of IV fluids containing oxytocin
- ✓ **Risk for Injury** (fetal) related to adverse drug effects of oxytocin (fetal bradycardia)
- ✓ **Pain** related to adverse reactions (abdominal cramping, nausea, headache)

absence of a fluid volume excess [oxytocin administration]), and an understanding of the treatment regimen.

IMPLEMENTATION

Promoting an Optimal Response to Therapy

OXYTOCIN. The patient receiving oxytocin to induce labor may have concern over the use of the drug to produce contractions. When given to induce or stimulate contractions, oxytocin may only be given intravenously (IV). The nurse explains the purpose of the IV infusion and the expected results to the patient. Because the patient receiving oxytocin must be closely supervised, the nurse spends time with the patient and offers encouragement and reassurance to help reduce anxiety.

When oxytocin is prescribed, the primary health care provider orders the type and amount of IV fluid, the number of units of oxytocin added to the IV solution, and the IV infusion rate. An electronic infusion device is used to control the infusion rate. The primary health care provider establishes guidelines for the administration of the oxytocin solution and for increasing or decreasing the flow rate or discontinuing the administration of oxytocin based on standards established by the Association of Women's Health, Obstetric, and Neonatal Nurses (AWHONN). Usually, the flow rate is increased every 20 to 30 minutes, but this may vary according to the patient's response. The strength, frequency, and duration of contractions and the FHR are monitored closely.

When administering oxytocin intranasally to facilitate the letdown of milk, the nurse places the patient in an upright position, and with the squeeze bottle held upright, administers the prescribed number of sprays to one or both nostrils. The patient then waits 2 to 3 minutes before breastfeeding the infant or pumping the breasts. If a breast pump is being used, the nurse records the amount of milk pumped from the breasts.

The nurse notifies the primary health care provider if milk drips from the breast before or after breastfeeding or if milk drips from the opposite breast during breastfeeding because there would be no need to continue drug therapy. The primary health care provider is notified if nasal irritation, palpations, or uterine cramping occurs.

ERGONOVINE AND METHYLERGONOVINE. The nurse administers ergonovine and methylergonovine at the direction of the primary health care provider. Ergonovine is usually given during the third stage of labor after the placenta has been delivered. Ergonovine is primarily administered IM, but in emergencies when quicker response is needed, the drug may be administered IV.

Methylergonovine is usually given IM at the time of the delivery of the anterior shoulder or after the delivery of the placenta. The drug is not given routinely IV because it may produce sudden hypertension and stroke. If the drug is given IV, the nurse administers the drug slowly during a period of 1 minute or more with close monitoring of the patient's blood pressure.

When ergonovine or methylergonovine is administered in the delivery room, the nurse briefly explains the purpose of the injection to the patient. If either of these drugs is given after delivery of the infant, the nurse explains the purpose of the drug (eg, to improve the tone of the uterus and to help the uterus to return to its [near] normal size).

Monitoring and Managing Adverse Reactions

OXYTOCIN. When oxytocin is administered, some adverse reactions must be tolerated or treated symptomatically until therapy is discontinued. For example, if the patient is nauseated, the nurse provides an emesis basin and perhaps a cool towel for the forehead. If vomiting occurs, the nurse notifies the primary health care provider.

If contractions are frequent, prolonged, or excessive, the infusion is stopped to prevent fetal anoxia or trauma to the uterus. Excessive stimulation of the uterus can cause uterine hypertonicity and possible uterine rupture. The nurse places the patient on her side and provides supplemental oxygen. The effects of the drug diminish rapidly because oxytocin is short acting.

When oxytocin is administered IV, there is a danger of a fluid volume excess (water intoxication) because oxytocin has an antidiuretic effect. The nurse measures the fluid intake and output. In some instances, hourly measurements of the output are necessary. The nurse observes the patient for signs of fluid overload (see Chap. 58). If any of these signs or symptoms is noted, the nurse should immediately discontinue the oxytocin infusion and run the primary IV line at the rate prescribed by the primary health care provider until the primary health care provider examines the patient.

ERGONOVINE AND METHYLERGONOVINE. When ergonovine or methylergonovine is administered for uterine atony and hemorrhage, abdominal cramping can occur and is usually an indication of drug effectiveness. The uterus is palpated in the lower abdomen as small, firm, and round. However, the nurse should report persistent or severe cramping to the primary health care provider.

※ **Nursing Alert**

In some patients who are calcium deficient, the uterus may not respond to ergonovine. The nurse immediately reports a lack of response to ergonovine. Administration of calcium by IV injection usually restores response to the drug.

Although rare, ergotism or ergot poisoning can occur with the administration of excessive amounts of ergonovine or methylergonovine.

 Nursing Alert

Symptoms of ergotism that must be reported immediately include coolness, numbness and tingling of extremities, dyspnea, nausea, confusion, tachycardia or bradycardia, chest pain, hallucinations, and convulsions. If these reactions occur, the nurse immediately reports them to the primary health care provider because use of the drug must be discontinued.

Educating the Patient and Family

The treatment regimen is explained to the patient and family (when appropriate). The nurse answers any questions the patient may have regarding treatment. The patient is instructed to report any adverse reactions. The patient and family are informed of therapeutic response during administration of the drug. If nasal spray is to be used, the patient is taught proper use.

EVALUATION

- The therapeutic effect is achieved, and normal labor is initiated.
- Adverse reactions are managed effectively.
- No evidence of a fluid volume excess (oxytocin administration) is seen.
- The patient is knowledgeable of the therapeutic regimen.

UTERINE RELAXANTS

Uterine relaxants are useful in the management of preterm labor. These drugs will decrease uterine activity and prolong the pregnancy to allow the fetus to develop more fully, thereby increasing the chance of neonatal survival. Ritodrine (Yutopar) and terbutaline (Brethine) are two drugs currently used as uterine relaxants in the management of preterm (or premature) labor.

ACTIONS AND USES

Ritodrine

Ritodrine has an effect on beta (β)$_2$-adrenergic receptors, principally those that innervate the uterus. Stimulation of these β_2-adrenergic receptors inhibits uterine smooth muscle contractions. The β_1-adrenergic receptors are located in the heart and are not stimulated by ritodrine when administered as prescribed. Ritodrine is used to manage preterm labor in pregnancies of greater than 20 weeks' gestation. Ritodrine administration requires hospitalization.

Terbutaline

Terbutaline (Brethine) is also classified as a β_2-adrenergic agonist (see Chap. 22) and is used primarily as a bronchodilator for patients with asthma and chronic obstructive pulmonary disease. Terbutaline is not approved by the Food and Drug Administration for treatment of preterm labor. Its use in the management of premature labor is investigational. However, many primary health care providers prefer terbutaline for the management of preterm labor, and it has proven to be highly effective for this purpose. When terbutaline is prescribed for the management of preterm labor, most agencies have the patient sign an informed consent before therapy is initiated.

ADVERSE REACTIONS

Ritodrine

Alterations in fetal and maternal heart rates and maternal blood pressure frequently occur when ritodrine is administered IV. Additional frequent adverse reactions associated with IV administration include nausea, vomiting, headache, palpitations, nervousness, restlessness, and emotional upset. A rare, but serious, adverse reaction is pulmonary edema.

Terbutaline

Adverse reactions observed with the administration of terbutaline include nervousness, restlessness, tremor, headache, anxiety, hypertension, hypokalemia (low serum potassium), arrhythmias, and palpitations. A serious, but rare, adverse reaction is pulmonary edema.

CONTRAINDICATIONS, PRECAUTIONS, AND INTERACTIONS

Ritodrine

Ritodrine is contraindicated in patients with known hypersensitivity to the drug, antepartum hemorrhage, eclampsia or severe preeclampsia, cardiac disease, pulmonary hypertension, uncontrolled diabetes mellitus, or bronchial asthma (patients treated with betamimetics or steroids), in pregnancies of less than 20 weeks' gestation, and in the event of intrauterine fetal death. Ritodrine is classified as a Pregnancy Category B drug

and is given cautiously during pregnancy. Because no adequate studies have been done in pregnant women before the 20th week of pregnancy, do not use this drug before the 20th week. Ritodrine is administered cautiously in patients with cardiac disease, migraine headaches, history of stroke, hyperthyroidism, and seizure disorders.

There is a decreased effectiveness of ritodrine when the drug is administered with a β-adrenergic blocking agent such as propranolol and an increased risk of pulmonary edema when administered with the corticosteroids. Co-administration of ritodrine with the sympathomimetics potentiates the effect of ritodrine. Cardiovascular effects (eg, arrhythmias or hypotension) of ritodrine may increase when the drug is administered with diazoxide, general anesthetics, magnesium sulfate, or meperidine.

Terbutaline

Terbutaline is contraindicated in patients with known hypersensitivity to the drug, severe cardiac problems (tachyarrhythmias), digitalis toxicity, or hypertension. Terbutaline is classified as a Pregnancy Category B drug and is given cautiously during pregnancy (after the 20th week of pregnancy only). Terbutaline is administered cautiously in patients with cardiac disease, history of stroke, hyperthyroidism, and seizure disorders. When terbutaline is administered with the anesthetic halothane, there is an increased risk of cardiac arrhythmias. Additional information about terbutaline can be found in Chapter 37.

NURSING PROCESS

● **The Patient Receiving a Uterine Relaxant**

ASSESSMENT

Preadministration Assessment
Before starting an IV infusion containing ritodrine or terbutaline, the nurse obtains the patient's vital signs. The nurse auscultates lung sounds to provide a baseline assessment. The nurse places the patient on a monitoring device to determine uterine contractions and the FHR before and during administration.

Ongoing Assessment
During the ongoing assessment of a patient receiving a uterine relaxant, the nurse performs the following tasks at 15- to 30-minute intervals:

● Obtains blood pressure, pulse, and respiratory rate.
● Monitors FHR.
● Checks the IV infusion rate.

- Examines the area around the IV needle insertion for signs of extravasation.
- Monitors uterine contractions (frequency, intensity, length).

NURSING DIAGNOSES

Drug-specific nursing diagnoses are highlighted in the Nursing Diagnoses Checklist. Other nursing diagnoses applicable to these drugs are discussed in depth in Chapter 4.

PLANNING

The expected outcomes of the patient may include an optimal response to therapy, a reduction in anxiety, and an understanding of the treatment of preterm labor.

IMPLEMENTATION

Promoting an Optimal Response to Therapy

Nursing management for ritodrine and terbutaline is similar. For IV administration, the nurse prepares the solution according to the primary health care provider's instructions. An infusion pump is used to control the rate of flow. Ritodrine or terbutaline may be piggy-backed to the primary line, allowing the primary line to maintain the patency of the IV should it be necessary to temporarily discontinue infusion of the drug. The primary health care provider may prescribe terbutaline for administration by the oral or the subcutaneous route throughout the treatment, rather than via the IV route. The nurse places a cardiac monitor on the patient. To minimize hypotension, the nurse positions the patient in a left lateral position unless the primary health care provider orders a different position.

The primary health care provider is kept informed of the patient's response to the drug because a dosage change may be necessary. The primary health care provider establishes guidelines for the regulation of the IV infusion rate, as well as the blood pressure and pulse ranges that require stopping the IV infusion.

Monitoring and Managing Adverse Reactions

The nurse monitors the maternal and fetal vital signs every 15 minutes during administrations of the drug. The nurse monitors uterine contractions frequently throughout infusion.

Nursing Alert

The nurse reports to the primary care provider a pulse rate of 140 bpm, persistent elevation of pulse rate, irregular pulse, or increase in respiratory rate of more than 20/min. The nurse assesses the respiratory status for symptoms of pulmonary edema (eg, dyspnea, tachycardia, increased respiratory rate, rales, and frothy sputum). If these reactions occur, the end result could mean pulmonary edema. The primary health care provider may decrease the dosage or discontinue the drug. The primary health care provider is notified immediately if any of these symptoms occur because use of the drug may be discontinued. After contractions cease, the nurse tapers the dosage to the lowest effective dose by decreasing the infusion rate of the drug at regular intervals prescribed by the primary health care provider. Continue the IV infusion for at least 12 hours after uterine contractions have ceased. Because the duration of treatment is short, mild adverse reactions must be tolerated. If adverse reactions are severe, use of the drug is discontinued or the dosage decreased.

Managing Anxiety

The patient in preterm labor may have many concerns about her pregnancy, as well as the effectiveness of drug therapy. The woman is encouraged to verbalize any fears or concerns. The nurse listens to the patient's concerns and carefully and accurately answers any questions she may have concerning drug therapy. In addition, the nurse offers emotional support and encouragement during the time the drug is being administered. If allowed by the institution, the presence of family members may decrease anxiety in the woman experiencing preterm labor.

Educating the Patient and Family

The nurse carefully explains the treatment regimen to the patient. The primary health care provider usually discusses the expected outcome of treatment with the patient and answers any questions regarding therapy. Although the patient is monitored closely during therapy, the patient is instructed to notify the nurse immediately if any of the following occur: nausea, vomiting, palpitations, or shortness of breath. If a patient is taking ritodrine, the nurse discusses the importance of lying on the left side during IV administration.

If oral terbutaline is prescribed for preterm labor, the patient is instructed on use of the drug and adverse reactions to report (excessive tremor, nervousness, drowsiness, headache, nausea, dizziness). If contractions resume during oral therapy, the patient is instructed to notify the primary health care provider if four to six contractions per hour occur.

EVALUATION

- The therapeutic drug effect is achieved.
- Adverse reactions are identified and reported to the primary health care provider.
- Anxiety is reduced.
- The patient demonstrates an understanding of in-hospital treatment.

● Critical Thinking Exercises

1. *Develop a nursing care plan for Ms. Morris, a 28-year-old woman who is admitted to the obstetric unit with premature labor during her third trimester. This is her second child, and she has had two miscarriages. She is prescribed ritodrine for preterm labor. Analyze what nursing diagnoses would have the highest priority. Discuss how you would explore and plan to meet her emotional needs.*

2. *Judith Watson, aged 28 years, is admitted to the obstetric unit and is to receive oxytocin to induce labor. This is her first child, and she is extremely anxious. Analyze what information would be necessary for her to receive from the nurse before the administration of oxytocin. What assessments would be important for the nurse to make during treatment with oxytocin?*

● Review Questions

1. When oxytocin is administered over a prolonged time, which of the following adverse reactions would be most likely to occur?

   A. Hyperglycemia
   B. Renal impairment
   C. Increased intracranial pressure
   D. Water intoxication

2. When the patient is receiving oxytocin, the nurse would notify the primary health care provider in which of the following conditions?

   A. Uterine contractions occur every 5 to 10 minutes.
   B. Uterine contractions last more than 60 seconds or contractions occur more frequently than every 2 to 3 minutes.
   C. Patient experiences pain during a uterine contraction.
   D. Patient experiences increased thirst.

3. Which of the following adverse reactions is most indicative of ergotism?

   A. Numbness, tingling of the extremities
   B. Headache, blurred vision
   C. Tachycardia and cardiac arrhythmias
   D. Diaphoresis, increased respirations

4. During administration of ritodrine, in what position would the nurse most probably place the patient?

   A. Supine
   B. Prone
   C. On the left side
   D. On the right side

● Medication Dosage Problems

1. Terbutaline 2.5 mg is prescribed. The drug is available in 5-mg tablets. The nurse administers _____.

2. Methylergonovine 0.2 mg IM is prescribed. The drug is available as 0.2 mg/mL. The nurse administers _____.

c h a p t e r **54**

Immunologic Agents

Key Terms

active immunity
antibody
antigen
antigen–antibody
  response
attenuated
booster
cell-mediated immunity

globulin
humoral immunity
immune globulin
immunity
passive immunity
toxin
toxoid
vaccine

Chapter Objectives

On completion of this chapter, the student will:

- Discuss humoral immunity and cell-mediated immunity.
- Distinguish between and define the different types of immunity.
- Discuss the use of vaccines, toxoids, immune globulins, and antivenins to provide immunity against disease.
- Discuss preadministration and ongoing assessments the nurse should perform on the patient receiving an immunologic agent.
- Identify nursing diagnoses particular to a patient receiving an immunologic agent.
- Discuss ways to promote an optimal response, management of common adverse reactions, special considerations, and important points to keep in mind when educating a patient taking an immunologic agent.

Immunity refers to the ability of the body to identify and resist microorganisms that are potentially harmful. This ability enables the body to fight or prevent infectious disease and inhibit tissue and organ damage. The immune system is not confined to any one part of the body. Immune stem cells, formed in the bone marrow, may remain in the bone marrow until maturation or migrate to different body sites for maturation. After maturation, most immune cells circulate into the body and exert specific effects. The immune system has two distinct, but overlapping, mechanisms with which to fight invading organisms:

- Cell-mediated defenses (cellular immunity)
- Antibody-mediated defenses (humoral immunity)

CELL-MEDIATED IMMUNITY

Cell-mediated immunity (CMI) is the result of the activity of many leukocyte actions, reactions, and interactions that range from simple to complex. This type of immunity is dependent on the actions of the T lymphocytes, which are responsible for a delayed type of immune response. The T lymphocyte becomes sensitized

by its first contact with a specific antigen. Subsequent exposure to an antigen stimulates multiple reactions aimed at destroying or inactivating the offending antigen. T lymphocytes and macrophages (large cells that surround, engulf, and digest microorganisms and cellular debris) work together in CMI to destroy the antigen. T lymphocytes attack the antigens directly, rather than produce antibodies (as is done in humoral immunity). Cellular reactions may also occur without macrophages.

Several T lymphocytes (T cells) are involved in CMI:

- Helper T4 cells—function within the bloodstream identifying and destroying antigens
- Helper T1 cells—increase B lymphocyte antibody production
- Helper T2 cells—increase activity of cytotoxic (killer) T cells, which attack the cell directly by altering the cell membrane and causing cell lysis (destruction)
- Suppressor T cells—suppress the immune response
- Memory T lymphocytes—recognize previous contact with antigens and activate an immune response

The T lymphocytes defend against viral infections, fungal infections, and some bacterial infections. If CMI is lost, as in the case of acquired immunodeficiency

Herbal Alert: Shiitake

The shiitake mushroom is an edible variety of mushroom and is not associated with severe adverse reactions. Mild side effects such as skin rashes or gastrointestinal upsets have been reported. The recommended dosage for general health maintenance:

- *3–4 fresh shiitake mushrooms*
- *1–5 capsules/day*
- *1 dropper two to three times a day*

Lentinan, a derivative of the shiitake mushroom, is proving to be valuable in boosting the body's immune system and may prolong the survival time of patients with cancer by supporting immunity. In Japan, lentinan is commonly used to treat cancer. Additional possible benefits of this herb are to lower cholesterol levels by increasing the rate at which cholesterol is excreted from the body. Under no circumstances should shiitake or lentinan be used for cancer or any serious illness without consulting a primary health care provider.

IMMUNOLOGIC AGENTS

Some immunologic agents capitalize on the body's natural defenses by stimulating the immune response, thereby creating within the body protection to a specific disease. Other immunologic agents supply ready-made antibodies to provide passive immunity. Examples of immunologic agents include vaccines, toxoids, and immune globulins.

ACTIONS AND USES

Vaccines and Toxoids

Antibody-producing tissues cannot distinguish between an antigen that is capable of causing disease (a live antigen), an attenuated antigen, or a killed antigen. Because of this phenomenon, vaccines, which contain either an attenuated or a killed antigen, have been developed to create immunity to certain diseases. The live antigens are either killed or weakened during the manufacturing process. Although the vaccine contains weakened or killed antigens, they do not have suffi-cient strength to cause disease. Although rare, vaccination with any vaccine may not result in a protective antibody response in all individuals given the vaccine.

A **toxin** is a poisonous substance produced by some bacteria, such as *Clostridium tetani,* the bacteria that cause tetanus. A toxin is capable of stimulating the body to produce antitoxins, which are substances that act in the same manner as antibodies. Toxins are powerful substances, and like other antigens, they can be attenuated. A toxin that is attenuated (or weakened) but still capable of stimulating the formation of antitoxins is called a **toxoid.**

Both vaccines and toxoids are administered to stimulate the immune response within the body to specific antigens or toxins. These agents must be administered before exposure to the pathogenic organism. The initiation of the immune response, in turn, produces resistance to a specific infectious disease. The immunity produced in this manner is active immunity. Display 54-5 gives examples of indications for use of toxoids and vaccines.

Immune Globulins and Antivenins

Globulins are proteins present in blood serum or plasma, which contain antibodies. **Immune globulins** are solutions obtained from human blood containing antibodies that have been formed by the body to specific antigens. Because they contain ready-made antibodies, they are given for passive immunity against disease. The immune globulins are administered to provide passive immunization to one or more infectious diseases. Those receiving immune globulins receive antibodies only to the diseases to which the donor blood is immune. The onset of protection is rapid but of short duration (1–3 months).

Antivenins are used for passive, transient protection from the toxic effects of bites by spiders (black widow and similar spiders) and snakes (rattlesnakes, copperhead and cottonmouth, and coral). The most effective response is obtained when the drug is administered within 4 hours after exposure.

DISPLAY 54-4 ● Example of Passive Immunity

An example of passive immunity is the administration of immune globulins (see Summary Drug Table: Agents for Passive Immunity), such as hepatitis B immune globulin. Administration of this vaccine is an attempt to prevent hepatitis B after the individual has been exposed to the virus.

DISPLAY 54-5 ● Uses of Vaccines and Toxoids

- Routine immunization of infants and children (see Fig. 54-1)
- Immunization of adults against tetanus
- Adults at high risk for certain diseases (eg, pneumococcal and influenza vaccines for individuals with serious respiratory disorders)
- Children or adults at risk for exposure to a particular disease (eg, hepatitis B for health care workers)
- Immunization of prepubertal girls or nonpregnant women of childbearing age against rubella

ADVERSE REACTIONS

Vaccines and Toxoids

Adverse reactions from the administration of vaccines or toxoids are usually mild. Chills, fever, muscular aches and pains, rash, and lethargy may be present. Pain and tenderness at the injection site may also occur. Although rare, a hypersensitivity reaction may occur. The Summary Drug Table: Agents for Active Immunization provides a listing of the more rare, but serious, adverse reactions.

Immune Globulins and Antivenins

Adverse reactions to immune globulins are rare. However, local tenderness and pain at the injection site may occur. The most common adverse reactions include urticaria, angioedema, erythema, malaise, nausea, diarrhea, headache, chills, and fever. Adverse reactions, if they occur, usually last for several hours. Systemic reactions are extremely rare.

The antivenins may cause various reactions, with hypersensitivity being the most severe. Some antivenins are prepared from horse serum, and if a patient is sensitive to horse serum, serious reactions and death may result. The immediate reactions usually occur within 30 minutes after administration of the antivenin. Symptoms include apprehension; flushing; itching; urticaria; edema of the face, tongue, and throat; cough; dyspnea; vomiting; cyanosis; and collapse. Other adverse reactions are included in the Summary Drug Table: Agents for Passive Immunity.

CONTRAINDICATIONS AND PRECAUTIONS

Vaccines and Toxoids

Immunologic agents are contraindicated in patients with known hypersensitivity to the agent or any component of it. The measles, mumps, rubella, and varicella vaccines are contraindicated in patients who have ever had an allergic reaction to gelatin, neomycin, or a previous dose of one of the vaccines. The measles, mumps, rubella, and varicella vaccines are contraindicated during pregnancy, especially during the first trimester, because of the danger of birth defects. Women are instructed to wait at least 3 months before getting pregnant after receiving these vaccines. Vaccines and toxoids are contraindicated during acute febrile illnesses, leukemia, lymphoma, immunosuppressive illness or drug therapy, and non-localized cancer. See Display 54-6 for additional infor-

---

DISPLAY 54-6 ● **Contraindications for Immunization**

- Moderate or severe illness, with or without fever
- Anaphylactoid reactions (eg, hives, swelling of the mouth and throat, difficulty breathing [dyspnea], hypotension, and shock)
- Known allergy to vaccine or vaccine constituents, particularly gelatin, eggs, or neomycin
- Individuals with an immunologic deficiency should not receive a vaccine (virus is transmissible to the immunocompromised individual).
- Immunizations are postponed during the administration of steroids, radiation therapy, and antineoplastic (anticancer) drug therapy.
- Virus vaccines against measles, rubella, and mumps should not be given to pregnant women.
- Patients who experience severe systemic or neurologic reactions after a previous dose of the vaccine should not be given any additional doses.

---

mation on the contraindications for immunologic agents.

The immunologic agents are used with extreme caution in individuals with a history of allergies. Sensitivity testing may be performed in individuals with a history of allergies. No adequate studies have been conducted in pregnant women, and it is not known whether these agents are excreted in breast milk. Thus, the immunologic agents (Pregnancy Category C) are used with caution in pregnant women and during lactation.

Immune Globulins and Antivenins

The immune globulins are contraindicated in patients with a history of allergic reactions after administration of human immunoglobulin preparations and individuals with isolated immunoglobulin A (IgA) deficiency (individuals could have an anaphylactic reaction to subsequent administration of blood products that contain IgA).

 Nursing Alert

Human immune globulin intravenous (IGIV) products have been associated with renal impairment, acute renal failure, osmotic nephrosis, and death. Individuals with a predisposition to acute renal failure, such as those with preexisting renal disease, diabetes mellitus, individuals older than 65 years, or patients receiving nephrotoxic drugs should not be given human IGIV products.

The antivenins are contraindicated in patients with hypersensitivity to horse serum or any other component of the serum.

The immune globulins and antivenins are administered cautiously during pregnancy (Pregnancy Category C) and lactation and in children.

INTERACTIONS

Vaccines and Toxoids

Vaccinations containing live organisms are not administered within 3 months of immune globulin administration because antibodies in the globulin preparation may interfere with the immune response to the vaccination. Corticosteroids, antineoplastic drugs, and radiation therapy depress the immune system to such a degree that insufficient numbers of antibodies are produced to prevent the disease. When the salicylates are administered with the varicella vaccination, there is an increased risk of Reye's syndrome developing.

Immune Globulins and Antivenins

Antibodies in the immune globulin preparations may interfere with the immune response to live virus vaccines, particularly measles, but also others, such as mumps and rubella. It is recommended that the live virus vaccines be administered 14 to 30 days before or 6 to 12 weeks after administration of immune globulins. No known interactions have been reported with antivenins.

NURSING PROCESS

● **The Patient Receiving an Immunologic Agent**

ASSESSMENT

Preadministration Assessment

Before the administration of any vaccine, the nurse obtains an allergy history. If the individual is known or thought to have allergies of any kind, the nurse tells the primary health care provider before the vaccine is given. Some vaccines contain antibodies obtained from animals, whereas other vaccines may contain proteins or preservatives to which the individual may be allergic. A highly allergic person may have an allergic reaction that could be serious and even fatal. If the patient has an allergy history, the primary health care provider may decide to perform skin tests for allergy to one or more of the components or proteins in the vaccine. The nurse also determines whether the patient has any conditions that contraindicate the administration of the agent (eg, cancer, leukemia, lymphoma, immunosuppressive drug therapy).

Ongoing Assessment

The patient is usually not hospitalized after administration of an immunologic agent. However, the patient may be asked to stay in the clinic or office for observation for about 30 minutes after the injection to observe for any

---

> **Nursing Diagnoses Checklist**
>
> ☑ **Risk of Injury** related to the development of infectious disease, hypersensitivity to the immunologic agent
>
> ☑ **Risk for Imbalanced Body Temperature** related to adverse reaction of vaccination
>
> ☑ **Pain** related to adverse reactions (pain and discomfort at the injection site, muscular aches and pain)

---

signs of hypersensitivity (eg, laryngeal edema, hives, pruritus, angioneurotic edema, and severe dyspnea [see Chap. 2 for additional information]). Emergency resuscitation equipment is kept available to be used in the event of a severe hypersensitivity reaction.

NURSING DIAGNOSES

Drug-specific nursing diagnoses are highlighted in the Nursing Diagnoses Checklist. Other nursing diagnoses applicable to these drugs are discussed in depth in Chapter 4.

PLANNING

The expected outcomes of the patient may include an optimal response to the immunologic agent, management of common adverse drug effects, and an understanding of and compliance with the prescribed immunization schedule.

IMPLEMENTATION

Promoting an Optimal Response to Therapy

If a vaccine is not in liquid form and must be reconstituted, the nurse must read the directions enclosed with the vaccine. It is important to follow the enclosed directions carefully. Package inserts also contain information regarding dosage, adverse reactions, method of administration, administration sites (when appropriate), and, when needed, recommended booster schedules.

On occasion, it may be necessary to postpone the regular immunization schedule, particularly for children. This is of special concern to parents. The decision to delay immunization because of illness or for other reasons must be discussed with the primary health care provider. However, the decision to administer or delay vaccination because of febrile illness (illness causing an elevated temperature) depends on the severity of the symptoms and the specific disorder. In general, all vaccines can be administered to those with minor illness, such as a cold virus and to those with a low-grade fever. However, moderate or severe febrile illness is a contraindication. In instances of moderate or severe febrile illness, vaccination is done as soon as the acute phase of the illness is over. Display 54-6 lists general contraindications for immunizations. Specific contraindications and precautions may be found in the package insert that comes with the drug.

The nurse documents the following information in the patient's chart or form provided by the institution:

● Date of vaccination
● Route and site, vaccine type, manufacturer
● Lot number and expiration date
● Name, address, and title of individual administering vaccine

Monitoring and Managing Adverse Reactions

Minor adverse reactions, such as fever, rashes, and aching of the joints, are possible with the administration of a vaccine. In most cases, these reactions subside within 48 hours.

☀ Nursing Alert

In most cases, the risk of serious adverse reactions from an immunization is much smaller than the risk of contracting the disease for which the immunizing agent is given.

General interventions, such as increasing the fluids in the diet, allowing for adequate rest, and keeping the atmosphere quiet and nonstimulating, may be beneficial. The primary health care provider may prescribe acetaminophen, every 4 hours, to control these reactions. Local irritation at the injection site may be treated with warm or cool compresses, depending on the patient's preference. A lump may be palpated at the injection site after a diphtheria, pertussis, tetanus (DPT) injection or other immunization. This is not abnormal and will resolve itself within several days to several months.

Vaccine Adverse Event Reporting System

The Vaccine Adverse Event Reporting System (VAERS) is a national vaccine safety surveillance program co-sponsored by the Centers for Disease Control and Prevention (CDC) and the Food and Drug Administration (FDA). VAERS collects and analyzes information from reports of adverse reactions after immunization. Anyone can report to VAERS, and reports are sent in by vaccine manufacturers, health care providers, and vaccine recipients and their parents or guardians. An example of the VAERS and instructions for completing the form are found in Appendix F. Any clinically significant adverse event that occurs after the administration of any vaccine should be reported. Individuals are encouraged to provide the information on the form even if the individual is uncertain if the event was related to the immunization. A copy of the form can be obtained by calling 1-800-822-7967 or by downloading it from the Internet at http://www.vaers.org.

Educating the Patient and Family

Because of the effectiveness of various types of vaccines in the prevention of disease, nurses must inform the public about the advantages of immunization. Parents are encouraged to have infants and young children receive the immunizations suggested by the primary health care provider.

The nurse advises those traveling to a foreign country to contact their primary health care provider or local health department well in advance of their departure date for information about the immunizations that will be needed. Immunizations should be given well in advance of departure because it may take several weeks to produce adequate immunity.

When an adult or child is receiving a vaccine for immunization, the nurse explains to the patient or a family member the possible reactions that may occur, for example, soreness at the injection site or fever.

Serious viral infections of the central nervous system and fatalities have been associated with the use of vaccines. Although the number of these incidents is small, a risk factor still remains when some vaccines are given. It is also important for the parents to understand that a risk is also associated with not receiving immunization against some infectious diseases. That risk may be higher and just as serious as the risk associated with the use of vaccines. It must also be remembered that when a large segment of the population is immunized, the small number of those not immunized are less likely to be exposed to and be infected with the disease-producing microorganism. However, when large numbers of the population are not immunized, there is a great increase in the chances of exposure to the infectious disease and a significant increase in the probability that the individual will experience the disease.

The nurse encourages the parents or guardians to report any adverse reactions or serious adverse events occurring after administration of a vaccine. It may be necessary to report the event to VAERS.

The following summarizes the information to be included when educating the parents of a child receiving a vaccination.

● Discuss briefly the risks of contracting vaccine-preventable diseases and the benefits of immunization.
● Instruct the parents to bring immunization records to all visits.
● Provide the date for return for the next vaccination.
● Discuss common adverse reactions (eg, fever, soreness at the injection site) and methods to combat these reactions (eg, acetaminophen, warm compresses).

● Instruct the parents to report any unusual or severe adverse reactions after the administration of a vaccination.

EVALUATION

● The therapeutic effect is achieved and the disease for which immunization is given does not present itself.
● Adverse drug reactions are managed successfully.
● The patient or parents/guardians comply with the immunization schedule.
● The patient and family express an understanding of the need for immunizations.

● *Critical Thinking Exercises*

1. *Ms. Wilson has brought her 2-month-old daughter, Michelle, to the clinic for the first of the series of three DPT and oral polio vaccine (OPV) immunizations. Ms. Wilson asks you to explain how a vaccination will keep her daughter from getting sick and why she has to have three injections. Discuss how you would address these topics with Ms. Wilson.*

2. *Jimmy, age 4 months, has a slight cold with a "runny nose" when he comes for his regular well-baby checkup. His mother tells the nurse that because Jimmy is sick, she does not think he needs his DPT injection at this time. She says that she will bring him in next month for this immunization. Analyze the situation to determine the best response to Jimmy's mother. Discuss any assessments that you think would be important to make before giving your response.*

● *Review Questions*

1. When discussing the possibility of adverse reactions after receiving a vaccine, the nurse tells the parents of a young child that _____.
   A. adverse reactions may be severe, and the child should be monitored closely for 24 hours
   B. adverse reactions are usually mild
   C. the child will likely experience a hypersensitivity reaction
   D. the most common adverse reaction is a severe headache

2. Which of the following statements made by the patient would alert the nurse to a possibility of an allergy to the measles vaccine? My daughter is allergic to _____.
   A. Jell-O
   B. peanut butter
   C. sugar
   D. corn

3. What type of immunity does an antivenin produce?
   A. Artificially acquired active immunity
   B. Naturally acquired active immunity
   C. Passive immunity
   D. Cell-mediated immunity

4. What type of immunity will be produced by the hepatitis B vaccine recombinant?
   A. Artificially acquired active immunity
   B. Naturally acquired active immunity
   C. Passive immunity
   D. Cell-mediated immunity

Antineoplastic Drugs

Key Terms

alopecia
anemia
anorexia
antineoplastic drugs
bone marrow
  suppression
chemotherapy

extravasation
leukopenia
oral mucositis
stomatitis
thrombocytopenia
vesicant

Chapter Objectives

On completion of this chapter, the student will:

- List the types of drugs used in the treatment of neoplastic diseases.
- Discuss the uses, general drug actions, general adverse reactions, contraindications, precautions, and interactions of the antineoplastic drugs.
- Discuss important preadministration and ongoing assessment activities the nurse should perform on the patient taking antineoplastic drugs.
- List some nursing diagnoses particular to a patient taking antineoplastic drugs.
- Discuss ways to promote an optimal response to therapy, how to manage common adverse reactions, and important points to keep in mind when educating patients about the use of an antineoplastic drug.

Antineoplastic drugs are used in the treatment of malignant diseases (cancer). These drugs can be used for cure, control, or palliative (relief of symptoms) therapy. Although these drugs may not always lead to a complete cure of the malignancy, they often slow the rate of tumor growth and delay metastasis (spreading of the cancer to other sites). Use of these drugs is one of the tools in the treatment of cancer. The term **chemotherapy** is often used to refer to therapy with antineoplastic drugs.

Many antineoplastic drugs are available to treat malignancies. The antineoplastic drugs covered in this chapter include the alkylating drugs, antibiotics, antimetabolites, hormones, mitotic inhibitors, and selected miscellaneous drugs. Many antineoplastic drugs not specifically discussed in this chapter are listed in the Summary Drug Table: Antineoplastic Drugs.

ACTIONS

Generally, most antineoplastic drugs affect cells that rapidly proliferate (divide and reproduce). Malignant neoplasms or cancerous tumors usually consist of rapidly proliferating aberrant (abnormal) cells. Cancer cells have no biological feedback controls that stop their aberrant growth or proliferation. Cancer cells are more sensitive to antineoplastic drugs when the cells are in the process of growing and dividing. Chemotherapy is administered at the time the cell population is dividing as part of a strategy to optimize cell death.

However, the normal cells that line the oral cavity and gastrointestinal tract, and cells of the gonads, bone marrow, hair follicles, and lymph tissue are also rapidly dividing cells and are usually affected by these drugs. Thus, antineoplastic drugs may affect normal as well as malignant (cancerous) cells.

Chemotherapy is administered in a series of cycles to allow for recovery of the normal cells and to destroy more of the malignant cells (Fig. 55-1). According to the cell kill theory, a drug regimen is intended to kill 90% of the cancer cells during the first course of treatment. The second course, according to this theory, targets the remaining cancer cells and reduces those cells by 90%. Further courses of chemotherapy continue to reduce the number of cancer cells, until all cells are killed. This theory is the rationale for using repeated doses of chemotherapy with several antineoplastic drugs. Every malignant cell must be destroyed for the cancer to be

(text continues on page 591)

583

SUMMARY DRUG TABLE ANTINEOPLASTIC DRUGS

GENERIC NAME	TRADE NAME*	USES	ADVERSE REACTIONS	DOSAGE RANGES
Alkylating Drugs				
busulfan *byoo-sul´-fan*	Busulfex, Myleran	Chronic myelogenous leukemia	Leukopenia, anemia, cataracts, anxiety, skin rash, thrombocytopenia, fever, anorexia, nausea, vomiting, diarrhea, stomatitis, constipation, tachycardia, hypertension, insomnia, dizziness	1–12 mg/d PO; 0.8 mg/kg IV
chlorambucil *klor-am´-byoo-sill*	Leukeran	Chronic lymphocytic leukemia, malignant lymphomas, Hodgkin's disease	Bone marrow depression, hyperuricemia, nausea, vomiting, diarrhea, hepatotoxicity, tremors	0.03–0.2 mg/kg/d PO
cyclophosphamide *sye-klo-foss´-fam-ide*	Cytoxan, Neosar	Malignant lymphomas, Hodgkin's disease, multiple myeloma, leukemia, carcinoma of the ovary and breast, neuroblastoma, retinoblastoma	Leukopenia, thrombocytopenia, anemia, anorexia, nausea, vomiting, diarrhea, cystitis, alopecia	Initial dose: 40–50 mg/kg IV; maintenance doses: 1–5 mg/kg/d PO; 3–15 mg/kg IV
ifosfamide *eye-fos´-fam-ide*	Ifex	Testicular cancer	Hemorrhagic cystitis, mental confusion, coma, alopecia, nausea, vomiting, anorexia, diarrhea, hematuria	1.2 g/m²/d IV
lomustine *loe-mus´-teen*	CeeNu	Brain tumors, Hodgkin's disease	Nausea, vomiting, diarrhea, thrombocytopenia, leukopenia, alopecia, anemia, stomatitis	100–300 mg/m² PO
mechlorethamine *me-klor-eth´-a-meen*	Mustargen	Hodgkin's disease, lymphosarcoma, bronchogenic carcinoma, leukemia, mycosis fungoides	Nausea, vomiting, jaundice, alopecia, lymphocytopenia, granulocytopenia, thrombocytopenia, skin rash, diarrhea	0.4 mg/kg IV as a total dose for a course of therapy, which may be given as a single dose or divided dose
melphalan *mel´-fa-lan*	Alkeran	Multiple myeloma, carcinoma of the ovary	Nausea, vomiting, bone marrow depression, skin rash, alopecia, diarrhea	6 mg/d PO; 16 mg/m² IV
thiotepa *thye-oh-tep´-a*	Thioplex, *generic*	Carcinoma of the breast, ovary, bladder, Hodgkin's disease, lymphosarcomas, intracavity effusions due to localized metastatic disease	Nausea, vomiting, pain at injection site, bone marrow depression, dermatitis, dysuria	0.3–0.4 mg/kg IV; dosage is higher for intracavity or intratumor administration; bladder instillation: 60 mg retained for 2 h
Antibiotics				
bleomycin sulfate *blee-oh-my´-sin*	Blenoxane	Carcinoma of the head and neck, lymphomas, testicular carcinoma	Pneumonitis, pulmonary fibrosis, erythema, rash, fever, chills, vomiting	0.25–0.5 U/kg IV, IM, SC
dactinomycin *dak-ti-no-my´-sin*	Cosmegen	Wilms' tumor, choriocarcinoma, Ewing's sarcoma, testicular carcinoma	Anorexia, alopecia, bone marrow depression, nausea, vomiting	Up to 15 mcg/kg/d IV; may also be given by isolation perfusion at 0.035–0.05 mg/kg
daunorubicin citrate liposomal *daw-noe-roo´-bi-sin*	DaunoXome	Kaposi's sarcoma	Fatigue, headache, diarrhea, nausea, cough, fever	40 mg/m² IV

SUMMARY DRUG TABLE ANTINEOPLASTIC DRUGS (*Continued*)

GENERIC NAME	TRADE NAME*	USES	ADVERSE REACTIONS	DOSAGE RANGES
daunorubicin HCl *daw-noe-roo′-bi-sin*	Generic	Leukemia	Bone marrow depression, alopecia, acute nausea and vomiting, fever, chills	25–45 mg/m^2/d IV
doxorubicin HCl *dox-oh-roo′-by-sin*	Adriamycin, Rubex	Acute leukemia, neuroblastoma, soft tissue and bone sarcomas, carcinomas of the breast, ovary, bladder, lymphomas, Wilms' tumor	Alopecia, acute nausea and vomiting, mucositis, chills, bone marrow depression, fever	25–75 mg/m^2/d IV
epirubicin *ep-ee-roo′-by-sin*	Ellence	Breast cancer	Alopecia, local toxicity, rash, itching, amenorrhea, hot flashes, nausea, vomiting, mucositis, leukopenia, neutropenia, anemia, thrombocytopenia, infection, lethargy, conjunctivitis	100–120 mg/m^2 IV
idarubicin HCl *eye-da-roo′-by-sin*	Idamycin	Leukemia	Congestive heart failure, arrhythmias, chest pain, myocardial infarction, nausea, vomiting, alopecia	12 mg/m^2 daily x 3 d IV
mitomycin *mye-toe-my′-sin*	Mutamycin	Adenocarcinoma of the stomach, pancreas	Bone marrow depression, anorexia, nausea, vomiting, headache, blurred vision, fever	10–20 mg/m^2/d IV
plicamycin *plye-ka-my′-sin*	Mithracin	Malignant tumors of the testes, hypercalcemia, and hypercalciuria associated with neoplasms	Hemorrhagic syndrome (epistaxis, hematemesis, widespread hemorrhage in the GI tract, generalized advanced bleeding), vomiting, diarrhea, anorexia, nausea, stomatitis	Testicular tumors: 25–30 mcg/kg/d IV; hypercalcemia, hypercalciuria: 25 mcg/kg/d IV for 3–4 d
valrubicin *val-roo′-by-sin*	ValStar	Bladder cancer	Bladder discomfort, dysuria, urinary frequency, urinary tract infection	800 mg intravesically weekly for 6 wk
Antimetabolites				
capecitabine *kap-ah-seat′-ah-bean*	Xeloda	Breast cancer	Dermatitis, diarrhea, nausea, vomiting, leukopenia, granulocytopenia, thrombocytopenia, hand and foot syndrome, stomatitis, abdominal pain, constipation, dyspnea, anemia, hyperbilirubinemia, fatigue, weakness, anorexia	2500 mg/m^2/d PO
cladribine *kla′-dri-bean*	Leustatin	Hairy cell leukemia	Neutropenia, fever, infection, fatigue, nausea, headache, rash, injection site reactions, nephrotoxicity, neurotoxicity	0.09 mg/kg/d IV
cytarabine *sye-tare′-a-bean*	Cytosar-U, generic	Acute myelocytic or lymphocytic leukemia	Bone marrow depression, nausea, vomiting, diarrhea, anorexia	100–200 mg/m^2/d IV, SC
fludarabine *floo-dar′-a-bean*	Fludara	Chronic lymphocytic leukemia	Bone marrow depression, fever, chills, infection, nausea, vomiting, rash, diarrhea	25 mg/m^2 IV
fluorouracil (5-FU) *flure-oh-yoor′-a-sill*	Adrucil, generic	Carcinoma of the breast, stomach, pancreas, colon, and rectum	Diarrhea, anorexia, nausea, vomiting, alopecia, bone marrow depression, angina, stomatitis	3–12 mg/kg/d IV

(continued)

SUMMARY DRUG TABLE ANTINEOPLASTIC DRUGS (*Continued*)

GENERIC NAME	TRADE NAME*	USES	ADVERSE REACTIONS	DOSAGE RANGES
gemcitabine HCl *jem-site´-ah-ben*	Gemzar	Pancreatic cancer, non–small-cell lung cancer	Anemia, proteinuria, nausea, vomiting, fever, rash, leukopenia, neutropenia, thrombocytopenia, diarrhea, constipation, alopecia	1000–1250 mg/m^2 IV
mercaptopurine (6-mercaptopurine, 6-MP) *mer-kap-toe-pyoor´-een*	Purinethol	Acute lymphatic leukemia, acute or chronic myelogenous leukemia	Bone marrow depression, hyperuricemia, hepatotoxicity, skin rash	2.5–5 mg/kg/d PO; do not exceed 5 mg/kg/d
methotrexate *meth-o-trex´-ate*	Rheumatrex, *generic,* Dose Pack	Lymphosarcoma, severe psoriasis, cancer of the head, neck, breast, lung, rheumatoid arthritis (RA)	Ulcerative stomatitis, nausea, rash, pruritus, renal failure, bone marrow depression, fatigue, fever, chills	Antineoplastic dosages vary widely depending on type of tumor; psoriasis: 10–50 mg/wk IV, IM, PO; RA: dose pack directed
pentostatin *pen´-toe-stat-in*	Nipent	Alpha-interferon-refractory hairy cell leukemia	Bone marrow depression, anemia, nausea, vomiting, diarrhea, rash, fever	4 mg/m^2 IV every other week
thioguanine (TG) *thye-oh-gwon´-een*	*generic*	Acute leukemias	Bone marrow depression, hepatic toxicity, nausea, vomiting, stomatitis, hyperuricemia	2–3 mg/kg/d PO

Mitotic Inhibitors (Antimitotic Agents)

docetaxel *dohs-eh-tax´-el*	Taxotere	Breast cancer, non–small-cell lung cancer	Nausea, skin rash, pruritus, stomatitis, vomiting, anemia, leukopenia, neutropenia, arthralgia, alopecia, asthenia, fever, infections	60–100 mg/m^2 IV
paclitaxel *pass-leh-tax´-ell*	Taxol	Ovarian cancer, breast cancer, AIDS-related Kaposi's sarcoma	Diarrhea, nausea, vomiting, flushing, myalgia, arthralgia, fever, peripheral neuropathy, opportunistic infections	135–175 mg/m^2 IV
vinblastine sulfate (VLB; LCR) *vin-blas´-teen*	Velban, *generic*	Hodgkin's disease, lymphocytic lymphoma, histiocytic lymphoma, mycosis fungoides, testicular cancer, Kaposi's sarcoma, breast cancer	Leukopenia, nausea, vomiting, paresthesias, malaise, weakness, mental depression, headache, hypertension, alopecia, diarrhea, constipation	3.7–18.4 mg/m^2 IV
vincristine sulfate (VCR; LRC) *vin-kris´-teen*	Oncovin, Vincasar PFS, *generic*	Acute leukemia, combination therapy for various cancers	Same as vinblastine	1.4 mg/m^2 IV

Hormones

Androgens

testolactone *tess-toe-lak´-tone*	Teslac	Palliative treatment of advanced disseminated metastatic breast carcinoma in postmenopausal women and premenopausal women whose ovarian function has been terminated	Paresthesia, glossitis, anorexia, nausea, vomiting, maculopapular erythema, aches, edema of the extremities, nail growth disturbances, increase in blood pressure, virilization	250 mg QID PO

GENERIC NAME	TRADE NAME*	USES	ADVERSE REACTIONS	DOSAGE RANGES
Antiandrogens				
bicalutamide *bye-cal-loo´-ta-mide*	Casodex	Prostate cancer	Hot flushes, hypertension, dizziness, paresthesia, insomnia, rash, constipation, nausea, diarrhea, nocturia, hematuria, peripheral edema, bone pain, dyspnea, general pain, back pain, asthenia, infection	50 mg once daily PO
flutamide *flu´-ta-mide*	Eulexin	Early stage and metastatic prostate cancer	Hot flashes, loss of libido, impotence, diarrhea, nausea, vomiting, gynecomastia	125 mg PO TID at 8-h intervals PO (up to 750 mg/d)
nilutamide *nah-loo´-ta-mide*	Nilandron	Metastatic prostate cancer	Pain, headache, asthenia, abdominal pain, chest pain, flu symptoms, fever, liver toxicity, insomnia, nausea, constipation, testicular atrophy, dyspnea, pain, asthenia	150–300 mg/d PO
Progestins				
medroxyprog-esterone *me-drox´-ee-proe-jess´-te-rone*	Depo-Provera	Endometrial or renal cancer	Breakthrough bleeding, spotting, change in menstrual flow, amenorrhea, rash with or without pruritus, acne, fluid retention, edema, increase or decrease in weight, sudden, partial, or complete loss of vision, migraine, nausea	400–1000 mg IM per week; if disease stabilizes 400 mg/month IM
megestrol acetate *me-jess´-trole*	Megace, *generic*	Breast or endometrial cancer	Same as medroxyprogesterone	Breast cancer: 160 mg/d PO; endometrial cancer: 40–320 mg/d in divided doses PO
Estrogens				
diethylstilbestrol diphosphate *dye-eth-il-stil-bess´-trole*	Stilphostrol	Inoperable prostatic carcinoma	Headache, dizziness, intolerance to contact lens, edema, thrombo-embolism, hypertension, nausea, weight changes, testicular atrophy, acne, breast tenderness, gynecomastia	Oral: 50–200 mg TID PO (not to exceed 1 g/d) Parenteral: 0.5–1 g/d IV
estramustine phosphate sodium estradiol and nitrogen mustard *ess-tra-muss´-teen*	Emcyt	Metastic or progressive prostatic carcinoma	Same as diethylstilbestrol and diarrhea, vomiting, decreased libido, sodium and water retention, skin rash	10–16 mg/kg/d PO in 3–4 divided doses
Antiestrogens				
tamoxifen citrate *ta-mox´-i-fen*	Nolvadex, *generic*	Breast cancer in menopausal women, preventative therapy for women at high risk for breast cancer	Fluid retension, vaginal discharge, nausea, vomiting, hypercalcemia, ophthalmic changes, hot flashes, vaginal bleeding and discharge	20–40 mg/d
toremifene citrate *tore-em´-ah-feen*	Fareston	Breast cancer	Hot flushes, nausea, vomiting, vaginal bleeding, vaginal discharge, menstrual irregularities, skin rash	60 mg once daily PO

(continued)

SUMMARY DRUG TABLE   ANTINEOPLASTIC DRUGS (*Continued*)

GENERIC NAME	TRADE NAME*	USES	ADVERSE REACTIONS	DOSAGE RANGES
Gonadotropin-Releasing Hormone Analogs				
goserelin acetate *goe´-se-rel-in*	Zoladex	Prostate cancer, endometriosis, advanced breast cancer, emdometrial thinning	Lethargy, dizziness, insomnia, anorexia, nausea, sexual dysfunction, headache, emotional lability, depression, sweating, acne, breast atrophy, peripheral edema, lower urinary tract symptoms, hot flashes, pain, edema, upper respiratory tract infection, rash	3.6 mg SC q28d or 10.8 mg q3 months into the upper abdominal wall
leuprolide acetate *loo-proe´-lide*	Lupron, Lupron Depot	Advanced prostatic carcinoma, endrometriosis, central precocious puberty, uterine leiomyomata	Edema, headache, dizziness, bone pain, nausea, vomiting, anorexia, ECG changes, hypertension	1 mg SC daily; Depot: 7.5–30 mg IM; endometriosis: Depot, 3.75 IM monthly; uterine leiomyomata: 3.75 IM monthly
triptorelin pamoate *trip-toe-rell´-in*	Trelstar Depot	Advanced prostate cancer	Hot flushes, skeletal pain, injection site pain, hypertension, headache, insomnia, dizziness, vomiting, diarrhea, impotence	3.75 mg IM
Aromastase Inhibitors				
anastrazole *an-ahs´-troh-zol*	Arimidex	Advanced breast cancer	Vasodilation, headache, dizziness, insomnia, GI disturbances, nausea, constipation, diarrhea, cough, increased dyspnea, hot flushes, asthenia, pain, back pain, peripheral edema, bone pain	1 mg once daily
exemestane *ex-ah´-mess-tane*	Aromasin	Advanced breast cancer	Depression, insomnia, anxiety, dizziness, nausea, vomiting, abdominal pain, anorexia, constipation, diarrhea, dyspnea, fatigue, hot flashes, pain, peripheral edema	25 mg/d PO
letrozole *le´-tro-zol*	Femara	Advanced breast cancer	Same as for anastrazole	2.5 mg once daily PO
Miscellaneous Anticancer Drugs				
Epipodophyllotoxins				
etoposide *e-toe-poe´-side*	Toposar, VePesid, *generic*	Testicular cancer, small-cell lung cancer	Nausea, vomiting, anorexia, diarrhea, constipation, alopecia, granulocytopenia	Testicular cancer: 50–100 mg/m² /d IV; small-cell lung cancer: 35–50 mg/m² /d IV (oral dose is 2 times the IV dose rounded to the nearest 50 mg)
teniposide (VM-26) *teh-nip-oh-side*	Vumon	Leukemia	Nausea, vomiting, anorexia, diarrhea, constipation, alopecia, rash, leukopenia, thrombocytopenia, anemia	165–250 mg/m² IV
Enzymes				
asparaginase *a-spare´-a-gi-nase*	Elspar	Leukemia	Hypersensitivity reactions (rash, urticaria, arthralgia, respiratory distress, acute anaphylaxis), depression, somnolence, fatigue, coma, anorexia, nausea, vomiting	200–1000 IU/kg/d IV; 6000 IU/m² /d IM

SUMMARY DRUG TABLE ANTINEOPLASTIC DRUGS (*Continued*)

GENERIC NAME	TRADE NAME*	USES	ADVERSE REACTIONS	DOSAGE RANGES
pegaspargase (PEG-asparaginase) *peg-ass-par´-jase*	Oncaspar	Acute lymphoblastic leukemia	Nausea, vomiting, fever, malaise, dyspnea, diarrhea, hypotension	2500 mg/m^2 IM or IV
Platinum Coordination Complex.				
carboplatin *kar´-boe-pla-tin*	Paraplatin	Advanced ovarian cancer	Peripheral neuritis; vomiting; nausea; abdominal pain; diarrhea; constipation; decreased serum sodium, magnesium, calcium, and potassium; increased blood urea nitrogen; visual disturbances; ototoxicity	360 mg/m^2 IV
cisplatin *sis´-pla-tin*	Platinol-AQ	Metastatic testicular tumors, advanced bladder cancer, ovarian tumors	Ototoxicity, peripheral neuropathies, nausea, vomiting, anorexia, bone marrow suppression, nephrotoxicity	20–70 mg/m^2 IV
Anthracenedione				
mitoxantrone HCl *mye-toe-zan´-trone*	Novantrone	Acute leukemias, bone pain in advanced prostatic cancer	Nausea, vomiting, diarrhea, headache, seizures, abdominal pain, mucositis, congestive heart failure, bone marrow depression	12 mg/m^2 IV
Substituted Ureas				
hydroxyurea *hye-drox-ee-yoor-ee´-ah*	Droxia, Hydrea	Melanoma, chronic myelocytic leukemia, ovarian cancer	Headache, dizziness, stomatitis, anorexia, nausea, vomiting, diarrhea, constipation, bone marrow depression, impaired renal tubular function, rash, mucositis, fever, chills, malaise	20–80 mg/kg PO
Methylhydrazine Derivatives				
procarbazine HCl *proe-kar´-ba-zeen*	Matulane	Hodgkin's disease	Leukopenia, anemia, nausea, vomiting, anorexia, thrombocytopenia	1–6 mg/kg PO
Cytoprotective Agents				
amifostine *am-ih-foss´-teen*	Ethyol	Renal toxicity associated with repeated administration of cisplatin in patients with advanced ovarian cancer	Nausea, vomiting, hypotension, fever, chills, dyspnea, skin rash, urticaria	910 mg/m^2 IV QID
dexrazoxane *dex-ray-zox´-ane*	Zinecard	Cardiomyopathy associated with doxorubicin administration in women with metastatic breast cancer	Alopecia, nausea, vomiting, fatigue, malaise, anorexia, stomatitis, fever, infection, diarrhea, neurotoxicity	500 mg/m^2 IV
DNA Topoisomerase Inhibitors				
irinotecan HCl *eh-rin-oh´-te-kan*	Camptosar	Metastatic carcinoma of the colon or rectum	Dizziness, somnolence, confusion, vasodilation, hypotension, thrombophlebitis, diarrhea, nausea, vomiting, abdominal pain, anorexia, constipation, mucositis, dyspnea, asthenia, pain, fever	125 mg/m^2 IV
topotecan HCl *toe-poh´-te-kan*	Hycamtin	Ovarian cancer, small-cell lung cancer	Alopecia, rash, nausea, vomiting, diarrhea, constipation, abdominal pain, stomatitis, anorexia, dyspnea, headache, fatigue, fever, pain, asthenia, bone marrow depression	1.5 mg/m^2 IV

(continued)

SUMMARY DRUG TABLE ANTINEOPLASTIC DRUGS (*Continued*)

GENERIC NAME	TRADE NAME*	USES	ADVERSE REACTIONS	DOSAGE RANGES
Biological Response Modifiers				
aldesleukin *al-dess-loo´-kin* (interleukin-2; IL-2)	Proleukin	Metastatic renal-cell carcinoma	Nausea, diarrhea, stomatitis, hypotension, anorexia, bone marrow depression, pulmonary congestion, dyspnea, oliguria	600,000 IU/kg IV q8h
BCG, intravesical	Pacis, TheraCys, TICE BCG	Carcinoma in situ of the bladder	Dysuria, urinary frequency, cystitis, hematuria, urinary incontinence	120 mg instilled in the bladder once a week for 6 wk
denileukin diftitox *deh-nih-loo´-kin diff´-tih-tox*	Ontak	Cutaneous T-cell lymphoma	Hypotension, vasodilation, tachycardia, dizziness, paresthesia, rash, pruritus, nausea, vomiting, anorexia, diarrhea	9–18 μg/kg/d IV
levamisole (HCl) *lev-am´-ih-sole*	Ergamisol	Combination therapy in patients with Dukes stage C colon cancer	Nausea, vomiting, diarrhea, stomatitis, anorexia	50 mg q8h PO
Retinoids				
tretinoin *tret´-i-noyn*	Vesanoid	Acute promylelocytic leukemia	Headache, fever, weakness, fatigue, skin/mucous membrane dryness, increased sweating, visual disturbances, ocular disturbances, alopecia, bone pain	45 mg/m^2/d PO
Rexinoids				
bexarotene *bex-air´-oh-teen*	Targretin	Cutaneous T-cell lymphoma	Elevated blood lipids, hypothyroidism, headache, asthenia, rash, leukopenia, anemia, nausea, infection, peripheral edema, abdominal pain, dry skin	300 mg/m^2/d PO
Monoclonal Antibodies				
alemtuzumab *ay-lem-tuh´-zoo-mab*	Campath	B-cell chronic lymphocytic leukemia	Hypotension, headache, dizziness, rash, bone marrow suppression, fever, chills, asthenia, nausea, vomiting, diarrhea, stomatitis, fatigue	3–30 mg IV
gemtuzumab ozogamicin *gem-too´-zoo-mab oh-zoh-gam´-ih-sin*	Mylotarg	Acute myeloid leukemia	Chills, fever, nausea, vomiting, headache, hypotension, hypertension, hypoxia, dyspnea, bone marrow depression	9 mg/m^2 IV
rituximab *rih-tuck-sih-mab*	Rituxan	Non-Hodgkin´s lymphoma	Infusion reactions, hypotension, dizziness, anxiety, night sweats, rash, pruritus, nausea, diarrhea, vomiting, bone marrow depression	375 mg/m^2 IV
ibritumomab tiuxetan *ib-ri-tu´-moe-mab tie-ux-eh´-tan*	Zevalin	Non-Hodgkin´s lymphoma	Infections, allergic reactions (bronchospasms and angiooedema), bone marrow depression, hemorrhage, anemia, nausea, vomiting, abdominal pain, diarrhea, increased cough, dyspnea, dizziness, arthralgia, anorexia, ecchymosis	250 mg/m^2 IV
trastuzumab *trass-to-zoo´-mab*	Herceptin	Breast cancer	Anemia, leukopenia, diarrhea, infection, nausea, vomiting, pain, headache, dizziness, dyspnea, hypotension, rash, asthenia, infusion reactions, pulmonary adverse effects	2–4 mg/kg IV

SUMMARY DRUG TABLE ANTINEOPLASTIC DRUGS (*Continued*)

GENERIC NAME	TRADE NAME*	USES	ADVERSE REACTIONS	DOSAGE RANGES
Unclassified Antineoplastics				
imatinib mesylate *eh-mat'-eh-nib*	Gleevec	Chronic myeloid leukemia, gastrointestinal stromal tumors, acute lymphocytic leukemia	Gastric irritation, arthralgia, muscle cramps, hemorrhage, pyrexia, weakness, epistaxis, fatigue, ecchymosis, fluid retention, night sweats	400–800 mg/d PO
porfimer sodium *poor-fi'-mer*	Photofrin	Esophageal cancer	Atrial fibrillation, insomnia, constipation, nausea, abdominal pain, vomiting, pleural effusion, dyspnea, pneumonia, pharyngitis, anemia, fever, chest pain, pain, photosensitivity	2 mg/kg IV
mitotane *mye'-toe-tane*	Lysodren	Adrenal cortical carcinoma	Leukocytosis, GI symptoms (nausea, vomiting, diarrhea, abdominal pain), fatigue, edema, hyperglycemia, dyspnea, cough, rash, or itching, headaches, dizziness	2–16 g/d PO

*The term *generic* indicates the drug is available in generic form.

cured. Each cycle of treatment with the antineoplastic drugs kills some, but by no means all, of the malignant cells. Therefore, repeated courses of chemotherapy are used to kill more and more of the malignant cells, until theoretically none are left.

Alkylating Drugs

Alkylating drugs interfere with the process of cell division of malignant and normal cells. The drug binds with DNA, causing breaks and preventing DNA replication.

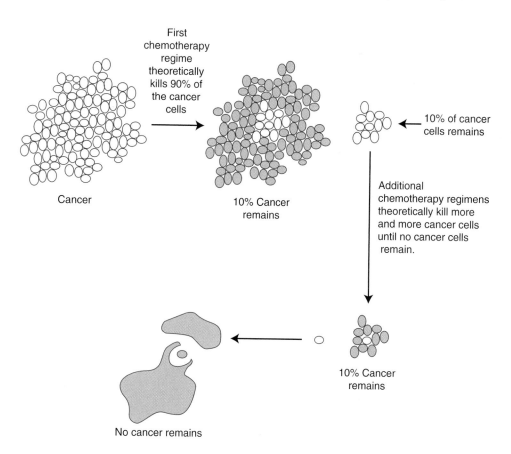

FIGURE 55-1. Cell kill theory describing activity of repeated chemotherapy regimens.

The malignant cells appear to be more susceptible to the effects of the alkylating drugs. Examples of alkylating drugs include busulfan (Myleran, Busulfex) and chlorambucil (Leukeran).

Antineoplastic Antibiotics

The antineoplastic antibiotics, unlike their anti-infection antibiotic relatives, do not have anti-infective (against infection) ability. Their action is similar to the alkylating drugs. Antineoplastic antibiotics appear to interfere with DNA and RNA synthesis and therefore delay or inhibit cell division, including the reproducing ability of malignant cells. Examples of antineoplastic antibiotics include bleomycin (Blenoxane), doxorubicin (Adriamycin), and plicamycin (Mithracin).

Antimetabolites

The antimetabolites interfere with various metabolic functions of cells, thereby disrupting normal cell functions. They inactivate enzymes or alter the structure of DNA, changing the DNA's ability to replicate. These drugs are most effective in the treatment of rapidly dividing neoplastic cells. Examples of the antimetabolites include methotrexate and fluorouracil (Adrucil).

Hormones

The exact method of antineoplastic action of hormones is unclear. These drugs also appear to counteract the effect of male or female hormones in hormone-dependent tumors (see Chap. 52). They appear to alter the hormonal environment of the cell. Examples of hormones used as neoplastic drugs include the androgen testolactone (Teslac), conjugate estrogens (see Chap. 52), and the progestin megestrol (Megace).

Gonadotropin-releasing hormone analogs, for example, goserelin (Zoladex), appear to act by inhibiting the anterior pituitary secretion of gonadotropins, thus suppressing the release of pituitary gonadotropins. These drugs primarily decrease serum testosterone levels and therefore are used in the treatment of advanced prostatic carcinomas.

Mitotic Inhibitors

Mitotic inhibitors (antimitotics) interfere with or stop cell division. Examples of mitotic inhibitors include paclitaxel (Taxol) and vincristine (Oncovin).

Miscellaneous Antineoplastic Drugs

The mechanism of action of this unrelated group of drugs is not entirely clear. Examples of miscellaneous antineoplastics include cisplatin (Platinol) and hydroxyurea (Hydrea).

USES

Antineoplastic drugs may be given alone or in combination with other antineoplastic drugs. In many instances, a combination of these drugs produces better results than the use of a single antineoplastic drug.

Although many antineoplastic drugs share a similar activity (ie, they interfere in some way with cell division), their uses are not necessarily similar. The more common uses of specific antineoplastic drugs are given in the Summary Drug Table.

ADVERSE REACTIONS

Antineoplastic drugs often produce a wide variety of adverse reactions. Some of these reactions are dose dependent; that is, their occurrence is more common or their intensity is more severe when higher doses are used. Other adverse reactions occur primarily because of the effect the drug has on many cells of the body. Because the antineoplastic drugs affect both cancer cells and rapidly proliferating normal cells (ie, cells in the bone marrow, gastrointestinal tract, reproductive tract, and the hair follicles), adverse reactions occur as the result of the action on these cells. Adverse reactions common to many of the antineoplastic drugs include bone marrow suppression, nausea, vomiting, stomatitis, diarrhea, and hair loss.

Some adverse reactions are desirable, for example, the depressing effect of certain antineoplastic drugs on the bone marrow because this adverse drug reaction is essential in the treatment of the leukemias. Other adverse reactions are not desirable, for example, severe vomiting or diarrhea.

Antineoplastic drugs are potentially toxic and their administration is often associated with many serious adverse reactions. At times, some of these adverse effects are allowed because the only alternative is to stop treatment of the malignancy. A treatment plan is developed that will prevent, lessen, or treat most or all of the symptoms of a specific adverse reaction. An example of prevention is giving an antiemetic before administering an antineoplastic drug known to cause severe nausea and vomiting. An example of treatment of the symptoms of an adverse reaction is the administration of an antiemetic and intravenous (IV) fluids and electrolytes when severe vomiting occurs.

Adverse reactions seen with the administration of these drugs may range from very mild to life threatening. Some of these reactions, such as the loss of hair (**alopecia**), may have little effect on the physical status of the patient but may definitely have a serious effect on the patient's mental health. Because nursing is concerned with the whole patient, these physically altering reactions that can have a profound effect on the patient must be considered when planning nursing management.

Some of the adverse reactions seen with antineoplastic drugs are listed in the Summary Drug Table: Antineoplastic Drugs. Appropriate references should be consulted when administering these drugs because there are a variety of uses, dose ranges, and, in some instances, many adverse reactions.

CONTRAINDICATIONS, PRECAUTIONS, AND INTERACTIONS

The information discussed in this section is general, and the contraindications, precautions, and interactions for each antineoplastic drug vary. The nurse should consult appropriate sources before administering any antineoplastic drug.

The antineoplastic drugs are contraindicated in patients with leukopenia, thrombocytopenia, anemia, serious infections, serious renal disease, or known hypersensitivity to the drug and during pregnancy (see Display 55-1 for pregnancy classifications of selected antineoplastic drugs).

Antineoplastic drugs are used cautiously in patients with renal or hepatic impairment, active infection, or other debilitating illnesses, or in those who have recently completed treatment with other antineoplastic drugs or radiation therapy.

The following sections give selected interactions of the alkylating drugs, antimetabolites, antibiotics, hormones, miotic inhibitors, and miscellaneous antineoplastic drugs. The nurse should consult appropriate sources for a more complete listing of interactions before any antineoplastic drug is administered.

Alkylating Drugs

The alkylating drugs may antagonize the effects of antigout drugs by increasing serum uric acid levels. Dosage adjustment of the antigout drug may be needed. If cisplatin is used concurrently with aminoglycosides, there may be an increase in nephrotoxicity and ototoxicity. When cisplatin is used concurrently with loop diuretics, there is an increased risk of ototoxicity. Administering live viral vaccines with cyclophosphamide may decrease the antibody response of the vaccine.

Antimetabolites

Antimetabolite drugs may antagonize the effects of antigout drugs by increasing the serum uric acid concentration. Toxicity from methotrexate may be increased by other nephrotoxic drugs. When the antimetabolites are administered with other antineoplastic drugs, bone marrow suppression is additive. Vitamin preparations containing folic acid may decrease the effects of methotrexate. Alcohol ingestion while taking methotrexate may increase the risk of hepatotoxicity. Concurrent use of methotrexate and the nonsteroidal anti-inflammatory drugs (NSAIDs) may cause severe methotrexate toxicity. Fluorouracil is not compatible with the diazepam, doxorubicin, and methotrexate. Food decreases the absorption of fluorouracil. Live viral vaccines should not be administered if the patient is receiving fluorouracil because a decrease in antibody production may occur, causing the vaccine to be ineffective. Severe cardiomyopathy with left ventricular failure has occurred when fluorouracil and cisplatin are given together.

Antineoplastic Antibiotics

Plasma digoxin levels may decrease when the drug is administered with bleomycin. When bleomycin is used with cisplatin, there is an increased risk of bleomycin toxicity. Pulmonary toxicity may occur when bleomycin is administered with other antineoplastic drugs. Plicamycin, mitomycin, mitoxantrone, and dactinomycin have an additive bone marrow depressant effect when administered with other antineoplastic drugs. In addition, mitomycin, mitoxantrone, and dactinomycin decrease antibody response to live virus vaccines. Dactinomycin potentiates or reactivates skin or gastrointestinal reactions of radiation therapy. There is an increased risk of bleeding when plicamycin is administered with aspirin, warfarin, heparin, and the NSAIDs.

Hormones

Bicalutamide may increase the effect of oral anticoagulants. Flutamide enhances the action of leuprolide. Additive antineoplastic effects may occur when leuprolide is administered with megestrol or flutamide. Estrogens decrease the effectiveness of tamoxifen.

DISPLAY 55-1 ● Pregnancy Classification for Selected Antineoplastic Drugs

PREGNANCY CATEGORY C

cyclophosphamide	asparaginase	pegaspargase
levamisole	dacarbazine	dactinomycin

PREGNANCY CATEGORY D

busulfan	idarubicin	vincristine
cladribine	mitomycin	anastrozole
chlorambucil	fluorouracil	mitoxantrone
cisplatin	toremifene	pentostatin
ifosfamide	hydroxyurea	teniposide
mechlorethamine	mercaptopurine	vinblastine
melphalan	thioguanine	bleomycin
procarbazine	mitoxantrone	epirubicin
thiotepa	flutamide	doxorubicin
daunorubicin	megestrol	teniposide
tamoxifen	etoposide	

PREGNANCY CATEGORY X

diethylstilbestrol	bicalutamide	goserelin
methotrexate	plicamycin	triptorelin

Miotic Inhibitors

Additive bone marrow depressive effects occur when the miotic inhibitor drugs are administered with other antineoplastic drugs or radiation therapy. Administration of vincristine with digoxin results in a decreased therapeutic effect of the digoxin and decreased plasma digoxin levels. There is a decrease in serum concentrations of phenytoin when administered with vinblastine.

Miscellaneous Antineoplastic Drugs

When asparaginase is administered to a patient with diabetes, the risk for hyperglycemia is increased; a dosage adjustment of the oral antidiabetic drug may be necessary. Glucocorticoids decrease the effectiveness of aldesleukin. When aldesleukin is administered with antihypertensive drugs, there is an additive hypotensive effect. Etoposide may decrease the immune response to live viral vaccines.

There is an increased risk for bone marrow suppression when levamisole or hydroxyurea are administered with other antineoplastic drugs. Use of levamisole with phenytoin increases the risk of phenytoin toxicity. Pegaspargase may alter drug response of the anticoagulants. When procarbazine is administered with other central nervous system (CNS) depressants, such as alcohol, antidepressants, antihistamines, opiates, or the sedatives, an additive CNS effect may be seen. Procarbazine may potentiate hypoglycemia when administered with insulin or oral antidiabetic drugs.

❋ Herbal Alert: Green Tea

Green tea and black teas come from the same plant. The difference is in the processing. Green tea is simply dried tea leaves, whereas black tea is fermented, giving it the dark color, the stronger flavor, and the lowest amount of tannins and polyphenols. The beneficial effects of green tea lie in the polyphenols, or flavonoids, that have antioxidant properties. Antioxidants are thought to play a major role in preventing disease (eg, colon cancer) and reducing the effects of aging. Green tea polyphenols are powerful antioxidants. The polyphenols are thought to act by inhibiting the reactions of free radicals within the body that are thought to play a role in aging. The benefits of green tea include an overall sense of well-being, cancer prevention, dental health, and maintenance of heart and liver health. Green tea taken as directed is safe and well tolerated. It contains as much as 50 mg of caffeine per cup. Decaffeinated green tea retains all of the polyphenol content. The recommended dosage is 2 to 5 cups a day. Standardized green tea extracts vary in strength, so dosages may need to be adjusted. The recommeded dosage is 250 to 400 mg/d of extract standardized to 90% polyphenols. Because green tea contains caffeine, nervousness, restlessness, insomnia, and gastrointestinal upset may occur. Green tea should be avoided during pregnancy because of its caffeine content. Patients with hypertension, cardiac conditions, anxiety, insomnia, diabetes, and ulcers should use green tea with caution.

● **The Patient Receiving an Antineoplastic Drug**

ASSESSMENT

Preadministration Assessment

The extent of the preadministration assessment depends on the type of malignancy and the patient's general physical condition. The initial assessment of the patient scheduled for chemotherapy may include:

- The type and location of the neoplastic lesion (as stated on the patient's chart)
- The stage of the disease, for example, early, metastatic, terminal
- The patient's general physical condition
- The patient's emotional response to the disease
- The anxiety or fears the patient may have regarding chemotherapy treatments
- Previous or concurrent treatments (if any), such as surgery, radiation therapy, other antineoplastic drugs
- Other current nonmalignant disease or disorder, for example, congestive heart failure or peptic ulcer, that may or may not be related to the malignant disease
- The patient's knowledge or understanding of the proposed chemotherapy regimen
- Other factors, such as the patient's age, financial problems that may be associated with a long-term illness, family cooperation and interest in the patient, and the adequacy of health insurance coverage (which may be of great concern to the patient)

Immediately before administering the first dose of an antineoplastic drug, the nurse takes the patient's vital signs. The nurse obtains a current weight because the dose of some antineoplastic drugs is based on the patient's weight in kilograms or pounds. The dosages of some antineoplastic drugs also may be based on body surface measurements and are stated as a specific amount of drug per square meter (m^2) of body surface. Additional physical assessments may be necessary for certain antineoplastic drugs.

A few antineoplastic drugs require treatment measures before administration. An example of preadministration treatment is hydration of the patient with 1 to 2 liters of IV fluid infused before administration of cisplatin (Platinol) or administration of an antiemetic before the administration of mechlorethamine. These measures are ordered by the primary health care provider and, in some instances, may vary slightly from the manufacturer's recommendations.

When an antineoplastic drug has a depressing effect on the bone marrow, laboratory tests, such as a complete blood count, are ordered to determine the effect of the previous drug dosage. Before the first dose of the drug is administered, pretreatment laboratory tests provide baseline data for future reference.

Ongoing Assessment

The patient who is acutely ill with many physical problems requires different ongoing assessment activities than does one who is ambulating and able to participate in the activities of daily living. Once the patient's general condition is assessed and needs identified, the nurse develops a care plan to meet those needs. Patients receiving chemotherapy can be at different stages of their disease; therefore, nurses must individualize the nursing care of each patient based on the patient's needs and not only on the type of drug administered.

In general, after the administration of an antineoplastic drug, the nurse bases the ongoing assessment on the following factors:

- The patient's general condition
- The patient's individual response to the drug
- Adverse reactions that may occur
- Guidelines established by the primary health care provider or hospital
- Results of periodic laboratory tests

Different types of laboratory tests may be used to monitor the patient's response to therapy. Some of these tests, for example, a complete blood count, may be used to determine the response of the bone marrow to an antineoplastic drug. Other tests, for example, liver function tests, may be used to detect liver toxicity, which may be an adverse reaction that can be seen with the administration of some of these drugs. Abnormal laboratory tests may also require a change in the nursing care plan. For example, a significant drop in the platelet count may result in bleeding episodes and require measures, such as prolonged pressure on injection sites, to prevent bleeding or bruising episodes.

The nurse reviews the results of all laboratory tests at the time they are reported. The primary health care provider is notified of the results before the administration of successive doses of an antineoplastic drug. If these tests indicate a severe depressant effect on the bone marrow or other test abnormalities, the primary health care provider may reduce the next drug dose or temporarily stop chemotherapy to allow the affected body systems to recover.

NURSING DIAGNOSES

The nursing diagnoses for the patient with a malignancy are usually extensive and are based on many factors, such as the patient's physical and emotional condition, the adverse reactions resulting from antineoplastic drug therapy, and the stage of the disease.

Nursing Diagnoses Checklist

✓ **Disturbed Body Image** related to adverse reactions of antineoplastic drugs (eg, alopecia, weight loss)

✓ **Imbalanced Nutrition: Less than Body Requirements** related to adverse drug reactions of antineoplastic drugs (eg, nausea, vomiting, anorexia)

✓ **Risk for Infection** related to adverse drug reactions of antineoplastic drugs (eg, bone marrow suppression)

✓ **Impaired Oral Mucous Membranes** related to adverse drug effects of the antineoplastic drugs (eg, stomatitis)

✓ **Diarrhea** related to adverse reactions of the antineoplastic drugs

✓ **Impaired Tissue Integrity** related to adverse reactions of the antineoplastic drugs (extravasation)

✓ **Anxiety** related to diagnosis, necessary treatment measures, the occurrence of adverse reactions, other factors

---

Drug-specific nursing diagnoses are highlighted in the Nursing Diagnoses Checklist. Other nursing diagnoses applicable to these drugs are discussed in depth in Chapter 4.

PLANNING

The expected outcomes of the patient may include an optimal response to therapy, management of common adverse reactions, a reduction in anxiety, and an understanding of the prescribed treatment modalities.

IMPLEMENTATION

Promoting an Optimal Response to Therapy

Care of the patient receiving an antineoplastic drug depends on factors such as the drug or combination of drugs given, the dosage of the drugs, the route of administration, the patient's physical response to therapy, the response of the tumor to chemotherapy, and the type and severity of adverse reactions. Some drugs may be administered by various routes, depending on the cancer being treated. For example, thiotepa may be administered by the intravenous route for breast cancer, intravesical route for superficial bladder cancer, intrapleural route for malignant pleural effusions, and by the intraperitoneal route for ovarian cancer.

Most hospitals and clinics require that nurses receive specialized training and standardized educational preparation before they are permitted to administer antineoplastic drugs. The Oncology Nursing Society has developed guidelines and educational tools for credentialing nurses for certification in administering chemotherapy.

In some hospitals, policies are established to provide nursing personnel with specific guidelines for the assessment and care of patients receiving a single or combination chemotherapeutic drug regimen. If guidelines are not provided, it is important for the nurse to review the drugs being given before their administration. The nurse consults appropriate references to obtain information regarding the preparation and administration of a particular drug, the average dose ranges, all the known adverse reactions, and the warnings and precautions given by the manufacturer.

ORAL ADMINISTRATION. A number of antineoplastic drugs are administered orally. The oral route is convenient, economical, noninvasive, and often less toxic. Most oral drugs are well absorbed when the gastrointestinal tract is functioning normally. Antineoplastic drugs such as melphalan, busulfan, and chlorambucil are usually given orally. (Melphalan and busulfan are also available as injectable products for specific indications.) Most oral drugs are administered by the patient in a home setting. The section on "Educating the Patient and Family" provides information to include in a teaching plan.

When an antineoplastic drug is administered orally, the nurse must handle the drug safely. Gloves are considered acceptable if physical contact with the tablet or capsule is necessary.

PARENTERAL ADMINISTRATION. Although some of these drugs are given orally, others are given by the parenteral route. Antineoplastic drugs may be administered subcutaneously, intramuscularly, and intravenously. When giving these drugs IM, the nurse gives the injection into the large muscles using the Z-track method (see Chap. 2) because administration can cause stinging or burning. When the SC method of administration is used, the injection should contain no more than 3 mL, and injections are given in the usual SC injection sites (see Chap. 2). If the injections are given frequently, the sites should be rotated and charted appropriately.

Goserelin (Zoladex), a hormonal antineoplastic drug used to treat breast cancer, is administered subcutaneously in an unusual way. The drug is contained in a dry pellet that is implanted in the soft tissue of the abdomen, where it is gradually absorbed during a period of 1 to 3 months. After a local anesthetic, such as lidocaine, is administered, a large needle (usually 16 gauge) is used to insert the pellet.

It is most important to follow the directions of the manufacturer or primary health care provider regarding the type of solution to be used for dilution or administration. When preparing an antineoplastic drug for parenteral administration, the nurse wears disposable plastic gloves. Some of these drugs can be absorbed through the skin of the individual preparing these drugs. Because antineoplastic drugs are highly toxic and can have an effect on many organs and systems of the body, nurses must use measures to prevent

absorption of the drug through the skin. It is important for the nurse to take precautions to prevent accidental spilling or spraying of the drug into the eyes or onto unprotected areas of the skin. The nurse thoroughly washes the hands before and after preparing and administering an antineoplastic drug. This is especially important when the drug is given by the parenteral route.

Special directions for administration, stated by either the primary health care provider or manufacturer, are also important. For example, cisplatin cannot be prepared or administered with needles or IV administration sets containing aluminum because aluminum reacts with cisplatin, causing formation of a precipitate and loss of potency.

ADMINISTERING ANTINEOPLASTIC DRUGS INTRAVENOUSLY. The intravenous route of drug delivery is the most common and most reliable method of drug delivery. Intravenous administration may be accomplished using a vascular access device, an Angiocath, or a butterfly needle. These devices have become a common method of drug delivery and depending on the patient's individual treatment regimen, may be inserted before therapy. Selection of the device depends on the type of therapy the patient is to receive, the condition of the veins, and how long the treatment regimen is to be continued. Instructions for monitoring the administration of intravenous antineoplastic drugs are given by the physician. Nurses who are certified in chemotherapy drug administration administer these drugs, but any nurse may be involved in monitoring patients receiving antineoplastic drugs.

Most antineoplastic drugs have specific recommended administration techniques. For example, an infusion pump is recommended for the administration of cisplatin, and plicamycin (Mithracin) is administered by slow IV infusion during a period of 4 to 6 hours. If administration guidelines are not provided by the primary health care provider or the hospital, the nurse checks with the appropriate authorities (physician, pharmacist) regarding the administration of a specific antineoplastic drug.

The nurse must read thoroughly the package insert supplied with the drug before the drug is prepared and administered. The manufacturer's recommendations may include information such as storage of the drug, reconstitution procedures, stability of the drug after reconstitution, the rate of administration, and the technique of administration.

Antineoplastic drugs are potentially toxic drugs that can cause a variety of effects during and after their administration. Display 55-2 summarizes important points to keep in mind when administering an antineoplastic drug.

DISPLAY 55-2 ● Important Points to Keep in Mind When Administering an Antineoplastic Drug

- Great care and accuracy are important in preparing and administering these drugs.
- Wear disposable plastic gloves when preparing any of these drugs for parenteral administration.
- Observe the patient closely before, during, and after the administration of an antineoplastic drug.
- Observe the IV site closely to detect any signs of **extravasation** (leakage into the surrounding tissues). Tissue necrosis can be a serious complication. Discontinue the infusion and notify the primary health care provider if discomfort, redness along the pathway of the vein, or infiltration occurs.
- Continually update nursing assessments, nursing diagnoses, and nursing care plans to meet the changing needs of the patient.
- Notify the primary health care provider of all changes in the patient's general condition, the appearance of adverse reactions, and changes in laboratory test results.
- Provide the patient and family with both physical and emotional support during treatment.

GUIDELINES ESTABLISHED BY THE PRIMARY HEALTH CARE PROVIDER OR HOSPITAL. During chemotherapy, the primary health care provider may write orders for certain nursing procedures, such as measuring fluid intake and output, monitoring the vital signs at specific intervals, and increasing the fluid intake to a certain amount. Even when orders are written, the nurse should increase the frequency of certain assessments, such as monitoring vital signs, if the patient's condition changes. Some hospitals have written guidelines for nursing management when the patient is receiving a specific antineoplastic drug. The nurse incorporates these guidelines into the nursing care plan with nursing observations and assessments geared to the individual. The nurse adds further assessments to the nursing care plan when the patient's condition changes.

Monitoring and Managing Adverse Drug Reactions

Not all patients have the same response to a specific antineoplastic drug. For example, an antineoplastic drug may cause vomiting, but the amount of fluid and electrolytes lost through vomiting may vary from patient to patient. One patient may require additional sips of water once nausea and vomiting have subsided, whereas another may require IV fluid and electrolyte replacement. Nursing management is geared not only to what may or what did happen, but also is based on the effects produced by a particular adverse reaction. In the example of the patient who is vomiting, it is important to accurately measure all fluid intake and all output from the gastrointestinal and urinary tracts, as well as to observe the patient for signs of dehydration and electrolyte imbalances. These measurements and observations aid the primary health care provider in determining if fluid replacement is necessary.

Knowing what adverse reactions may occur allows the nurse to prepare for any event that will happen. For example, a hemorrhagic syndrome may be seen with the administration of plicamycin. Knowing this, assessments for hemorrhage are incorporated in the nursing care plan. Another example is the development of hyperuricemia (elevated blood uric acid levels), which may be seen with drugs, such as melphalan (Alkeran) or mercaptopurine (Purinethol). When this adverse reaction is known to occur, fluid intake and output measurements, as well as encouragement to increase fluid intake to at least 2000 mL of oral fluid per day, are included in the nursing care plan. Other antineoplastic drugs are nephrotoxic. Therefore, blood urea nitrogen levels and serum creatinine are monitored closely during therapy.

❄ Gerontologic Alert

Older adults are at increased risk for adverse reactions from the antineoplastic drugs because of the increased incidence of chronic disease, particularly renal impairment or cardiovascular disease. When renal impairment is present, a lower dosage of the antineoplastic may be indicated. Creatinine clearance is used to monitor renal function in the older adult. Blood creatinine levels are likely to be inaccurate because of a decreased muscle mass in the older adult.

MANAGING ALOPECIA. Alopecia (loss of hair) is a common adverse reaction associated with some of the antineoplastic drugs. Some drugs cause severe hair loss, whereas others cause gradual thinning. Examples of drugs commonly associated with severe hair loss are doxorubicin and vinblastine. Methotrexate, bleomycin, vincristine, and etoposide are associated with gradual hair loss.

If hair loss is associated with the antineoplastic drug being given, the nurse informs the patient that hair loss may occur. This problem occurs 10 to 21 days after the treatment cycle is completed. Hair loss is temporary, and hair will grow again when the drug therapy is completed. The nurse warns the patient that hair loss may occur suddenly and in large amounts. Although it is not life threatening, alopecia can lower self-esteem and serve as a reminder that the individual is undergoing treatment for cancer.

Depending on the patient, the nurse may need to make plans for the purchase of a wig or cap to disguise the hair loss until the hair grows back. Although this may seem to be a minor problem when compared with the serious reactions that may be seen during chemotherapy, the loss of hair is a personal problem for most patients and requires significant nursing consideration.

MANAGING ANOREXIA. **Anorexia** (loss of appetite resulting in the inability to eat) is a common occurrence with the antineoplastic drugs. Is it not uncommon for the patient to report alterations in the sense of taste during the course of chemotherapy. The nurse assesses the nutritional status of the patient before and during treatment. Small, frequent meals (five to six meals daily) are usually better tolerated than are three large meals. Breakfast is often the best tolerated meal of the day. The nurse stresses the importance of eating meals high in nutritive value, particularly protein (eg, eggs, milk products, tuna, beans, peas, and lentils). Some patients are able to eat high-protein finger foods such as cheese or peanut butter and crackers. Nutritional supplements may also be prescribed. The nurse monitors the patient's body weight weekly (or more often if necessary) and reports any weight loss. If the patient continues to lose weight, a feeding tube may be used to administer a nutritionally complete liquid. While this is not ideal, the patient who is malnourished and weak may benefit from this intervention.

MANAGING BONE MARROW SUPPRESSION. **Bone marrow suppression** is a potentially dangerous adverse reaction resulting in decreased production of blood cells. Bone marrow suppression is manifested by abnormal laboratory test results and clinical evidence of leukopenia, thrombocytopenia, or anemia. For example, there is a decrease in the white blood cells or leukocytes **(leukopenia),** a decrease in the thrombocytes **(thrombocytopenia),** and a decrease in the red blood cells, resulting in anemia. Patients with leukopenia have a decreased resistance to infection, and the nurse must monitor them closely for any signs of infection.

> ### Nursing Alert
>
> *The nurse should report any of the following signs of infection to the health care provider immediately: temperature of 100.4°F (38°C) or higher, cough, sore throat, chills, frequent urination, or a white blood cell count of less than 2500 mm³.*

Thrombocytopenia is characterized by a decrease in the platelet count ($<100,000/mm^3$). The nurse monitors patients with thrombocytopenia for bleeding tendencies and takes precautions to prevent bleeding. Injections are avoided but, if necessary, the nurse applies pressure to the injection site for 3 to 5 minutes to prevent bleeding into the tissue and the formation of a hematoma. The nurse informs the patient to avoid the use of electric razors, nail trimmers, dental floss, firm toothbrushes, or any sharp objects. The patient is monitored closely for easy bruising, skin lesions, and bleeding from any orifice (opening) of the body.

> ### Nursing Alert
>
> *The nurse reports any of the following to the health care provider immediately: bleeding gums, easy bruising, petechiae (pinpoint hemorrhages), increased menstrual bleeding, tarry stools, bloody urine, or coffee-ground emesis.*

Anemia occurs as the result of a decreased production of red blood cells in the bone marrow and is characterized by fatigue, dizziness, shortness of breath, and palpitations. On occasion, the administration of blood transfusions may be necessary to correct the anemia.

MANAGING NAUSEA AND VOMITING. Nausea and vomiting are common adverse reactions to the antineoplastic drugs. The primary health care provider may order an antiemetic about 30 minutes before treatment with the antineoplastic drug begins and continue the antiemetic for several days after administration of the chemotherapy. The nurse provides small, frequent meals to coincide with the patient's tolerance for food. Greasy or fatty foods and unpleasant sights, smells, and tastes are avoided. Cold foods, dry foods, and salty foods may be better tolerated. It is a good idea to provide diversional activities, such as music, television, and books. Relaxation, visualization, guided imagery, hypnosis, and other nonpharmacologic measures have been helpful to some patients.

MANAGING STOMATITIS. Because the cells in the mouth grow rapidly, they are particularly sensitive to the effects of the antineoplastic drugs. **Stomatitis** (inflammation of the mouth) or **oral mucositis** (inflammation of the oral mucous membranes) may occur 5 to 7 days after chemotherapy and continue up to 10 days after therapy. This adverse reaction is particularly uncomfortable because irritation of the oral mucous membranes affects the nutritional aspects of care. The patient must avoid any foods or products that are irritating to the mouth, such as alcoholic beverages, spices, strong mouthwashes, or toothpaste. The nurse provides soft or liquid food high in nutritive value. The oral cavity is inspected for increased irritation. The nurse reports any white patches on the tongue, throat, or gums; any burning sensation; and bleeding from the mouth or gums. Good mouth care is provided every 4 hours with normal saline or alcohol-free mouthwash. Lemon/glycerin swabs are avoided because they tend to irritate the oral mucosa and complicate stomatitis. The primary health care provider may order a topical viscous anesthetic, such as lidocaine viscous, before meals to decrease discomfort when eating.

MANAGING DIARRHEA. Measures to manage diarrhea include a low-residue diet while the bowel rests. Electrolytes are monitored and supplemented as needed. Adequate hydration must be maintained; intravenous fluids may be necessary. If diarrhea is severe, therapy may be delayed or stopped or the dose decreased.

MAINTAINING TISSUE INTEGRITY. Some antineoplastic drugs are **vesicants** (ie, they cause tissue necrosis if they infiltrate or extravasate out of the blood vessel and into the soft tissue). If extravasation occurs, underlying tissue is damaged. The damage can be severe, causing physical deformity or loss of vascularity or tendon function. Examples of vesicant drugs are daunorubicin, doxorubicin, and vinblastine.

☀ Nursing Alert

Patients at risk for extravasation are those unable to communicate to the nurse about the pain of extravasation, the elderly, debilitated or confused patient, and any patient with fragile veins.

When the patient is receiving a vesicant, the nurse monitors the IV site continuously and checks for blood return frequently (every 1–2 mL). Extravasation may occur without warning, or signs may be detected by an alert nurse. The earlier the extravasation is detected, the less likely soft-tissue damage will occur.

☀ Nursing Alert

Signs of an extravasation include:
- *Swelling (most common)*
- *Stinging, burning, or pain at the injection site (not always present)*
- *Redness*
- *Lack of blood return (if this is the only symptom, the IV should be re-evaluated)*

A lack of blood return alone is not always indicative of an extravasation, and an extravasation can occur even if a blood return is present. If an extravasation is suspected, the infusion is stopped immediately and the extravasation reported to the primary health care provider.

If a vesicant is prescribed as an infusion, it is given through a central line only and checked every 1 to 2 hours. The nurse keeps an extravasation kit containing all materials necessary to manage an extravasation available, along with the extravasation policy and procedure guidelines.

Managing Anxiety

Patients and family members are usually devastated by the diagnosis of a malignancy. The emotional impact of the disease may be forgotten or put aside by members of the medical team as they plan and institute therapy to control the disease. Patients undergoing chemotherapy require a great deal of emotional support from all members of the medical team. Kindness and gentleness in giving care and an understanding of the strain placed on the patient and the family may help reduce some of the fear and anxiety experienced during treatment.

Educating the Patient and Family

When the patient is hospitalized, the nurse explains all treatments and possible adverse effects to the patient before the initiation of therapy. The primary health care provider usually discusses the proposed treatment and possible adverse drug reactions with the patient and family members. The nurse briefly reviews these explanations immediately before parenteral administration of a drug.

Some of these drugs are taken orally at home. The areas included in a patient and family teaching plan for this type of treatment regimen are based on the drug prescribed, the primary health care provider's explanation of the chemotherapy regimen and instructions for taking the drug, and the needs of the individual. Some hospitals or primary health care providers give printed instructions to the patient. The nurse reviews these instructions after the patient has read them and allows time for the patient or family member to ask questions. The patient has a right to know the dangers associated with these drugs and what adverse reactions may occur.

Some patients are given antineoplastic drugs in the medical office or outpatient clinic. Before the institution of therapy, the treatment regimen is explained thoroughly to the patient and family. In some instances, a drug to prevent nausea may be prescribed to be taken before administration of the drugs in the medical office or clinic. To obtain the best possible effects, the nurse stresses to the patient that the drug must be taken at the time specified by the primary health care provider. It is important for the patient to comply with the treatment regimen to maximize a therapeutic effect. Most patients are compliant with therapy; however, some patients might decide to omit a dose in order to feel better temporarily. The nurse must stress the importance of maintaining the dosing schedule exactly as prescribed. A calendar indicating the doses to take, dates the drug is to be taken, and space to record each dose is often given to the patient. The patient is instructed to bring the treatment calendar to each appointment, and the patient is questioned about any omitted or delayed doses. One course of therapy is generally prescribed at a time to avoid inadvertent overdosing that could be life threatening.

The nurse includes the following points in a patient and family teaching plan when oral therapy is prescribed:

- Take the drug only as directed on the prescription container. Unless otherwise indicated, take the drug on a empty stomach with water to enhance absorption. However, the patient should follow specific directions, such as "take on an empty stomach" or "take at the same time each day"; they are extremely important.
- Familiarize yourself with the brand or trade name and the generic name to avoid confusion.
- Never increase, decrease, or omit a dose unless advised to do so by the primary health care provider.
- If any problems (adverse reactions) occur, no matter how minor, contact the primary health care provider immediately.
- All recommendations given by the primary health care provider, such as increasing the fluid intake, eating, or avoiding certain foods are important.
- The effectiveness or action of the drug could be altered if these directions are ignored. Other recommendations, such as checking the mouth for sores, rinsing the mouth thoroughly after eating or drinking, or drinking extra fluids, are given to identify or minimize some of the effects these drugs have on the body. It is important to follow these recommendations.
- Keep all appointments for chemotherapy. These drugs must be given at certain intervals to be effective.
- Do not take any nonprescription drug unless the use of a specific drug has been approved by the primary health care provider.
- Avoid drinking alcoholic beverages unless the primary health care provider has approved their use.
- Always inform other physicians, dentists, and medical personnel of therapy with this drug.
- Keep all appointments for the laboratory tests ordered by the primary health care provider. If unable to keep a laboratory appointment, notify the primary health care provider immediately.

EVALUATION

- The therapeutic effect is achieved.
- Adverse reactions are identified, reported to the primary health care provider, and managed using nursing interventions.
- Anxiety is reduced.
- The patient verbalizes an understanding of the dosage regimen.
- The patient verbalizes an understanding of treatment modalities and the importance of continued follow-up care.
- The patient verbalizes the importance of complying with the prescribed therapeutic regimen.

● *Critical Thinking Exercises*

1. *Dennis, age 10 years, has leukemia and is to begin chemotherapy with chlorambucil (Leukeran). Discuss what information would be important to discuss with Dennis and his parents before beginning the treatment regimen.*
2. *Ms. Thompson has cancer of the lung and will begin a treatment regimen with methotrexate. Discuss important preadministration assessments you would perform before beginning therapy with methotrexate.*
3. *Patients with a malignant disease need special consideration, understanding, and emotional support. On occasion, these needs are unrecognized by members of the medical profession. Suppose you recently received a diagnosis of cancer. Discuss some of the feelings you would experience at this time. Describe what you would want the nurse to do for you at this time. Analyze your thoughts about your future. Discuss what you would want to know or not know. As you think about this or discuss these questions, remember that any patient may have these same emotional responses and may need the same things you would expect from the nurse or other members of the medical profession.*

● *Review Questions*

1. Which of the following findings would be most indicative to the nurse that the patient has thrombocytopenia?

   A. Nausea
   B. Blurred vision
   C. Headaches
   D. Easy bruising

2. Which of the following is the most common symptom of extravasation?

   A. Swelling around the injection site
   B. Redness along the vein and around the injection site
   C. Pain at the injection site
   D. Tenderness along the path of the vein

3. Which of the following adverse reactions to the antineoplastic drugs is most likely to affect the patient's mental health and self-esteem?

   A. Hematuria
   B. Alopecia
   C. Nausea
   D. Diarrhea

4. When assessing the patient for leukopenia the nurse _____.

   A. checks the patient every 8 hours for hematuria
   B. monitors the patient for fever, sore throat, chills

C. checks female patients for increased menstrual bleeding

D. reports a WBC count of 5000 mm^3

5. Which of the following interventions would be most helpful for a patient with stomatitis?

A. Mouth care should be provided at least once daily.

B. Swab the mouth with lemon glycerin swabs every 4 hours.

C. Provide frequent mouth care with normal saline or alcohol-free mouthwash.

D. Use a hard bristle toothbrush to thoroughly cleanse the mouth and teeth of debris.

● Medication Dosage Problems

1. Chlorambucil (Leukeran) dosage is calculated based on the patient's body weight. Mrs. Garcia weighs 142 pounds. The prescribed dosage of chlorambucil is 0.2 mg/kg of body weight per day. What is the correct daily dosage for Mrs. Garcia?

2. A patient weighing 120 pounds is to receive bleomycin sulfate (Blenoxane) 0.25 units per kilogram of body weight. What is the correct dosage of bleomycin?

chapter 56

Topical Drugs Used in the Treatment of Skin Disorders

Key Terms

antipsoriatics
antiseptic
bactericidal
bacteriostatic
dermis
epidermis
germicide
hypersensitivity

immunocompromised
keratolytic
necrotic
proteolysis
proteolytic
purulent exudates
superinfection

Chapter Objectives

On completion of this chapter, the student will:

- List the types of drugs used in the treatment of skin disorders.
- Discuss the general drug actions, uses, and reactions of and any contraindications, precautions, and interactions associated with drugs used in the treatment of skin disorders.
- Discuss important preadministration and ongoing assessment activities the nurse should perform on patients receiving a drug used to treat skin disorders.
- List some nursing diagnoses particular to a patient using a drug to treat a skin disorder.
- Discuss ways to promote an optimal response to therapy and important points to keep in mind when educating the patient about a skin disorder.

The skin forms a barrier between the outside environment and the structures located beneath the skin. The **epidermis** is the outermost layer of the skin. Immediately below the epidermis is the dermis. The **dermis** contains small capillaries, which supply nourishment to the dermis and epidermis, sebaceous (oil-secreting) glands, sweat glands, nerve fibers, and hair follicles. Because of the skin's proximity to the outside environment, it is subject to various types of injury and trauma, as well as changes in the skin itself. Each of the following sections discusses only select topical drugs. See the Summary Drug Table: Dermatologic Drugs for a more complete listing of the drugs and additional information.

TOPICAL ANTI-INFECTIVES

Localized skin infections may require the use of a topical anti-infective. The topical anti-infectives include antibiotic, antifungal, and antiviral drugs.

ACTIONS AND USES

Topical Antibiotic Drugs

Topical antibiotics exert a direct local effect on specific microorganisms and may be bactericidal or bacteriostatic. Bacitracin (Baciguent) inhibits the cell wall synthesis. Bacitracin, gentamicin (G-myticin), erythromycin (Emgel), and neomycin are examples of topical antibiotics. These drugs are used to prevent superficial infections in minor cuts, wounds, skin abrasions, and minor burns. Erythromycin is also indicated for treatment of acne vulgaris.

Topical Antifungal Drugs

Antifungal drugs exert a local effect by inhibiting growth of the fungi. Examples of antifungal drugs and their uses are:

- Amphotericin B (Fungizone)—used for treatment of mycotic infections (fungal)

SUMMARY DRUG TABLE DERMATOLOGIC DRUGS

GENERIC NAME	TRADE NAME*	USES	ADVERSE REACTIONS	DOSAGE RANGES
Antibiotic Drugs				
azelaic acid *az-e-lak'*	Azelex	Acne vulgaris	Mild and transient pruritus, burning, stinging, erythema	Apply twice daily
bacitracin *ba-ci-tra'-sin*	Baciguent, *generic*	Relief of skin infections	Rare; occasionally redness, burning, pruritus, stinging	Apply 1–5 times daily
benzoyl peroxide *been'-zoyl per-ox'-ide*	Acne-5, Benzac, Desquam-X 10% Wash, Dryox Wash, Exact, Laroxide Neutrogena, Acne Mask, *generic*	Mild to moderate acne vulgaris and oily skin	Excessive drying, stinging, peeling, erythema, possible edema, allergic dermatitis	Use once to three times daily
clindamycin, topical *clin'-da-my-sin*	Cleocin T, Clinda-Derm, Clindets, C/T/S, *generic*	Acne vulgaris	Dryness, erythema, burning, peeling, oiliness/oily skin, diarrhea, bloody diarrhea, abdominal pains, colitis	Apply a thin film twice daily to affected area
erythromycin *ee-rith-ro-my'-sin*	Akne-Mycin, Emgel, Erygel	Acne vulgaris	Skin irritation, tenderness, pruritus, erythema, peeling, oiliness and burning sensations	Clean affected area twice daily
gentamicin *jen-ta-my'-sin*	G-myticin, *generic*	Relief of primary skin infections	Mild and transient pruritus, burning, stinging, erythema, photosensitivity	Apply 1–5 times daily to affected area
metronidazole *meh-trow-nye'-dah-zoll*	Metro-Gel, MetroLotion, Noritate	Rosacea	Watery (tearing) eyes, transient redness, mild dryness, burning, skin irritation	Apply a thin film twice daily to affected areas
mupirocin *mew'-pie-ro-sin*	Bactroban	Impetigo, infections caused by *Staphylococcus aureus* and *S. pyogenes*	Ointment: burning, stinging, pain, itching, rash, nausea, erythema, dry skin Cream: headache, rash, nausea, abdominal pain, burning at application site, dermatitis Nasal: headache, rhinitis, respiratory disorders, such as pharyngitis, taste perversion, burning, stinging, cough	Ointment: apply 3 times daily for 3–5 d Cream: apply 3 times daily for 10 d Nasal: divide the single-use tube between both nostrils and apply twice daily for 5 d
neomycin *knee-oh-my'-sin*	Myciguent, *generic*	Relief of skin infections	Mild and transient pruritus, burning, stinging, erythema	Apply 1–3 times daily
sulfacetamide sodium *sul-fah-see'-ta-mide*	Sebizon	Seborrheic dermatitis, seborrhea sicca (dandruff), bacterial infections of the skin	Rare: skin rash, nausea, vomiting	Apply 2–4 times daily
Antifungal Drugs				
amphotericin B *am-fo-ter'-eye-sin*	Fungizone	Mycotic infections	Rare; drying effect, local irritation, including erythema, pruritus, burning sensation	Apply liberally to lesions 2–4 times daily for 2–4 wk
butenafine HCl *beu-ten'-ah-feen*	Mentax	Dermatologic infections	Burning, stinging, itching, worsening of the condition, contact dermatis, erythema, irritation	Apply 1 time daily for 4 wk

SUMMARY DRUG TABLE DERMATOLOGIC DRUGS (*Continued*)

GENERIC NAME	TRADE NAME*	USES	ADVERSE REACTIONS	DOSAGE RANGES
ciclopirox *sic-lo-peer'-ox*	Loprox, Penlac Nail Lacquer	Loprox: tinea pedis (athelete's foot), tinea cruris (jock itch), tinea corporis (ringworm), cutaneous candidiasis Penlac: mild to moderate onychomycosis of fingernails and toenails	Pruritus, burning, worsening of clinical signs and symptoms, periungual erythema, nail disorders, irritation, ingrown toenail, burning of the skin	Apply to affected areas 1–2 times daily
clioquinol *kli-oh-qwe'-knol*	*Generic*	Tinea pedis, tinea cruris, and other skin infections caused by ringworm	Burning, itching, erythema, worsening of the condition	Apply thin layer to affected areas BID for 4 wk
econazole nitrate *ee-kon'-a-zole*	Spectazole	Tinea pedis, tinea cruris, tinea corporis, cutaneous candidiasis, tinea versicolor	Local burning, itching, stinging, erythema, pruritic rash	Apply to affected areas 1–2 times daily
gentian violet *jen'-shun*	*Generic*	External treatment of abrasions, minor cuts, surface injuries, superficial fungus, infections of the skin	Local irritation or sensitivity reactions	Apply locally BID
haloprogin *ha-lo-pro'-jin*	Halotex	Tinea pedis, tinea cruris, tinea corporis, tinea manuum	Local irritation, burning sensation, vesicle formation, erythema, scaling, itching, pruritus	Apply twice daily for 2–4 wk
ketoconazole *kee-toe-koe'-na-zole*	Nizoral, *generic*	Cream: tinea cruris, tinea corporis, and tinea versicolor Shampoo: reductions of scaling due to dandruff	Local burning, itching, stinging, erythema, pruritic rash	Cream: once daily to affected areas for 2 wk Shampoo: twice a week for 4 wk with at least 3 d between each shampoo
miconazole nitrate *mi-kon'-a-zole*	Fungoid-HC Creme, Lotrimin, Micatin, Monistat-Derm Cream, Tetterine, *generic*	Tinea pedis, tinea cruris, tinea corporis, cutaneous candidiasis	Local irritation, burning, maceration, allergic contact dermatitis	Cover affected areas twice daily
naftifine HCl *naf'-ti-feen*	Naftin	Topical treatment of tinea pedis, tinea cruris, tinea corporis	Burning, stinging, erythema, itching, local irritation, rash, tenderness	Apply BID for 4 wk
nystatin *nye-stat'-in*	Mycostatin, Nystex, *generic*	Mycotic infections caused by *Candida albicans,* and other *Candida* species	Virtually nontoxic and nonsensitizing; well tolerated by all age groups, even with prolonged administration; if irritation occurs, discontinue use	Apply 2–3 times daily until healing is complete
oxiconazole *ox-ee-kon'-ah-zole*	Oxistat	Tinea pedis, tinea cruris, tinea corporis	Pruritus, burning, stinging, irritation, contact dermatitis, scaling, tingling	Apply daily to BID 1 month
suconazole nitrate *sue-kon'-ah-zole*	Exelderm	Same as oxiconazole	Pruritus, burning, stinging, irritation	Apply 1–2 times daily for 2 wk
terbinafine HCl *ter-ben'-a-feen*	Lamisil	Same as oxiconazole	Same as oxiconazole	Apply twice daily until infection clears (1–4 wk)

(continued)

SUMMARY DRUG TABLE DERMATOLOGIC DRUGS (*Continued*)

GENERIC NAME	TRADE NAME*	USES	ADVERSE REACTIONS	DOSAGE RANGES
tolnaftate *tole-naf'-tate*	Aftate, Genaspor, Tinactin, Ting, *generic*	Same as oxiconazole	Same as oxiconazole	Apply twice daily for 2–3 wk (4–6 wk may be needed)
Antiviral Drugs				
acyclovir *ay-sye'-kloe-veer*	Zovirax, *generic*	Herpes genitalis, herpes simplex virus infections	Mild pain with transient burning/stinging, pruritus, rash, vulvitis, edema or pain at application site	Apply to all lesions q3h 6 times daily for 1 wk
penciclovir *pen-sye'-kloe-veer*	Denavir	Herpes labialis (cold sores)	Irritation at application site, headache, mild erythema, rash, taste perversion	Apply q2h for 4 d
Antiseptic and Germicides				
benzalkonium chloride (BAC) *benz-al-cone'-e-um*	Benza, Mycocide NS, Ony-Clear, Zephiran, *generic*	Asepsis of skin, mucous membranes, and wounds; preoperative preparation of the skin; surgeon's hand and arm soaks; preservation of ophthalmic solutions; irrigations of the eye; vaginal douching	Well tolerated in most individuals; occasionally mild sensitivity reaction	Varies, depending on administration
chlorhexidine gluconate *klor-hex'-e-deen*	Bacto Shield 2, Betasept, Exidine-2 Scrub, Hibiclens	Surgical scrub, skin cleanser, preoperative skin preparation, skin wound cleanser, preoperative showering and bathing	Irritation, dermatitis, photosensitivity (rare), deafness, mild sensitivity reactions	Varies, depending on administration
povidone-iodine *pov-e-don*	Acu-Dyne, Aerodine, Betadine, *generic*	Microbicidal against bacteria, fungi, viruses, spores, protozoa, yeasts	Dermatitis, irritation, burning, sensitivity reactions	Varies, depending on administration
triclosan *trye'-klo-san*	Clearasil Daily Face Wash	Skin cleanser, and skin degermer	None significant	5 mL on hands or face and rub thoroughly for 30 seconds, rinse thoroughly, pat dry
Corticosteroids, Topical				
alclometasone dipropionate *al-kloe-met-a-sone die-pro'-pee-oh-nate*	Aclovate	Treatment of various allergic/immunologic skin problems	Allergic contact dermatitis, burning, dryness, edema, irritation	Apply 1–6 times daily according to directions
amcinonide *am-sin'-oh-nide*	Cyclocort	Same as alclometasone	Same as alclometasone	Apply 1–6 times daily according to directions
augmented betamethasone dipropionate *bay-ta-meth'-a-sone*	Diprolene	Same as alclometasone	Same as alclometasone	Apply 1–4 times daily according to directions
betamethasone dipropionate *bay-ta-meth'-a-sone*	Alphatrex, Diprosone, Maxivate, *generic*	Same as alclometasone	Same as alclometasone	Apply 1–4 times daily according to directions

SUMMARY DRUG TABLE DERMATOLOGIC DRUGS (*Continued*)

GENERIC NAME	TRADE NAME*	USES	ADVERSE REACTIONS	DOSAGE RANGES
betamethasone valerate *bay-ta-meth´-a-sone-val´-eh-rate*	Betatrex, *generic*	Same as alclometasone	Same as alclometasone	Apply 1−4 times daily according to directions
desoximetasone *dess-ox-i-met´-a-sone*	Topicort, *generic*	Same as alclometasone	Same as alclometasone	Apply 1−4 times daily according to directions
dexamethasone sodium phosphate *dex-a-meth´-a-sone*	Decadron Phosphate	Same as alclometasone	Same as alclometasone	Apply 1−4 times daily according to directions
diflorasone diacetate *dye-flor´-a-sone*	Florone, Maxiflor	Same as alclometasone	Same as alclometasone	Apply 1−4 times daily according to directions
fluocinolone acetonide *floo-oh-sin´-oh-lone*	Fluonid, Flurosyn, Synalar, *generic*	Same as alclometasone	Same as alclometasone	Apply 1−4 times daily according to directions
fluocinonide *floo-oh-sin´-oh-nide*	Lidex, *generic*	Same as alclometasone	Same as alclometasone	Apply 1−4 times daily according to directions
flurandrenolide *floor-an-dren´-oh-lide*	Cordran, *generic*	Same as alclometasone	Same as alclometasone	Apply 1−4 times daily according to directions
hydrocortisone *hye-droe-kor´-ti-sone*	Bactine Hydrocortisone, Cort-Dome, Hytone, *generic*	Same as alclometasone	Same as alclometasone	Apply 1−4 times daily according to directions
hydrocortisone buteprate *hye-droe-kor´-ti-sone*	Pandel	Psoriasis and other deep-seated dermatoses	Same as alclometasone	Apply once or twice daily
hydrocortisone butyrate *hye-droe-kor´-ti-sone*	Locoid	Same as alclometasone	Same as alclometasone	Apply 2−3 times daily
triamcinolone acetonide *trye-am-sin´-oh-lone*	Aristocort, Flutex, Kenalog, Triacet, *generic*	Same as alclometasone	Same as alclometasone	Apply 1−4 times daily according to directions
Anti-psoriatic Drugs				
ammoniated mercury *ah-mo´-ne-at-ed mer-ku-re*	Emersal	Psoriasis	Ammoniated mercury is a potential sensitizer that can cause allergic reactions	Apply 1−2 times daily
anthralin *an-thra´-lin*	Anthra-Derm Dritho Creme, Miconal	Psoriasis	Few; transient irritation of normal skin or uninvolved skin	Apply once a day
calcipotriene *cal-cip-o-tri-een*	Dovonex	Psoriasis	Burning, itching, skin irritation, erythema, dry skin, peeling, rash, worsening of psoriasis, dermatitis, hyperpigmentation	Apply twice daily
selenium sulfide *se-le´-ne-um*	Exsel Head and Shoulders Intensive Treatment Dandruff Shampoo, Selsun Blue, *generic*	Treatment of dandruff, seborrheic dermatitis of the scalp, and tinea versicolor	None significant. Rare, some skin irritation	Massage 5−10 mL into wet scalp and allow to remain on scalp for 2−3 minutes, rinse

(continued)

SUMMARY DRUG TABLE DERMATOLOGIC DRUGS (*Continued*)

GENERIC NAME	TRADE NAME*	USES	ADVERSE REACTIONS	DOSAGE RANGES
Enzyme Preparations				
collagenase *koll-ah-gen´-ase*	Santyl, *generic*	For debriding chronic dermal ulcers and severely burned areas	Well tolerated and nonirritating; transient burning sensation may occur	Apply once daily according to directions
enzyme combinations	Accuzyme, Granulderm, Granulex, Panafil	Debridement of necrotic tissue and liquefication of slough in acute and chronic lesions such as decubitus ulcers, varicose and diabetic ulcers, burns, wounds, pilonidal cyst wounds, and miscellaneous trauma of infected wounds	Well tolerated and nonirritating; transient burning sensation may occur	Apply once or twice daily
Keratolytic Drugs				
diclofenac sodium *dye-kloe´-fen-ak*	Solaraze	Actinic keratoses	Usually well tolerated; transient burning sensation, rash, dry skin, scaling, flu syndrome	Apply twice daily
masoprocol *ma-so-pro-kol*	Actinex	Actinic keratoses	Erythema, flaking, dryness, itching, edema, burning, soreness, bleeding, crusting, skin roughness	Apply twice daily
salicylic acid *sal-i-sill´-ik*	DuoFilm, Wart Remover, Fostex, Fung-O, Mosco, Panscol	Aids in the removal of excessive keratin in hyperkeratotic skin disorders, including warts, psoriasis, calluses, and corns	Local irritation	Apply as directed in individual product labeling
Local Anesthetics				
benzocaine *benz-o-kaine´*	Lanacane	For topical anesthesia in local skin disorders	Rare; hypersensitivity, local burning, stinging, tenderness, sloughing	Apply to affected area
dibucaine *di-bu-kaine´*	Nupercainal, *generic*	For topical anesthesia in local skin disorders, local anesthesia of accessible mucous membranes	Same as benzocaine	Topical: apply to affected area as needed; mucous membranes: dosage varies and depends on the area to be anesthetized
lidocaine *lie´-doe-kaine*	ELA-Max, Lidocaine Viscous, Xylocaine, *generic*	For topical anesthesia in local skin disorders, local anesthesia of accessible mucous membranes	Same as benzocaine	Topical: apply to affected area as needed; mucous membranes: dosage varies and depends on the area to be anesthetized
lidocaine HCl *lie´-doe-kaine*	Dentipatch	Topical anesthesia of accessible mucous membranes of the mouth before dental procedures	Rare; local burning, stinging, tenderness	Apply to affected area
butamben picrate *byoo´-tam-ben*	*Generic*	Topical anesthesia	Rare; local burning, stinging, tenderness	Apply to affected area

*The term *generic* indicates the drug is available in generic form.

- Miconazole (Micatin), ciclopirox (Loprox), and econazole (Spectazole)—used for treatment of tinea pedis (athlete's foot), tinea cruris (jock itch), tinea corporis (ringworm), and superficial candidiasis
- Clioquinol—used for eczema, athlete's foot, and other fungal infections

Topical Antiviral Drugs

Acyclovir (Zovirax) and penciclovir (Denavir) are the only topical antiviral drugs currently available. These drugs inhibit viral replication. Acyclovir is used in the treatment of initial episodes of genital herpes, as well as herpes simplex virus infections in **immunocompromised** patients (patients with an immune system incapable of fighting infection). Penciclovir is used for the treatment of recurrent herpes labialis (cold sores) in adults.

ADVERSE REACTIONS

Adverse reactions to topical anti-infectives are usually mild. Occasionally, the patient may experience a skin rash, itching, urticaria (hives), dermatitis, irritation, or redness, which may indicate a **hypersensitivity** (allergic) reaction to the drug. Prolonged use of topical antibiotic preparations may result in a superficial **superinfection** (an overgrowth of bacterial or fungal microorganisms not affected by the antibiotic being administered).

CONTRAINDICATIONS, PRECAUTIONS, AND INTERACTIONS

These drugs are contraindicated in patients with known hypersensitivity to the drugs or any components of the drug. Because neomycin toxicity can cause nephrotoxicity and ototoxicity, neomycin is used cautiously in patients with extensive burns or trophic ulceration when extensive absorption can occur.

The topical antibiotics are Pregnancy Category C drugs and are used cautiously during pregnancy and lactation. Acyclovir and penciclovir are Pregnancy Category B drugs and are used cautiously during pregnancy and lactation. The pregnancy categories of the antifungals are unknown except for econazole nitrate, which is Pregnancy Category C, and ciclopirox, which is Pregnancy Category B; both are used with caution during pregnancy and lactation. There are no significant interactions for the topical anti-infectives.

TOPICAL ANTISEPTICS AND GERMICIDES

An **antiseptic** is a drug that stops, slows, or prevents the growth of microorganisms. A **germicide** is a drug that kills bacteria.

ACTIONS

The exact mechanism of action of topical antiseptics and germicides is not well understood. These drugs affect a variety of microorganisms. Some of these drugs have a short duration of action, whereas others have a long duration of action. The action of these drugs may depend on the strength used and the time the drug is in contact with the skin or mucous membrane.

Benzalkonium

Benzalkonium (Zephiran) is a rapid-acting preparation with a moderately long duration of action. It is active against bacteria and some viruses, fungi, and protozoa. Benzalkonium solutions are **bacteriostatic** (slow or retard the multiplication of bacteria) or **bactericidal** (destroy bacteria), depending on their concentration.

Chlorhexidine

Chlorhexidine gluconate (Hibiclens) affects a wide range of microorganisms, including gram-positive and gram-negative bacteria.

Iodine

Iodine has anti-infective action against many bacteria, fungi, viruses, yeasts, and protozoa. Povidone-iodine (Betadine) is a combination of iodine and povidone, which liberates free iodine. Povidone-iodine is often preferred over iodine solution or tincture because it is less irritating to the skin. Unlike with the use of iodine, treated areas may be bandaged or taped.

USES

Topical antiseptics and germicides are primarily used to reduce the number of bacteria on skin surfaces. Some of these drugs, such as chlorhexidine gluconate, may be used as a surgical scrub, as a preoperative skin cleanser, for washing the hands before and after caring for patients, and in the home to cleanse the skin. Others may be applied to minor cuts and abrasions to prevent infection. Some of these drugs may also be used on mucous membranes.

ADVERSE REACTIONS

Topical antiseptics and germicides have few adverse reactions. Occasionally, an individual may be allergic to the drug, and a skin rash or itching may occur. If an allergic reaction is noted, use of the topical drug is discontinued.

CONTRAINDICATIONS, PRECAUTIONS, AND INTERACTIONS

These drugs are contraindicated in patients with known hypersensitivity to the individual drug or any component of the preparation. There are no significant precautions or interactions when used as directed.

TOPICAL CORTICOSTEROIDS

Topical corticosteroids vary in potency, depending on the concentration of the drug (percentage), the vehicle in which the drug is suspended (lotion, cream, aerosol spray), and the area to which the drug is applied (open or denuded skin, unbroken skin, thickness of the skin over the treated area).

Examples of topical corticosteroids include amcinonide (Cyclocort), betamethasone dipropionate (Diprosone), fluocinolone acetonide (Flurosyn), hydrocortisone (Cort-Dome), and triamcinolone acetate (Aristocort).

ACTIONS AND USES

Topical corticosteroids exert localized anti-inflammatory activity. When applied to inflamed skin, they reduce itching, redness, and swelling. These drugs are useful in treating skin disorders, such as psoriasis, dermatitis, rashes, eczema, insect bite reactions, and first- and second-degree burns, including sunburns.

ADVERSE REACTIONS

Localized reactions may include burning, itching, irritation, redness, dryness of the skin, and secondary infection.

CONTRAINDICATIONS, PRECAUTIONS, AND INTERACTIONS

The topical corticosteroids are contraindicated in patients with known hypersensitivity to the drug or any component of the drug; as monotherapy for bacterial skin infections; for use on the face, groin, or axilla (only the high-potency corticosteroids); and for ophthalmic use (may cause steroid-induced glaucoma or cataracts). The topical corticosteroids are Pregnancy Category C drugs and are used cautiously during pregnancy and lactation. There are no significant interactions when administered as directed.

TOPICAL ANTIPSORIATICS

ACTION AND USES

Topical **antipsoriatics** are drugs used in the treatment of psoriasis (a chronic skin disease manifested by bright red patches covered with silvery scales or plaques). These drugs help remove the plaques associated with this disorder. Examples of antipsoriatics include anthralin (Anthra-Derm) and calcipotriene (Dovonex).

ADVERSE REACTIONS

These drugs may cause burning, itching, and skin irritation. Anthralin may cause skin irritation, as well as temporary discoloration of the hair and fingernails.

CONTRAINDICATIONS, PRECAUTIONS, AND INTERACTIONS

These drugs are contraindicated in patients with known hypersensitivity to the drugs. Anthralin and calcipotriene are Pregnancy Category C drugs and are used cautiously during pregnancy and lactation.

TOPICAL ENZYMES

ACTIONS AND USES

A topical enzyme aids in the removal of dead soft tissues by hastening the reduction of proteins into simpler substances. This is called **proteolysis** or a **proteolytic** action. The components of certain types of wounds, namely **necrotic** (dead) tissues and **purulent exudates** (pus-containing fluid), prevent proper wound healing. Removal of this type of debris by application of a topical enzyme aids in healing. Examples of conditions that may respond to application of a topical enzyme include second- and third-degree burns, pressure ulcers, and ulcers caused by peripheral vascular disease. An example of a topical enzyme is collagenase (Santyl).

ADVERSE REACTIONS

The application of collagenase may cause mild, transient pain. Numbness and dermatitis also may be seen. Collagenase has a low incidence of adverse reactions.

CONTRAINDICATIONS, PRECAUTIONS, AND INTERACTIONS

The topical enzyme preparations are contraindicated in patients with known hypersensitivity to the drugs, in wounds in contact with major body cavities or where nerves are exposed, and in fungating neoplastic ulcers. These drugs are Pregnancy Category B drugs and are used cautiously during pregnancy and lactation. Enzymatic activity may be impaired when these agents are administered with several detergents and antiseptics (benzalkonium chloride, hexachlorophene, iodine, and nitrofurazone).

KERATOLYTICS

ACTIONS AND USES

A **keratolytic** is a drug that removes excess growth of the epidermis (top layer of skin) in disorders such as warts. These drugs are used to remove warts, calluses, corns, and seborrheic keratoses (benign variously colored skin growths arising from oil glands of the skin). Examples of keratolytics include salicylic acid, masoprocol (Actinex), and diclofenac (Solaraze). Some strengths of salicylic acid are available as nonprescription products for the removal of warts on the hands and feet.

ADVERSE REACTIONS

These drugs are usually well tolerated. Occasionally a transient burning sensation, rash, dry skin, scaling, or flu-like syndrome may occur.

CONTRAINDICATIONS, PRECAUTIONS, AND INTERACTIONS

The keratolytics are contraindicated in patients with known hypersensitivity to the drugs and for use on moles, birthmarks, or warts with hair growing from them, on genital or facial warts, on warts on mucous membranes, or on infected skin. Prolonged use of the keratolytics in infants or patients with diabetes or impaired circulation is contraindicated. Salicylic acid

may cause salicylate toxicity (see Chap. 17) with prolonged use. These drugs are Pregnancy Category C drugs and are used cautiously during pregnancy and lactation.

TOPICAL LOCAL ANESTHETICS

A topical anesthetic may be applied to the skin or mucous membranes.

ACTIONS AND USES

Topical anesthetics temporarily inhibit the conduction of impulses from sensory nerve fibers. These drugs may be used to relieve itching and pain due to skin conditions, such as minor burns, fungus infections, insect bites, rashes, sunburn, and plant poisoning, such as poison ivy. Some are applied to mucous membranes as local anesthetics. Examples of local anesthetics include benzocaine (Lanacane), dibucaine (Nupercainal), and lidocaine (Xylocaine).

ADVERSE REACTIONS

Occasionally, local irritation, dermatitis, rash, burning, stinging, and tenderness may be noted.

CONTRAINDICATIONS, PRECAUTIONS, AND INTERACTIONS

These drugs are contraindicated in those with a known hypersensitivity to any component of the preparation. The topical anesthetics are used cautiously in patients receiving Class I antiarrhythmic drugs such as tocainide and mexiletine because the toxic effects are additive and potentially synergistic.

❋ Herbal Alert: Aloe Vera

Aloe is used to prevent infection and promote healing of minor burns (eg, sunburn) and wounds. When used externally, the herb helps repair skin tissue and reduce inflammation. Aloe gel is naturally thick when taken from the leaf but quickly becomes watery because of the action of enzymes in the plant. Commercially available preparations have additive thickeners to make the aloe appear like the fresh gel. The herb can be applied directly from the fresh leaf by cutting the leaf in half lengthwise and gently rubbing the inner gel directly onto the skin. Commercially prepared products are applied externally as needed. Rare reports of allergy have been reported with the external use of aloe. Although available as an oral juice, its benefits have not been confirmed. Some individuals have reported the oral juice effective in healing and preventing stomach ulcers.

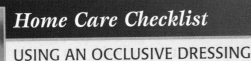

Home Care Checklist

USING AN OCCLUSIVE DRESSING

In certain circumstances, the patient who requires a topical drug must also apply an occlusive dressing to enhance the drug's effectiveness. Although commercial-type occlusive dressings are available, they are expensive, especially if your patient requires frequent dressing changes at home. So, if appropriate, suggest these less costly home alternatives:

✓ Plastic food wrap such as Saran wrap

✓ Plastic food storage bags

After your patient gathers the necessary supplies, instruct him or her to do the following:

✓ Wash hands before beginning care.

✓ Remove the old dressing.

✓ Cleanse the area as directed.

✓ Apply the topical drug as ordered.

✓ Cover the area with a dry gauze dressing.

✓ Apply a skin adhesive to the area around the gauze dressing.

✓ Cover the gauze dressing with the occlusive dressing, making sure that the occlusive dressing is approximately 1 inch larger than the gauze dressing on all sides. For example, if the gauze dressing is 4 inches × 4 inches, then the occlusive dressing should be 5 inches × 5 inches.

✓ Check to make sure that the occlusive dressing lies flat without wrinkles.

✓ Run fingers around all the edges of the occlusive dressing to ensure good adhesion.

✓ Tape the edges of the occlusive dressing on all sides, preferably with paper tape, to secure it.

- Discontinue use of the drug and contact the primary health care provider if rash, burning, itching, redness, pain, or other skin problems occur.
- Gentamicin may cause photosensitivity. Take measures to protect the skin from ultraviolet rays (eg, wear protective clothing and use a sunscreen when out in the sun).

EVALUATION

- The therapeutic drug response is achieved.
- The patient or family member demonstrates an understanding of the use and application of the prescribed or recommended drug.

● *Critical Thinking Exercises*

1. *A nurse tells you that she is upset because she was reprimanded about the labeling of a topical antiseptic used for cleaning a pressure ulcer and for leaving the solution*

at the patient's bedside. She thinks her supervisor is unfair and the entire situation is not as serious as the supervisor contends. Analyze the situation to determine what you would say to this nurse.

2. *Discuss the ongoing assessment activities you would include in the daily assessment of a patient prescribed a topical drug.*

3. *Describe important preadministration assessments that the nurse would make before administering a topical corticosteroid.*

● *Review Questions*

1. What reaction could occur with prolonged use of the topical antibiotics?
   - **A.** Water intoxication
   - **B.** Superficial superinfection
   - **C.** An outbreak of eczema
   - **D.** Cellulitis

2. Which of the following drugs has a proteolytic action?

   A. Amcinonide (Cyclocort)
   B. Collagenase (Santyl)
   C. Bacitracin (Baciguent)
   D. Ciclopirox (Loprox)

3. A keratolytic agent would be safe to use on which of the following skin conditions?

   A. Moles
   B. Birthmarks
   C. Facial warts
   D. Calluses

4. What type of action do the corticosteroids have when used topically?

   A. Bacteriocidal activity
   B. Anti-inflammatory activity
   C. Antifungal activity
   D. Antiviral activity

5. Which of the following drugs is best suited to be used as a topical antiseptic?

   A. Amphotericin B
   B. Benzocaine
   C. Iodine
   D. Povidone-iodine

Otic and Ophthalmic Preparations

The eyes and ears are subject to various disorders, which range from mild to serious. Because the eyes and ears provide an interpretation of our outside environment, any disease or injury that has the potential for partial or total loss of function of these organs must be treated.

OTIC PREPARATIONS

ACTIONS

Various types of preparations are used for the treatment of **otic** (ear) disorders. Otic preparations can be divided into three categories: (1) antibiotics; (2) antibiotic and steroid combinations; and (3) miscellaneous preparations. The miscellaneous preparations usually contain one or more of the following ingredients:

- Benzocaine—a local anesthetic
- Phenylephrine—a vasoconstrictor decongestant
- Hydrocortisone, desonide—corticosteroids for anti-inflammatory and antipruritic effects
- Glycerin—an emollient and a solvent
- Antipyrine—an analgesic

- Acetic acid, boric acid, benzalkonium chloride, aluminum acetate, benzethonium chloride—provide antifungal or antibacterial action
- Carbamide peroxide—aids in removing earwax by softening and breaking up the wax

Examples of otic preparations are given in the Summary Drug Table: Otic Preparations.

USES

Otic preparations are instilled in the external auditory canal and may be used to relieve pain, treat infection and inflammation, and aid in the removal of earwax. When the patient has an inner ear infection, systemic antibiotic therapy is indicated.

ADVERSE REACTIONS

When otic drugs are applied topically, the amount of drug that enters the systemic circulation is not sufficient to produce adverse reactions. Prolonged use of otic

SUMMARY DRUG TABLE OTIC PREPARATIONS

GENERIC COMBINATIONS	TRADE NAME*	USES	ADVERSE REACTIONS	DOSAGE RANGES
Steroid and Antibiotic Combinations, Solutions				
1% hydrocortisone, 5 mg neomycin sulfate, 10,000 units polymyxin B	Antibiotic Ear Solution, AntibiOtic, Cortisporin Otic, Drotic, Ear-Eze, Otic-Care, Oticair, Otocort, Otosporin	Bacterial infections of the external auditory canal	Few; when used for prolonged periods there is a danger of a superinfection	4 gtt instilled TID, QID
0.5% hydrocortisone, 10,000 units polymyxin B	Otobiotic Otic	Same as hydrocortisone, above	Same as hydrocortisone, above	4 gtt instilled TID, QID
Steroid and Antibiotic Combinations, Suspensions				
1% hydrocortisone, 5 mg neomycin sulfate, 10,000 units polymyxin B	AK-Spore, AntibiOtic, Antibiotic Ear Suspension, Otocort, UAD Otic	Same as hydrocortisone, above	Same as hydrocortisone, above	4 gtt instilled TID, QID
1% hydrocortisone, 4.71 mg neomycin sulfate	Coly-Mycin S Otic	Same as hydrocortisone, above	Same as hydrocortisone, above	4 gtt instilled TID, QID
1% hydrocortisone, 3.3 mg neomycin sulfate	Cortisporin-TC Otic	Same as hydrocortisone, above	Same as hydrocortisone, above	4 gtt instilled TID, QID
2 mg ciprofloxacin, 10 mg hydrocortisone/mL	Cipro HC Otic	Same as hydrocortisone, above	Same as hydrocortisone, above	4 gtt instilled TID, QID
Otic Antibiotics				
Chloramphenicol	Chloromycetin Otic	Treatment of superficial infections involving the external auditory canal	Local irritation (itching, burning, angioneurotic edema, urticaria, vesicular and maculopapular dermatitis)	2–3 gtt into the ear TID
Select Miscellaneous Preparations				
1% hydrocortisone, 2% acetic acid, 3% propylene glycol diacetate, 0.015% sodium acetate, 0.02% benzethonium chloride	Acetasol HC, VoSoL HC Otic	Relieve pain, inflammation, and irritation in the external auditory canal	Local irritation, itching, burning	Insert wick, use 3–5 gtt q4–6h × 24 h; remove wick, instill 5 gtt TID, QID
1% hydrocortisone, 1% pramoxine HCl, 0.1% chloroxylenol, 3% propylene glycol diacetate and benzalkonium chloride	Cortic	Same as hydrocortisone, above	Same as hydrocortisone, above	Insert saturated wick into the ear; leave in for 24 h, keeping moist with 3–5 gtt q4–6h; remove wick and instill 5 gtt TID, QID

(continued)

SUMMARY DRUG TABLE OTIC PREPARATIONS *(Continued)*

GENERIC COMBINATIONS	TRADE NAME*	USES	ADVERSE REACTIONS	DOSAGE RANGES
1% hydrocortisone, 2% acetic acid glacial, 3% propylene glycol diacetate, 0.02% benzethonium Cl, 0.015% sodium acetate, 0.2% citric acid	AA-HC Otic	Same as hydrocortisone, above	Same as hydrocortisone, above	Insert saturated wick into the ear; leave in for 24 h, keeping moist with 3–5 gtt q4–6h; remove wick and instill 5 gtt TID, QID
1.4% benzocaine, 5.4% antipyrine glycerin	Allergen Ear Drops, Auralgan Otic, Auroto Otic, Ear Drops, Otocalm Ear	Same as hydrocortisone, above	Same as hydrocortisone, above	Fill ear canal with 2–4 gtt; insert saturated cotton pledget; repeat TID, QID or q1–2h
20% benzocaine, 0.1% benzethonium chloride, 1% glycerin, PEG 300	Americaine Otic, Otocain	Same as hydrocortisone, above	Same as hydrocortisone, above	Instill 4–5 gtt; insert cotton pledget; repeat every 1–2h
10% triethanolamine polypeptide oleate-condensate, 0.5% chlorobutanol in propylene glycol	Cerumenex Drops	Aid in the removal of ear wax	Local irritation, itching, burning	Fill ear canal, insert cotton plug, allow to remain 15–30 min; flush ear
1 mg chloroxylenol, 10 mg hydrocortisone, 10 mg/mL pramoxine HCl	Otomar-HC	Relieve pain and irritation in the external auditory canal	Local irritation, itching, burning	Instill 5 gtt into affected ear TID, QID
2% acetic acid in aluminum acetate solution	Burow's Otic, Otic Domeboro, *generic*	Relieve pain and irritation in the external auditory canal	Local irritation, itching, burning	Insert saturated wick; keep moist for 24 h; instill 4–6 gtt every 2–3 h

*The term *generic* indicates the drug is available in generic form.

preparations containing an antibiotic may result in a **superinfection** (an overgrowth of bacterial or fungal microorganisms not affected by the antibiotic being administered).

CONTRAINDICATIONS, PRECAUTIONS, AND INTERACTIONS

These drugs are contraindicated in patients with a known hypersensitivity to the drugs. The otic drugs are used with caution during pregnancy and lactation. The pregnancy category of these drugs is unknown when they are used as otic drugs. Otic drugs available in dropper bottles may be dangerous if ingested by young children. Therefore, the drugs are stored safely out of the reach of children. Drugs to remove cerumen are not used if ear drainage, discharge, pain, or irritation is present; if the eardrum is perforated; or after ear surgery. Although rare, bone marrow hypoplasia including

aplastic anemia has been reported with local application of chloramphenicol. No significant interactions have been reported with use of the otic preparations.

NURSING PROCESS

● **The Patient Receiving an Otic Preparation**

ASSESSMENT

Preadministration Assessment
Before administration of an otic preparation, the primary health care provider examines the ear and external structures surrounding the ear and prescribes the drug indicated to treat the disorder. The nurse may be responsible for examining the outer structures of the ear, namely the earlobe and the skin around the ear. The nurse documents a description of any drainage or the presence of impacted cerumen.

Nursing Diagnoses Checklist

☑ **Risk for Infection** related to prolonged use of the anti-infective otic drug

☑ **Anxiety** related to ear pain or discomfort, changes in hearing, diagnosis, other factors

☑ **Risk for Ineffective Therapeutic Regimen Management** related to lack of knowledge of correct technique for instilling ear drug, therapeutic regimen

Ongoing Assessment

The nurse assesses the patient's response to therapy. For example, a decrease in pain or inflammation should occur. The nurse examines the outer ear and ear canal for any local redness or irritation that may indicate sensitivity to the drug.

NURSING DIAGNOSES

Drug-specific nursing diagnoses are highlighted in the Nursing Diagnoses Checklist. Other nursing diagnoses applicable to these drugs are discussed in depth in Chapter 4.

PLANNING

The expected outcomes of the patient may include an optimal response to the drug, a reduction in anxiety, and an understanding of the application and use of an otic preparation.

IMPLEMENTATION

Promoting an Optimal Response to Therapy

Before instillation of otic preparations, the nurse holds the container in the hand for a few minutes to warm it to body temperature. Cold and warm (above body temperature) preparations may cause dizziness or other sensations after being instilled into the ear.

> ✳ **Nursing Alert**
>
> *Only preparations labeled as otic are instilled in the ear. The nurse must check the label of the preparation carefully for the name of the drug and a statement indicating that the preparation is for otic use.*

Special instructions for specific ear preparations are found in the Summary Drug Table: Otic Preparations. When instilling ear drops, the nurse has the patient lie on his or her side with the ear toward the ceiling. If the patient wishes to remain in an upright position, the head is tilted toward the untreated side with the ear toward the ceiling (Fig. 57-1). In the adult, the earlobe is pulled up and back. In children, the earlobe is pulled down and back. The nurse instills the prescribed number of drops into the ear canal. If the primary health

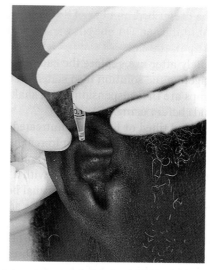

FIGURE 57-1. Instilling ear drops. With the head turned toward the unaffected side, the nurse pulls the cartilaginous portion of the outer ear (pinna) up and back in the adult pictured and instills the prescribed number of drops on the side of the auditory canal.

care provider has not ordered a soft cotton plug to be placed in the opening of the external ear canal, the patient is kept lying on the untreated side for 2 to 3 minutes. Once the patient is upright, the solution running out of the ear may be gently removed with gauze.

Drugs that loosen cerumen work by softening the dried earwax inside the ear canal. Cerumenex is available by prescription and is not allowed to stay in the ear canal more than 30 minutes before irrigation. When Cerumenex is administered, the ear canal is filled with the solution and a cotton plug is inserted. The drug is allowed to remain in the ear for 15 to 30 minutes, and then the ear is flushed with warm water using a soft rubber bulb ear syringe.

Managing Anxiety

Ear disorders may result in symptoms such as pain, a feeling of fullness in the ear, tinnitus, dizziness, or a change in hearing. Patients with an ear disorder or injury usually have great concern over the effect the problem will have on their hearing. The nurse reassures the patient that every effort is being made to treat the disorder and relieve the symptoms. Before instilling an otic solution, the nurse informs the patient that a feeling of fullness may be felt in the ear and that hearing in the treated ear may be impaired while the solution remains in the ear canal.

Educating the Patient and Family

The nurse gives the patient or a family member instructions or a demonstration of the instillation technique of an otic preparation. The following information may be given to the patient when an ear ointment or solution is prescribed:

● Wash the hands thoroughly before cleansing the area around the ear (when necessary) and instilling ear drops or ointment.

SUMMARY DRUG TABLE   SELECT OPHTHALMIC PREPARATIONS (*Continued*)

GENERIC NAME	TRADE NAME*	USES	DOSAGE RANGES
pilocarpine nitrate	Pilagan	Elevated IOP	1–2 gtt in affected eye(s) 2–4 times daily
pilocarpine ocular therapeutic system	Ocusert Pilo-20, Ocusert Pilo-40	Elevated IOP	See package insert
Miotics, Cholinesterase Inhibitors			
demecarium bromide *deh-meh-care´-ee-uhm broe´-mide*	Humorsol	Glaucoma and strabismus	1–2 gtt/wk, up to 1–2 gtt/d
echothiophate iodide *eck-oh-thigh´-oh-fate eye-oh-dide*	Phospholine Iodide	Chronic open-angle glaucoma	2 doses/d in the morning and at HS or one dose every other day
Carbonic Anhydrase inhibitors			
brinzolamide *brin-zoe´-lah-mide*	Azopt	Elevated IOP	1 gtt in affected eye(s) TID
dorzolamide HCl *dore-zole-lah-mide*	TruSopt	Elevated IOP	1 gtt in affected eye(s) TID
Prostaglandin Agonist			
latanoprost *lah-tan´-oh-prahst*	Xalatan	Elevated IOP	1 gtt in affected eye(s) QD in the evening
travoprost	Travatan	Elevated IOP	1 gtt in affected eye(s) QD in the evening
bimatoprost	Lumigan	Elevated IOP	1 gtt in affected eye(s) QD in the evening
unoprostone isopropyl *yoo-noh-prost´-ohn*	Rescula	Elevated IOP	1 gtt in affected eye(s) BID
Combinations Used, to Treat Glaucoma			
pilocarpine and epinephrine	E-Pilo-1, E-Pilo-2, E-Pilo-4, E-Pilo-6, P_1E_1, P_4E_1	Glaucoma	1–2 gtt in the affected eye(s) 1–4 times daily
dorzolamide HCl and timolol maleate *dore-zole´-ah-mide*	Cosopt	Elevated IOP	1 gtt into the affected eye(s) BID
Mast Cell Stabilizer			
nedocromil sodium *neh-doe-kroe´-mill*	Alocril	Allergic conjunctivitis	1–2 gtt in each eye BID
pemirolast potassium *peh-mihr-oh´-last*	Alamast	Allergic conjunctivitis	1–2 gtt in each eye QID
Nonsteroidal Anti-inflammatory Drugs			
diclofenac sodium *di-klo´-fen-ak*	Voltaren, *generic*	Postoperative inflammation after cataract surgery	1 drop QID
flurbiprofen sodium *flure-bi´-pro-fen*	Ocufen, *generic*	Inhibition of intraoperative miosis	1 gtt q 30 min beginning 2 h before surgery (total of 4 gtt)
ketorolac tromethamine *ke-tor´-o-lac*	Acular	Relief of ocular itching due to seasonal allergies	1 drop QID

SUMMARY DRUG TABLE SELECT OPHTHALMIC PREPARATIONS *(Continued)*

GENERIC NAME	TRADE NAME*	USES	DOSAGE RANGES
Corticosteroids			
dexamethasone phosphate *dex-a-meth′-a-sone*	AK-Dex, Maxidex, *generic*	Treatment of inflammatory conditions of the conjunctiva, lid, cornea, anterior segment of the eye	Solution: 1−2 gtt qh during the day and q2h at night, reduced to 1 gtt q4h when response noted, then 1 gtt TID−QID Ointment: thin coating in lower conjunctival sac 3−4 times/d
fluorometholone *flure-oh-meth′-oh-lone*	Flarex, Fluor-Op, *generic*	Treatment of inflammatory conditions of the conjunctiva, lid, cornea, anterior segment of the eye	Suspension: 1−2 gtt 2−4 times/d, may increase to 2 gtt q2h; ointment: thin coating in lower conjunctival sac 1−3 times/d (up to 1 application q4h)
loteprednol etabonate *low-teh′-pred′-nol ett-ab′-ohn-ate*	Alrex, Lotemex	Allergic conjunctivitis	1−2 gtt QID
prednisolone *pred-niss′-oh-lone*	AK-Pred, Pred Forte, Pred Mild, *generic*	Treatment of inflammatory conditions of the conjunctiva, lid, cornea, anterior segment of the eye	1−2 gtt qh during the day and q2h at night, reduced to 1 drop q4h, then 1 gtt TID or QID. Suspensions: 1−2 gtt 2−4 times daily
Antibiotics			
bacitracin *bass-i-tray′-sin*	AK-Tracin	Treatment of eye infections	See package insert
erythromycin *er-ith-roe-mye′-sin*	Ilotycin, *generic*	Treatment of eye infections	See package insert
gentamicin *jen-ta-mye′-sin*	Garamycin, *generic*	Treatment of eye infections	See package insert
tobramycin *toe-bra-mye′-sin*	Tobrex, *generic*	Treatment of eye infections	See package insert
Sulfonamides			
sodium sulfacetamide *sul-fa-see′-ta-mide*	AK-Sulf, *generic*	Treatment of conjunctivitis, corneal ulcer, other superficial eye infections	1−2 gtt q1−3h
Silver			
silver nitrate *nye-trate*	*generic*	Prevention of ophthalmia neonatorum	2 gtt of 1% solution in each eye
Antiviral Drugs			
idoxuridine *eye-dox-yoor′-i-deen*	Herplex	Treatment of herpes simplex keratitis	1 gtt qh during the day and q2h at night
vidarabine *vye-dare′-a-been*	Vira-A	Treatment of herpes simplex keratitis and conjunctivitis	0.5 inch of ointment into lower conjunctival sac 5 times/d at 3-h intervals
Antifungal Drugs			
natamycin *na-ta-mye′-sin*	Natacyn	Treatment of fungal infections of the eye	1 gtt q1−2h

(continued)

SUMMARY DRUG TABLE SELECT OPHTHALMIC PREPARATIONS (*Continued*)

GENERIC NAME	TRADE NAME*	USES	DOSAGE RANGES
Vasoconstrictors/Mydriatics			
oxymetazoline hydrochloride *ox-i-met-az´-oh-leen*	Ocuclear, Visine L. R.	Relief of redness of eye due to minor irritation	1−2 gtt q3−4h up to QID
phenylephrine hydrochloride *fen-ill-ef´-rin*	AK-Dilate 2.5%, Neo-Synephrine 10%	0.12% for relief of redness of eye due to minor irritation; 2.5% and 10% treatment of uveitis, glaucoma; refraction procedures, before eye surgery	0.12% 1−2 gtt up to 4 times/d; 2.5% and 10%, 1 gtt
tetrahydrozoline hydrochloride *tet-ra-hyd-drozz´-a-leen*	Murine Plus Eye Drops, Visine, *generic*	Relief of redness of eye due to minor irritation	1−2 gtt up to 4 times/d
Cycloplegic/Mydriatics			
atropine sulfate *a´-troe-peen*	Isopto-Atropine, *generic*	Eye refraction, treatment of acute inflammatory conditions of iris, uveal tract	1−2 gtt up to 4 times/d
homatropine hydrobromide *hoe-ma´-troe-peen*	Isopto Homatropine	Eye refraction, treatment of inflammatory conditions of uveal tract	1−2 gtt q3−4h
Artificial Tears			
benzalkonium chloride *benz-al-koe´-nee-um*	Artificial Tears	Treatment of dry eyes	1−2 gtt 3−4 times/d
glycerin, sodium chloride	Eye-Lube-A	Treatment of dry eyes	1−2 gtt 3−4 times/d

*The term *generic* indicates the drug is available in generic form.

Sympathomimetic Drugs

Sympathomimetics have alpha (α)- and beta (β)-adrenergic activity (see Chap. 22 for a detailed discussion of adrenergic drugs). These drugs lower the **intraocular pressure** (IOP) (the pressure within the eye) by increasing the outflow of aqueous humor in the eye and are used to treat glaucoma. Apraclonidine is used to control or prevent postoperative elevations in IOP. The Summary Drug Table: Select Ophthalmic Preparations provides additional information about these drugs.

Alpha-Adrenergic Blocking Drugs

Dapiprazole acts by blocking the α-adrenergic receptor in smooth muscle and produces miosis through an effect on the dilator muscle of the iris. The drug is used primarily after ophthalmic examinations to reverse the diagnostic **mydriasis** (dilation of the pupil).

Beta-Adrenergic Blocking Drugs

The β-adrenergic blocking drugs decrease the rate of production of aqueous humor and thereby lower the IOP. These drugs are used to treat glaucoma.

Miotics, Direct Acting

Miotics contract the pupil of the eye (miosis), resulting in an increase in the space through which the aqueous humor flows. This increased space and improved flow results in a decrease in the IOP. Miotics may be used in the treatment of glaucoma (see Chap. 22). The miotics were, for a number of years, the drug of choice for glaucoma. These drugs have lost that first choice treatment status to the β-adrenergic blocking drugs.

Miotics, Cholinesterase Inhibitors

The cholinesterase inhibitors are more potent and longer acting than the direct-acting miotics and are used to treat open-angle glaucoma. When administered into the eye, these drugs produce intense **miosis** (constriction of the pupil) and muscle contractions, causing a decreased resistance to aqueous outflow.

Carbonic Anhydrase Inhibitors

Except for dorzolamide and brinzolamide, carbonic anhydrase inhibitors are administered systemically. Carbonic anhydrase is an enzyme found in many tissues of the body, including the eye. Inhibition of carbonic anhydrase in the eye decreases aqueous humor secretion, resulting in a decrease of IOP. These drugs are used in the treatment of elevated IOP seen in open-angle glaucoma.

Prostaglandin Agonists

The prostaglandin agonists are used to lower IOP in patients with open-angle glaucoma and ocular hypertension in patients who do not tolerate other IOP-lowering medications or have an insufficient response to these medications. These drugs act to lower IOP by increasing the outflow of aqueous humor through the trabecular meshwork.

Mast Cell Stabilizers

The mast cell stabilizers currently for ophthalmic use are nedocromil and pemirolast. These drugs are used for the prevention of eye itching caused by allergic conjunctivitis. The mast cell stabilizers act by inhibiting the antigen-induced release of inflammatory mediators (eg, histamine) from human mast cells.

Nonsteroidal Anti-inflammatory Drugs (NSAIDs)

The NSAIDs inhibit prostaglandin synthesis (see Chap. 18 for a discussion of the NSAIDs), thereby exerting anti-inflammatory action. These drugs are used to treat postoperative inflammation after cataract surgery (diclofenac), for the relief of itching of the eyes caused by seasonal allergies (ketorolac), and during eye surgery to prevent miosis (flurbiprofen).

Corticosteroids

These drugs possess anti-inflammatory activity and are used for inflammatory conditions, such as allergic conjunctivitis, keratitis, herpes zoster keratitis, and inflammation of the iris. Corticosteroids also may be used after injury to the cornea or after corneal transplants to prevent rejection.

Antibiotics and Sulfonamides

Antibiotics possess antibacterial activity and are used in the treatment of eye infections. Sulfonamides possess a bacteriostatic effect against a wide range of gram-positive and gram-negative microorganisms. They are used in the treatment of conjunctivitis, corneal ulcer, and other superficial infections of the eye. See the Summary Drug Table: Select Ophthalmic Preparations and Chapter 6 for additional information on the sulfonamides.

Silver

Silver possesses antibacterial activity against gram-positive and gram-negative microorganisms. Silver protein, mild, is occasionally used in the treatment of eye infections. Silver nitrate is occasionally used to prevent gonorrheal ophthalmia neonatorum (gonorrhea infection of the newborn's eyes). Ophthalmic tetracycline and erythromycin have largely replaced the use of silver nitrate in newborns.

Antiviral Drugs

Antiviral drugs interfere with viral reproduction by altering DNA synthesis. These drugs are used in the treatment of herpes simplex infections of the eye, treatment in immunocompromised patients with cytomegalovirus (CMV) retinitis, and for the prevention of CMV retinitis in patients undergoing transplant.

Antifungal Drugs

Natamycin is the only ophthalmic antifungal in use. This drug possesses antifungal activity against a variety of yeast and fungi.

Vasoconstrictors/Mydriatics

These drugs dilate the pupil (mydriasis), constrict superficial blood vessels of the sclera, and decrease the formation of aqueous humor. Depending on the specific drug and strength, these drugs may be used before eye surgery in the treatment of glaucoma, for relief of minor eye irritation, and to dilate the pupil for examination of the eye.

Cycloplegic Mydriatics

Cycloplegic mydriatics cause mydriasis and **cycloplegia** (paralysis of the ciliary muscle, resulting in an inability to focus the eye). These drugs (see Chap. 25) are used in the treatment of inflammatory conditions of the iris and uveal tract of the eye and for examination of the eye.

Artificial Tear Solutions

These products lubricate the eyes and are used for conditions such as dry eyes and eye irritation caused by inadequate tear production.

Inactive ingredients may be found in some preparations. Examples of these drugs include preservatives, antioxidants, which prevent deterioration of the product, and drugs that slow drainage of the drug from the eye into the tear duct. Examples of the types of eye preparations are found in the Summary Drug Table: Select Ophthalmic Preparations.

ADVERSE REACTIONS

Alpha$_2$-Adrenergic Drugs

Although side effects are usually mild, treatment with brimonidine tartrate includes oral dryness, ocular hyperemia, burning and stinging, headache, visual blurring, foreign body sensation, fatigue, drowsiness, ovular allergic reactions, and ocular pruritus.

Sympathomimetic Drugs

These drugs may cause transient local reactions such as burning and stinging, eye pain, brow ache, headache, allergic lip reactions, and ocular irritation. With prolonged use adrenochrome (a red pigment contained in epinephrine) deposits may occur in the conjunctiva and cornea. Although rare, systemic reactions may occur such as headache, palpitations, tachycardia, extrasystoles, cardiac arrhythmia, hypertension, and faintness. Dipivefrin appears to be better tolerated and has fewer adverse reactions than the other sympathomimetic drugs used to lower IOP.

Alpha-Adrenergic Blocking Drugs

The drug may cause burning in the eye, ptosis (drooping of the upper eyelid), lid edema, itching, corneal edema, browache, photophobia, dryness of the eye, tearing, and blurring of vision.

Beta-Adrenergic Blocking Drugs

Adverse reactions associated with the β-adrenergic blocking drugs include eye irritation, burning, tearing, conjunctivitis, decreased night vision, ptosis, abnormal corneal staining, and corneal sensitivity. Systemic reactions, although rare, include arrhythmias, palpitation, headache, nausea, and dizziness. (See Chap. 23 for additional systemic adverse reactions.)

Miotic, Direct Acting

The direct-acting miotics may cause stinging on instillation, transient burning, tearing, headache, browache, and decreased night vision. Systemic adverse reactions included hypotension, flushing, breathing difficulties, nausea, vomiting, diarrhea, cardiac arrhythmias, and frequent urge to urinate.

Miotics, Cholinesterase Inhibitors

Adverse reactions and systemic toxicity are more common in the cholinesterase inhibitor ophthalmic preparations than in the direct-acting miotics. Ophthalmic adverse reactions include the development of iris cysts, burning, lacrimation, lid muscle twitching, conjunctivitis and ciliary redness, browache, headache, activation of latent iritis or uveitis (an inner-eye inflammation), retinal detachment, and conjunctival thickening. Systemic adverse reactions include nausea, vomiting, abdominal cramps, diarrhea, urinary incontinence, fainting, salivation, difficulty breathing, and cardiac irregularities. Iris cysts may form, enlarge, and obstruct vision. The iris cyst usually shrinks upon discontinuation of use of the drug or after a reduction in strength of the drops or frequency of instillation.

Carbonic Anhydrase Inhibitors

Adverse reactions associated with use of the carbonic anyhdrase inhibitors include ocular burning, stinging, or discomfort immediately after administration, bitter taste, ocular allergic reaction, blurred vision, tearing, dryness, dermatitis, foreign body sensation, ocular discomfort, photophobia, and headache.

Prostaglandin Agonists

Adverse reactions associated with the prostaglandin agonists include blurred vision, burning and stinging, foreign body sensation, itching, increased pigmentation of the iris, dry eye, excessive tearing, lid discomfort and pain, and photophobia.

Mast Cell Stabilizers

Although mild, the adverse reactions associated with the mast cell inhibitors include headache, rhinitis, unpleasant taste, asthma, and cold/flu symptoms. These drugs may also cause ocular burning or irritation, dry eye, eye redness, foreign body sensation, and ocular discomfort.

Nonsteroidal Anti-inflammatory Drugs

The most common adverse reactions associated with the NSAIDs include transient burning and stinging upon instillation and other minor ocular irritation.

Corticosteroids

Adverse reactions associated with administration of the corticosteroid ophthalmic preparations include elevated IOP with optic nerve damage, loss of visual acuity, cataract formation, delayed wound healing, secondary ocular infection, exacerbation of corneal infections, dry eyes, ptosis, blurred vision, discharge, ocular pain, foreign body sensation, and pruritus.

Antibiotics, Sulfonamides, and Silver

The antibiotic and sulfonamide ophthalmics are usually well tolerated, and few adverse reactions are seen. Occasional transient irritation, burning, itching, stinging, inflammation, or blurring of vision may occur. With prolonged or repeated use, a superinfection may occur.

Antiviral Drugs

The administration of the antiviral ophthalmics may cause occasional irritation, pain, pruritus, inflammation, or edema of the eyes or lids; allergic reactions; foreign body sensation; photophobia; and corneal clouding.

Antifungal Drugs

Adverse reactions are rare. Occasional local irritation to the eye may occur.

Vasoconstrictors/Mydriatics

Adverse reactions include transitory stinging on initial instillation, blurring of vision, mydriasis, increased redness, irritation, discomfort, and increased IOP. Systemic adverse reactions include headache, browache, palpitations, tachycardia, arrhythmias, hypertension, myocardial infarction, and stroke.

Cycloplegic Mydriatics

Local adverse reactions associated with administration of the cycloplegic mydriatics include increased IOP, transient stinging or burning, and irritation with prolonged use (eg, conjunctivitis, edema, exudates). Systemic adverse reactions include dryness of the mouth and skin, blurred vision, photophobia, corneal staining, tachycardia, headache, parasympathetic stimulation, and somnolence.

Artificial Tear Solutions

Adverse reactions are rare, but on occasion redness or irritation may occur.

CONTRAINDICATIONS, PRECAUTIONS, AND INTERACTIONS

Alpha$_2$-Adrenergic Drugs

The drug is contraindicated in patients with hypersensitivity to the drug or any component of the drug and in patients taking the monoamine oxidase inhibitors (MAOIs). Patients should wait at least 15 minutes after instilling brimonidine before inserting soft contact lenses because the preservative in the drug may be absorbed by soft contact lenses. The drug is used cautiously during pregnancy (Pregnancy Category B) and lactation and in patients with cardiovascular disease, depression, cerebral or coronary insufficiency, orthostatic hypotension, or Raynaud's phenomenon. When brimonidine is used with central nervous system (CNS) depressants such as alcohol, barbiturates, opiates, sedatives, or anesthetics, there is a risk for an additive CNS depressant effect. Use the drug cautiously in combination with the beta blockers, antihypertensive drugs, and cardiac glycosides because a synergistic effect may occur.

Sympathomimetic Drugs

These drugs are contraindicated in patients with hypersensitivity to the drug or any component of the drug. Epinephrine is contraindicated in patients with narrow angle glaucoma, or patients with a narrow angle, but no glaucoma, aphakia (absence of the crystalline lens of the eye). Epinephrine should not be used while wearing soft contact lenses (discoloration of the lenses may occur).

These drugs are used cautiously during pregnancy (epinephrine and apraclonidine, Pregnancy Category C; dipivefrin, Pregnancy Category B) and lactation and in patients with hypertension, diabetes, hyperthyroidism, heart disease, cerebral arteriosclerosis, or bronchial asthma. Some of these drugs contain sulfites that may cause allergic-like reactions (hives, wheezing, anaphylaxis) in patients with sulfite sensitivity. See Chapter 22 for information on interactions.

Alpha-Adrenergic Blocking Drugs

The drug is contraindicated in patients with hypersensitivity to the drug or any component of the drug, in conditions in which pupil constriction is not desirable, such as in acute iritis (inflammation of the iris), and in the treatment of IOP in open-angle glaucoma. This drug is used cautiously during pregnancy (Pregnancy Category B) and lactation. No significant drug interactions have been reported.

Beta-Adrenergic Blocking Drugs

The β-adrenergic blocking drugs are contraindicated in patients with bronchial asthma, obstructive pulmonary disease, sinus bradycardia, heart block, cardiac failure, or cardiogenic shock and in patients with hypersensitivity to the drug or any components of the drug. These drugs are Pregnancy Category C and are used cautiously during pregnancy and lactation and in patients with cardiovascular disease, diabetes (may mask the symptoms of hypoglycemia), and hyperthyroidism (may mask symptoms of hyperthyroidism). The patient taking β-adrenergic blocking drugs for ophthalmic reasons may experience increased or additive effects when the drugs are administered with the oral beta blockers. Co-administration of timolol maleate and calcium antagonists may cause hypotension, left ventricular failure, and condition disturbances within the heart. There is a potential additive hypotensive effect when the beta-blocking ophthalmic drugs are administered with the phenothiazines.

Miotic, Direct Acting

These drugs are contraindicated in patients with hypersensitivity to the drug or any component of the drug and in conditions where constriction is undesirable (eg, iritis, uveitis, and acute inflammatory disease of the anterior chamber). The drugs are used cautiously in patients with corneal abrasion, pregnancy (Pregnancy Category C), lactation, cardiac failure, bronchial asthma, peptic ulcer, hyperthyroidism, gastrointestinal spasm, urinary tract infection, Parkinson's disease, recent myocardial infarction, hypotension, or hypertension. These drugs are also used cautiously in patients with angle closure glaucoma because miotics can, occasionally, precipitate angle closure glaucoma by increasing the resistance to aqueous flow from posterior to anterior chamber. See Chapter 24 for information on interactions.

Miotics, Cholinesterase Inhibitors

The cholinesterase inhibitors are contraindicated in patients with hypersensitivity to the drug or any components of the drug. Some of these products contain sulfites, and patients with sulfite sensitivity may experience allergic-type reactions. The drugs are also contraindicated in patients with any active inflammatory disease of the eye and during pregnancy (demecarium, Pregnancy Category X; echothiophate iodine, Pregnancy Category C) and lactation. The cholinesterase inhibitors are used cautiously in patients with myasthenia gravis (may cause additive adverse effects), before and after surgery, and in patients with chronic angle-closure (narrow angle) glaucoma or those with narrow angles (may cause papillary block and increase the angle blockage). When the cholinesterase inhibitors are administered with systemic anticholinesterase drugs, there is a risk for additive effects. Individuals, such as farmers, warehouse workers, or gardeners, working with carbamate/organophosphate insecticides or pesticides are at risk for systemic effects of the cholinesterase inhibitors from absorption of the pesticide or insecticide through the respiratory tract or the skin. Individuals working with pesticides or insecticides containing carbamate/organophosphate and taking a cholinesterase inhibitor should be advised to wear respiratory masks, change clothes frequently, and wash exposed clothes thoroughly.

Carbonic Anhydrase Inhibitors

Use of the carbonic anhydrase inhibitors is contraindicated in patients with hypersensitivity to the drug or any components of the drug and during pregnancy (Pregnancy Category C) and lactation. The drugs are used cautiously in patients with renal and hepatic impairment. When high doses of the salicylates are administered concurrently, toxic levels of the carbonic anhydrase inhibitors have been reported. See Chapter 46 for more information on interactions when administering the carbonic anhydrase inhibitors.

Prostaglandin Agonists

These drugs are contraindicated in patients with hypersensitivity to the drug or any component of the drug and during pregnancy (Pregnancy Category C). The drugs are used cautiously in lactating women and in patients with active intraocular inflammation, those wearing contact lenses (contact lenses must be removed and left out for at least 15 minutes after administration of the drug), and those with macular edema.

Mast Cell Stabilizers

These drugs are contraindicated in patients with a hypersensitivity to the drug or any component of the drug. The mast cell stabilizers are used cautiously in patients who wear contact lenses (preservative may be absorbed by the soft contact lenses) and during pregnancy (pemirolast, Pregnancy Category C; nedocromil, Pregnancy Category B) and lactation. There have been no significant drug–drug interactions associated with these drugs.

Nonsteroidal Anti-inflammatory Drugs

These drugs are contraindicated in individuals with known hypersensitivity to an individual drug or any components of the drug. The NSAID flurbiprofen is contraindicated in patients with herpes simplex keratitis. Diclofenac and ketorolac are contraindicated in patients who wear soft contact lenses (may cause ocular irritation).

The NSAIDs are used cautiously during pregnancy (Pregnancy Category C, flurbiprofen, ketorolac; Pregnancy Category B, diclofenac) and lactation. The NSAIDs are used cautiously in patients with bleeding tendencies. When used topically there is less risk of interactions with drugs or other substances. There is a possibility of a cross-sensitivity reaction when the NSAIDs are administered to patients allergic to the salicylates. The corticosteroids and the antibiotics are used cautiously in patients with sulfite sensitivity because an allergic-type reaction may result. Co-administration of idoxuridine with solutions containing boric acid may cause irritation. The sulfonamides are incompatible with silver nitrate.

Corticosteroids

The corticosteroid ophthalmic preparations are contraindicated in patients with acute superficial herpes simplex keratitis, fungal disease of the eye, or viral diseases of the eye, and after removal of a superficial corneal foreign body.

The corticosteroid ophthalmic preparations are used cautiously in patients with infectious conditions of the eye. These drugs are Pregnancy Category C drugs and are used cautiously during pregnancy and lactation. Prolonged use of the corticosteroids may result in elevated IOP and optic nerve damage.

Antibiotics and Sulfonamides

The antibiotic and sulfonamide ophthalmics are contraindicated in patients with a hypersensitivity to the drug or any component of the drug. These drugs are also contraindicated in patients with epithelial herpes simplex keratitis, varicella, mycobacterial infection of the eye, and fungal diseases of the eye. There are no significant precautions or interactions when the drugs are administered as directed by the primary health care provider.

Antiviral Drugs

These drugs are contraindicated in patients with hypersensitivity to the drug or any component of the drug. These drugs are used cautiously in immunocompromised patients and during pregnancy and lactation. Some of these solutions contain boric acid and may result in a precipitate that causes irritation.

Antifungal Drugs

Natamycin is contraindicated in patients with hypersensitivity to the drug or any component of the drug. The drug is a Pregnancy Category C drug and is used cautiously during pregnancy and lactation. If use of the drug for 7 to 10 days does not result in improvement, the infection may be attributable to another microorganism not susceptible to natamycin.

Vasoconstrictors/Mydriatics

These drugs are contraindicated in individuals with hypersensitivity to the drug or any component of the drug and in patients with narrow angle glaucoma or anatomically narrow angle and no glaucoma and in patients with a sulfite sensitivity (some of these products contain sulfite). The drugs are used cautiously in patients with hypertension, diabetes, hyperthyroidism, cardiovascular disease, and arteriosclerosis. Local anesthetics can increase absorption of topical drugs. Systemic adverse reactions may occur more frequently when these drugs are administered with the β-adrenergic blocking drugs. When the **mydriatics** (drugs that dilate the pupil) are administered with the MAOIs or as long as 21 days after MAOI administration, exaggerated adrenergic effects may occur.

Cycloplegic Mydriatics

These drugs are contraindicated in patients with a hypersensitivity to the drug or any component of the drug and in patients with glaucoma. Some of these preparations contain sulfite, and individuals who are allergic to sulfites may exhibit allergic-like symptoms. The cycloplegic mydriatics are used cautiously in elderly patients and during pregnancy (Pregnancy Category C) and lactation. No significant interactions have been reported when the drugs are given topically.

Artificial Tear Solutions

Artificial tears are contraindicated in patients who are allergic to any component of the solution. No precautions or interactions have been reported.

❁ Herbal Alert: Bilberry

Bilberry, also known as whortleberry, blueberry, trackleberry, and huckleberry, is a shrub with bluish flowers that appear in early spring and ripen in July and August. Although bilberry is given to improve capillary strength and flexibility and as an antioxidant, the most beneficial use appears to be in promoting healthy eyes. Bilberry is thought to increase production of the enzymes responsible for energy production in the eye and promote capillary blood flow in the eyes, hands, and feet. Bilberry extract has been shown to increase the flexibility of the cell walls of both red blood cells and endothelial cells, making the cells better able to stretch and squeeze through tighter spaces. By increasing the flexibility of the red blood cells, more oxygen reaches the tissues, including the retina of the eye. A component of bilberry also speeds the regeneration of rhodopsin (visual purple), which is a critical protein found in the rods of the eye.

Bilberry fruit is a safe food herb with no known adverse reactions or toxicity. There are no known contraindications to its use as directed. The dosage of standard extract is 160 to 320 mg a day.

NURSING PROCESS

● **The Patient Receiving an Ophthalmic Preparation**

ASSESSMENT

Preadministration Assessment

The primary health care provider examines the eye and external structures surrounding the eye and prescribes the drug indicated to treat the disorder. The nurse examines the eye for irritation, redness, and the presence of any exudate and carefully documents the findings in the patient's record. A purulent discharge is often found with infection of the eye. Pruritus (itching) is often present with allergic conditions of the eye. It is also important to determine if any visual impairment is present because this would indicate the need for assistance with ambulation and possibly activities of daily living.

Ongoing Assessment

During the ongoing assessment the nurse observes for a therapeutic drug effect and reports any increase in symptoms and the presence of any redness, irritation, or pain in the eye. Patients admitted for treatment of acute glaucoma should be assessed every 2 hours for relief of pain. Pain in the eye may indicate increased IOP.

NURSING DIAGNOSES

Drug-specific nursing diagnoses are highlighted in the Nursing Diagnoses Checklist. Other nursing diagnoses applicable to these drugs are discussed in depth in Chapter 4.

PLANNING

The expected outcomes of the patient depend on the reason for administration but may include an optimal response to therapy, management of adverse reactions,

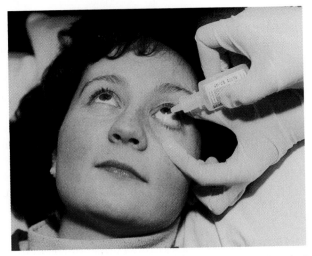

FIGURE 57-2. Instilling eye medication. While the patient looks upward, the nurse gently pulls the lower lid down and instills the correct number of drops into the lower conjunctival sac.

minimized anxiety, and an understanding of the application and use of an ophthalmic preparation.

IMPLEMENTATION

Promoting an Optimal Response to Therapy

Before instillation, ophthalmic solutions and ointments can be warmed in the hand for a few minutes. Ophthalmic ointments are applied to the eyelids or dropped into the lower conjunctival sac; ophthalmic solutions are dropped into the middle of the lower conjunctival sac (Fig. 57-2). When eye solutions are instilled, the nurse applies gentle pressure on the inner canthus to delay drainage of the drug down the tear duct. The primary health care provider is consulted regarding use of this technique before the first dose is instilled because this technique can be potentially dangerous in some eye conditions, such as recent eye surgery. When two eye drops are prescribed for use at the same time, the nurse waits at least 5 minutes before instilling the second drug. This help prevents dilution of the drug and loss of some therapeutic effect from tearing.

Some ophthalmic drugs produce blurring of vision, which can result in falls and other injuries. The nurse warns patients to exercise care when getting out of bed when the vision is impaired by these drugs. Patients using the pilocarpine ocular therapeutic system must have the system replaced every 7 days (see Chap. 24). The system is inserted at bedtime because **myopia** (nearsightedness) occurs for several hours after insertion.

When a patient is scheduled for eye surgery, it is most important that the eye drops ordered by the primary health care provider are instilled at the correct time. This is especially important when the purpose of the drug is to change the size of the pupil.

Nursing Diagnoses Checklist

☑ **Sensory-Perceptual Alteration: Impaired Vision** related to adverse drug effects or disease condition

☑ **Risk for Injury** related to adverse reactions to drug therapy (blurring of the vision)

☑ **Impaired Physical Mobility** related to visual impairment from drug therapy

☑ **Anxiety** related to eye pain or discomfort, diagnosis, other factors

☑ **Risk for Ineffective Regimen Management** related to lack of knowledge of technique of instilling an eye drug

Nursing Alert

Only preparations labeled as ophthalmic are instilled in the eye. The nurse must check the label of the preparation carefully for the name of the drug, the percentage of the preparation, and a statement indicating that the preparation is for ophthalmic use.

Monitoring and Managing Adverse Reactions

Although adverse reactions are rare, these drugs can cause visual impairment such as blurring of vision and local irritation and burning. These reactions are most often self-limiting and will resolve if the patient waits a few minutes. However, if visual impairment does not resolve itself or occurs as a consequence of an eye disorder, the nurse provides assistance with ambulation to prevent injury from falls. In addition, assistance with activities of daily living may also be needed. Visual impairment that does not clear within 30 minutes after therapy is reported to the primary health care provider.

Gerontologic Alert

Older adults, in particular, are at risk for exacerbation of existing disorders such as hypertension, tachycardia, or arrhythmias if systemic absorption of sympathomimetic ophthalmic drugs occurs.

Managing Anxiety

Eye injuries and some eye infections are very painful. Other eye conditions may result in discomfort or a loss of or change in vision. The patient with an eye disorder or injury usually has great concern about the effect the problem will have on his or her vision. The nurse reassures the patient that every effort is being made to treat the disorder.

Educating the Patient and Family

The patient or a family member will require instruction in the technique of instilling an ophthalmic preparation (see Home Care Checklist: Instilling an Ophthalmic Preparation). In addition, the nurse may give the following information to the patient and family member when an eye ointment or solution is prescribed:

- Eye preparations may cause a momentary stinging or burning sensation; this is normal.
- Temporary blurring of vision may occur. Avoid activities requiring visual acuity until vision returns to normal.
- If more than one topical ophthalmic drug is being used, administer the drugs at least 5 to 10 minutes apart or as directed by the physician.
- Complete a full course of treatment with the prescribed drug to achieve satisfactory results.
- Do not rub the eyes, and keep hands away from the eyes.

- Do not use nonprescription eye products during or after treatment unless such use has been approved by the primary health care provider.
- Some of these preparations cause sensitivity (photophobia) to light; to minimize this, wear sunglasses.
- Notify the primary health care provider if symptoms do not improve or if they worsen.
- Brimonidine—patients should wait at least 15 minutes after instilling brimonidine before inserting soft contact lenses.

PROSTAGLANDIN AGONISTS

- Remove contact lenses before administration and leave out at least 15 minutes before reinserting them.
- The color of the iris may change because of an increase of the brown pigment and cause different eye coloration. This may be more noticeable in patients with blue, green, or gray brown or other light-colored eyes.

EVALUATION

- The therapeutic effect is achieved.
- Adverse reactions are managed.
- Anxiety is reduced.
- The patient demonstrates the ability to instill an ophthalmic preparation in eye.
- The patient and family demonstrate an understanding of the drug regimen.
- The patient verbalizes knowledge of and the importance of the treatment regimen.

● *Critical Thinking Exercises*

1. *Prepare a teaching plan for a patient prescribed Cerumenex for removal of earwax.*
2. *Ms. Stone, age 76 years, has glaucoma and is prescribed timolol (Timoptic) eye drops. Your initial assessment reveals that she has severe arthritis and appears to have difficulty following instructions. Discuss any further investigations you feel are important to make before developing a teaching plan for this patient.*
3. *Mr. Caravel, age 38 years, is prescribed tobramycin ophthalmic (Tobrex) for bacterial conjunctivitis. Discuss preadministration assessments the nurse would perform before instilling the drug.*

● *Review Questions*

1. What is the rationale for warming an otic solution that has been refrigerated before instilling the drops into the patient's ear?
   A. The drug becomes thick when refrigerated, and warming liquefies the solution.
   B. It helps to prevent dizziness on instillation.
   C. A cold solution can significantly increase the patient's blood pressure.

Home Care Checklist

INSTILLING AN OPHTHALMIC PREPARATION

Because of shortened hospital stays and increases in the number of ambulatory surgeries for many eye problems, the patient may be required to instill eye drops or ointment at home. If the patient is unable to do so, a family member or friend may have to instill the preparation. The nurse uses the following guide to evaluate that the patient or caregiver can properly instill the eye drops or ointment:

✓ Washes hands thoroughly before beginning.

✓ Holds bottle (drops) or tube (ointment) in hand for a few minutes before using.

✓ Cleanses the area around the eye of any secretions.

✓ Squeezes the eye dropper bulb to release and then refill the dropper, squeezes the bottle to fill the drop chamber, or squeezes ointment to tip of the tube.

✓ Tilts head slightly backward and toward the eye to be treated.

✓ Pulls affected lower lid down.

✓ Positions dropper, bottle, or tube over lower conjunctival sac.

✓ Steadies hand by resting fingers against cheek or by resting base of hand on cheek.

✓ Looks up at ceiling and squeezes dropper, bottle, or tube.

✓ Drops ordered number of drops into the middle of lower conjunctival sac; instills prescribed amount of ointment to eyelid or lower conjunctival sac.

✓ Closes eye briefly and gently and releases lower lid (does not squeeze eyes shut after instilling the drug).

✓ Places finger on inner canthus to avoid absorption via the tear duct (when instilling drops and only if ordered).

✓ Repeats procedure with other eye (if ordered).

✓ If more than one type of ophthalmic preparation is being instilled, waits the recommended time interval before instilling the second drug (usually 5 minutes for drops and 10–15 minutes for ointment).

✓ Replaces the cap of the eye preparation immediately after instilling the eye drops or ointment. Does not touch the tip of the dropper, bottle, or tube.

D. A cold solution could damage the tympanic membrane.

2. Which of the following adverse reactions would the nurse suspect in a patient receiving prolonged treatment with an antibiotic otic drug?

A. Congestive heart failure
B. Superinfection
C. Anemia
D. Hypersensitivity reactions

3. When administering an ophthalmic solution the drug is instilled into the ___.

A. inner canthus
B. upper conjunctival sac

C. lower conjunctival sac
D. upper canthus

4. Which of the following instructions would be included in a teaching plan for the patient prescribed an ophthalmic solution?

A. Squeeze the eyes tightly after the solution is instilled.
B. Immediately wipe the eye using pressure to squeeze out excess medication.
C. After the drug is instilled, remain upright with the head bent slightly forward for about 2 minutes.
D. A temporary stinging or burning may be felt at the time the drug is instilled.

Fluids and Electrolytes

The composition of body fluids remains relatively constant despite the many demands placed on the body each day. On occasion, these demands cannot be met, and electrolytes and fluids must be given in an attempt to restore equilibrium. The solutions used in the management of body fluids discussed in this chapter include blood plasma, plasma protein fractions, protein substrates, energy substrates, plasma proteins, electrolytes, and miscellaneous replacement fluids. **Electrolytes** are electrically charged particles (ions) that are essential for normal cell function and are involved in various metabolic activities. This chapter discusses the use of electrolytes to replace one or more electrolytes that may be lost by the body. The last section of this chapter gives a brief overview of total parenteral nutrition (TPN).

SOLUTIONS USED IN THE MANAGEMENT OF BODY FLUIDS

Parenteral nutrients are used to correct nutritional or fluid deficiencies, as well as to treat certain diseases and conditions.

ACTION AND USES

Blood Plasma

Blood plasma is the liquid part of blood, containing water, sugar, electrolytes, fats, gases, proteins, bile pigment, and clotting factors. Human plasma, also called human pooled plasma, is obtained from donated blood. Although whole blood must be typed and crossmatched because it contains red blood cells carrying blood type and Rh factors, human plasma does not require this procedure. Because of this, plasma can be given in acute emergencies. Plasma administered intravenously (IV) is used to increase blood volume when severe hemorrhage has occurred and it is necessary to partially restore blood volume while waiting for whole blood to be typed and crossmatched. Another use of plasma is in treating conditions when plasma alone has been lost, as may be seen in severe burns.

Plasma Protein Fractions

Plasma protein fractions include human plasma protein fraction 5% and normal serum albumin 5% (Albuminar-5, Buminate 5%) and 25% (Albuminar-25, Buminate 25%). Plasma protein fraction 5% is an IV solution containing 5% human plasma proteins. Serum albumin is obtained from donated whole blood and is a protein found in plasma. The albumin fraction of human blood acts to maintain plasma colloid osmotic pressure and as a carrier of intermediate metabolites in the transport and exchange of tissue products. It is critical in regulating the volume of circulating blood. When blood is lost from shock, such as in hemorrhage, there is a reduced plasma volume. When blood volume is reduced, albumin quickly restores the volume in most situations.

Plasma protein fractions are used to treat hypovolemic (low blood volume) shock that occurs as the result of burns, trauma, surgery, and infections, or in conditions where shock is not currently present but likely to occur. Plasma protein fractions are also used to treat hypoproteinemia (a deficiency of protein in the blood), as might be seen in patients with nephrotic syndrome and hepatic cirrhosis, as well as other diseases or disorders. As with human pooled plasma, blood type and crossmatch is not needed when plasma protein fractions are given.

Protein Substrates

A **substrate** is a substance that is the basic component of an organism. Protein substrates are amino acids, which are essential to life. **Protein substrates** are amino acid preparations that act to promote the production of proteins (anabolism). Amino acids are necessary to promote synthesis of structural components, reduce the rate of protein breakdown (catabolism), promote wound healing, and act as buffers in the extracellular and intracellular fluids. Crystalline amino acid preparations are hypertonic solutions of balanced essential and nonessential amino acid concentrations that provide substrates for protein synthesis or act to conserve existing body protein.

Amino acids promote the production of proteins, enhance tissue repair and wound healing, and reduce the rate of protein breakdown. Amino acids are used in certain disease states, such as severe kidney and liver disease, as well as in TPN solutions. (See the last section of this chapter for a more detailed discussion of TPN.) TPN may be used in patients with conditions such as impairment of gastrointestinal absorption of protein, in patients with an increased requirement for protein, as seen in those with extensive burns or infections, and in patients with no available oral route for nutritional intake.

Energy Substrates

Dextrose & Lipids

Energy substrates include dextrose solutions and fat emulsion. Solutions used to supply energy and fluid include dextrose (glucose) in water or sodium chloride, alcohol in dextrose, and IV fat emulsion. Dextrose is a carbohydrate used to provide a source of calories and fluid. Alcohol (as alcohol in dextrose) also provides calories. Dextrose is available in various strengths (or percent of the carbohydrate) in a fluid, which may be water or sodium chloride (saline). Dextrose and dextrose in alcohol are available in various strengths (or percent of the carbohydrate and percent of the alcohol) in water. Dextrose solutions also are available with electrolytes, for example, Plasma-Lyte 56 and 5% Dextrose. Calories provided by dextrose and dextrose and alcohol solutions are listed in Table 58-1.

An IV fat emulsion contains soybean or safflower oil and a mixture of natural triglycerides, predominately unsaturated fatty acids. It is used in the prevention and treatment of essential fatty acid deficiency. It also provides nonprotein calories for those receiving TPN when calorie requirements cannot be met by glucose. Examples of intravenous fat emulsion include Intralipid 10% and 20%, Liposyn II 10% and 20%, and Liposyn III 10% and 20%. Fat emulsion is used as a source of calories and essential fatty acids for

sepsis?

Table 58-1	Calories Provided in Intravenous Carbohydrate Solutions	
CARBOHYDRATE	**PERCENTAGE**	**CALORIES/1,000 ML**
Dextrose	2.5%	85
Dextrose	5%	170
Dextrose	10%	340
Dextrose	20%	680
Dextrose	50%	1,700
Dextrose	70%	2,380
Alcohol in dextrose	5% alcohol and 5% dextrose	450
	10% alcohol and 5% dextrose	720

patients requiring parenteral nutrition for extended periods (usually more than 5 days). No more than 60% of the patient's total caloric intake should come from fat emulsion, with carbohydrates and amino acids comprising the remaining 40% or more of caloric intake.

Plasma Expanders

The IV solutions of plasma expanders include hetastarch (Hespan), low–molecular-weight dextran (Dextran 40), and high–molecular-weight dextran (Dextran 70, Dextran 75). Plasma expanders are used to expand plasma volume when shock is caused by burns, hemorrhage, surgery, and other trauma and for prophylaxis of venous thrombosis and thromboembolism. When used in the treatment of shock, plasma expanders are not a substitute for whole blood or plasma, but they are of value as emergency measures until the latter substances can be used.

Intravenous Replacement Solutions

Intravenous replacement solutions are a source of electrolytes and water for hydration (Normosol M Ringer's Injection, Lactated Ringer's, Plasma-Lyte R), and used to facilitate amino acid utilization and maintain electrolyte balance (Lypholyte, Multilyte, TPN Electrolytes). Dextrose and electrolyte solutions such as Plasma-Lyte R and 5% dextrose are used as a parenteral source of electrolytes, calories, or water for hydration. Invert sugar-electrolyte solutions, such as Multiple Electrolytes and Travert 5% and 10%, contain equal parts of dextrose and fructose and are used as a source of calories and hydration.

ADVERSE REACTIONS, CONTRAINDICATIONS, PRECAUTIONS, AND INTERACTIONS ●

Blood Plasma

Solutions used in the management of body fluids are contraindicated in patients with hypersensitivity to any component of the solution. All solutions used to manage body fluids discussed in this chapter are Pregnancy Category C drugs and are used cautiously during pregnancy and lactation. No interactions have been reported.

Plasma Protein Fractions

Adverse reactions are rare when plasma protein fractions are administered, but nausea, chills, fever, urticaria, and hypotensive episodes may occasionally be seen.

Plasma proteins are contraindicated in those with a history of allergic reactions to albumin, severe anemia, or cardiac failure; in the presence of normal or increased intravascular volume; and in patients on cardiopulmonary bypass. Plasma protein fractions are used cautiously in patients who are in shock or dehydrated and in those with congestive cardiac failure or hepatic or renal failure. These solutions are Pregnancy Category C drugs and are used cautiously during pregnancy and lactation.

Most IV solutions should not be combined with any other solutions or drugs but should be administered alone. The nurse should consult the drug insert or other appropriate sources before combining any drug with any plasma protein fraction.

Protein Substrates

Administration of protein substrates (amino acids) may result in nausea, fever, flushing of the skin, metabolic acidosis or alkalosis, and decreased phosphorus and calcium blood levels.

Solutions used in the management of body fluids are contraindicated in patients with hypersensitivity to any component of the solution. Plasma expanders are used cautiously in patients with renal disease, congestive heart failure, pulmonary edema, and severe bleeding disorders. These solutions are Pregnancy Category C drugs and are used cautiously during pregnancy and lactation. Protein substrates should not be combined with any other solutions or drugs without consulting the drug insert or other appropriate sources.

Energy Substrates

Low– or high–molecular-weight dextran administration may result in allergic reactions, which are evidenced by urticaria, hypotension, nausea, vomiting, headache, dyspnea, fever, tightness of the chest, and wheezing. Hyperglycemia and phlebitis may be seen with administration of glucose.

The energy substrates are contraindicated in patients with hypersensitivity to any component of the solution. Dextrose solutions are contraindicated in patients with diabetic coma with excessively high blood sugar. Concentrated dextrose solutions are contraindicated in patients with increased intracranial pressure, delirium tremens (if patient is dehydrated), hepatic coma, or glucose–galactose malabsorption syndrome. Alcohol dextrose solutions are contraindicated in patients with epilepsy, urinary tract infections, alcoholism, and diabetic coma.

Alcohol dextrose solutions are used cautiously in patients with hepatic and renal impairment, vitamin deficiency (may cause or potentate vitamin deficiency), diabetes, or shock; during postpartum hemorrhage; and after cranial surgery. The nurse should consult the drug insert or other appropriate sources before combining any drug with an IV solution. Dextrose solutions are used cautiously in patients receiving a corticosteroid or corticotropin. Dextrose and alcohol dextrose solutions are incompatible with blood (may cause hemolysis).

The most common adverse reaction associated with the administration of fat emulsion is sepsis caused by administration equipment and thrombophlebitis caused by vein irritations from concurrently administering hypertonic solutions. Less frequently occurring adverse reactions include dyspnea, cyanosis, hyperlipidemia, hypercoagulability, nausea, vomiting, headache, flushing, increase in temperature, sweating, sleepiness, chest and back pain, slight pressure over the eyes, and dizziness.

IV fat emulsions are contraindicated in conditions that interfere with normal fat metabolism (eg, acute pancreatitis) and in patients allergic to eggs. IV fat emulsions are used with caution in those with severe liver impairment, pulmonary disease, anemia, and blood coagulation disorders. These solutions are Pregnancy Category C drugs and are used cautiously during pregnancy and lactation. In general, fat emulsions should not be combined with any other solutions or drugs, except when combined in TPN. The nurse should consult appropriate sources before combining any drug with a fat emulsion.

Plasma Expanders

Administration of hetastarch, a plasma expander, may be accompanied by vomiting, a mild temperature elevation, itching, and allergic reactions. Allergic reactions are evidenced by wheezing, edema around the eyes (periorbital edema), and urticaria. Other plasma expanders may result in mild cutaneous eruptions, generalized urticaria, hypotension, nausea, vomiting, headache, dyspnea, fever, tightness of the chest, bronchospasm, wheezing, and rarely, anaphylactic shock.

Plasma expanders are contraindicated in patients with hypersensitivity to any component of the solution and those with severe bleeding disorders, severe cardiac failure, renal failure with oliguria, or anuria. Plasma expanders are used cautiously in patients with renal disease, congestive heart failure, pulmonary edema, and severe bleeding disorders. Plasma expanders are Pregnancy Category C drugs and are used cautiously during pregnancy and lactation. The nurse should consult the drug insert or other appropriate sources before combining a plasma expander with another drug for IV administration.

Fluid Overload

One adverse reaction common to all solutions administered by the parenteral route is fluid overload, that is, the administration of more fluid than the body is able to

---

DISPLAY 58-1 ● **Signs and Symptoms of Fluid Overload**

- Headache
- Weakness
- Blurred vision
- Behavioral changes (confusion, disorientation, delirium, drowsiness)
- Weight gain
- Isolated muscle twitching
- Hyponatremia
- Rapid breathing
- Wheezing
- Coughing
- Rise in blood pressure
- Distended neck veins
- Elevated central venous pressure
- Convulsions

---

handle. The term **fluid overload** (circulatory overload) is not a specific amount of fluid that is given. It describes a condition when the body's fluid requirements are met and the administration of fluid occurs at a rate that is greater than the rate at which the body can use or eliminate the fluid. Thus, the amount of fluid and the rate of administration of fluid that will cause fluid overload depend on several factors, such as the patient's cardiac status and adequacy of renal function. The signs and symptoms of fluid overload are listed in Display 58-1.

NURSING PROCESS

● **The Patient Receiving a Solution for Management of Body Fluids**

ASSESSMENT

Preadministration Assessment

Solutions used to manage body fluids are often administered IV. Before administering an IV solution, the nurse assesses the patient's general status, reviews recent laboratory test results (when appropriate), weighs the patient (when appropriate), and takes the vital signs. Blood pressure, pulse, and respiratory rate provide a baseline, which is especially important when the patient is receiving blood plasma, plasma expanders, or plasma protein fractions for shock or other serious disorders.

Ongoing Assessment

During the ongoing assessment, the nurse checks the needle site every 15 to 30 minutes or more frequently if the patient is restless or confused. When one of these preparations is given with a regular IV infusion set, the nurse checks the infusion rate every 15 minutes. The needle site is inspected for signs of **extravasation** (escape of fluid from a blood vessel into surrounding tissues) or **infiltration** (the collection of fluid into tissues).

If signs of extravasation or infiltration are apparent, the nurse restarts the infusion in another vein.

When these solutions are given, a central venous pressure line may be inserted to monitor the patient's response to therapy. Central venous pressure readings are taken as ordered. During administration, the nurse takes the blood pressure, pulse, and respiratory rate as ordered or at intervals determined by the patient's clinical condition. For example, a patient in shock and receiving a plasma expander may require monitoring of the blood pressure and pulse rate every 5 to 15 minutes, whereas the patient receiving dextrose 3 days after surgery may require monitoring every 30 to 60 minutes.

The nurse observes patients receiving IV solutions at frequent intervals for signs of fluid overload. If signs of fluid overload (see Display 58-1) are observed, the nurse slows the IV infusion rate and immediately notifies the primary health care provider.

 Gerontologic Alert

Older adults are at increased risk for fluid overload because of the increased incidence of cardiac disease and decreased renal function that may accompany old age. Careful monitoring for signs and symptoms of fluid overload (see Table 58-2) is extremely important when administering fluids to older adults.

FAT EMULSIONS. When a fat emulsion is administered, the nurse must monitor the patient's ability to eliminate the infused fat from the circulation. The lipidemia must clear between daily infusions. The nurse monitors for lipidemia through assessing the result of the following laboratory exams: hemogram, blood coagulation, liver function tests, plasma lipid profile, and platelet count. The nurse reports an increase in any of these laboratory examinations as abnormal.

NURSING DIAGNOSES

Drug-specific nursing diagnoses are highlighted in the Nursing Diagnoses Checklist. Other nursing diagnoses applicable to these drugs are discussed in depth in Chapter 4.

Nursing Diagnoses Checklist

✔ **Excess Fluid Volume** related to adverse effects resulting from too rapid intravenous infusion

✔ **Deficient Fluid Volume** related to inability to take oral fluids, abnormal fluid loss, other factors (specify cause of deficient fluid volume)

✔ **Imbalanced Nutrition: Less than Body Requirements** related to inability to eat, recent surgery, other factors (specify cause of altered nutrition)

PLANNING

The expected outcomes of the patient may include an optimal response to therapy, prevention of fluid overload, correction of the fluid volume deficit (where appropriate), improved oral nutrition (where appropriate), and an understanding of the administration procedure.

IMPLEMENTATION

Promoting an Optimal Response to Therapy

Patients receiving an IV fluid should be made as comfortable as possible, although under some circumstances this may be difficult. The extremity used for administration should be made comfortable and supported as needed by a small pillow or other device. An IV infusion pump may be ordered for the administration of these solutions. The nurse sets the alarm of the infusion pump and checks the functioning of the unit at frequent intervals.

 Nursing Alert

The nurse must administer all IV solutions with great care. At no time should any IV solution be infused at a rapid rate, unless there is a specific written order to do so.

Unless otherwise directed, the IV solution should be administered at room temperature. If the solution is refrigerated, the nurse allows the solution to warm by exposing it to room temperature 30 to 45 minutes before use. The average length of time for infusion of 1000 mL of an IV solution is 4 to 8 hours. The only exception is when there is a written or verbal order by the primary health care provider to give the solution at a rapid rate because of an emergency. In this instance, the order must specifically state the rate of administration as drops per minute, milliliters per minute, or the period of time over which a specific amount of fluid is to be infused (eg, 125 mL/h or 1000 mL in 8 hours). Calculation of IV flow rates is discussed in Chapter 3.

LIPID SOLUTIONS. Fat solutions (emulsions) should be handled with care to decrease the risk of separation or "breaking out of the oil." Separation can be identified by yellowish streaking or the accumulation of yellowish droplets in the emulsion. Fat solutions are administered to adults at a rate no greater than 1 to 2 mL/min.

 Nursing Alert

During the first 30 minutes of infusion of a fat solution, the nurse carefully observes the patient for difficulty in breathing, headache, flushing, nausea, vomiting, or signs of a hypersensitivity reaction. If any of these reactions occur, the nurse discontinues the infusion and immediately notifies the primary health care provider.

AMINO ACIDS. A microscopic filter is attached to the IV line when amino acid solutions are administered. The filter prevents microscopic aggregates (particles that may form in the IV bag) from entering the bloodstream where they could cause massive emboli.

Managing Fluid Volume Deficit and Nutritional Imbalances

Many times the solutions used in the management of body fluids are given to correct a fluid volume deficit and to supply carbohydrates (nutrition). The nurse reviews the patient's chart for a full understanding of the rationale for administration of the specific solution.

When appropriate, nursing measures that may be instituted to correct a fluid volume and carbohydrate deficit may be included in a plan of care. Examples of these measures include offering oral fluids at frequent intervals and encouraging the patient to take small amounts of nourishment between meals and to eat as much as possible at mealtime.

Educating the Patient and Family

The nurse gives the patient or family a brief explanation of the reason for and the method of administration of an IV solution. Sometimes, patients and families tamper with or adjust the rate of flow of IV administration sets. The nurse emphasizes the importance of not touching the IV administration set or the equipment used to administer IV fluids.

EVALUATION

- The therapeutic effect of the drug is achieved.
- The fluid volume deficit is corrected.
- The nutrition deficit is corrected.
- The patient and family demonstrate an understanding of the procedure.

ELECTROLYTES

Along with a disturbance in fluid volume (eg, loss of plasma, blood, or water) or a need for providing parenteral nutrition with the previously discussed solutions, an electrolyte imbalance may exist. An electrolyte is an electrically charged substance essential to the normal functioning of all cells. Electrolytes circulate in the blood at specific levels where they are available for use when needed by the cells. An electrolyte imbalance occurs when the concentration of an electrolyte in the blood is either too high or too low. In some instances, an electrolyte imbalance may be present without an appreciable disturbance in fluid balance. For example, a patient taking a diuretic is able to maintain fluid balance by an adequate oral intake of water, which

replaces the water lost through diuresis. However, the patient is likely to be unable to replace the potassium that is also lost during diuresis. When the potassium concentration in the blood is too low, as may occur with the administration of a diuretic, an imbalance may occur that requires the addition of potassium. Commonly used electrolytes are listed in the Summary Drug Table: Electrolytes.

ACTIONS AND USES

Bicarbonate (HCO$_3^-$)

This electrolyte plays a vital role in the acid-base balance of the body. Bicarbonate may be given IV as sodium bicarbonate (NaHCO$_3$) in the treatment of metabolic acidosis, a state of imbalance that may be seen in diseases or situations such as severe shock, diabetic acidosis, severe diarrhea, extracorporeal circulation of blood, severe renal disease, and cardiac arrest. Oral sodium bicarbonate is used as a gastric and urinary alkalinizer. It may be used as a single drug or may be found as one of the ingredients in some antacid preparations. It is also useful in treating severe diarrhea accompanied by bicarbonate loss.

Bicarbonate is no longer used as the first line treatment during cardiopulmonary resuscitation following cardiac arrest. Recent evidence suggests little benefit, and the drug may actually be detrimental to resuscitation. According to the American Heart Association, bicarbonate is used when all other treatment options have failed.

Calcium (Ca^{++})

Calcium is necessary for the functioning of nerves and muscles, the clotting of blood (see Chap. 44), the building of bones and teeth, and other physiologic processes. Examples of calcium salts are calcium gluconate and calcium carbonate. Calcium may be given for the treatment of **hypocalcemia** (low blood calcium), which may be seen in those with parathyroid disease or after accidental removal of the parathyroid glands during surgery of the thyroid gland. Calcium may also be given during cardiopulmonary resuscitation, particularly after open heart surgery, when epinephrine fails to improve weak or ineffective myocardial contractions. Calcium may be used as adjunct therapy of insect bites or stings to reduce muscle cramping, such as occurs with black widow spider bites. Calcium may also be recommended for those eating a diet low in calcium or as a dietary supplement when there is an increased need for calcium, such as during pregnancy.

SUMMARY DRUG TABLE **ELECTROLYTES**

GENERIC NAME	TRADE NAME*	USES	ADVERSE REACTIONS	DOSAGE RANGES
calcium acetate	PhosLo	Control of hyperphosphatemia in end-stage renal disease	See Display 58-2	3–4 tablets PO with each meal
calcium carbonate	Calcium-600, Caltrate, Oyster Shell Calcium Tums, Tums E-X, Tums Ultra, *generic*	Dietary supplement for prevention or treatment of calcium deficiency, osteoporosis, osteomalcia, rickets, latent tetany	Rare; see Display 58-2 for signs of hypercalcemia	500–2000 mg/d PO
calcium citrate	Citracal, Citracal Liquitab, *generic*	Same as calcium carbonate; premenstrual syndrome	Same as calcium carbonate	500–2000 mg/d PO
calcium gluconate	*Generic*	Same as calcium carbonate; premenstrual syndrome	Same as calcium carbonate	500–2000 mg/d PO
calcium lactate	*Generic*	Same as calcium carbonate	Same as calcium carbonate	500–2000 mg/d PO
oral electrolyte mixtures	Infalyte Oral Solution, Naturalyte, Pedialyte, Pedialyte Electrolyte, Pedialyte Freezer Pops, Rehydralyte, Resol	Maintenance of water and electrolytes after corrective parenteral therapy of severe diarrhea; maintenance to replace mild to moderate fluid losses when food and liquid intake are discontinued, to restore fluid and minerals lost in diarrhea and vomiting in infants and children	Rare	Individualize dosage following the guidelines on the product labeling
magnesium	Almora, Magonate, Mag-Ox 400, Magtrate, Mag-200, Slow-Mag, Uro-Mag, *generic*	Dietary supplement, hypomagnesemia	Rare; see Display 58-2 for signs of hypermagnesemia	54–483 mg/d PO
potassium replacements	Effer K, K+10, Kaon Cl, K-Dur, Klor-Con, K-Lyte, K-Tab, Micro-K, Slow-K, *generic*	Hypokalemia	See Display 58-2; most common: nausea, vomiting, diarrhea, flatulence, abdominal discomfort, skin rash	40–150 mEq/d PO
sodium chloride	*generic*	Prevention or treatment of extracellular volume depletion, dehydration, sodium depletion, aid in the prevention of heat prostration	Nausea, vomiting, diarrhea, abdominal cramps, edema, irritability, restlessness, weakness, hypertension, tachycardia, fluid accumulation, pulmonary edema, respiratory arrest (see Display 58-2)	Individualize dosage

*The term *generic* indicates the drug is available in generic form.

Magnesium (Mg⁺⁺)

Magnesium plays an important role in the transmission of nerve impulses. It is also important in the activity of many enzyme reactions, for example, carbohydrate metabolism. Magnesium sulfate is used as replacement therapy in hypomagnesemia. Magnesium sulfate ($MgSO_4$) is used in the prevention and control of seizures in obstetric patients with pregnancy-induced hypertension (PIH, also referred to as eclampsia and preeclampsia). It may also be added to TPN mixtures.

Potassium (K⁺)

Potassium is necessary for the transmission of impulses; the contraction of smooth, cardiac, and skeletal muscles; and other important physiologic processes. Potassium as a drug is available as potassium chloride (KCl) and potassium gluconate, and is measured in milliequivalents (mEq), for example, 40 mEq in 20 mL or 8 mEq controlled-release tablet. Potassium may be given for **hypokalemia** (low blood potassium). Examples of causes of hypokalemia are a marked loss of gastrointestinal fluids (severe vomiting, diarrhea, nasogastric suction, draining intestinal fistulas), diabetic acidosis, marked diuresis, and severe malnutrition.

Sodium (Na⁺)

Sodium is essential for the maintenance of normal heart action and in the regulation of osmotic pressure in body cells. Sodium, as sodium chloride (NaCl), may be given IV. A solution containing 0.9% NaCl is called **normal saline,** and a solution containing 0.45% NaCl is called **half-normal saline.** Sodium also is available combined with dextrose, for example, dextrose 5% and sodium chloride 0.9%.

Sodium is administered for **hyponatremia** (low blood sodium). Examples of causes of hyponatremia are excessive diaphoresis, severe vomiting or diarrhea, excessive diuresis, and draining intestinal fistulas.

Combined Electrolyte Solutions

Combined electrolyte solutions are available for oral and IV administration. The IV solutions contain various electrolytes and dextrose. The amount of electrolytes, given as milliequivalents per liter (mEq/L), also varies. The IV solutions are used to replace fluid and electrolytes that have been lost and to provide calories by means of their carbohydrate content. Examples of IV electrolyte solutions are dextrose 5% with 0.9% NaCl, lactated Ringer's injection, Plasma-Lyte, and 10% Travert (invert sugar—a combination of equal parts of fructose and dextrose) and Electrolyte No. 2.

The primary health care provider selects the type of combined electrolyte solution that will meet the patient's needs.

Oral electrolyte solutions contain a carbohydrate and various electrolytes. Examples of combined oral electrolyte solutions are Pedialyte and Rehydralyte. Oral electrolyte solutions are most often used to replace lost electrolytes, carbohydrates, and fluid in conditions such as severe vomiting or diarrhea.

ADVERSE REACTIONS, CONTRAINDICATIONS, PRECAUTIONS, AND INTERACTIONS ●

Bicarbonate (HCO₃⁻)

In some instances, excessive oral use may produce nausea and vomiting. Some individuals may use sodium bicarbonate (baking soda) for the relief of gastric disturbances, such as pain, discomfort, symptoms of indigestion, and gas. Prolonged use of oral sodium bicarbonate or excessive doses of IV sodium bicarbonate may result in systemic alkalosis.

Bicarbonate is contraindicated in patients losing chloride by continuous gastrointestinal suction or through vomiting, in patients with metabolic or respiratory alkalosis, hypocalcemia, renal failure, or severe abdominal pain of unknown cause, and in those on sodium-restricted diets. Bicarbonate is used cautiously in patients with congestive heart failure or renal impairment and with glucocorticoid therapy. Bicarbonate is a Pregnancy Category C drug and is used cautiously during pregnancy.

Oral administration of bicarbonate may decrease the absorption of ketoconazole. Increased blood levels of quinidine, flecainide, or sympathomimetics may occur when these agents are administered with bicarbonate. There is an increased risk of crystalluria when bicarbonate is administered with the fluoroquinolones. Possible decreased effects of lithium, methotrexate, chlorpropamide, salicylates, and tetracyclines may occur when these drugs are administered with sodium bicarbonate. Sodium bicarbonate is not administered within 2 hours of enteric-coated drugs; the protective enteric coating may disintegrate before the drug reaches the intestine.

Calcium (Ca⁺⁺)

Irritation of the vein used for administration, tingling, a metallic or chalky taste, and "heat waves" may occur when calcium is given IV. Rapid IV administration (calcium gluconate) may result in bradycardia, vasodilation, decreased blood pressure, cardiac arrhythmias, and cardiac arrest. Oral administration may result in gastrointestinal disturbances. Administration of calcium chloride may cause peripheral vasodilation, temporary fall in blood pressure, and a local burning. Display 58-2 gives adverse reactions associated with hyper- and hypocalcemia.

Calcium is contraindicated in patients with hypercalcemia or ventricular fibrillation and in patients taking digitalis. Calcium is used cautiously in patients with cardiac disease. Hypercalcemia may occur when calcium is administered with the thiazide diuretics. When calcium is administered with atenolol there is a decrease in the effect of atenolol, possibly resulting in decreased beta blockade. There is an increased risk of digitalis toxicity when digitalis preparations are administered with calcium. The clinical effect of verapamil may be decreased when the drug is administered with calcium. Concurrent ingestion of spinach or cereal may decrease the absorption of calcium supplements.

Magnesium (Mg^{++})

Adverse reactions seen with magnesium administration are rare. If they do occur, they are most likely related to overdose and may include flushing, sweating, hypotension, depressed reflexes, muscle weakness, and circulatory collapse (see Display 58-2).

Magnesium sulfate is contraindicated in patients with heart block or myocardial damage and in women with PIH during the 2 hours before delivery. Magnesium is a Pregnancy Category A drug, and studies indicate no increased risk of fetal abnormalities if the agent is used during pregnancy. Nevertheless, caution is used when administering magnesium during pregnancy. In addition, magnesium chloride is contraindicated in patients with renal impairment or marked myocardial disease and those in a coma. Magnesium (sulfate) is used with caution in patients with renal function impairment. Prolonged respiratory depression and apnea may occur when magnesium is administered with the neuromuscular blocking agents.

Potassium (K$^+$)

Nausea, vomiting, diarrhea, abdominal pain, and phlebitis have been seen with oral and IV administration of potassium. Adverse reactions related to hypo- or hyperkalemia are listed in Display 58-2.

If extravasation of the IV solution should occur, local tissue necrosis (death of tissue) may be seen. If extravasation occurs, the primary health care provider is contacted immediately and the infusion slowed to a rate that keeps the vein open.

Potassium is contraindicated in patients who are at risk for experiencing hyperkalemia, such as those with renal failure, oliguria, or azotemia (the presence of nitrogen-containing compounds in the blood), anuria, severe hemolytic reactions, untreated Addison's disease (see Chap. 50), acute dehydration, heat cramps, and any form of hyperkalemia. Potassium is used cautiously in patients with renal impairment or adrenal insufficiency, heart disease, metabolic acidosis, or prolonged or severe diarrhea. Concurrent use of potassium with angiotensin-converting enzyme (ACE) inhibitors may result in elevated serum potassium. Potassium-sparing diuretics and salt substitutes used with potassium can produce severe hyperkalemia. The use of digitalis with potassium increases the risk of digoxin toxicity.

Sodium (Na⁺)

Sodium as the salt (eg, NaCl) has no adverse reactions except those related to overdose (see Display 58-2). In some instances, excessive oral use may produce nausea and vomiting.

Sodium is contraindicated in patients with hypernatremia, fluid retention, and when the administration of sodium or chloride could be detrimental. Sodium is used cautiously in surgical patients and those with circulatory insufficiency, hypoproteinemia, urinary tract obstruction, congestive heart failure, edema, and renal impairment. Sodium is a Pregnancy Category C drug and is used cautiously during pregnancy.

NURSING PROCESS

● The Patient Receiving an Electrolyte

ASSESSMENT

Preadministration Assessment

Before administering any electrolyte, electrolyte salt, or a combined electrolyte solution, the nurse assesses the patient for signs of an electrolyte imbalance (see Display 58-2). All recent laboratory and diagnostic tests appropriate to the imbalance are reviewed. The nurse obtains vital signs to provide a database.

Ongoing Assessment

During therapy, the nurse periodically obtains (daily or more frequently) serum electrolyte or bicarbonate studies to monitor therapy.

BICARBONATE. When given in the treatment of metabolic acidosis, the drug may be added to the IV fluid or given as a prepared IV sodium bicarbonate solution. Frequent laboratory monitoring of the blood pH and blood gases is usually ordered because dosage and length of therapy depend on test results. The nurse frequently observes the patient for signs of clinical improvement and monitors the blood pressure, pulse, and respiratory rate every 15 to 30 minutes or as ordered by the primary health care provider. Extravasation of the drug requires selection of another needle site because the drug is irritating to the tissues.

CALCIUM. Before, during, and after the administration of IV calcium, the nurse monitors the blood pressure,

pulse, and respiratory rate every 30 minutes until the patient's condition has stabilized. After administration of calcium, the nurse observes the patient for signs of hypercalcemia (see Display 58-2).

> ### Nursing Alert
>
> *Systemic overloading of calcium ions in the systemic circulation results in acute hypercalcemic syndrome. Symptoms of hypercalcemic syndrome include elevated plasma calcium, weakness, lethargy, severe nausea and vomiting, coma, and, if left untreated, death. The nurse reports any signs of hypercalcemic syndrome immediately to the primary health care provider.*

To combat this syndrome the physician may prescribe IV sodium chloride and a potent diuretic, such as furosemide. When used together these two drugs markedly increase calcium renal clearance and reduce hypercalcemia.

POTASSIUM. Patients receiving oral potassium should have their blood pressure and pulse monitored every 4 hours, especially during early therapy. The nurse also observes the patient for signs of hyperkalemia (see Display 58-2), which would indicate that the dose of potassium is too high. Signs of hypokalemia may also occur during therapy and may indicate that the dose of potassium is too low and must be increased. If signs of hypokalemia or hyperkalemia are apparent or suspected, the nurse notifies the primary health care provider. In some instances, frequent laboratory monitoring of the serum potassium may be ordered.

The nurse inspects the IV needle site every 30 minutes for signs of extravasation. Potassium is irritating to the tissues. If extravasation occurs, the nurse discontinues the IV immediately and notifies the primary health care provider. The acutely ill patient and the patient with severe hypokalemia will require monitoring of the blood pressure and pulse rate every 15 to 30 minutes during the time of the IV infusion. The nurse measures the intake and output every 8 hours. The infusion rate is slowed to keep the vein open, and the primary health care provider is notified if an irregular pulse is noted.

MAGNESIUM. When magnesium sulfate is ordered to treat convulsions or severe hypomagnesemia, the patient requires constant observation. The nurse obtains the patient's blood pressure, pulse, and respiratory rate immediately before the drug is administered, as well as every 5 to 10 minutes during the time of IV infusion or after the drug is given direct IV. The nurse continues monitoring these vital signs at frequent intervals until the patient's condition has stabilized. Because magnesium is eliminated by the kidneys, it is used with caution in patients with renal impairment. The nurse monitors the urine output for at least 100 mL every 4 hours. Voiding less than 100 mL of urine every 4 hours is reported to the primary health care provider.

The nurse observes the patient for early signs of hypermagnesemia (see Display 58-2) and contacts the primary health care provider immediately if this imbalance is suspected. Frequent plasma magnesium levels are usually ordered. The nurse notifies the primary health care provider if the magnesium level is higher or lower than the normal range.

> ### ☀ Nursing Alert
>
> *As plasma magnesium levels rise above 4 mEq/L, the deep tendon reflexes are first decreased and then absent as the plasma levels reach 10 mEq/L. The knee jerk reflex is tested before each dose of magnesium sulfate. If the reflex is absent or a slow response is obtained, the nurse withholds the dosage and notifies the primary health care provider.*

SODIUM. When NaCl is administered by IV infusion, the nurse observes the patient during and after administration for signs of hypernatremia (see Display 58-2). The nurse checks the rate of IV infusion as ordered by the primary health care provider, usually every 15 to 30 minutes. More frequent monitoring of the infusion rate may be necessary when the patient is restless or confused. To minimize venous irritation during administration of sodium or any electrolyte solution, the nurse uses a small bore needle placed well within the lumen of a large vein.

Patients receiving a 3% or 5% NaCl solution by IV infusion are observed closely for signs of pulmonary edema (dyspnea, cough, restlessness, bradycardia). If any one or more of these symptoms should occur, the IV infusion is slowed to keep the vein open, and the primary health care provider is contacted immediately. Patients receiving NaCl by the IV route have their intake and output measured every 8 hours. The nurse observes the patient for signs of hypernatremia every 3 to 4 hours and contacts the primary health care provider if this condition is suspected.

NURSING DIAGNOSES

Drug-specific nursing diagnoses are highlighted in the Nursing Diagnoses Checklist. Other nursing diagnoses applicable to these drugs are discussed in depth in Chapter 4.

PLANNING

The expected outcomes of the patient depend on the specific drug, dose, route of administration, and reason for administration of an electrolyte but may include an

---

> ### Nursing Diagnoses Checklist
>
> ☑ **Imbalanced Nutrition: Less than Body Requirements** related to adverse drug reaction (nausea, vomiting)
>
> ☑ **Risk for Injury** related to adverse drug effects (muscular weakness)
>
> ☑ **Disturbed Thought Processes** related to adverse drug effects
>
> ☑ **Risk for Decreased Cardiac Output** related to adverse drug effects (cardiac arrhythmias)

optimal response to therapy, compliance with the prescribed therapeutic regimen, and an understanding of the drug regimen and adverse drug effects.

IMPLEMENTATION

Promoting an Optimal Response to Therapy

In some situations, electrolytes are administered when an electrolyte imbalance may potentially occur. For example, the patient with nasogastric suction is prescribed one or more electrolytes added to an IV solution, such as 5% dextrose or a combined electrolyte solution, to be given IV to make up for the electrolytes that are lost through nasogastric suction. In other instances, electrolytes are given to replace those already lost, such as the patient admitted to the hospital with severe vomiting and diarrhea of several days' duration.

When electrolytes are administered parenterally, the dosage is expressed in milliequivalents (mEq), for example, calcium gluconate 7 mEq IV. When administered orally, sodium bicarbonate, calcium, and magnesium dosages are expressed in milligrams (mg). Potassium liquids and effervescent tablet dosages are expressed in milliequivalents; capsule or tablet dosages may be expressed as milliequivalents or milligrams.

Electrolyte disturbances can cause varying degrees of confusion, muscular weakness, nausea, vomiting, and cardiac irregularities (see Display 58-2 for specific symptoms). Serum electrolyte blood levels have a very narrow therapeutic range. Careful monitoring is needed to determine if blood levels fall above or below normal. Normal values may vary with the laboratory, but a general range of normal values for each electrolyte is found in Display 58-2. Adverse reactions are usually controlled by maintaining blood levels of the various electrolytes within the normal range.

ADMINISTERING BICARBONATE. The nurse gives oral sodium bicarbonate tablets with a full glass of water; the powdered form is dissolved in a full glass of water. If oral sodium bicarbonate is used to alkalinize the urine, the nurse checks the urine pH two or three times a day or as ordered by the primary health care provider. If the urine remains acidic, the nurse notifies the primary health care provider because an increase in the dose of the drug may be necessary. IV sodium bicarbonate is given in emergency situations, such as metabolic acidosis or certain types of drug overdose when alkalinization of the urine is necessary to hasten drug elimination.

ADMINISTERING CALCIUM. When calcium is administered IV, the solution is warmed to body temperature immediately before administration, and the drug is administered slowly. In some clinical situations, the primary health care provider may order the patient to have a cardiac monitor because additional drug administration may be determined by electrocardiographic changes.

ADMINISTERING POTASSIUM. When given orally, potassium may cause gastrointestinal distress. Therefore, it is given immediately after meals or with food and a full glass of water. Oral potassium must not be crushed or chewed. If the patient has difficulty swallowing, the nurse consults the primary health care provider regarding the use of a solution or an effervescent tablet, which effervesces (fizzes) and dissolves on contact with water. Potassium in the form of effervescent tablets, powder, or liquid must be thoroughly mixed with 4 to 8 oz of cold water, juice, or other beverage. Effervescent tablets must stop fizzing before the solution is sipped slowly during a period of 5 to 15 minutes. Oral liquids and soluble powders that have been mixed and dissolved in cold water or juice are also sipped slowly during a period of 5 to 15 minutes. The nurse advises patients that liquid potassium solutions have a salty taste. Some of these products have a flavoring added, which makes the solution more palatable.

The primary health care provider orders the dose of the potassium salt (in mEq) and the amount and type of IV solution, as well as the time interval during which the solution is to be infused. After the drug is added to the IV container, the container is gently rotated to ensure mixture of the solution. A large vein is used for administration; the veins on the back of the hand should be avoided. An IV containing potassium should infuse in no less than 3 to 4 hours. This necessitates frequent monitoring of the IV infusion rate, even when an IV infusion pump is used.

Nursing Alert

Concentrated potassium solutions are for IV mixtures only and should never be used undiluted. Direct IV injection of potassium could result in sudden death. When potassium is given IV, it is always diluted in 500 to 1000 mL of an IV solution. The maximum recommended concentration of potassium is 80 mEq in 1000 mL of IV solution (although in acute emergency situations a higher concentration of potassium may be required).

ADMINISTERING MAGNESIUM. Magnesium sulfate may be ordered intramuscularly, IV, or by IV infusion diluted in a specified type and amount of IV solution. When ordered to be given intramuscularly, this drug is given undiluted as a 50% solution for adults and a 20% solution for children. Magnesium sulfate is given deep intramuscularly in a large muscle mass, such as the gluteus muscle.

Gerontologic Alert

Older adults may need a reduced dosage of magnesium because of decreased renal function. The nurse should closely monitor serum magnesium levels when magnesium is administered to older adults.

Monitoring and Managing Adverse Reactions

When electrolyte solutions are administered, adverse reactions are most often related to overdose. Correcting the imbalance by decreasing the dosage or discontinuing the solution usually works, and the adverse reactions subside within a short period of time. Frequent serum electrolyte levels are used to monitor blood levels.

If gastrointestinal disturbances occur from oral administration, taking the drug with meals may decrease the nausea. Should the patient become disoriented or confused, the nurse gently reorients the individual. Frequent observation and quickly answering the call light helps to maintain the patient's safety. If weakness or muscular cramping occurs, the nurse assists the patient when ambulating to prevent falls or other injury.

Some electrolytes may cause cardiac irregularities. The nurse checks the pulse rate at regular intervals, usually every 4 hours or more often if an irregularity in the heart rate is observed. Depending on the patient's condition, cardiac monitoring may be indicated when administering the electrolytes (particularly when administering potassium or calcium). For example, if potassium is administered to a patient with cardiac disease, a cardiac monitor is needed to continuously monitor the heart rate and rhythm during therapy.

Nursing Alert

Mild (5.5–6.5 mEq/L) to moderate (6.5–8 mEq/L) potassium blood level increases may be asymptomatic and manifested only by increased serum potassium concentrations and characteristic ECG changes, such as disappearance of P waves or spreading (widening) of the QRS complex.

Educating the Patient and Family

To ensure accurate compliance with the prescribed drug regimen, the nurse carefully explains the dose and time intervals to the patient or a family member. Because overdose (which can be serious) may occur if the patient does not adhere to the prescribed dosage and schedule, it is most important that the patient completely understands how much and when to take the drug. The nurse stresses the importance of adhering to the prescribed dosage schedule during patient teaching.

The primary health care provider may order periodic laboratory and diagnostic tests for some patients receiving oral electrolytes. The nurse encourages the patient to keep all appointments for these tests, as well as primary health care provider or clinic visits. Persons with a history of using sodium bicarbonate (baking soda) as an antacid are warned that overuse can result in alkalosis and could disguise a more serious problem. Those with a history of using salt tablets (sodium chloride) are advised not to do so during hot weather unless it is recommended by a primary health care provider. Excessive use of salt tablets can result in a serious electrolyte imbalance.

The nurse includes the following points for specific electrolytes in a patient teaching plan.

CALCIUM

- Contact the primary health care provider if the following occur: nausea, vomiting, anorexia, constipation, abdominal pain, dry mouth, thirst, or polyuria (symptoms of hypercalcemia).
- Do not exceed the dosage recommendations.

POTASSIUM

- Take the drug exactly as directed on the prescription container. Do not increase, decrease, or omit doses of the drug unless advised to do so by the primary health care provider. Take the drug immediately after meals or with food and a full glass of water. Avoid the use of nonprescription drugs and salt substitutes (many contain potassium) unless use of a specific drug or product has been approved by the primary health care provider.
- Contact the primary health care provider if tingling of the hands or feet, a feeling of heaviness in the legs, vomiting, nausea, abdominal pain, or black stools should occur.
- If the tablet has a coating (enteric-coated tablets), swallow it whole. Do not chew or crush the tablet.
- If effervescent tablets are prescribed, place the tablet in 4 to 8 oz of cold water or juice. Wait until the fizzing stops before drinking. Sip the liquid during a period of 5 to 10 minutes.
- If an oral liquid or a powder is prescribed, add the dose to 4 to 8 oz of cold water or juice and sip slowly during a period of 5 to 10 minutes. Measure the dose accurately.

MAGNESIUM

- Do not take oral magnesium sulfate when abdominal pain, nausea, or vomiting is present. If diarrhea and abdominal cramping occur, discontinue the drug.

EVALUATION

- The therapeutic effect of the drug is achieved.
- The patient complies with the prescribed drug regimen.
- The patient and family demonstrate an understanding of the drug regimen.
- The patient verbalizes the importance of complying with the prescribed therapeutic regimen.

TOTAL PARENTERAL NUTRITION

When normal enteral feeding in not possible or is inadequate to meet an individual's nutritional needs, intravenous (IV) nutritional therapy or total parenteral nutrition (TPN) is required. Products used to meet the IV nutritional requirements of the patient include protein substrates (amino acids), energy substrates (dextrose and fat emulsions), fluids, electrolytes, and trace minerals (see the Summary Drug Table: Electrolytes).

TPN is used to prevent nitrogen and weight loss or to treat negative nitrogen (mineral component in protein and amino acids) balance (a situation in which more nitrogen is used by the body than is taken in) in the following situations:

- When the oral, gastrostomy, or jejunostomy route cannot or should not be used
- Gastrointestinal (GI) absorption of protein is impaired by obstruction
- Inflammatory disease or antineoplastic therapy prevents normal GI functioning
- Bowel rest is needed (eg, after bowel surgery)
- Metabolic requirements for protein are significantly increased (eg, in hypermetabolic states such as serious burns, infections, or trauma)
- Morbidity and mortality may be reduced by replacing amino acids lost from tissue breakdown (eg, renal failure)
- When tube feeding alone cannot provide adequate nutrition

TPN may be administered through a peripheral vein or through a central venous catheter. Peripheral TPN is used for patients requiring parenteral nutrition for relatively short periods of time (no more than 5–14 days) and when the central venous route is not possible or necessary. Peripheral TPN is used when the patient's caloric needs are minimal and can be partially met by normal means (through the alimentary tract). Peripheral TPN prevents protein catabolism (breakdown of cells) in patients who have adequate body fat and no clinically significant protein malnutrition. An example of a solution used in TPN is amino acids with electrolytes. These solutions may be used alone or combined with dextrose (5% or 10%) solutions.

TPN through a central vein is indicated in patients to promote protein synthesis in those who are severely hypercatabolic, severely depleted of nutrients, or require long-term nutritional parenteral nutrition. For example, amino acids combined with hypertonic dextrose and IV fat emulsions are infused through a central venous catheter to promote protein systhesis. Vitamins, trace minerals, and electrolytes may be added to the TPN mixture to meet the patient's individual needs. The daily dose depends on the patient's daily protein requirement and the patient's metabolic state and clinical responses. Various laboratory studies and assessments are required before and during administration of TPN. For example baseline studies done before beginning treatment include complete blood count, prothrombin time, body weight, electrolytes, blood urea nitrogen, glucose, creatinine, cholesterol, triglycerides (if on fat emulsion), uric acid, and various other tests. Daily assessments during stabalization of the therapy (3–5 days) include urine glucose, acetone and ketones, intake/output, electrolytes, CO_2 levels, creatinine, and blood urea nitrogen. Thereafter baseline laboratory assessments are made every 2 to 3 days or weekly as the patient's condition indicates.

✳ Nursing Alert

Hyperglycemia is the most common metabolic complication. A too rapid infusion of amino acid–carbohydrate mixtures may result in hyperglycemia, glycosuria, mental confusion, and loss of consciousness. Blood glucose levels may be obtained every 4 to 6 hours to monitor for hyperglycemia and guide the dosage of dextrose and insulin (if required). To minimize these complications, the primary health care provider may decrease the rate of administration, reduce the dextrose concentration, or administer insulin.

To prevent a rebound hypoglycemic reaction from the sudden withdrawal of TPN containing a concentrated dose of dextrose, the rate of administration is slowly reduced or the concentration of dextrose gradually decreased. If TPN must be abruptly withdrawn, a solution of 5% or 10% dextrose is begun to gradually reduce the amount of dextrose administered.

● *Critical Thinking Exercises*

1. *Ms. Land is receiving 20 mEq of potassium chloride (KCl) added to 1000 mL of 5% dextrose and water.*

Discuss preadministration and ongoing assessments you would make while her IV is infusing.

2. *Mr. Kendall is prescribed an oral potassium chloride liquid. Discuss the instructions you should give to Mr. Kendall regarding preparing and taking the drug.*
3. *Ms. Hartsel is to receive an IV fat emulsion. Discuss special precautions the nurse should take when administering the solution.*

● *Review Questions*

1. Which of the following is a symptom of fluid overload?

   A. Tinnitus
   B. Hypotension
   C. Decreased body temperature
   D. Behavioral changes

2. Which of the following symptoms would indicate hypocalcemia?

   A. Tetany
   B. Constipation
   C. Muscle weakness
   D. Hypertension

3. Which of the following potassium plasma concentration laboratory results would the nurse report immediately to the physician?

   A. 3.5 mEq/L
   B. 4.0 mEq/L
   C. 4.5 mEq/L
   D. 5.5 mEq/mL

4. Which of the following symptoms would most likely indicate hypernatremia?

   A. Fever, increased thirst
   B. Cold, clammy skin
   C. Decreased skin turgor
   D. Hypotension

5. Which of the following is the most common metabolic complication of TPN?

   A. Hypomagnesemia
   B. Hypermagnesemia
   C. Hypoglycemia
   D. Hyperglycemia

● *Medication Dosage Problems*

1. Mr. Parker is to receive 1000 mL of 5% dextrose and water during a period of 10 hours. Calculate how many milliliters should infuse each hour (see Chap. 3 for additional information on calculation).
2. The patient is prescribed potassium 40 mEq orally. The drug is available from the pharmacy in a solution of 20 mEq/15 mL. The nurse administers _____.

Abbreviations

A

aa	of each
abd	abdomen, abdominal
ABG	arterial blood gas
ac	before meals
ADH	antidiuretic hormone
ADL	activities of daily living
ad lib	as much as desired
ADT	alternate-day therapy
AIDS	acquired immunodeficiency syndrome
ALT	alanine aminotransferase
AMA	against medical advice
AMI	acute myocardial infarction
AODM	adult-onset diabetes mellitus
ARC	AIDS-related complex
ASAP	as soon as possible
ASHD	arteriosclerotic heart disease
AST	aspartate aminotransferase

B

BE	barium enema; base excess
bid	twice a day
bili	bilirubin
BM	bowel movement
BMR	basal metabolic rate
B&O	belladonna and opium
BP	blood pressure
BPH	benign prostatic hypertrophy
BRP	bathroom privileges
BUN	blood urea nitrogen

C

c̄	with
Ca	cancer; calcium
C&A	clinitest and acetest
CAD	coronary artery disease
caps	capsules
CBC	complete blood count
CC	chief complaint
CCU	Coronary Care Unit
CHF	congestive heart failure
CHO	carbohydrate
chol	cholesterol
CLL	chronic lymphocytic leukemia
CNS	central nervous system
C/O	complains of
COPD	chronic obstructive pulmonary disease
CPK	creatine phosphokinase
CRF	chronic renal failure
C&S	culture and sensitivity
CTZ	chemoreceptor trigger zone
CVA	cerebrovascular accident
CVP	central venous pressure
CXR	chest x-ray

D

/d	per day
d	daily
DC (D/C)	discontinue
Diff	differential blood count
DJD	degenerative joint disease
DM	diabetes mellitus
DOE	dyspnea on exertion
DT	delirium tremens
Dx	diagnosis

E

ECG	electrocardiogram
ECT	electroconvulsive therapy
EENT	eyes, ears, nose, and throat
EKG	electrocardiogram
ENT	eyes, nose, and throat
ER	emergency room
ESR	erythrocyte sedimentation rate (sed rate)
et	and

F

F	Fahrenheit
FBS	fasting blood sugar
fl	fluid
fx	fracture; fraction

G

g	gram
GB	gallbladder

GERD	gastroesophageal reflux disease
GFR	glomerular filtration rate
GI	gastrointestinal
gtt	drop
GU	genitourinary

H

h	hour
HA	headache
Hct	hematocrit
Hgb	hemoglobin
hs	hour of sleep
HNT	hypertension
Hx	history

I

ICU	intensive care unit
IM	imtramuscular
I&O	intake and output
IOP	intraocular pressure
IPPB	intermittent positive pressure breathing
IU	international units
IV	intravenous
IVP	intravenous pyelogram
IVPB	intravenous piggyback

J

JRA	juvenile rheumatoid arthritis

K

K	potassium
KUB	kidney, ureters, and bladder
KVO	keep vein open

L

LDH	lactic dehydrogenase
LDL	low-density lipoproteins
LOC	level of consciousness
LP	lumbar puncture
lytes	electrolytes

M

mcg	microgram
MI	myocardial infarction (heart attack)
mL	mililiter
MOM	milk of magnesia
MS	morphine sulfate; multiple sclerosis; mitral stenosis

N

N	normal
NG	nasogastric
NPO	nothing by mouth
NS	normal saline
NGT	nitroglycerin
NVD	nausea, vomiting, diarrhea; neck vein distension

O

O_2	oxygen
OD	right eye
OOB	out of bed
OR	operating room
OU	both eyes
OTC	over the counter (nonprescription)
OS	left eye

P

PAT	paroxysmal atrial tachycardia
PBI	protein-bound iodine
PC	after meals
PERRLA	pupils equal, round, react to light and accommodation
PERL	pupils equal and react to light
PID	pelvic inflammatory disease
PKU	phenylketonuria
PND	paroxymal noctural dyspnea
PO	by mouth
postop	after surgery
preop	before surgery
prn	as needed
PT	physical therapy; prothrombin time
PZI	protamine zinc insulin

Q

qd	every day
qh	every hour (q2h, q3h, etc.—every 2 hours, every 3 hours, etc.)
qid	four times a day
qod	every other day

R

RA	rheumatoid arthritis; right atrium
RBC	red blood cell
REM	rapid eye movement
RF	rheumatoid factor
RHD	rheumatic heart disease; renal hypertensive disease
ROM	range of motion
RR	recovery room

S

$\overline{s}$	without
SC	subcutaneous
sed rate	erythrocyte sedimentation rate (ESR)
SGOT	serum glutamic oxaloacetic transaminase
SGPT	serum glutamic pyruvic transaminase
SL	sublingual
SOB	shortness of breath
SR	sedimentation rate (ESR)
STAT	as soon as possible

T

t	temperature
T_3	triiodothyronine
T_4	thyroxine
T&A	tonsillectomy and adenoidectomy
TB	tuberculosis
TEDS	elastic stockings
TIA	transient ischemic attack
tid	three times a day
TKO	to keep open

TLC	tender loving care
TM	tympanic membrane
TPN	total parenteral nutrition
TPR	temperature, pulse, respiration
TSH	thyroid-stimulating hormone

U

UGI	upper gastrointestinal
ung	ointment
URI	upper respiratory infection
UTI	urinary tract infection

V

VS	vital signs

W

WNL	within normal limits
Wt	weight

Glossary

A

abstinence syndrome: symptoms that occur if a drug causing physical or psychological dependence is suddenly discontinued

achalasia: failure to relax; usually referring to the smooth muscle fibers of the gastrointestinal tract, especially failure of the lower esophagus to relax when swallowing causing difficulty swallowing and a feeling of fullness in the sternal region

active immunity: type of immunity that occurs when the person is exposed to a disease and develops the disease, and the body makes antibodies to provide future protection against the disease

addiction: a compulsive desire or craving to use a drug or chemical with a resultant physical dependence

adrenergic drug: a drug that acts like or mimics the actions of the sympathetic nervous system

aerobic: organisms that require oxygen to live

afferent nerve fiber: a sensory nerve that carries an impulse toward the brain

agonist: drug that binds with a receptor to produce a therapeutic response

agonist-antagonist: drug with both agonist and antagonist properties

agranulocytosis: a decrease or lack of granulocytes (a type of white blood cell)

akathisia: extreme restlessness and increased motor activity

aldosterone: hormone secreted by the adrenal cortex and contributing to a rise in blood pressure

alopecia: abnormal loss of hair; baldness

amenorrhea: absence or suppression of menstruation

anabolism: tissue-building process

anaerobic: organisms that do not require oxygen to live

analgesic: a drug that relieves pain

anaphylactic reaction: a sudden, severe hypersensitivity reaction with symptoms that progress rapidly and may result in death if not treated

anemia: a decrease in the number of red blood cells and hemoglobin value below normal

androgens: testosterone and its derivatives

angina pectoris (angina): acute pain in the chest resulting from decreased blood supply to the heart muscle

angioedema: localized wheals or swellings in subcutaneous tissues or mucous membranes, which may be due to an allergic response; also called angioneurotic edema

anorexia: loss of appetite

anorexiant: a drug used to suppress the appetite

antagonist: drugs that join with a receptor to prevent the action of an agonist

anthelmintic: a drug used to treat helminthiasis (worms)

antibacterial: active against bacteria

antibody: molecule with the ability to bind with a specific antigen responsible for the immune response

antiemetic: drug that is used to treat or prevent nausea

antiflatulent: drug that works against flatus (gas)

antigen: substance that is capable of inducing a specific immune response

anti-infective: a drug used to treat infection

antipsoriatics: drugs used to treat psoriasis

antipyretic: a drug that lowers an elevated body temperature

antiseptic: an agent that stops or slows, or prevents the growth of microorganisms

anxiolytics: term used to describe the antianxiety drugs

aplastic anemia: a blood disorder caused by damage to the bone marrow resulting in a marked reduction in the number of red blood cells and some white blood cells

arrhythmia: abnormal heart rate or rhythm; also called dysrhythmia

assessment: the collection of subjective and objective data

asthenia: weakness; loss of strength

ataxia: unsteady gait; muscular incoordination

atherosclerosis: a disease characterized by deposits of fatty plaques on the inner walls of arteries

atrial fibrillation: quivering of the atria of the heart

attenuate: weaken

aura: sense preceding a sudden attack, as in the aura that occurs before a convulsion

auscultation: the process of listening for sounds within the body

autonomic nervous system: a division of the peripheral nervous system concerned with functions essential to the life of the organism and not consciously controlled (ie, blood pressure, heart rate, gastrointestinal activity)

azotemia: retention of excessive amounts of nitrogenous compounds in the blood caused by failure of the kidney to remove urea from the blood

B

bactericidal: a drug or agent that destroys or kills bacteria

bacteriostatic: a drug or agent that slows or retards the multiplication of bacteria

bigeminy: an irregular pulse rate consisting or two beats followed by a pause before the next two paired beats

biliary colic: pain caused by the pressure of passing gallstones

blepharospasm: a twitching or spasm of the eyelid

blood–brain barrier: ability of the nervous system to prohibit large and potentially harmful molecules form crossing into the brain

bone marrow suppression: a decreased production of all blood cells

booster: an immunogen injected following a specified interval; often after the primary immunization to stimulate and sustain the immune response

brachial plexus: a network of spinal nerves affecting the arm, forearm, and the hand

bradycardia: slow heart rate, usually at a rate below 60 beats per minute

bronchospasm: spasm or constriction of the bronchi resulting in difficulty breathing

bulla: blister or skin vesicle filled with fluid

bursa: pad-like sac found in connecting tissue usually located in the joint area

C

candidiasis: infection of the skin or mucous membrane with the species *Candida*

cardiac output: amount of blood discharged from the left or right ventricle per minute

catabolism: tissue-depleting process

catalyst: substance that accelerates a chemical reaction without itself undergoing a change

central nervous system: one of two main divisions of the nervous system consisting of the brain and spinal cord

cervical mucorrhea: increased cervical discharge

chelating agent: a substance that selectively and chemically binds the ion of a metal to itself, thus aiding in the elimination of the metallic ion from the body

cheilosis: cracking of the edges of the lips

chemoreceptor trigger zone: a group of nerve fibers located on the surface of the fourth ventricle of the brain that, when stimulated, results in vomiting

chemotherapy: drug therapy with a chemical, often used when referring to treatment with an antineoplastic drug

cholesterol: a fat-like substance produced mostly in the liver of animals

chorea: continuous rapid, jerky, involuntary movements

choreiform movements: involuntary muscular twitching of the limbs or facial muscles

chylomicrons: small particles of fat in the blood

cinchonism: quinidine toxicity or poisoning

conjunctivitis: inflammation of the conjunctiva (mucous membrane lining the inner surfaces of the eye)

convulsions: paroxysm (occurring suddenly) of involuntary muscular contractions and relaxations

Crohn's disease: inflammation of the terminal portion of the ileum

cross-allergenicity: allergy to drugs in the same or related groups

cross-sensitivity: see cross allergenicity

crystalluria: formation of crystals in the urine

cumulative drug effect: occurs when the body is unable to metabolize and excrete one dose of a drug before the next dose is given

Cushing's syndrome: a disease caused by the overproduction of endogenous glucocorticoids

cyanosis: bluish, grayish, or dark purple discoloration of the skin due to abnormal amounts of reduced hemoglobin in the blood

cycloplegia: paralysis of the ciliary muscle resulting in an inability to focus the eye

cytomegalovirus (CMV): any of a group of herpes viruses infecting man, monkeys, or rodents; the human CMV is found in the salivary glands and causes cytomegalic inclusion disease

cystinuria: the presence of cystine, an amino acid, in the urine

D

debridement: removal of all foreign material and dead or damaged tissue from a wound or infected lesion

decaliter: 10 liters or 10,000 mL

delirium tremens: signs and symptoms of withdrawal from a drug or chemical including tremors, weakness, anxiety, restlessness, excessive perspiration, nausea, and vomiting

dermis: a layer of skin immediately below the epidermis

diabetes insipidus: a disease resulting in the failure of the pituitary to secrete vasopressin or from the surgical removal of the pituitary gland

diaphoresis: increased sweating or perspiration

digitalization: administration of digitalis at intervals to produce and maintain a therapeutic blood level

diluent: a fluid that dilutes

dioplopia: double vision

diuretic drug: drug that produces urine secretion

dyscrasia: disease or disorder

dyskinesia: impairment of voluntary movement

dyspnea: labored or difficult breathing

dystonia: prolonged muscle contractions that may cause twisting and repetitive movements of abnormal posture

dysuria: painful or difficult urination

E

efferent: carrying away from a central organ or section

edema: accumulation of excess water in the body

emetic: drug that induces vomiting

endogenous: normally occurring within the organism or in the community

endorphins: naturally occurring analgesic produced by the body in response to certain stimulus (ie, exercise)

enkephalins: neurotransmitter within the brain involved with pain perception, mood, movement, and behavior

epidermis: outermost layer of the skin

epidural: outside or above the dura mater

epilepsy: a permanent, recurring seizure disorder

epiphysis: a center of ossification (conversion of tissue to bone) at each extremity of long bone

epistaxis: nosebleed

erythrocytes: red blood cells; one of several formed elements in the blood

Escherichia coli: a nonpathogenic colon bacillus; when found outside of the colon may cause infection

estrogens: female hormones

euthyroid: normal thyroid function

evaluation: a decision-making process determining the effectiveness of nursing action or intervention

exacerbation: increase in severity

exfoliative dermatitis: reddish rash in which scaling occurs following the erythema

exogenous: normally occurring outside of the organism or community

expectorant: drug that aids in raising thick, tenacious mucus from the respiratory tract

extrapulmonary: occurring outside of the respiratory systems (ie, lungs)

extrapyramidal effects: a group of adverse reactions occurring on the extrapyramidal portion of the nervous system causing abnormal muscle movements, especially akathisia and dystonia

extravasation: escape of fluid from a blood vessel into surrounding tissue

F

fat soluble: dissolves in fat

febrile: related to fever (elevated body temperature)

fibrolytic: term used to describe a drug that dissolves clots already formed within the vessel walls

G

germicide: an agent that kills bacteria

gingival hyperplasia: overgrowth of gum tissue

gingivitis: inflammation of the gums

glaucoma: a group of diseases of the eye characterized by increased intraocular pressure; results in changes within the eye, visual field defects, and eventually blindness (if left untreated)

globulin: proteins that are insoluble in water and present in the plasma

glossitis: inflammation of the tongue

glucagon: hormone secreted by the alpha cells of the pancreas that increase the concentration of glucose in the blood

goiter: enlargement of the thyroid gland causing a swelling in the front part of the neck, usually caused by a lack of iodine in the diet

gonadotropin: hormone that stimulates the sex glands (gonads)

gonad: glands responsible for sexual activity and characteristics

granulocytopenia: a reduction or decrease in the number of granulocytes (a type of white blood cell)

gynecomastia: breast enlargement in the male

H

habituation: a desire to continually use a drug or chemical for the desired effect with no physical dependence but some psychological dependence

hallucinogen: drug capable of producing a state of delirium characterized by visual or sensory disturbances

helminthiasis: invasion by helminths (worms)

hemolytic anemia: disorder characterized by chronic premature destruction of red blood cells

herb: plant used in medicine or as seasoning

high-density lipoproteins (HDL): macromolecules that carry cholesterol from the body cells to the liver to be excreted

hirsutism: excessive growth of hair or hair growth in unusual places, usually in women

histamine: a substance found in various parts of the body (ie, liver, lungs, intestines, skin) and produced in excess in response to a substance to which the body is sensitive

humoral immunity: antibody-mediated immune response of the body

hyperglycemia: high blood glucose (sugar) level

hyperinsulinism: elevated levels of insulin in the body

hyperkalemia: increase in potassium levels in the blood

hyperlipidemia: an increase in the lipids in the blood

hypersensitivity reaction: allergic reaction to a drug or other substance

hypertension: high blood pressure

hypnotic: drug that induces sleep

hypoglycemia: low blood glucose (sugar) level

hypoinsulinism: low levels of insulin in the body

hypokalemia: low blood potassium level

hyponatremia: low blood sodium level

hypotension: abnormally low blood pressure

hypotension, orthostatic: a decrease in blood pressure occurring after standing in one place for an extended period

hypotension, postural: a decrease in blood pressure after a sudden change in body position

hypoxia: inadequate oxygen at the cellular level

I

idiosyncrasy: unusual or abnormal drug response

immunocompromised: having a immune system incapable of fighting an infection

implementation: the carrying out of a plan of action

infiltration: the collection of fluid into tissue

inotropic: affecting the force of muscular contractions

intraocular pressure: the pressure within the eye

intrinsic factor: substance produced by the cells in the stomach and necessary for the absorption of vitamin B_{12}

iritis: inflammation of the iris of the eye

J

jaundice: yellow discoloration of the skin

K

keratolyte: an agent that removes excessive growth of the epidermis (top layer of skin)

ketoacidosis: a type of metabolic acidosis caused by an accumulation of ketone bodies in the blood

ketonuria: presence of ketones in the blood

L

laryngospasm: spasm of the larynx resulting in dyspnea and noisy respirations

lethargic: sluggish, difficult to rouse

leukopenia: a decrease in the number of leukocytes (white blood cells)

lipids: a group of fats or fat-like substances

lipodystrophy: atrophy of subcutaneous fat

lipoproteins: a macromolecule consisting of a lipid (fat) and protein; the method by which fats are transported in the blood

low-density lipoproteins (LDL): macromolecules that carry cholesterol from the liver to the body cells

lumen: inside diameter, the space or opening within an artery

lupus erythematosus: A chronic inflammatory connective tissue disease affecting the skin, joints, kidneys, nervous system, and mucous membranes. A butterfly rash or erythema may be seen on the face, particularly across the nose

M

malaise: discomfort, uneasiness

megacolon: dilatation and hypertrophy of the colon

megaloblastic anemia: anemia characterized by the presence of large, abnormal, immature erythrocytes circulating in the blood

melasma: discoloration of the skin

melena: blood in the stools

merozoites: cells formed as the result of asexual reproduction

methemoglobinemia: clinical condition in which more than 1% of hemoglobin in the blood has been oxidized to the ferric form

micturition: voiding of urine

miosis: constriction of the pupils

mucolytic: drug that loosens and thins respiratory secretions (lessens the viscosity of the secretions)

myasthenia gravis: condition characterized by weakness and fatigability of the muscles

mycotic: pertaining to a fungus or fungal infection

mydriasis: dilation of the pupil

myocardial infarction: heart attack

myopia: nearsightedness

myxedema: condition caused by hypothyroidism or deficiency of thyroxine and characterized by swelling of the face, periorbital tissues, hands, and feet.

N

narcolepsy: a chronic disorder that results in recurrent attacks of drowsiness and sleep during daytime

necrosis: death of tissue (as adjective, necrotic)

nephrotoxic: harmful to the kidney

nephrotoxicity: damage to the kidneys by a toxic substance

neurohypophysis: posterior lobe of the pituitary gland

neuroleptic: drug that causes an altered state of consciousness (ie, antipsychotic)

neuromuscular blockade: acute muscle paralysis and apnea

neurotoxicity: damage to the nervous system of a toxic substance

neurotransmitter: chemical substances released at the nerve ending that facilitate the transmission of nerve impulses

neutropenia: abnormally small number of neutrophil cells (type of white blood cell)

nonsteroidial: not a steroid

nursing process: a framework for nursing action, consisting of a series of problem-solving steps, that helps members of the health care team provide effective and consistent patient care

nystagmus: an involuntary and constant movement of the eyeball

O

objective data: information obtained by means of a physical assessment or physical examination

oliguria: a decrease in urinary output

ophthalmic: pertaining to the eye

opportunistic infection: infection resulting from microorganisms commonly found in the environment, which normally do not cause an infection unless there is an impaired immune system

orthostatic hypotension: see hypotension, orthostatic

osteomalacia: a softening of the bones

osteoporosis: a loss of calcium from the bones, resulting in a decrease in bone density

otic: pertaining to the ear

ototoxic: harmful to the ear

ototoxicity: damage to the organs of hearing by a toxic substance

overt: not hidden, clearly evident

oxytocic: agent that stimulates contractions of the uterus resulting in labor

P

palliative: therapy designed to treat symptoms, not to produce a cure

pancytopenia: a reduction in all cellular elements of the blood

paralytic ileus: paralysis of the bowel resulting in lack of movement of the bowel contents

parasite: an organism living in or on another organism (the host) without contributing to the survival or well-being of the host

parasympathetic nervous system: part of the autonomic nervous system concerned with conserving body energy (ie, slowing the heart rate, digesting food, and eliminating waste)

parenteral: administration of a substance, such as a drug, by any route other than the oral route

paresthesia: an abnormal sensation such as numbness, tingling, prickling, or heightened sensitivity

parkinsonism: referring to the symptoms of Parkinson's disease (ie, fine tremors, slowing of the voluntary movements, and muscular weakness)

passive immunity: a type of immunity occurring from the administration of ready-made antibodies from another individual or animal

pathogenic: disease producing

peripheral: pertaining to the outward surface; away from the center

petechiae: tine purple or red spots that appear on the skin as a result of pinpoint hemorrhages within the outer layers of the skin

phenochromocytoma: tumor of the adrenal medulla characterized by hypersecretion of epinephrine and norepinephrine

phlebitis: inflammation of a vein

phenylketonuria (PKU): a congenital disease due to a defect in the metabolism of phenylalanine (an amino acid); results from the lack of an enzyme necessary for the conversion of phenylalanine into tyrosine; untreated, the condition leads to mental retardation

photophobia: an aversion to or intolerance of light

photosensitivity: exaggerated sunburn reaction when the skin is exposed to sunlight or ultraviolet light

physical dependence: compulsive need to use a substance repeatedly to avoid withdrawal symptoms

plasma expanders: intravenous solutions used to expand plasma volume with shock due to burns, hemorrhage, or other trauma

polydipsia: excessive thirst

polyphagia: eating large amounts of food

polypharmacy: taking a large number of drugs (may be prescribed or over-the-counter drugs)

polyposis: numerous polyps

postural hypotension: see hypotension, postural

prepubertal: before puberty

progesterone: a female hormone produced by the corpus luteum that works in the uterus (along with estrogen) to prepare the uterus for possible conception

progestins: natural and synthetic progesterones

prophylaxis: prevention

prostaglandins: a fatty acid derivative found in almost every tissue of the body and body fluid that affects the uterus and other smooth muscles; also thought to increase the sensation of peripheral pain receptors to painful stimuli

prostatic hypertrophy: abnormal enlargement of the prostate gland

protein substrates: amino acids essential to life

pruritus: itching

pseudomembranous colitis: a severe, life-threatening form of diarrhea

psychological dependence: compulsion to use a substance to obtain a pleasurable experience

ptosis: drooping of the upper eyelid

purpura: condition characterized by various degrees of hemorrhaging into the skin and/or mucous membranes producing ecchymoses (bruises) and petechiae (small red patches) on the skin

R

rales: abnormal lung sounds often described as crackles

REM: (rapid eye movement) the dreaming stage of sleep

remission: periods of partial or complete disappearance of signs and symptoms

retinitis: inflammation of the retina of the eye

Reye's syndrome: acute and potentially fatal disease of childhood; associated with a previous viral infection

rheumatic fever: a disease associated with a delayed response to a prior streptococca infection in the body and characterized by fever and pain in the joints

rheumatoid arthritis: a type of arthritis marked by inflammation, degeneration, and derangement of the joints and related structures resulting in contractures and deformities of the joints

rhinitis: inflammation of the nasal passages resulting in increased nasal secretions

S

sedative: a drug producing a relaxing, calming effect

somatotropic hormone: growth hormone produced by the anterior pituitary gland

somnolence: prolonged drowsiness; sleepiness

soporific: substance or procedure that causes sleep

sprue: a disease characterized by weakness, anemia, weight loss, and malabsorption of essential nutrients

Standard Precautions: see Universal Precautions

status epilepticus: an emergency situation characterized by continual seizure activity

Stevens-Johnson syndrome: fever, cough, muscular aches and pains, headache, and lesions of the skin, mucous membranes, and eyes. The lesions appear as red wheals or blisters, often starting on the face, in the mouth, or on the lips, neck, and extremities.

stomatitis: inflammation of the mouth

striae: lines or bands elevated above or depressed below surrounding tissue, or differing in color or texture

subjective data: information supplied by the patient or family

sublingual: under the tongue

sulfonylurea: a type of drug used to lower blood sugar in persons with non–insulin-dependent diabetes

superinfection: an overgrowth of bacterial or fungal microorganism not affected by the antibiotic being administered

sympathomimetic: acting like the sympathetic nervous system

synergistic: a drug interaction occurring when two drugs interact to produce an effect that is greater than the sum of their separate actions

T

tachycardia: heart rate above 100 beats/minute

tardive dyskinesia: rhythmic, involuntary movements of the tongue, face, mouth, jaw, and sometimes the extremities

testosterone: the most prominent male sex hormone that acts to stimulate development of the male reproductive organ and the secondary sex characteristics

tetany: nervous condition characterized by sharp flexion of the wrist and ankle joints, muscle twitching, cramps, and possible convulsions, usually caused by abnormal levels of calcium, vitamin D, and alkalosis

thrombocytopenia: low platelet count

thrombus: a blood clot (pl. thrombi)

thyroid storm: see thyrotoxicosis

thrombocytopenia: low number of the platelets in the blood

thyrotoxicosis: severe hyperthyroidism that is characterized by symptoms such as high fever, extreme tachycardia, and altered mental status (also called thyroid storm)

tinnitus: ringing in the ears

tolerance: decreased response to a drug, usually requiring an increase in the dosage to give the desired effect

tonic-clonic seizure: generalized seizure activity consisting of alternate contraction (tonic) and relaxation of muscles (clonic)

toxicity: poisonous or harmful

toxoid: an attenuated toxin that is capable of stimulating the formation of antitoxins

transient ischemic attack (TIA): temporary interference with blood supply to the brain causing symptoms related to the portion of the brain affected (ie, temporary blindness, aphasia, dizziness, numbness, difficulty swallowing or paresthesias); may last from a few moments to several hours, after which no residual neurologic damage is evident

trigeminy: an irregular pulse rate consisting of three beats followed by a pause before the next three beats

tyramine: substance found in most cheeses and in beer, bean pods, yeast, wine, and chicken liver; individuals taking the antidepressant MAOIs and eating foods containing tyramine may experience severe hypertension

U

Universal Precautions: guidelines set forth by the Centers for Disease Control (CDC) to control the spread of disease

urticaria: hives; itchy wheals on the skin resulting from contact with or ingestion of an allergic substance or food

uveitis: a nonspecific term for any intraocular inflammatory disorder

V

vaccine: substance with either weakened or killed antigens developed for the purpose of creating resistance to disease

vasodilatation: an increase in the size of the blood vessels, which when widespread results in a rise in blood pressure

venous: pertaining to the veins

vertigo: a feeling of a spinning or rotation-type motion

vitamin: organic substance needed by the body in small amounts for normal growth and nutrition

von Willebrand's disease: a congenital bleeding disorder manifested at an early age by epistaxis and easy bruising; symptoms usually decrease in severity with age

W

water soluble: dissolves in water

U.S. Department of Health and Human Services

MEDWATCH

The FDA Safety Information and Adverse Event Reporting Program

For **VOLUNTARY** reporting of adverse events and product problems

Form Approved: OMB No. 0910-0291 Expires: 04/30/03
See OMB statement on reverse

FDA Use Only

Triage unit sequence #

Page ____ of ____

A. Patient information

1. Patient identifier	2. Age at time of event: or _____ Date of birth:	3. Sex ☐ female ☐ male	4. Weight ____ lbs or ____ kgs
In confidence			

B. Adverse event or product problem

1. ☐ **Adverse event** and/or ☐ **Product problem** (e.g., defects/malfunctions)

2. **Outcomes attributed to adverse event** (check all that apply)
☐ death _____ (mo/day/yr)
☐ life-threatening
☐ hospitalization - initial or prolonged
☐ disability
☐ congenital anomaly
☐ required intervention to prevent permanent impairment/damage
☐ other: _____

3. Date of event (mo/day/yr)	4. Date of this report (mo/day/yr)

5. **Describe event or problem**

6. **Relevant tests/laboratory data, including dates**

7. **Other relevant history, including preexisting medical conditions** (e.g., allergies, race, pregnancy, smoking and alcohol use, hepatic/renal dysfunction, etc.)

PLEASE TYPE OR USE BLACK INK

C. Suspect medication(s)

1. **Name** (give labeled strength & mfr/labeler, if known)
#1
#2

2. Dose, frequency & route used #1 #2	3. Therapy dates (if unknown, give duration) from/to (or best estimate) #1 #2

4. **Diagnosis for use** (indication)
#1
#2

5. **Event abated after use stopped or dose reduced**
#1 ☐ yes ☐ no ☐ doesn't apply
#2 ☐ yes ☐ no ☐ doesn't apply

6. Lot # (if known) #1 #2	7. Exp. date (if known) #1 #2

8. **Event reappeared after reintroduction**
#1 ☐ yes ☐ no ☐ doesn't apply
#2 ☐ yes ☐ no ☐ doesn't apply

9. **NDC #** (for product problems only)
- -

10. **Concomitant medical products** and therapy dates (exclude treatment of event)

D. Suspect medical device

1. **Brand name**

2. **Type of device**

3. **Manufacturer name & address**

4. **Operator of device**
☐ health professional
☐ lay user/patient
☐ other: _____

5. **Expiration date** (mo/day/yr)

6.
model # _____
catalog # _____
serial # _____
lot # _____
other # _____

7. **If implanted, give date** (mo/day/yr)

8. **If explanted, give date** (mo/day/yr)

9. **Device available for evaluation?** (Do not send to FDA)
☐ yes ☐ no ☐ returned to manufacturer on _____ (mo/day/yr)

10. **Concomitant medical products** and therapy dates (exclude treatment of event)

E. Reporter (see confidentiality section on back)

1. Name & address	phone #

2. Health professional?	3. Occupation	4. Also reported to
☐ yes ☐ no		☐ manufacturer ☐ user facility ☐ distributor

5. If you do NOT want your identity disclosed to the manufacturer, place an " X " in this box. ☐

FDA

Mail to: **MEDWATCH**
5600 Fishers Lane
Rockville, MD 20852-9787

or FAX to:
1-800-FDA-0178

FDA Form 3500

Submission of a report does not constitute an admission that medical personnel or the product caused or contributed to the event.

ADVICE ABOUT VOLUNTARY REPORTING

Report adverse experiences with:
- medications (drugs or biologics)
- medical devices (including in-vitro diagnostics)
- special nutritional products (dietary supplements, medical foods, infant formulas)
- cosmetics
- medication errors

Report product problems – quality, performance or safety concerns such as:
- suspected contamination
- questionable stability
- defective components
- poor packaging or labeling
- therapeutic failures

Report SERIOUS adverse events. An event is serious when the patient outcome is:
- death
- life-threatening (real risk of dying)
- hospitalization (initial or prolonged)
- disability (significant, persistent or permanent)
- congenital anomaly
- required intervention to prevent permanent impairment or damage

Report even if:
- you're not certain the product caused the event
- you don't have all the details

How to report:
- just fill in the sections that apply to your report
- use section C for all products except medical devices
- attach additional blank pages if needed
- use a separate form for each patient
- report either to FDA or the manufacturer (or both)

Confidentiality: The patient's identity is held in strict confidence by FDA and protected to the fullest extent of the law. FDA will not disclose the reporter's identity in response to a request from the public, pursuant to the Freedom of Information Act. The reporter's identity, including the identity of a self-reporter, may be shared with the manufacturer unless requested otherwise.

If your report involves a serious adverse event with a device and it occurred in a facility outside a doctor's office, that facility may be legally required to report to FDA and/or the manufacturer. Please notify the person in that facility who would handle such reporting.

Important numbers:
- 1-800-FDA-0178 to FAX report
- 1-800-FDA-1088 to report by phone or for more information
- 1-800-822-7967 for a VAERS form for vaccines

To Report via the Internet:
https://www.accessdata.fda.gov/scripts/medwatch/

The public reporting burden for this collection of information has been estimated to average 30 minutes per response, including the time for reviewing instructions, searching existing data sources, gathering and maintaining the data needed, and completing and reviewing the collection of information. Send comments regarding this burden estimate or any other aspect of this collection of information, including suggestions for reducing this burden to:

DHHS Reports Clearance Office
Paperwork Reduction Project (0910-0291)
Hubert H. Humphrey Building, Room 531-H
200 Independence Avenue, S.W.
Washington, DC 20201

Please DO NOT
RETURN this form
to this address.

U.S. DEPARTMENT OF HEALTH AND HUMAN SERVICES
Public Health Service • Food and Drug Administration

FDA Form 3500-back   **Please Use Address Provided Below – Just Fold In Thirds, Tape and Mail**

**Department of
Health and Human Services**

Public Health Service
Food and Drug Administration
Rockville, MD 20857

Official Business
Penalty for Private Use $300

NO POSTAGE
NECESSARY
IF MAILED
IN THE
UNITED STATES
OR APO/FPO

BUSINESS REPLY MAIL
FIRST CLASS MAIL   PERMIT NO. 946 ROCKVILLE, MD

POSTAGE WILL BE PAID BY FOOD AND DRUG ADMINISTRATION

MedWatch

The FDA Safety Information and Adverse Event Reporting Program
Food and Drug Administration
5600 Fishers Lane
Rockville, MD 20852-9787

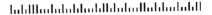

Select Herbs and Natural Products Used for Medicinal Purposes

COMMON NAME (S)	SCIENTIFIC NAME	USES	ADVERSE REACTIONS	SIGNIFICANT CONSIDERATIONS
Aloe vera	*Aloe vera*	Inhibits infection and promotes healing of minor burns and wounds	None significant if used as directed; may cause burning sensation in wound	Rare reports of delayed healing when used in the gel form on a wound. Taken internally, aloe gel may have laxative effect.
Billberry	*Vaccinium myrtillus*	Vision enhancement and eye health, microcirculation, spider veins and varicose veins, capillary strengthening before surgery	No adverse effects have been reported in clinical studies.	None significant.
Black Cohosh, (black snakeroot, squawroot)	*Cimicifuga racemosa*	Management of some symptoms of menopause and as an alternative to hormone replacement therapy; may be beneficial for hypercholesterolemia or peripheral vascular disease	Overdose causes nausea, dizziness, nervous system and visual disturbances, decreased pulse rate and increased perspiration	Should not be used during pregnancy. Possible interactions with hormone therapy.
Chamomile	*Matricaria chamomilla*	As a tea for gastrointestinal disturbances, as a sedative, and as an anti-inflammatory agent	Possible contact dermatitis and, in rare instances, anaphylaxis	Chamomile is a member of the ragweed family and those allergic to ragweed should not take the herb.
Chondroitin	Chondroitin sulfate, chondroitin sulfuric acid, chonsurid	Arthritis	None significant if used as directed	Because chondroitin is concentrated in cartilage, theoretically it produces no toxic or teratogenic effects.
Cranberry	*Vaccinium macrocarpon*	Urinary tract infection (UTI)	Large doses can produce gastrointestinal symptoms (ie, diarrhea)	None significant.
Echinacea (American coneflower, black susans)	*Echinacea angustifolia*	Prevents and shortens symptoms and duration of upper respiratory Infections (URIs) including colds	Rare. Nausea and mild gastrointestinal (GI) upsets	Should not be used by individuals with autoimmune diseases such as tuberculosis, collagenosis, multiple sclerosis, AIDS, and HIV infection.

(continued)

Select Herbs and Natural Products Used for Medicinal Purposes (Continued)

COMMON NAME (S)	SCIENTIFIC NAME	USES	ADVERSE REACTIONS	SIGNIFICANT CONSIDERATIONS
Ephedra (sea grape, ma-huang, yellow horse)	ephedra sinica	Relieves colds, improves respiratory function, headaches, diuretic effects	Skin eruptions, hypertension, irregular heart rate, psychosis	Ephedra should only be used after consulting with the physician. Many restrictions apply and the herb can cause serious reactions. Do not use with cardiac glycosides, monoamine oxidase inhibitors (MAOIs), halothane, guanethidine, or oxytocin. Do not use with St. John's wort or in weight loss formulas.
Garlic	Allium sativum	Lowers blood sugar, cholesterol, and lipids	May cause abnormal blood glucose levels	Increased risk of bleeding in patients taking the coumarins, salicylates, or antiplatelet drugs.
Ginger (ginger root, black ginger)	Zingiber officinale	Antiemetic, cardiotonic, antithrombotic, antibacterial, antioxidant, antitussive, anti-inflammatory, GI disturbances, lower cholesterol, prophylaxis for nausea and vomiting, colic, bronchitis	Excessive doses may cause CNS depression and interfere with cardiac functioning or anticoagulant activity.	Theoretically, ginger could enhance the effects of the antiplatelet drugs, such as coumarin.
Ginkgo (maiden hair tree, kew tree)	Ginkgo biloba	Raynauds disease, cerebral insufficiency anxiety, stress, tinnitus, dementias, circulatory problems, asthma	Rare if used as directed; possible effects include headache, dizziness, heart palpitations, GI effects, rash, allergic dermatitis	Do not take with antidepressant drugs, such as the MAOIs, or the antiplatelet drugs such as coumarin, unless advised to do so by the primary care provider.
Ginseng	Panax quinquefolius, Panax ginseng	Popular but un-proven uses: Anti-neoplastic, enhances immune function, improves cardiovascular or CNS function	Most common: nervousness, excitation, hypoglycemia; rare: diffuse mammary nodularity, vaginal bleeding	Taking ginseng in combination with stimulants such as caffeine is not advised. Do not use for longer than 3 months. (Some herbalists recommend use for 1 month followed by nonuse for 2 months.)
Goldenseal	Hydrastis canadensis	Antiseptic for skin (topical), astringent for mucous membranes (mouthwash), wash for inflamed eyes, sinus infections, peptic ulcers, colitis, gastritis	Large doses may cause dry or irritated mucous membranes and injury to the gastrointestinal system; may reduce the beneficial bacteria in the intestines.	Should not be taken for more than 3-7 days.
Glucosamine (chitosamine)	2-Amino-2-deoxyglucose	Antiarthritic in osteoarthritis	Well-tolerated	No direct toxic effects have been reported.
Green tea	Camellia sinensis	Reduces cancer, lowers lipid levels, helps prevent dental caries, antimicrobial and antioxidative effects	Contains caffeine (may cause mild stimulant effects such as anxiety, nervousness, heart irregularities, restlessness, insomnia, and digestive irritation)	Contains caffeine and should be avoided during pregnancy, by individuals with hypertension, anxiety, eating disorders, insomnia, diabetes, and ulcers.

Select Herbs and Natural Products Used for Medicinal Purposes (*Continued*)

COMMON NAME (S)	SCIENTIFIC NAME	USES	ADVERSE REACTIONS	SIGNIFICANT CONSIDERATIONS
Kava (kawa, kava-kava, awa yangona)	*Piper methysticum*	Mild to moderate anxiety and as a sedative	Scaly skin rash, disturbances in visual accommodation, habituation	Limit use to no more than 3 months.
Lemon balm (balm, melissa, sweet balm)	*Melissa officinalis*	Graves' disease, sedative, antispasmodic, cold sores (topical)	None significant.	None significant.
Passion Flower (passion fruit, granadilla, water lemon, apricot vine)	*Passiflora incarnata*	Promotes sleep, treatment for pain and nervous exhaustion	None if used as directed. Excessively large doses may cause CNS depression.	May interact with anticoagulants and MAOIs.
Saw palmetto (cabbage palm, fan palm, scrub palm)	*Serenoa repens*	Symptoms of benign prostatic hyperplasia	Generally well-tolerated; occasional gastrointestinal effects	May interact with hormones such as oral contraceptive drugs and hormone replacement therapy.
St. John's wort (Klamath weed, goatweed, rosin rose)	*Hypericum perforatum*	Antidepressant and antiviral	Usually mild. May cause dry mouth, dizziness, constipation, other GI symptoms, photosensitivity	May decrease efficacy of theophylline, warfarin, and digoxin; use with other prescriptions is not recommended.
Tea tree oil	*Melaleuca alternifolia*	Topical antimicrobial	Contact dermatitis	For topical use only; do not take orally.
Valerian	*Valeriana officinalis*	Restlessness, sleep disorders	Rare if used as directed.	May interact with the barbiturates (eg, phenobarbital), the benzodiazepines (eg, diazepam) and the opiates, (eg, morphine).
Willow bark (weidenrinde, white willow, purple osier willow, crack willow)	*Salix alba, S. purpurea, S. fragilis*	Analgesic	Adverse reactions are those associated with the salicylates	Do not use with aspirin or other NSAIDs. Do not use in patients with peptic ulcers and other medical conditions in which the salicylates are contraindicated.

USP MEDICATION ERRORS REPORTING PROGRAM
Presented in cooperation with the Institute for Safe Medication Practices
The USP Practitioners' Reporting Network℠ is an FDA MEDWATCH partner

MEDI-CATION ERRORS

REPORTING PROGRAM

❏ ACTUAL ERROR   ❏ POTENTIAL ERROR

Please describe the error. Include sequence of events, personnel involved, and work environment (e.g., code situation, change of shift, short staffing, no 24-hr. pharmacy, floor stock). If more space is needed, please attach separate page.

Was the medication administered to or used by the patient? ❏ No ❏ Yes   Date and time of event: _____

What type of staff or health care practitioner made the initial error? _____

Describe outcome (e.g., death, type of injury, adverse reaction). _____

If the medication did not reach the patient, describe the intervention. _____

Who discovered the error? _____

When and how was error discovered? _____

Where did the error occur (e.g., hospital, outpatient or retail pharmacy, nursing home, patient's home)? _____

Was another practitioner involved in the error ? ❏ No ❏ Yes If yes, what type of practitioner? _____

Was patient counseling provided? ❏ No ❏ Yes If yes, before or after error was discovered? _____

If a product was involved, please complete the following:

	Product #1	Product #2
Brand name of product involved		
Generic name		
Manufacturer		
Labeler (if different from mfr.)		
Dosage form		
Strength/concentration		
Type and size of container		
NDC number		

If available, please provide relevant patient information (age, gender, diagnosis, etc.). Patient identification not required.

Reports are most useful when relevant materials such as product label, copy of prescription/order, etc. can be reviewed.
Can these materials be provided? ❏ No ❏ Yes If yes, please specify. _____

Suggest any recommendations you have to prevent recurrence of this error or describe policies or procedures you have instituted to prevent future similar errors.

A copy of this report is routinely sent to the Institute for Safe Medication Practices (ISMP), to the manufacturer/labeler, and to the Food and Drug Administration (FDA). **USP may release my identity to: (check boxes that apply)**

❏ ISMP ❏ The manufacturer and/or labeler as listed above ❏ FDA ❏ Other persons requesting a copy of this report   ❏ Anonymous to all

Your name and title

Your facility name, address, and ZIP

Telephone number
(include area code)

Signature   Date

Return to the attention of:
Diane D. Cousins, R.Ph.
USP PRN
12601 Twinbrook Parkway
Rockville, MD 20852-1790

Call Toll Free: **800-23-ERROR** (800-233-7767)
or FAX 301-816-8532
USP home page: http://www.usp.org/prn
Electronic reporting forms are available. Please call for
additional information and/or your free diskette.

Date Received by USP: File Access Number:

C-194
8/5/97

Additional forms can be found in the *USP DI Vol. I* and *Vol. III* and in all monthly *Updates.*

MEDICATION ERRORS REPORTING PROGRAM

Medication Errors Do Occur

Medication errors can occur anywhere, any time along the drug therapy course, from prescribing through transcribing, dispensing, administering, and monitoring. An error can cause confusion, alarm, and frustration for the health care provider and for the patient. And YES, an error can even cause a death or injury to your patient. The causes of errors are many; for example, lack of product knowledge or training; poor communication; ambiguities in product names, directions for use, medical abbreviations, handwriting, or labeling; job stress; poor procedures or techniques; or patient misuse. Along this continuum, any health care professional may be the cause of or contribute to an actual or potential error.

A Safer Environment for Your Patients

It is important to recognize that health care providers learn from medication errors. By sharing your experience through the nationwide USP Medication Errors Reporting (MER) Program you help your colleagues to gain an understanding of why errors occur and how to prevent them. You can also have a positive impact on the quality of patient care and influence drug standards and information. When others are informed about an error, the chance of recurrence may be lessened. Education regarding medication errors assists health care professionals to avoid errors by recognizing the circumstances and causes of actual and potential errors.

Easy Access

Just call 800-233-7767 to reach a USP health care professional, who will take your report and respond to your concerns. Reports may also be submitted in writing or faxed. All reports are forwarded to the Food and Drug Administration, the product manufacturer/labeler when appropriate, the ISMP, and the USP Divisions of Standards and Information Development. If you wish to remain anonymous to any of these sources, the USP will act as your intermediary in all correspondence. While including your identity is optional, it does allow for appropriate follow-up with you to discuss your observations or provide feedback.

USP: A Partner in MEDWATCH

The USP Practitioners' Reporting Network is a partner in MEDWATCH, the FDA's medical products reporting program. As a partner, USP PRN contributes to the FDA's efforts to protect the public health by helping to identify serious adverse events for the agency. This means that your reported information is shared with the FDA on a daily basis, or immediately if necessary.

 The USP PRN® is designed to collect experiences and observations from health care providers through four separate reporting programs:

- The USP Drug Product Problem Reporting Program
- The USP Medication Errors Reporting Program
- The USP Drug Product Problem Reporting Program for Radiopharmaceuticals
- The USP Veterinary Practitioners' Reporting Program

The Institute for Safe Medication Practices, the Society of Nuclear Medicine, and the American Veterinary Medical Association cooperate in presenting the USP PRN.

Your Input Could Make the Difference!
USP PRN...CALL US WHEN YOU NEED US.

SINCE 1820
U.S. Pharmacopeia
12601 Twinbrook Parkway,
Rockville, MD 20852-1790

NO POSTAGE
NECESSARY
IF MAILED
IN THE
UNITED STATES

BUSINESS REPLY MAIL
FIRST-CLASS MAIL PERMIT NO 39 ROCKVILLE MD

POSTAGE WILL BE PAID BY ADDRESSEE:
DIANE D COUSINS RPh
THE USP PRACTITIONERS' REPORTING NETWORK
12601 TWINBROOK PARKWAY
ROCKVILLE MD 20897-5211

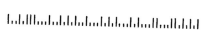

"Fold in thirds, tape & mail - DO NOT STAPLE FORM"

||||

BUSINESS REPLY MAIL
FIRST-CLASS MAIL   PERMIT NO. 1895   ROCKVILLE, MD

POSTAGE WILL BE PAID BY ADDRESSEE

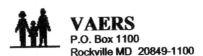 **VAERS**
P.O. Box 1100
Rockville MD 20849-1100

DIRECTIONS FOR COMPLETING FORM

(Additional pages may be attached if more space is needed)

GENERAL

Use a separate form for each patient. Complete the form to the best of your abilities. Items 3, 4, 7, 8, 10, 11, and 13 are considered essential and should be completed whenever possible. Parents/Guardians may need to consult the facility where the vaccine was administered for some of the information (such as manufacturer, lot number or laboratory data.)

Refer to the Reportable Events Table (RET) for events mandated for reporting by law. Reporting for other serious events felt to be related but not on the RET is encouraged.

Health care providers other than the vaccine administrator (VA) treating a patient for a suspected adverse event should notify the VA and provide the information about the adverse event to allow the VA to complete the form to meet the VA's legal responsibility. These data will be used to increase understanding of adverse events following vaccination and will become part of CDC Privacy Act System 09-20-0136, "Epidemiologic Studies and Surveillance of Disease Problems". Information identifying the person who received the vaccine or that person's legal representative will not be made available to the public, but may be available to the vaccinee or legal representative.

Postage will be paid by addressee. Forms may be photocopied (must be front & back on same sheet).

SPECIFIC INSTRUCTIONS

Form Completed By: To be used by parents/guardians, vaccine manufacturers/distributors, vaccine administrators, and/or the person completing the form on behalf of the patient or the health professional who administered the vaccine.

Item 7:   Describe the suspected adverse event. Such things as temperature, local and general signs and symptoms, time course, duration of symptoms diagnosis, treatment and recovery should be noted.

Item 9:   Check "YES" if the patient's health condition is the same as it was prior to the vaccine, "NO" if the patient has not returned to the pre-vaccination state of health, or "UNKNOWN" if the patient's condition is not known.

Item 10:   Give dates and times as specifically as you can remember. If you do not know the exact time, please

Item 11:   indicate "AM" or "PM" when possible if this information is known. If more than one adverse event, give the onset date and time for the most serious event.

Item 12:   Include "negative" or "normal" results of any relevant tests performed as well as abnormal findings.

Item 13:   List ONLY those vaccines given on the day listed in Item 10.

Item 14:   List any other vaccines that the patient received within 4 weeks prior to the date listed in Item 10.

Item 16:   This section refers to how the person who gave the vaccine purchased it, not to the patient's insurance.

Item 17:   List any prescription or non-prescription medications the patient was taking when the vaccine(s) was given.

Item 18:   List any short term illnesses the patient had on the date the vaccine(s) was given (i.e., cold, flu, ear infection).

Item 19:   List any pre-existing physician-diagnosed allergies, birth defects, medical conditions (including developmental and/or neurologic disorders) for the patient.

Item 21:   List any suspected adverse events the patient, or the patient's brothers or sisters, may have had to previous vaccinations. If more than one brother or sister, or if the patient has reacted to more than one prior vaccine, use additional pages to explain completely. For the onset age of a patient, provide the age in months if less than two years old.

Item 26:   This space is for manufacturers' use only.

Answers to Review Questions and Medication Dosage Problems

UNIT I FOUNDATIONS OF CLINICAL PHARMACOLOGY

Chapter 1 General Principles of Pharmacology

Review Questions

1. a
2. b
3. b
4. d
5. d
6. a

Chapter 2 The Administration of Drugs

Review Questions

1. c
2. c
3. d
4. b
5. b

Chapter 3 Review of Arithmetic and Calculation of Drug Dosages

Answers are in the chapter.

Chapter 4 The Nursing Process

Review Questions

1. d
2. c
3. a

Chapter 5 Patient and Family Teaching

Review Questions

1. d
2. a
3. b
4. c

UNIT II ANTI-INFECTIVES

Chapter 6 Sulfonamides

Review Questions

1. b
2. d
3. c
4. b

Medication Dosage Problems

1. 10 mL or 2 teaspoons
2. 2 tablets

Chapter 7 Penicillins

Review Questions

1. b
2. b
3. b
4. d

Medication Dosage Problems

1. 1 teaspoon (t) = 250 mg of Amoxil (1 t = 5 mL) The nurse will administer 2 teaspoons (t) or 10 mL of Amoxil.
2. Ninety (90 mL) milliters of water needed for reconstitution.

Directions for reconstitution: Tap bottle until all powder flows freely. Add approximately 2/3 of the 90 mL of water; shake vigorously to wet powder. Add remaining water and shake vigorously again.

Strength of reconstituted solution is 125 mg/ 5 mL.

The nurse would administer 20 mL.

Chapter 8 Cephalosporins

Review Questions

1. b
2. a
3. d
4. c

Medication Dosage Problems

1. 2 tablets
2. 4 mL

Chapter 9 Tetracyclines, Macrolides, and Lincosamides

Review Questions

1. c
2. b
3. d
4. a

Medication Dosage Problems

1. 2 tablets, 1 tablet
2. 2 mL
3. 20 mL

Chapter 10 Fluoroquinolones and Aminoglycosides

Review Questions

1. c
2. c
3. b
4. a
5. c

Medication Dosage Problems

1. 1 mL
2. 2 tablets

Chapter 11 Miscellaneous Anti-Infectives

Review Questions

1. b
2. c
3. a
4. b

Medication Dosage Problems

1. 1 tablet
2. 1 mL
3. 20 mL

Chapter 12 Antitubercular Drugs

Review Questions

1. a
2. d
3. c
4. b
5. d

Medication Dosage Problems

1. 6 mL
2. 4 tablets

Chapter 13 Leprostatic Drugs

Review Questions

1. d
2. c
3. a
4. b

Medication Dosage Problems

1. 6 tablets
2. ½ tablet

Chapter 14 Antiviral Drugs

Review Questions

1. a
2. a
3. a
4. b

Medication Dosage Problems

1. 2 tablets
2. 10 mg
3. 10 mL

Chapter 15 Antifungal Drugs

Review Questions

1. a
2. c
3. a
4. d

Medication Dosage Problems

1. 63.6 kg, 95.4 mg or 95 if rounded to the nearest whole number
2. 2 tablets

Chapter 16 Antiparasitic Drugs

Review Questions

1. b
2. b
3. c
4. a

Medication Dosage Problems

1. 2 tablets
2. 2 tablets

UNIT III DRUGS USED TO MANAGE PAIN

Chapter 17 Nonnarcotic Analgesics: Salicylates and Nonsalicylates

Review Questions

1. c
2. a
3. c
4. c
5. c
6. b

Medication Dosage Problems

1. 1.5 or 1½ mL
2. 2 tablets

Chapter 18 Nonnarcotic Analgesics: Nonsteroidal Anti-Inflammatory Drugs

Review Questions

1. a
2. a
3. d
4. b

Medication Dosage Problems

1. 10 mL
2. 2 tablets

Chapter 19 Narcotic Analgesics

Review Questions

1. d
2. c
3. b
4. c
5. a

Medication Dosage Problems

1. 1.2 mL
2. 1 mL

Chapter 20 Narcotic Antagonists

Review Questions

1. b
2. c
3. d

Medication Dosage Problems

1. 0.8 mL
2. ½ tablet

UNIT IV DRUGS THAT AFFECT THE NEUROMUSCULAR SYSTEM

Chapter 21 Drugs That Affect the Musculoskeletal System

Review Questions

1. c
2. a
3. c
4. d
5. d

Medication Dosage Problems

1. 3 tablets
2. 3 tablets

Chapter 22 Adrenergic Drugs

Review Questions

1. b
2. a

3. d
4. d
5. b

Medication Dosage Problems

1. $^{1}/_{2}$ tablet
2. $^{1}/_{2}$ mL

Chapter 23 Adrenergic Blocking Drugs

Review Questions

1. d
2. d
3. a
4. b

Medication Dosage Problems

1. 15 mL
2. 4 tablets

Chapter 24 Cholinergic Drugs

Review Questions

1. a
2. b
3. b

Medication Dosage Problems

1. 68.2 kg (weight), 1.5 mg (dosage)
2. $^{1}/_{2}$ mL

Chapter 25 Cholinergic Blocking Drugs

Review Questions

1. b
2. b
3. d
4. b

Medication Dosage Problems

1. $^{1}/_{2}$ mL
2. 10 mL

Chapter 26 Sedatives and Hypnotics

Review Questions

1. a
2. c
3. a
4. d
5. c

Medication Dosage Problems

1. $^{1}/_{2}$ tablet
2. 2 tablets

Chapter 27 Central Nervous System Stimulants

Review Questions

1. c
2. a
3. d
4. d

Medication Dosage Problems

1. 24 mg, yes
2. 2 tablets

Chapter 28 Anticonvulsants

Review Questions

1. d
2. b
3. a
4. c
5. b

Medication Dosage Problems

1. 3.3 mL
2. 2 tablets
3. 10 mL

Chapter 29 Antiparkinsonism Drugs

Review Questions

1. a
2. b
3. d
4. b

Medication Dosage Problems

1. one 500-mg tablet and one 250-mg tablet
2. 3 tablets

Chapter 30 Antianxiety Drugs

Review Questions

1. a
2. d
3. b
4. c

Medication Dosage Problems

1. 1 mL
2. 2 tablets

Chapter 31 Antidepressant Drugs

Review Questions

1. d
2. c
3. c
4. b

Medication Dosage Problems

1. 3 tablets
2. 25 mL

Chapter 32 Antipsychotic Drugs

Review Questions

1. c
2. b
3. c
4. b

Medication Dosage Problems

1. 1.5 mL
2. 2 tablets
3. 2 tablets

Chapter 33 Cholinesterase Inhibitors

Review Questions

1. b
2. c
3. a
4. d

Medication Dosage Problems

1. 3 mL
2. ½ tablet

Chapter 34 Antiemetic and Antivertigo Drugs

Review Questions

1. b
2. c
3. b
4. d

Medication Dosage Problems

1. 2 mL

2. 2 tablets
3. ½ tablet

Chapter 35 Anesthetic Drugs

Review Questions

1. b
2. c
3. a
4. b

Medication Dosage Problems

1. 1 mL
2. 0.3 mg

UNIT V DRUGS THAT AFFECT THE RESPIRATORY SYSTEM

Chapter 36 Antihistamines and Decongestants

Review Questions

1. a
2. c
3. b
4. c

Medication Dosage Problems

1. 10 mL
2. 2 tablets

Chapter 37 Bronchodilators and Antiasthma Drugs

Review Questions

1. d
2. d
3. d
4. a
5. a

Medication Dosage Problems

1. 0.25 mL
2. 2 tablets

Chapter 38 Antitussives, Mucolytics, and Expectorants

Review Questions

1. a
2. a

3. d
4. a

Medication Dosage Problems

1. 5 mL
2. 5 mL

UNIT VI DRUGS THAT AFFECT THE CARDIOVASCULAR SYSTEM

Chapter 39 Cardiotonics and Miscellaneous Inotropic Drugs

Review Questions

1. b
2. d
3. a
4. a
5. c

Medication Dosage Problems

1. one 0.5-mg tablet and one 0.25-mg tablet
2. ½ mL

Chapter 40 Antiarrhythmic Drugs

Review Questions

1. a
2. a
3. a
4. d
5. c

Medication Dosage Problems

1. 1.5 mL
2. 2 tablets

Chapter 41 Antianginal and Peripheral Dilating Drugs

Review Questions

1. b
2. b
3. c
4. b
5. a
6. d

Medication Dosage Problems

1. 3 tablets
2. 2 tablets

Chapter 42 Antihypertensives

Review Questions

1. c
2. c
3. d
4. b
5. b

Medication Dosage Problems

1. 4 tablets
2. 90-mg tablets and give 2 tablets

Chapter 43 Antihyperlipidemic Drugs

Review Questions

1. c
2. a
3. a
4. b
5. c

Medication Dosage Problems

1. 2 tablets
2. No, notify the primary health care provider

UNIT VII DRUGS THAT AFFECT THE HEMATOLOGICAL SYSTEM

Chapter 44 Anticoagulant and Thrombolytic Drugs

Review Questions

1. d
2. d
3. b
4. a
5. b

Medication Dosage Problems

1. 0.67 mL or 0.7 mL
2. 2 tablets

Chapter 45 Agents Used in the Treatment of Anemia

Review Questions

1. a
2. a
3. c
4. a
5. c

Medication Dosage Problems

1. ½ mL
2. 0.2 mL

UNIT VIII DRUGS THAT AFFECT THE GASTROINTESTINAL AND URINARY SYSTEM

Chapter 46 Diuretics

Review Questions

1. b
2. b
3. c
4. b
5. d
6. c

Medication Dosage Problems

1. 2 tablets
2. 2.5 mL

Chapter 47 Urinary Anti-infectives and Miscellaneous Urinary Drugs

Review Questions

1. a
2. d
3. c
4. d

Medication Dosage Problems

1. 2 tablets
2. 10 mL

Chapter 48 Drugs That Affect the Gastrointestinal System

Review Questions

1. c
2. c
3. a
4. b
5. d
6. a

Medication Dosage Problems

1. 2 tablets
2. 15 mL

UNIT IX DRUGS THAT AFFECT THE ENDOCRINE SYSTEM

Chapter 49 Antidiabetic Drugs

Review Questions

1. c
2. d
3. c
4. b
5. c

Medication Dosage Problems

1. Draw an arrow to the number 45.
2. 2 tablets at each dose; total daily dose 2000 mg
3. 4 tablets
4. Label B

Chapter 50 Pituitary and Adrenocortical Hormones

Review Questions

1. b
2. c
3. a
4. b
5. c

Medication Dosage Problems

1. 2 mL
2. 20 mL

Chapter 51 Thyroid and Antithyroid Drugs

Review Questions

1. b
2. c
3. a
4. c

Medication Dosage Problems

1. 6 tablets
2. 2 tablets

Chapter 52 Male and Female Hormones

Review Questions

1. c
2. d

3. c
4. a
5. b

Medication Dosage Problems

1. 1.6 mL
2. 1 mL

Chapter 53 Drugs Acting on the Uterus

Review Questions

1. d
2. b
3. a
4. c

Medication Dosage Problems

1. ¹/₂ tablet
2. 1 mL

UNIT X DRUGS THAT AFFECT THE IMMUNE SYSTEM

Chapter 54 Immunologic Agents

Review Questions

1. b
2. a
3. c
4. a

Chapter 55 Antineoplastic Drugs

Review Questions

1. d
2. a
3. b
4. b
5. c

Medication Dosage Problems

1. 13.7 mg/d
2. 1.375 or 1.4 U

UNIT XI DRUGS THAT AFFECT OTHER BODY SYSTEMS

Chapter 56 Topical Drugs Used in the Treatment of Skin Disorders

Review Questions

1. b
2. b
3. d
4. b
5. d

Chapter 57 Otic and Ophthalmic Preparations

Review Questions

1. b
2. b
3. c
4. d

Chapter 58 Fluids and Electrolytes

Review Questions

1. d
2. a
3. d
4. a
5. d

Medication Dosage Problems

1. 100 mL/hr
2. 30 mL

Examples of Combination Drugs

Antacid Combinations

Acid-X—calcium carbonate, acetaminophen

Advanced Formula Di-Gel—magnesium hydroxide, calcium carbonate, simethicone, sucrose

Alamag Plus—aluminum hydroxide, magnesium hydroxide, simethicone, parabens, sorbitol, saccharin

Alamag Suspension—aluminum hydroxide, magnesium hydroxide, sorbitol, sucrose, parabens

Alenic Alka—aluminum hydroxide, magnesium trisilicate, sodium bicarbonate, calcium stearate, sugar

Almacone—aluminum hydroxide, magnesium hydroxide, simethicone

Bromo-Seltzer Effervescent Granules—sodium bicarbonate, acetaminophen, citric acid, sugar

Calcium Rich Rolaids—magnesium hydroxide, calcium carbonate

Citrocarbonate Effervescent Granules—sodium bicarbonate, sodium citrate anhydrous

Di-Gel Liquid—aluminum hydroxide, simethicone, saccharin, sorbitol, parabens

Extra Strength Maalox Suspension—aluminum hydroxide, magnesium hydroxide, simethicone, parabens, sorbitol, saccharin

Gas-Ban—simethicone, calcium carbonate

Gas-Ban DS Liquid—aluminum hydroxide, magnesium hydroxide, simethicone

Gaviscon Extra Strength Reliever Formula Liquid—aluminum hydroxide, magnesium carbonate, parabens, EDTA, saccharin, sorbitol, simethicone, sodium alginate

Gaviscon Liquid—magnesium carbonate, parabens, EDTA, saccharin, sorbitol, sodium alginate

Gelusil—aluminum hydroxide, magnesium hydroxide, simethicone, dextrose, saccharin, sorbitol, sugar

Lowslum Plus Liquid—magaldrate, simethicone

Maalox—aluminum, magnesium hydroxide

Maalox Plus—aluminum hydroxide, magnesium hydroxide, simethicone, sugar

Maalox Suspension—aluminum hydroxide, magnesium hydroxide, saccharin, sorbitol, parabens

Marblen—magnesium carbonate, calcium carbonate

Marblen Liquid—calcium carbonate, magnesium carbonate

Mintox—aluminum, magnesium hydroxide

Mintox Plus—aluminum hydroxide, magnesium hydroxide, simethicone, saccharin, sorbitol, sugar

Mintox Suspension—aluminum hydroxide, magnesium hydroxide, parabens, sorbitol, saccharin

Mylagen Liquid—simethicone, parabens, sorbitol, sucrose

Mylanta—aluminum hydroxide, magnesium hydroxide, simethicone, sorbitol

Mylanta Gelcaps—calcium carbonate, magnesium carbonate, parabens

Mylanta Liquid—simethicone, sorbitol

Nephrox Liquid—aluminum hydroxide, mineral oil

Original Alka-Seltzer Effervescent Tablets—sodium bicarbonate, aspirin, citric acid, phenylalanine

Riopan Plus—magaldrate, simethicone, sorbitol, sucrose

Riopan Plus Suspension—magaldrate, simethicone, saccharin, sorbitol

Rulox # 2—aluminum, magnesium hydroxide, simethicone

Rulox Plus—aluminum hydroxide, magnesium hydroxide, simethicone, sugar, saccharin, dextrose

Rulox Suspension—aluminum hydroxide, magnesium hydroxide, parabens, sorbitol, saccharin

Simaal Gel 2 Liquid—aluminum hydroxide, magnesium hydroxide, simethicone

Tempo—aluminum hydroxide, magnesium hydroxide, calcium carbonate, simethicone, sorbitol, corn syrup

Antiasthmatic Combinations

Bronchial Capsules—theophylline, guaifenesin

Brondelate Elixir—theophylline, oxtriphylline, guaifenesin

Dilor-G Tablets—dyphylline, guaifenesin

Dyflex-G Tablets—dyphylline, guaifenesin

Glyceryl-T Liquid—theophylline, guaifenesin

Hydrophed Tablets—theophylline, hydroxyzine, ephedrine sulfate

Lufyllin-EPG Tablets—dyphylline, ephedrine HCl, guaifenesin, phenobarbitol

Marax Tablets—theophylline, hydroxyzine, ephedrine sulfate

Mundrane GG Tablets—theophylline, guaifenesin, aminophylline anhydrous, ephedrine HCl, phenobarbital

Primatene Dual Action Tablets—theophylline, ephedrine, guaifenesin

Primatene Tablets—theophylline, phenobarbital, ephedrine HCl

Quadrinal Tablets—theophylline, theophylline calcium salicylate, ephedrine HCl, potassium iodide, phenobarbital

Quibron Capsules—theophylline, guaifenesin

Slo-Phyllin GG Capsules—theophylline, guaifenesin

Slo-Phyllin GG Syrup—theophylline, guaifenesin

Tedrigen Tablets—theophylline, Phenobarbital, ephedrine HCl

Theodrine Tablets—theophylline, ephedrine HCl

Theolate Liquid—theophylline, guaifenesin

Antidiarrheal Combinations

Diasorb—activated attapulgite, sorbitol

Donnagel—attapulgite, saccharin

Kaodene Non-Narcotic—kaolin, pectin, bismuth subsalicylate, sucrose

Kaolin w/ Pectin—kaolin, pectin

Kaopectate Maximum Strength—attapulgite, sucrose

Kapectolin—kaolin, pectin

K-C—kaolin, pectin, bismuth subcarbonate, peppermint flavor

Antihistamine and Analgesic Combinations

Aceta-Gesic Tablets—phenyltoloxamine citrate, acetaminophen

Coricidin HBP Cold and Flu Tablets—chlorpheniramine maleate, acetaminophen

Ed-Flex Capsules—phenyltoloxamine citrate, acetaminophen, salicylamide

Major-Gesic Tablets—phenyltoloxamine citrate, acetaminophen

Percogesic—phenyltoloxamine citrate, acetaminophen

Percogesic Extra Strength Tablets—diphenhydramine HCl, acetaminophen

Phenylgesic Tablets—phenyltoloxamine citrate, acetaminophen

Tylenol PM Extra Strength Tablets—diphenhydramine HCl, acetaminophen

Tylenol Severe Allergy Tablets—diphenhydramine HCl, acetaminophen

Antihypertensive Combinations

Aldoclor—chlorothiazide, methyldopa

Aldoril—hydrochlorothiazide, methyldopa

Apresazide—hydrochlorothiazide, hydralazine

Avalide—hydrochlorothiazide, irbesartan

Capozide—hydrochlorothiazide, captopril

Chloroserpine—chlorothiazide, reserpine

Combipres—clonidine, chlorthalidone

Corzide—bendroflumethiazide, nadolol

Demi-Regroton Tablets—chlorthalidone, reserpine

Diovan HCT—hydrochlorothiazide, valsartan

Diutensen-R Tablets—methyclothiazide, reserpine

Enduronyl—methyclothiazide, desperidine

Esimil—hydrochlorothiazide, guanethidine monosulfate

Hydrap-ES—hydrochlorothiazide, reserpine, hydralazine HCl

Hydropres-50—hydrochlorothiazide, reserpine

Hydro-Serp—hydrochlorothiazide, reserpine

Hydroserpine #1 Tablets—hydrochlorothiazide, reserpine

Hydroserpine #2 Tablets—hydrochlorothiazide, reserpine

Hyzaar—hydrochlorothiazide, losartan potassium

Inderide—hydrochlorothiazide, propranolol HCl

Inderide LA—hydrochlorothiazide, propranolol HCl

Lexxel Extended-Release—enalapril maleate, felodipine

Lopressor—hydrochlorothiazide, metoprolol

Lotensin HCT—hydrochlorothiazide, benazepril

Lotrel—amlodopine, benazepril

Marpres—hydrochlorothiazide, reserpine, hydralazine HCl

Metatensin Tablets—trichlormethiazide, reserpine

Minizide—polythiazide, prazosin

Prinzide—hydrochlorothiazide, lisinopril

Rauzide Tablets—rauwolfia, bendroflumethiazide

Regroton—chlorthalidone, reserpine

Salutensin Tablets—hydroflumethiazide, reserpine

Salutensin-Demi—hydrochlorothiazide, reserpine

Ser-Ap-Es—hydrochlorothiazide, reserpine, hydralazine HCl

Tarka—trandolapril, verapamil

Teczem Extended-Release—diltiazem maleate, enalapril maleate

Tenoretic—chlorthalidone, atenolol

Timolide—hydrochlorothiazide, timolol maleate

Tri-Hydroserpine—hydrochlorothiazide, reserpine, hydralazine HCl

Uniretic—hydrochlorothiazide, moexipril HCl

Vaseretic—hydrochlorothiazide, enalapril maleate

Zestoretic—hydrochlorothiazide, lisinopril

Ziac—hydrochlorothiazide, bisoprolol fumarate

Antitussive Combinations

Alka-Seltzer Plus Cold and Flu Liqui-Gels—dextromethorphan HBr, pseudoephedrine HCl, acetaminophen

Bromatane DX—dextromethorphan HBr, brompheniramine maleate, pseudoephedrine HCl

Cardec DM—dextromethorphan HBr, carbinoxamine maleate, pseudoephedrine HCl

Coricidin HBP Cough & Cold Tablets—dextromethorphan HBr, chlorpheniramine, acetaminophen

Dimetane-DX Cough—dextromethorphan HBr, brompheniramine maleate, pseudoephedrine HCl

Hycodan Tablets or Syrup—hydrocodone bitartrate, homatropine MBr

Hydromide Syrup—hydrocodone bitartrate, homatropine MBr

Nucofed Capsules—codeine phosphate, pseudoephedrine HCl

Promethazaine HCl/w Codeine Cough Syrup—codeine phosphate, promethazine HCl

Quad Tann Tablets—carbetapentane tannate, chlorpheniramine tannate, phenylephrine tannate, ephedrine tannate

Robitussin Maximun Strength—dextromethorphan HBr, pseudoephedrine HCl

Rynatuss Tablets—carbetapentane tannate, chlorpheniramine tannate, phenylephrine tannate, ephedrine tannate

Sudafed Non-Drowsy Severe Cold Formula Maximum Strength Tablets—dextromethorphan HBr, pseudoephedrine HCl, acetaminophen

Tannic-12 Tablets—carbetapentane tannate, chlorpheniramine tannate

Tricodeine Cough & Cold Liquid—codeine phosphate, pyrilamine maleate

Trionate Tablets—carbetapentane tannate, chlorpheniramine tannate

Tussafed Syrup—dextromethorphan HBr, carbinoxamine maleate, pseudoephedrine HCl

Tussend Tablets—hydrocodone bitartrate, chlorpheniramine, pseudoephedrine HCl

Vanex HD Liquid—hydrocodone bitartrate, chlorpheniramine, phenylephrine HCl

Decongestant and Expectorant Combinations

Allegra-D Tablets—pseudoephedrine HCl, fexofenadine HCl

Allerfrim Syrup—pseudoephedrine HCl, triprolidine HCl

Aprodine Tablets—pseudoephedrine HCl, triprolidine HCl

Benadryl Allergy & Sinus Tablets—pseudoephedrine HCl, diphenhydramine citrate, diphenhydramine HCl

Bromfed Capsules—pseudoephedrine HCl, brompheniramine maleate

Bromfed Syrup—pseudoephedrine HCl, brompheniramine maleate

Claritin D—pseudoephedrine HCl, loratadine

Deconamine Syrup—pseudoephedrine HCl, chlorpheniramine maleate

Dynex Tablets—pseudoephedrine, guaifenesin

Ed A Hist Tablets—phenylephrine HCl, chlorpheniramine maleate

Genac Tablets—pseudoephedrine HCl, triprolidine HCl

Guaifed Capsules—pseudoephedrine, guaifenesin

Guiatuss PE Liquid—pseudoephedrine, guaifenesin

Histade Capsules—pseudoephedrine HCl, chlorpheniramine maleate

Histatab Plus Tablets—phenylephrine HCl, chlorpheniramine maleate

Histex Liquid—pseudoephedrine HCl, chlorpheniramine maleate

Lodrane Liquid—pseudoephedrine HCl, brompheniramine maleate

Phenergan VC Syrup—phenylephrine HCl, promethazine

Profen II Tablets—pseudoephedrine, guaifenesin

Pseudovent Capsules—pseudoephedrine, guaifenesin

Respahist Capsules—pseudoephedrine HCl, brompheniramine maleate

Respaire-60 SR Capsules—pseudoephedrine, guaifenesin

Rinade B.I.D. Capsules—pseudoephedrine HCl, chlorpheniramine maleate

Robafen PE Liquid—pseudoephedrine, guaifenesin

Robitussin Cold Sinus and Congestion—pseudoephedrine, guaifenesin, acetaminophen

Robitussin PE Liquid—pseudoephedrine, guaifenesin

Rondec Tablets—pseudoephedrine HCl, carbinoxamine maleate

Ryna Liquid—pseudoephedrine HCl, chlorpheniramine maleate

Rynatan Tablets—phenylephrine tannate, chlorpheniramine tannate

Severe Congestion Tussin Softgels—pseudoephedrine, guaifenesin

Sinutab Nondrying Liquid Caps—pseudoephedrine, guaifenesin

Sudafed Cold and Allergy Maximum Strength—pseudoephedrine HCl, chlorpheniramine maleate

Tanafed Suspension—pseudoephedrine, chlorpheniramine tannate

Versacaps Capsules—pseudoephedrine, guaifenesin

Decongestant, Antihistamine, and Analgesic Combinations

Alka-Seltzer Plus Cold Medicine—phenylephrine HCl, chlorpheniramine maleate, acetaminophen

Decodult Tablets—pseudoephedrine HCl, chlorpheniramine maleate, acetaminophen

Kolephrin Tablets—pseudoephedrine HCl, chlorpheniramine maleate, acetaminophen

Simplet Tablets—pseudoephedrine HCl, chlorpheniramine, acetaminophen

Sinutab Sinus Allergy, Maximum Strength—pseudoephedrine HCl, chlorpheniramine maleate, acetaminophen

Tavist Allergy/Sinus/Headache Tablets—pseudoephedrine HCl, clemastine fumarate, acetaminophen

TheraFlu Flu and Cold Medicine Original Formula Powder—pseudoephedrine HCl, chlorpheniramine maleate, acetaminophen

Triaminic Cold, Allergy, Sinus Medicine—pseudoephedrine HCl, chlorpheniramine maleate, acetaminophen

Tylenol Sinus NightTime Maximum Strength Tablets—pseudoephedrine HCl, diphenhydramine HCl, acetaminophen

Decongestant, Antihistamine, and Anticholinergic Combinations

AH-Chew Tablets—phenylephrine HCl, chlorpheniramine maleate, methscopolamine nitrate

D.A. Chewable Tablets—phenylephrine HCl, chlorpheniramine maleate, methscopolamine nitrate

Dallergy Syrup or Tablets—phenylephrine HCl, chlorpheniramine maleate, methscopolamine nitrate

Dehistine Syrup—phenylephrine HCl, chlorpheniramine maleate, methscopolamine nitrate

Extendryl Syrup—phenylephrine HCl, chlorpheniramine maleate, methscopolamine nitrate

Pannaz Tablets or Syrup—phenylephrine HCl, chlorpheniramine maleate, methscopolamine nitrate

Rescon-MX Tablets—phenylephrine HCl, chlorpheniramine maleate, methscopolamine nitrate

Diuretic Combinations

Aldactazide—spironolactone, hydrochlorothiazide
Amiloride/hydrochlorothiazide—generic
Dyazide—triamterene, hydrochlorothiazide
Maxzide—triamterene, hydrochlorothiazide
Maxzide-25MG—triamterene, hydrochlorothiazide
Modiuretic—amiloride, hydrochlorothiazide
Spironolactone/hydrochlorothiazide—generic
Triamterene/hydrochlorothiazide—generic

Estrogen and Progestin Combinations

Activella—estradiol, norethindrone acetate
CombiPatch—estradiol, norethindrone
Femhrt—ethinyl estradiol, norethindrone acetate
Ortho-Prefest—estradiol, norgestimate
Premephase—conjugated estrogens, medroxyprogesterone acetate
Prempro—conjugated estrogens, medroxyprogesterone acetate

Estrogen and Androgen Combinations, Oral and Parenteral

Depo-Testadiol—estradiol cypionate, testosterone cypionate

Depotestogen—estradiol cypionate, testosterone cypionate

Duo-Cyp—estradiol cypionate, testosterone cypionate
Estratest—esterified estrogens, methyltestosterone
Estratest H.S.—esterified estrogens, methyltestosterone

Valertest No. 1—estradiol valerate, testosterone enanthate

Glaucoma Combinations

E-Pilo—pilocarpine, epinephrine
E-Pilo-2—pilocarpine, epinephrine
E-Pilo-4—pilocarpine, epinephrine
P6E1—pilocarpine, epinephrine

Gastrointestinal Anticholinergic Combinations

Antrocol Elixir—atropine sulfate, phenobarbital, alcohol

Barbidonna—atropine, scopolamine HBr, hyoscyamine sulfate, phenobarbital

Bellacane Elixir—atropine, scopolamine HBr, hyoscyamine HBr or sulfate, phenobarbital, alcohol, tartrazine

Bellacane SR Tablets—l-alkaloids of belladonna, phenobarbital, ergotamine tartrate

Bellergal-S Tablets—l-alkaloids of belladonna, phenobarbital, ergotamine tartrate

Butibel Elixir—belladonna extract, butabarbital sodium, alcohol, sucrose, saccharin

Butibel Tablets—belladonna extract, butabarbitol

Chardonna-2 Tablets—belladonna extract, phenobarbital

Donnatal Elixir—atropine, scopolamine HBr, hyoscyamine HBr or sulfate, phenobarbital, alcohol, sucrose, saccharin

Donnatal Capsules and Tablets—atropine, scopolamine HBr, hyoscyamine sulfate, phenobarbital

Folergot-DF Tablets—l-alkaloids of belladonna, phenobarbital, ergotamine tartrate

Hyosophen Tablets—atropine, scopolamine HBr, hyoscyamine sulfate, phenobarbital

Librax Capsules—clindinium, chlordiazepoxide HCl

Phenerbel-S Tablets—l-alkaloids of belladonna, phenobarbital, ergotamine tartrate

Spasmolin Tablets—atropine, scopolamine HBr, hyoscyamine sulfate, phenobarbital

Isoniazid Combinations

Rifamate—rifampin, isoniazid
Rifater—rifampin, isoniazid, pyrazinamide

Laxative Combinations

DDS 100 Plus Capsules—docusate, casanthranol
Doxidan Capsules—docusate, casanthranol, sorbitol
Nature's Remedy—cascara sagrada, aloe, lactose
Peri-Colace—docusate, casanthranol, sorbitol, parabens
Senokot-S tablets—docusate, senna concentrate, lactose

Ophthalmic Decongestant and Antihistamine Combinations

Naphcon-A Solution—naphazoline HCl, pheniramine maleate

Vasocon-A Solution—naphazoline HCl, antazoline phosphate

Ophthalmic Antibiotic Combinations

AK-Poly-Bac Ophthalmic Ointment—polymyxin B sulfate, bacitracin zinc

AK-Spore—polymyxin B Sulfate, neomycin, bacitracin zinc

Neosporin Ophthalmic Ointment—polymyxin B sulfate, neomycin, bacitracin zinc

Polysporin Ophthalmic Ointment—polymyxin B sulfate, bacitracin zinc

Polytrim Ophthalmic Solution—polymyxin B sulfate, trimethoprim sulfate

Peripheral Vasodilator Combinations

Lipo-Nicin—niacin, niacinamide, vitamins C, B_1, B_2, B_6

Sedative and Hypnotic Combinations

Tuinal—amobarbital, secobarbitol

Skeletal Muscle Relaxant Combinations

Carisoprodol Compound—carisoprodol, aspirin

Flexaphen—chlorzoxazone, acetaminophen

Lobac—salicylamide, phenyltoloxamine, acetaminophen

Norgesic Forte—orphenadrine citrate, aspirin, caffeine

Norgesic—orphenadrine citrate, aspirin, caffeine

Robaxisal—methocarbamol, aspirin

Sodol Compound—carisoprodol, aspirin

Soma Compound—carisoprodol, aspirin

Index

Note: Page numbers followed by f, t, and d indicate figures, tables, and display material, respectively.

A

AA-HC Otic. *see* 1% Hydrocortisone, 2% acetic acid glacial, 3% propylene glycol diacetate, 0.02% benzethonium chloride, 0.015% sodium acetate, 0.2% citric acid
Abacavir sulfate, 121t
Abbokinase. *see* Urokinase
Abdominal distention, 520–521
Abelcet. *see* Amphotericin B
Abreva. *see* Docosanol
Absence seizure, 253
Absorption, 6
Abstinence syndrome, 176d
Acarbose, 500t
Accolate. *see* Zafirlukast
Accupril. *see* Quinapril hydrochloride
Acebutolol, 211t, 371t, 398t
Aceon. *see* Perindopril erbumine
Acetaminophen
  actions of, 153
  adverse reactions of, 153–154, 156
  characteristics of, 152t
  contraindications, precautions, and interactions, 154
  patient education regarding, 158
  toxicity, 154, 156
  uses of, 153
Acetasol HC. *see* 1% Hydrocortisone, 2% acetic acid, 3% propylene glycol diacetate, 0.015% sodium acetate, 0.02% benzethonium chloride
Acetazolamide, 444t, 446–447, 450t
Acetohexamide, 500t
Acetylcholine, 221, 304
Acetylcholinesterase, 221
Acetylcysteine, 351t, 353–355
Acetylsalicylic acid, 4
Aciphex. *see* Rabeprazole sodium
Aclovate. *see* Alclometasone dipropionate
Acne-5. *see* Benzoyl peroxide
Acquired immunodeficiency syndrome, 3
Acthar. *see* Corticotropin
ActHB. *see* Haemophilus influenzae type b conjugate and hepatitis B vaccine
Actigall. *see* Ursodiol
Actinex. *see* Masoprocol
Action potential, 368
Actiq. *see* Fentanyl transmucosal
Activase. *see* Alteplase
Active absorption, 6
Active immunity, 568
Activella. *see* Estrogen and progestin
Actonel. *see* Risedronate sodium
Actos. *see* Pioglitazone hydrochloride
Acu-Dyne. *see* Povidone-iodine
Acular. *see* Ketorolac
Acute pain, 150
Acute renal failure, 504
Acyclovir

adverse reactions of, 123, 126
characteristics of, 121t, 606t
contraindications, 124
nursing process for, 125
patient education regarding, 127
uses of, 609
Adalat. *see* Nifedipine
Additive drug reaction, 11
Administration of drugs. *see* Drug administration
Adrenalin chloride. *see* Epinephrine
Adrenal insufficiency, 527
Adrenergic blocking drugs. *see also* Sympathomimetics
  α-
    actions of, 210
    adverse reactions of, 213, 217–218
    contraindications, precautions, and interactions, 213
    definition of, 210
    types of, 211t
    uses of, 210, 213
  α/β-
    actions of, 215
    adverse reactions of, 215, 217–218, 215
    contraindications, precautions, and interactions, 215
    definition of, 210
    types of, 212t
    uses of, 215
  β-
    actions of, 213–214
    adverse reactions of, 217–218
    antihypertensive uses of, 398t–399t
    contraindications, precautions, and interactions, 214
    definition of, 210
    elderly use of, 214
    types of, 211t–212t, 213–214
    uses of, 214
  classification of, 210
  family/patient education, 218–219
  nursing process for, 216–219
Adrenergic drugs. *see also specific drug*
  actions of, 200–201
  adverse reactions of, 204, 207–208
  contraindications, 204
  description of, 200
  elderly use of, 207
  family/patient education, 208–209
  hemodynamic status improved using, 204
  interactions, 205
  nursing process for, 205–209
  precautions, 205
  shock treated using, 203–204, 204t
  uses of, 201, 203–204
Adrenergic nerve receptors, 200, 203t
Adrenocorticotropic hormone, 516–518
Adriamycin. *see* Doxorubicin hydrochloride
Adrucil. *see* Fluorouracil

Adsorbocarpine. *see* Pilocarpine hydrochloride
Adverse reactions. *see also specific drug, adverse reactions of*
  description of, 8, 12
  patient teaching regarding, 56
  reporting of, 2d
Advil. *see* Ibuprofen
AeroBid/AeroBid-M, *see* Flunisolide
Aerodine. *see* Povidone-iodine
Affective domain of learning, 52–53
Afrin. *see* Oxymetazoline hydrochloride
Aftate. *see* Tolnaftate
Agenerase. *see* Amprenavir
Age of patient, 11
Agonist(s)
  adverse reactions of, 171
  definition of, 8, 167
  narcotic, 169t
Agonist-antagonist
  adverse reactions of, 171
  definition of, 169
  interactions, 171–172
Agoral. *see* Sennosides
Agranulocytosis, 61
Akarpine. *see* Pilocarpine hydrochloride
Akathisia, 297d
AKBeta. *see* Levobunolol hydrochloride
AK-Dex. *see* Dexamethasone
Akineton. *see* Biperiden
Akne-Mycin. *see* Erythromycin
AKPro. *see* Dipivefrin hydrochloride
AK-Spore. *see* 1% Hydrocortisone, 5 mg neomycin sulfate, 10,000 units polymyxin B
AK-Sulf. *see* Sodium sulfacetamide
AK-Tracin. *see* Bacitracin
Alanine aminotransferase, 308
Albendazole, 138–139, 139t
Albenza. *see* Albendazole
Albuterol sulfate, 335t
Alclometasone dipropionate, 606t
Alconefrin. *see* Phenylephrine hydrochloride
Aldactone. *see* Spironolactone
Aldara. *see* Imiquimod
Aldesleukin, 590t
Aldomet. *see* Methyldopa
Aldosterone, 396, 524
Alemtuzumab, 590t
Alendronate sodium, 18, 188t, 195, 197
Aleve. *see* Naproxen
Alfenta. *see* Alfentanil hydrochloride
Alfentanil hydrochloride, 168t
Alkeran. *see* Melphalan
Allegra. *see* Fexofenadine
Aller-Chlor. *see* Chlorpheniramine maleate
Allergen Ear Drops. *see* 1.4% Benzocaine, 5.4% antipyrine glycerin
Allergic drug reactions, 8–9
Allopurinol, 187, 189t, 449
Almora. *see* Magnesium

P